# Clinical
# &Immunology
# Serology

## A LABORATORY PERSPECTIVE

**THIRD EDITION**

# Clinical &Immunology Serology

## A LABORATORY PERSPECTIVE

**THIRD EDITION**

Christine Dorresteyn Stevens, EdD, MT(ASCP)
Professor Emeritus of Clinical Laboratory Sciences
Western Carolina University
Cullowhee, North Carolina

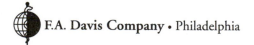
F.A. Davis Company · Philadelphia

F.A. Davis Company
1915 Arch Street
Philadelphia, PA 19103
www.fadavis.com

Printed in the United States of America

Last digit indicates print number: 10 9 8 7 6 5 4 3

*Senior Acquisitions Editor:* Christa Fratantoro
*Manager of Content Development:* George W. Lang
*Developmental Editor:* Sarah Granlund and Grace Caputo
*Art and Design Manager:* Carolyn O'Brien

As new scientific information becomes available through basic and clinical research, recommended treatments and drug therapies undergo changes. The author(s) and publisher have done everything possible to make this book accurate, up to date, and in accord with accepted standards at the time of publication. The author(s), editors, and publisher are not responsible for errors or omissions or for consequences from application of the book, and make no warranty, expressed or implied, in regard to the contents of the book. Any practice described in this book should be applied by the reader in accordance with professional standards of care used in regard to the unique circumstances that may apply in each situation. The reader is advised always to check product information (package inserts) for changes and new information regarding dose and contraindications before administering any drug. Caution is especially urged when using new or infrequently ordered drugs.

**Library of Congress Cataloging-in-Publication Data**

Stevens, Christine Dorresteyn.
  Clinical immunology and serology : a laboratory perspective / Christine Dorresteyn Stevens. — 3rd ed.
    p. ; cm.
  Includes bibliographical references and index.
  ISBN 978-0-8036-1814-5
  1. Immunodiagnosis—Laboratory manuals. 2. Serodiagnosis—Laboratory manuals. 3. Clinical immunology. I. Title.
  [DNLM: 1. Immunity—physiology. 2. Immune System Diseases—diagnosis. 3.
Immunologic Techniques. 4. Immunologic Tests. 5. Serologic Tests. QW 540 S844c 2010]
  RB46.5.S73 2010
  616.07'56—dc22

2009022707

To my wonderful family:
Eric, Kathy, and Hannah,
and Kevin, Melissa, and Turner

# Preface

The third edition of *Clinical Immunology and Serology: A Laboratory Perspective* is built on the success of the first two editions. This text is tailored to meet the needs of clinical laboratory students on both the two and four year levels. It combines practical information about laboratory testing with a concise discussion of the theory behind the testing. For practicing laboratorians and other allied health professionals, the book may serve as a valuable reference about new developments in the field of immunology. All chapters have been updated to include new information about the immune system as well as new treatments for immunological diseases. Two new chapters have been added. They include: automated assays, emphasizing flow cytometry (Chapter 12), and serology of bacterial infections (Chapter 19). The chapter on fungal and parasitic infections has been expanded (Chapter 20), as well as the chapter on molecular techniques (Chapter 19). All the features that readers enjoyed have been retained and strengthened. The number of illustrations has increased, and new case studies have been added.

The book remains a practical introduction to the field of clinical immunology that combines essential theoretic principles with serologic techniques commonly used in the clinical laboratory. The theory is comprehensive but concise, and the emphasis is on direct application to the clinical laboratory. The text is readable and user-friendly, with learning objectives, chapter outlines, and a glossary of all key terms. Each chapter is a complete learning module that contains theoretic principles, illustrations, definitions of relevant terminology, procedures for simulated clinical testing, and questions and case studies that help to evaluate learning.

The organization of the chapters is based on the experience of many years of teaching immunology to clinical laboratory science students. This book has been designed to provide the necessary balance of theory with practical application because it is essential for the practitioner to have a thorough understanding of the theoretic basis for testing methodologies. For the instructor, suggested laboratory exercises are included where applicable. While some of the exercises are not used in an actual clinical laboratory, they serve to illustrate and reinforce principles discussed in the chapters. Since most clinical laboratory science programs do not have extensive technology available in the academic setting, exercises have been designed to be performed with minimal equipment. Because the field of immunology is expanding so rapidly, the challenge in writing this book has been to ensure adequate coverage but to keep it on an introductory level. Every chapter has been revised to include current practices as of the time of writing. It is hoped that this book will kindle an interest in both students and laboratory professionals in this exciting and dynamic field.

# Contributors

Thomas S. Alexander, PhD, D(ABMLI)
Immunologist
Dept. of Pathology and Laboratory Medicine
Summa Health System
Akron, Ohio

Diane L. Davis, PhD
Professor and Clinical Coordinator
Clinical Lab Science Program/Health Sciences Dept
Salisbury University
Salisbury, Maryland

Dorothy J. Fike, MS, MT(ASCP)SBB
Professor
Clinical Laboratory Sciences
Marshall University
Huntington, West Virginia

Candace Golightly, MS, MLT(ASCP)
Associate Clinical Professor
School of Medicine
Stony Brook University
Stony Brook, New York

Marc G. Golightly, PhD
Professor of Pathology
Director and Head of Flow Cytometry
    and Clinical Immunology
Dept of Pathology
School of Medicine
Stony Brook University
Stony Brook, New York

Maureane Hoffman, MD, PhD
Professor of Pathology and Immunology
Duke University and Durham Medical Centers
Durham, North Carolina

Patsy C. Jarreau, MHS, CLS(NCA), MT(ASCP)
Associate Professor
Department of Clinical Laboratory Sciences
Louisiana State University Health Sciences Center
New Orleans, Louisiana

Donald C. Lehman, EdD, MT(ASCP), SM(NRM)
Associate Professor
Department of Medical Technology
University of Delaware
Newark, Delaware

Linda E. Miller, PhD, I,MP(ASCP)SI
Professor
Department of Clinical Laboratory Science, College
    of Health Professions
SUNY Upstate Medical University
Syracuse, New York

Susan M. Orton, PhD, MT(ASCP), D(ABMLI)
Assistant Professor, Division of Clinical Laboratory Science
Department of Allied Health Sciences
    School of Medicine
The University of North Carolina
Chapel Hill, North Carolina

John L. Schmitz, PhD, D(ABMLI, ABHI)
Associate Professor, Pathology and Laboratory Medicine
UNC Chapel Hill
Director, Histocompatibility, Flow Cytometry Laboratories
UNC Hospitals
Chapel Hill, North Carolina

Timothy Stegall, PhD
Assistant Professor
Clinical Laboratory Science Program
Western Carolina University
Cullowhee, North Carolina

Susan King Strasinger, DA, MT(ASCP)
Faculty Associate
Clinical Laboratory Science
The University of West Florida
Pensacola, Florida

# Reviewers

Hassan Aziz, PhD, CLS(NCA)
Associate Professor and Department Head
Armstrong Atlantic State University
Medical Technology Department
Savannah, Georgia

Maribeth Laude Flaws, PhD, SM(ASCP)SI
Associate Chairman and Associate Professor
Rush University Medical Center
Clinical Laboratory Sciences Department
Chicago, Illinois

Abraham Furman, PhD, MT(ASCP)
Assistant Professor
Oregon Institute of Technology / Oregon Health
and Science University
Clinical Laboratory Science Department
Portland, Oregon

Karen A. Golemboski, PhD, MT(ASCP)
Assistant Professor and Program Director
Bellarmine University
Clinical Laboratory Science Department
Louisville, Kentucky

Phyllis Gutowski, MT(ASCP), MS
Director
Housatonic Community College
CLT Program
Bridgeport, Connecticut

Kay Harris, MS, MT(ASCP)NM
Director and Department Chair
Northeastern Oklahoma A and M College
Allied Health Department
Medical Lab Tech Program
Miami, Oklahoma

Kathy Heidrick, MT(ASCP)
Instructor
Barton County Community College
MLT Department
Great Bend, Kansas

Paulette Howarth, MS, CLS
Professor
Bristol Community College
Clinical Laboratory Science Department
Fall River, Massachusetts

Stephen M. Johnson, MS, MT(ASCP)
Program Director
Saint Vincent Health Center
School of Medical Technology
Erie, Pennsylvania

Donald C. Lehman, EdD, MT(ASCP), SM(NRM)
Assistant Professor
University of Delaware
Medical Technology Department
Newark, Delaware

Karen Jean McClure, PhD, CLS(NCA),
MT(ASCP)SBB
Assistant Professor and Director
University of Texas M.D. Anderson Cancer Center
The School of Health Sciences
Clinical Laboratory Science Program
Houston, Texas

Wendy Miller, MS, CLS(NCA), MT(ASCP)SI
Program Director
Elgin Community College
Clinical Laboratory Technology department
Elgin, Illinois

Marguerite E. Neita, PhD, MT(ASCP)
Chairperson and Program Director
Howard University
Department of Clinical Laboratory Science
Washington, DC

# Acknowledgments

I am grateful for the assistance I received from a number of sources during the preparation of this third edition. A special thank you to Linda Miller, who not only contributed two chapters, but who also served as the section editor for Serological Diagnosis of Infectoius Diseases. My other contributors, whose expertise enriched this book are : Tom Alexander, Diane Davis, Dorothy Fike, Marc Golightly, Candace Golightly, Patsy Jarreau, Donald Lehman, Susan Orton, John Schmitz, Tim Stegall, and Sue Strasinger. I would also like to thank the reviewers whose additional sets of eyes and thoughtful suggestions helped to strengthen the chapters.

Finally I would like to acknowledge all the folks at F.A. Davis for their hard work in making this third edition a reality. To the Senior Acquisitions Editor for Health Professions, Christa Fratantoro, as usual you made the task of writing almost fun, and you were a gentle taskmaster who kept me going. I also appreciate the efforts of Sarah Granlund and Grace Caputo who served as Developmental Editors, and Sam Rondinelli, David Orzechowski, George Lang, Marsha Hall, and all the others who helped this book come to life.

My immunology students, past, present, and future, are the reason for writing this book. My hope is that this text will help make a very complex subject a little easier to understand. I appreciate and learn as much or more from your curiosity and your questioning as you do from me.

A thank you to friends whose encouragement and understanding helped me to stay on task. Finally, to my two wonderful sons Eric and Kevin, their wives Kathy and Melissa, and my grandchildren Hannah and Turner, you are my inspiration and my source of strength.

# Contents

# Color Plates

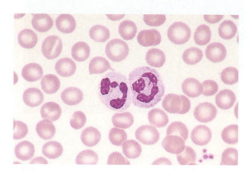

COLOR PLATE 1. Photo of Neutrophils. (From Harmening, D. Clinical Hematology and Fundamentals of Hemostasis, ed. 4. FA Davis, Philadelphia, 2002. Color Plate 10.) See Figure 1–1 in the text.

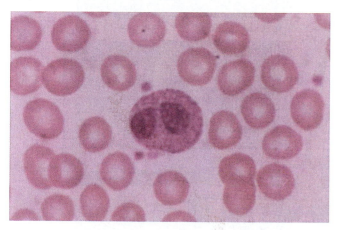

COLOR PLATE 2. Photo of an eosinophil. (From Harmening, D. Clinical Hematology and Fundamentals of Hemostasis, ed. 4. FA Davis, Philadelphia, 2002. Color Plate 12.) See Figure 1–2 in the text.

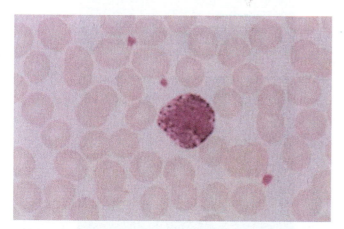

COLOR PLATE 3. Photo of a basophil. (From Harmening, D. Clinical Hematology and Fundamentals of Hemostasis, ed. 4. FA Davis, Philadelphia, 2002. Color Plate 13.) See Figure 1–3 in the text.

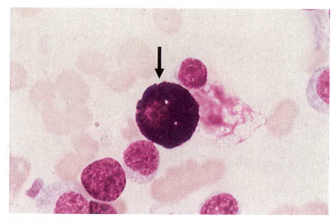

COLOR PLATE 4. Photo of a mast cell. (From Harmening, D. Clinical Hematology and Fundamentals of Hemostasis, ed. 4. FA Davis, Philadelphia, 2002. Color Plate 42.) See Figure 1–4 in the text.

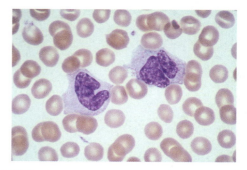

COLOR PLATE 5. Photo of two monocytes. (From Harmening, D. Clinical Hematology and Fundamentals of Hemostasis, ed. 4. FA Davis, Philadelphia, 2002. Color Plate 17.) See Figure 1–5 in the text.

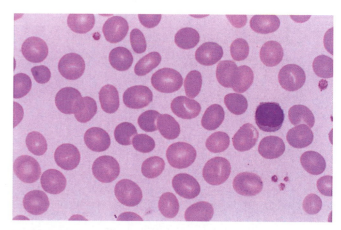

COLOR PLATE 6. Typical lymphocyte found in peripheral blood. (From Harr, R: Clinical Laboratory Science Review, FA Davis, Philadelphia, 2000, Color Plate 31.) See Figure 2–1 in the text.

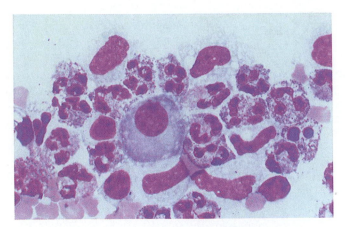

COLOR PLATE 7. A typical plasma cell. (From Harr, R: Clinical Laboratory Science Review, FA Davis, Philadelphia, 2000, Color Plate 28.) See Figure 2–8 in the text.

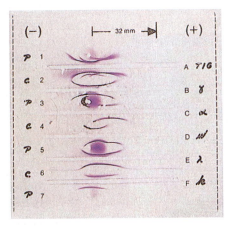

COLOR PLATE 8. Immunoelectrophoresis film showing normal controls (odd-numbered wells) and patient serum (even-numbered wells). (From Harr, R: Clinical Laboratory Science Review, ed. 2, FA Davis, Philadelphia, 2000, Color Plate 4, with permission.) See Figure 8–7 in the text.

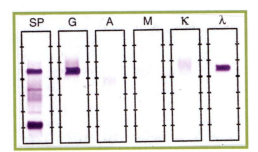

COLOR PLATE 9. Immunofixation electrophoresis. (Courtesy of Helena Laboratories, Beaumont, TX. ) See Figure 8–8 in the text.

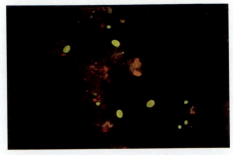

COLOR PLATE 10. Direct fluorescent antibody test for *Giardia* and *Cryptosporidium* in stool. Larger oval bodies are *Giardia lamblia* cysts, and the smaller round bodies are *Cryptosporidium sp.* cysts. (Courtesy of Meridian Bioscience, Cincinnati, Ohio.) See Figure 10-5 in the text.

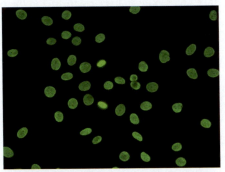

homogeneous pattern

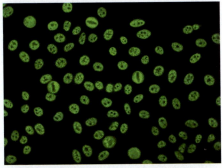

speckled pattern

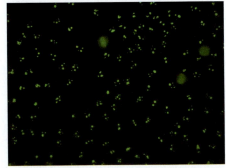

nucleolar pattern

COLOR PLATE 11. Patterns of immunofluorescent staining for anti-nuclear antibodies. (Courtesy of DiaSorin, Inc., with permission.) See Figure 14–2 in the text.

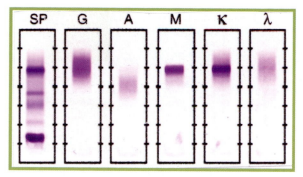

**COLOR PLATE 12.** Agarose gel immunofixation electrophoresis of serum. (Courtesy of Helena Laboratories.) See Figure 15–2 in the text.

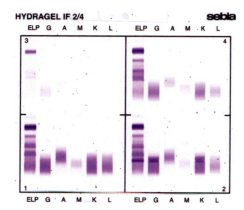

**COLOR PLATE 13.** Four different patient immunofixation patterns. See Figure 16-2 in the text.

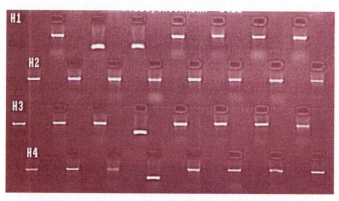

**COLOR PLATE 14.** An example of a PCR with sequence specific primers (PCR-SSP) analysis of the HLA-DQB1 locus. See Figure 17–3 in the text.

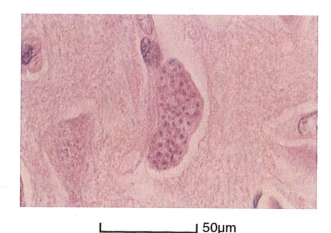

**COLOR PLATE 15.** Pseudocyst of Toxoplasma gondii seen in a brain section. (From Leventhal, R and Cheadle, RF. Medical Parasitology:A Self-Instructional Text. Ed 5. FA Davis, Philadelphia, color plate 127, 2002, with permission.) See Figure 20-1 in the text.

# Nature of the Immune System

# 1 Introduction and Natural Immunity

## LEARNING OBJECTIVES

*After finishing this chapter, the reader will be able to:*

1. Discuss how immunology as a science began with the study of immunity.
2. Describe Jenner's role in discovering the phenomenon of cross-immunity in relation to smallpox.
3. Discuss Pasteur's work with attenuated vaccines.
4. Explain how the controversy over humoral versus cellular immunity contributed to expanding knowledge in the field of immunology.
5. Explain what an antibody is.
6. Differentiate between the external and internal defense systems.
7. Distinguish natural from acquired immunity.
8. Discuss the role of acute-phase reactants in the innate or natural immune response.
9. Describe the types of white blood cells capable of phagocytosis.
10. List the steps in the process of phagocytosis.
11. Explain the importance of phagocytosis in both natural and acquired immunity.
12. Discuss the intracellular mechanism for destruction of foreign particles during the process of phagocytosis.
13. Describe the process of inflammation.
14. Recognize false-positive and false-negative reactions in the latex agglutination test for C-reactive protein.
15. Determine the significance of abnormal levels of acute-phase reactants.

## KEY TERMS

____ Acquired immunity
____ Acute-phase reactant
____ Antibody
____ Antigen
____ Chemotaxin
____ Complement
____ C-reactive protein
____ Cross-immunity
____ Diapedesis
____ External defense system
____ Humoral immunity
____ Immunity
____ Immunology
____ Inflammation
____ Internal defense system
____ Natural immunity
____ Opsonin
____ Phagocytosis
____ Phagolysosome
____ Phagosome
____ Respiratory burst
____ Toll-like receptors

# CHAPTER OUTLINE

While humans have been trying for many centuries to unravel the secrets of preventing disease, the field of immunology is a relatively new science. Virtually the entire history of immunology has been recorded within the last 100 years, and it is only in the recent past that the most significant part of this history has been written. It was not until the 1960s that the cells responsible for the immune response were identified and characterized. At the same time, pioneering techniques to measure small amounts of substances using antibodies with radioactive or enzyme tags were developed. These discoveries have impacted testing in every area of the laboratory and have played a significant role in the diagnosis and treatment of disease.

## IMMUNITY AND IMMUNIZATION

**Immunology** can be defined as the study of a host's reactions when foreign substances are introduced into the body. A foreign substance that induces such an immune response is called an **antigen.**

Immunology as a science has its roots in the study of **immunity,** the condition of being resistant to infection. The first written records of immunological experimentation date back to the 1500s, when the Chinese developed a practice of inhaling powder made from smallpox scabs in order to produce protection against this dreaded disease. This practice of deliberately exposing an individual to material from smallpox lesions was known as *variolation.* The theory was that if a healthy individual was exposed as a child or young adult, the effects of the disease would be minimized. However, this was not always the case.

Further refinements did not occur until the late 1700s, when an English country doctor by the name of Edward Jenner discovered a remarkable relationship between exposure to cowpox and immunity to smallpox. After observing the fact that milkmaids who were exposed to cowpox had apparent immunity to smallpox, he deliberately injected individuals with material from a cowpox lesion and then exposed them to smallpox. He thus proved that immunity to cowpox, a very mild disease, provided protection against smallpox. This procedure of injecting cellular material became known as *vaccination,* from *vacca,* the Latin word for "cow." The phenomenon in which exposure to one agent produces protection against another agent is known as **cross-immunity.** Within 50 years of this discovery, most of the European countries had initiated a compulsory vaccination program.[1]

In working with the bacteria that caused chicken cholera, Louis Pasteur, a key figure in the development of both microbiology and immunology, accidentally found that old cultures would not cause disease in chickens.[2] Subsequent injections of more virulent organisms had no effect on the birds that had been previously exposed to the older cultures. In this manner, the first attenuated vaccine was discovered. Attenuation, or change, may occur through heat, aging, or chemical means, and it remains the basis for many of the immunizations that are used today. Pasteur applied this same principle of attenuation to the prevention of rabies, a fatal disease at that time. Although he did not know the causative agent, he recognized that the central nervous system was affected, and thus he studied spinal cords from rabid animals. He noted that spinal cords left to dry for a few days were less infectious to laboratory animals than fresh spinal cords. In 1885, when a boy who was severely bitten by a rabid dog was brought to his home, Pasteur tried out his new procedure. The boy received a series of 12 injections beginning with material from the least infectious cords and progressing to the fresher, more infectious material. Miraculously, the boy survived, and a modification of this procedure is the standard treatment for rabies today.

## CELLULAR VERSUS HUMORAL IMMUNITY

In the late 1800s, scientists turned to identifying the actual mechanisms that produce immunity in a host.[2] Elie Metchnikoff, a Russian scientist, observed that foreign objects introduced into transparent starfish larvae became surrounded by motile cells that attempted to destroy these invaders. He called this process **phagocytosis,** meaning cells that eat cells.[2] He hypothesized that immunity to disease was based on the action of these scavenger cells.

Other researchers contended that noncellular elements in the blood were responsible for protection from microorganisms. The theory of **humoral immunity** was thus born, and this set off a long-lasting dispute over the relative importance of cellular versus humoral immunity.

In 1903, an English physician named Almoth Wright linked the two theories by showing that the immune response involved both cellular and humoral elements. He observed that certain humoral, or circulating, factors called *opsonins* acted to coat bacteria so that they became more susceptible to ingestion by phagocytic cells.[3] These serum factors include specific proteins known as **antibodies** and nonspecific factors called *acute-phase reactants* that increase nonspecifically in any infection. This chapter will consider the branch of immunity know as *natural immunity*, while other chapters will focus on the more specific response known as *acquired immunity*.

**Natural, or innate, immunity** is the ability of the individual to resist infection by means of normally present body functions. These are considered nonadaptive or nonspecific and are the same for all pathogens or foreign substances to which one is exposed. No prior exposure is required, and the response does not change with subsequent exposures. Many of these mechanisms are subject to influence by such factors as nutrition, age, fatigue, stress, and genetic determinants. **Acquired immunity,** in contrast, is a type of resistance that is characterized by specificity for each individual pathogen, or microbial agent, and the ability to remember a prior exposure, which results in an increased response upon repeated exposure. Both systems are essential to maintain good health; in fact, they operate in concert and are dependent upon one another for maximal effectiveness.

The natural defense system is composed of two parts: the external defense system and the internal defense system. The external defense system is designed to keep microorganisms from entering the body. If these defenses are overcome, then the internal defense system must clear invaders as quickly as possible. Internal defenses can be categorized into cellular mechanisms and humoral factors. Both of these systems work together to promote phagocytosis, which results in the destruction of foreign cells and organisms. The process of inflammation brings cells and humoral factors to the area in need of healing. If the healing process is begun and resolved as quickly as possible, the tissues are less likely to be damaged.

## EXTERNAL DEFENSE SYSTEM

The **external defense system** is composed of structural barriers that prevent most infectious agents from entering the body. First and foremost is the unbroken skin and the mucosal membrane surfaces. To understand how important a role these play, one has only to consider how vulnerable victims of severe burns are to infection. Not only does the skin serve as a major structural barrier, but also the presence of several secretions discourages the growth of microorganisms. Lactic acid in sweat, for instance, and fatty acids from sebaceous glands maintain the skin at a pH of approximately 5.6. This acid pH keeps most microorganisms from growing.

Additionally, each of the various organ systems in the body has its own unique mechanisms. In the respiratory tract, mucous secretions and the motion of cilia lining the nasopharyngeal passages clear away almost 90 percent of the deposited material. The flushing action of urine, plus its slight acidity, helps to remove many potential pathogens from the genitourinary tract. Lactic acid production in the female genital tract keeps the vagina at a pH of about 5, another means of preventing invasion of pathogens. In the digestive tract, acidity of the stomach, which is due to production of hydrochloric acid, keeps the pH as low as 1 and serves to halt microbial growth. Lysozyme is an enzyme found in many secretions such as tears and saliva, and it attacks the cell walls of microorganisms, especially those that are gram-positive.

In many locations of the body, there is normal flora that often keeps pathogens from establishing themselves in these areas. This phenomenon is known as *competitive exclusion*. The significance of the presence of normal flora is readily demonstrated by looking at the side effects of antimicrobial therapy. Frequently, yeast infections due to *Candida albicans* occur, the result of wiping out normal flora that would ordinarily compete with such opportunists.

## INTERNAL DEFENSE SYSTEM

The second part of natural immunity is the **internal defense system,** in which both cells and soluble factors play essential parts. The internal defense system is designed to recognize molecules that are unique to infectious organisms.[4] This typically involves recognizing a carbohydrate such as mannose that is found in microorganisms and is not evident on human cells. White blood cells seek out and destroy foreign cells by participating in phagocytosis, which is the engulfment of cells or particulate matter by leukocytes, macrophages, and other cells. This process destroys most of the foreign invaders that enter the body, and it is the most important function of the internal defense system. Phagocytosis is enhanced by soluble factors called *acute-phase reactants*.

### Acute-Phase Reactants

**Acute-phase reactants** are normal serum constituents that increase rapidly by at least 25 percent due to infection, injury, or trauma to the tissues.[5] Some of the most important ones are C-reactive protein, serum amyloid A, complement components, mannose-binding protein, alpha$_1$-antitrypsin, haptoglobin, fibrinogen, and ceruloplasmin.[5,6] They are produced primarily by hepatocytes (liver parenchymal cells) within 12 to 24 hours in response to an increase in certain intercellular signaling polypeptides called *cytokines* (see Chapter 5 for a complete discussion of cytokines). These cell messengers, most notably interleukin-1β (IL-1β), interleukin-6 (IL-6), and tumor necrosis factor-alpha (TNF-α) are mainly produced by monocytes and macrophages at the sites of inflammation.[7,8] **Table 1-1** summarizes characteristics of the main acute-phase reactants.

| Table 1-1. Characteristics of Acute-Phase Reactants | | | | |
|---|---|---|---|---|
| **PROTEIN** | **RESPONSE TIME (HR)** | **NORMAL CONCENTRATION (MG/DL)** | **INCREASE** | **FUNCTION** |
| C-reactive protein | 6–10 | 0.5 | 1000× | Opsonization, complement activation |
| Serum amyloid A | 24 | 3.0 | 1000× | Removal of cholesterol |
| Alpha₁-antitrypsin | 24 | 200–400 | 2–5× | Protease inhibitor |
| Fibrinogen | 24 | 110–400 | 2–5× | Clot formation |
| Haptoglobin | 24 | 40–200 | 2–10× | Binds hemoglobin |
| Ceruloplasmin | 48–72 | 20–40 | 2× | Binds copper and oxidizes iron |
| Complement C3 | 48–72 | 60–140 | 2× | Opsonization, lysis |
| Mannose-binding protein | ? | 0.15–1.0 | ? | Complement activation |

## C-Reactive Protein

**C-reactive protein (CRP)** is a trace constituent of serum originally thought to be an antibody to the c-polysaccharide of pneumococci. It increases rapidly within 4 to 6 hours following infection, surgery, or other trauma to the body. Levels increase dramatically as much as a hundredfold to a thousandfold, reaching a peak value within 48 hours.[9,10] They also decline rapidly with cessation of the stimulus. CRP has a plasma half-life of about 19 hours.[9] Elevated levels are found in conditions such as bacterial infections, rheumatic fever, viral infections, malignant diseases, tuberculosis, and after a heart attack. The median CRP value for an individual increases with age, reflecting an increase in subclinical inflammatory conditions.[11]

C-reactive protein is a homogeneous molecule with a molecular weight of 118,000 daltons and a structure that consists of five identical subunits held together by noncovalent bonds. It is a member of the family known as the pentraxins, all of which are proteins with five subunits. CRP acts somewhat like an antibody, as it is capable of opsonization (the coating of foreign particles), agglutination, precipitation, and activation of complement by the classical pathway. However, binding is calcium-dependent and nonspecific, and the main substrate is phosphocholine, a common constituent of microbial membranes. It also binds to small ribonuclear proteins; phospholipids; peptidoglycan; and other constituents of bacteria, fungi, and parasites.[9] In addition, CRP binds to specific receptors found on monocytes, macrophages, and neutrophils, which promotes phagocytosis. Thus, CRP can be thought of as a primitive, nonspecific form of antibody molecule that is able to act as a defense against microorganisms or foreign cells until specific antibodies can be produced.

Because the levels rise and then decline so rapidly, CRP is the most widely used indicator of acute inflammation. Although CRP is a nonspecific indicator of disease or trauma, monitoring of its levels can be useful clinically to follow a disease process and observe the response to treatment of inflammation and infection.[9] It is also a noninvasive means of following the course of malignancy and organ transplantation, because a rise in the level may mean a return of the malignancy, or in the case of transplantation, the beginning of organ rejection.

In accord with the finding that atherosclerosis, or coronary artery disease, is the result of a chronic inflammatory process,[10,12] recent research indicates that an increased level of CRP is a significant risk factor for myocardial infarction and ischemic stroke in men and women who have no previous history of cardiovascular disease.[13–16] A concentration of more than 2 mg/L has been defined as the threshold for high cardiovascular risk.[16] Normal levels in adults range from approximately 1.5 mg/L for men to 2.5 mg/L for women.[17,18] Thus, monitoring CRP may be an important preventative measure in determining the potential risk of heart attack or stroke, although only automated, high-sensitivity tests for CRP are useful for this purpose. High-sensitivity CRP testing has a lower level of detection of 0.01 mg/dL, allowing for measurement of much smaller increases than the traditional latex agglutination screening test.[9]

## Serum Amyloid A

Serum amyloid A is the other major protein whose concentration can increase almost a thousandfold, as is the case in CRP. It is an apolipoprotein that is synthesized in the liver and has a molecular weight of 11,685 daltons. Normal circulating levels are approximately 30ug/ml. In plasma, it is associated with HDL cholesterol, and it is thought to play a role in metabolism of cholesterol.[19] By removing cholesterol from cholesterol-filled macrophages at the site of tissue injury, serum amyloid A contributes to the cleaning up of the area.[19] This also facilitates recycling of cell membrane cholesterol and phospholipids for reuse in building membranes of new cells required during acute inflammation.[20] It has been found to increase significantly more in bacterial infections than in viral infections.[21]

## Complement

**Complement** refers to a series of serum proteins that are normally present and whose overall function is mediation of inflammation. There are nine such proteins that are activated by bound antibodies in a sequence known as the *classical cascade;* an additional number are involved in the alternate pathway that is triggered by microorganisms. The major functions of complement are opsonization, chemotaxis, and lysis of cells. Complement is discussed more fully in Chapter 6.

## Mannose-Binding Protein

Mannose-binding protein (MPB), also called *mannose-binding lectin,* is a trimer that acts as an opsonin, which is calcium-dependent. It is able to recognize foreign carbohydrates such as mannose and several other sugars found primarily on bacteria, some yeasts, viruses, and several parasites.[22] It is widely distributed on mucosal surfaces throughout the body. It has many similarities to the complement component C1q, as binding activates the complement cascade and helps to promote phagocytosis.[22] Normal concentrations are up to 10 ug/ml. Lack of MBP has been associated with recurrent yeast infections.[22]

## Alpha₁-Antitrypsin

Alpha$_1$-antitrypsin (AAT) is the major component of the alpha band when serum is electrophoresed. Although the name implies that it acts against trypsin, it is a general plasma inhibitor of proteases released from leukocytes, especially elastase.[6] Elastase is an endogenous enzyme that can degrade elastin and collagen. In chronic pulmonary inflammation, lung tissue is damaged because of its activity. Thus, alpha$_1$-antitrypsin acts to "mop up" or counteract the effects of neutrophil invasion during an inflammatory response. It also regulates expression of proinflammatory cytokines such as tumor necrosis factor-alpha, interleukin-1β, and interleukin-6, mentioned previously.

Alpha$_1$-antitrypsin deficiency can result in premature emphysema, especially in individuals who smoke or who are exposed to a noxious occupational environment.[6,23] In such a deficiency, uninhibited proteases remain in the lower respiratory tract, leading to destruction of parenchymal cells in the lungs and to development of emphysema or idiopathic pulmonary fibrosis. It has been estimated that as many as 60,000 Americans suffer from this deficiency.[24] There are at least 17 alleles of the gene coding for AAT that are associated with low production of the enzyme.[6] One particular variant gene for alpha$_1$-antitrypsin is associated with lack of its secretion from the liver, and such individuals are at risk of developing liver disease and emphysema.[6] Homozygous inheritance of this most severe variant gene may lead to development of cirrhosis, hepatitis, or hepatoma in early childhood.[6]

Alpha$_1$-antitrypsin can also react with any serine protease, such as those generated by triggering of the complement cascade or fibrinolysis. Once bound to alpha$_1$-antitrypsin, the protease is completely inactivated and is subsequently removed from the area of tissue damage and catabolized.

## Haptoglobin

Haptoglobin is an alpha$_2$-globulin with a molecular weight of 100,000 daltons. Its primary function is to bind irreversibly to free hemoglobin released by intravascular hemolysis. Once bound, the complex is cleared rapidly by Kupffer and parenchymal cells in the liver, thus preventing loss of free hemoglobin.[25,26] The rise in plasma haptoglobin is due to de novo synthesis by the liver and does not represent release of previously formed haptoglobin from other sites.[6] A twofold to tenfold increase in haptoglobin can be seen following inflammation, stress, or tissue necrosis. Early in the inflammatory response, however, haptoglobin levels may drop because of intravascular hemolysis, consequently masking the protein's behavior as an acute-phase reactant. Thus, plasma levels must be interpreted in light of other acute-phase reactants. Normal plasma concentrations range from 40 to 290 mg/dL.[6,25] Haptoglobin plays an important role in protecting the kidney from damage and in preventing the loss of iron by urinary excretion. However, its most important function may be to provide protection against oxidative damage mediated by free hemoglobin, a powerful oxidizing agent that can generate peroxides and hydroxyl radicals.[26,27] It may also bind to partially unfolded and damaged proteins to prevent them from aggregating in blood vessels.

## Fibrinogen

Fibrinogen is the most abundant of the coagulation factors in plasma, and it forms the fibrin clot.[6] The molecule is a dimer with a molecular weight of 340,000 daltons. Normal levels range from 100 to 400 mg/dL.[6] A small portion is cleaved by thrombin to form fibrils that make up a fibrin clot. This increases the strength of a wound and stimulates endothelial cell adhesion and proliferation, which are critical to the healing process.[5] Formation of a clot also creates a barrier that helps prevent the spread of microorganisms further into the body. Fibrinogen also serves to promote aggregation of red blood cells, and increased levels contribute to an increased risk for developing coronary artery disease, especially in women.[28,29]

## Ceruloplasmin

Ceruloplasmin consists of a single polypeptide chain with a molecular weight of 132,000 daltons.[6] It is the principal copper-transporting protein in human plasma, binding 90 to 95 percent of the copper found in plasma by attaching six cupric ions per molecule. Additionally, ceruloplasmin acts as a ferroxidase, oxidizing iron from $Fe^{2+}$ to $Fe^{3+}$. This may serve as a means of releasing iron from ferritin for binding to transferrin.[6]

A depletion of ceruloplasmin is found in Wilson's disease, an autosomal recessive genetic disorder characterized by a massive increase of copper in the tissues. Normally, circulating copper is absorbed out by the liver and either combined with ceruloplasmin and returned to the plasma or excreted into the bile duct. In Wilson's disease, copper accumulates in the liver and subsequently in other tissues such as the brain, cornea, kidneys, and bones.[30,31]

## Cellular Defense Mechanisms

There are five principal types of leukocytes, or white blood cells, in peripheral blood: neutrophils, eosinophils, basophils, monocytes, and lymphocytes. Some of these white blood cells participate in the process of phagocytosis; these are known as the *myeloid line* and arise from a common precursor in the marrow. These can be further divided into granulocytes and monocytes, or mononuclear cells. Neutrophils, eosinophils, and basophils are considered granulocytes. Each of these cell types is described in this chapter. Several cell lines that are found in the tissues, namely mast cells, macrophages, and dendritic cells, will also be discussed in this chapter, as they all contribute to the process of natural immunity. Lymphocytes form the basis of the acquired immune response and are discussed in Chapter 2.

### Neutrophils

The neutrophil, or polymorphonuclear neutrophilic (PMN) leukocyte, represents approximately 50 to 70 percent of the total peripheral white blood cells. These are around 10 to 15 µm in diameter, with a nucleus that has between two and five lobes (**Fig. 1–1**). They contain a large number of neutral staining granules, which are classified as primary, secondary, and tertiary granules. Primary granules, also called *azurophilic granules*, contain enzymes such as myeloperoxidase; elastase; proteinase 3; lysozyme; cathepsin G; and defensins, small proteins that have antibacterial activity.[25,32] Secondary granules are characterized by the presence of collagenase, lactoferrin, lysozyme, reduced nicotinamide adenine dinucleotide phosphate (NADPH) oxidase, and other membrane proteins normally associated with the plasma membrane.[25,32] Newly discovered tertiary granules contain gelatinase and plasminogen activator.[25,32] Acid hydrolases are found in separate compartments called *lysosomes.*[32,33]

Normally, half of the total neutrophil population is found in a marginating pool on blood vessel walls, while the rest circulate freely for approximately 6 to 10 hours. There is a continuous interchange, however, between the marginating and the circulating pools. Marginating occurs to allow neutrophils to move from the circulating blood to the tissues through a process known as **diapedesis,** or movement through blood vessel walls. Receptors known as *selectins* help make neutrophils sticky and enhance adherence to endothelial cells that make up the vessel wall.[34] Neutrophils then form pseudopods, which squeeze through junctions of the

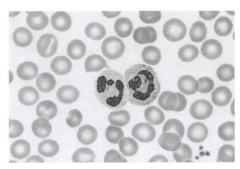

FIGURE 1–1. Photo of neutrophils. *(From Harmening, D. Clinical Hematology and Fundamentals of Hemostasis, ed 4. F. A. Davis, Philadelphia, 2002. Color Plate 10.) See Color Plate 1.*

endothelial cells. They are attracted to a specific area by chemotactic factors. **Chemotaxins** are chemical messengers that cause cells to migrate in a particular direction. Factors that are chemotactic for neutrophils include complement components; proteins from the coagulation cascade; products from bacteria and viruses; platelet activating factor; and secretions from mast cells, lymphocytes, macrophages, and other neutrophils. Once in the tissues, neutrophils have a life span of about 5 days.[35] Normally, the input of neutrophils from the bone marrow equals the output from the blood to the tissues to maintain a steady state. However, in the case of acute infection, an increase of neutrophils in the circulating blood can occur almost immediately.[25]

### Eosinophils

Eosinophils are approximately 12 to 15 µm in diameter, and they normally make up between 1 and 3 percent of the circulating white blood cells in a nonallergic person. Their number increases in an allergic reaction or in response to many parasitic infections. The nucleus is usually bilobed or ellipsoidal and is often eccentrically located (**Fig. 1–2**). Eosinophils take up the acid eosin dye, and the cytoplasm is filled with large orange to reddish orange granules.

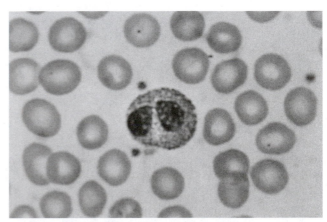

FIGURE 1–2. Photo of an eosinophil. *(From Harmening, D. Clinical Hematology and Fundamentals of Hemostasis, ed 4. F. A. Davis, Philadelphia, 2002. Color Plate 12.) See Color Plate 2.*

Primary granules contain acid phosphatase and arylsulfatase, while eosinophil-specific granules contain several different proteins: major basic protein, eosinophil cationic protein, eosinophil peroxidase, and eosinophil-derived neurotoxin.[25] These cells are capable of phagocytosis but are much less efficient than neutrophils because of the smaller numbers present and their lack of digestive enzymes.[35] Their most important role is neutralizing basophil and mast cell products and killing certain parasites (discussed in Chapter 20).

## Basophils

Basophils are found in very small numbers, representing less than 1 percent of all circulating white blood cells. The smallest of the granulocytes, they are between 10 to 15 μm in diameter and contain coarse, densely staining deep-bluish-purple granules that often obscure the nucleus[35] **(Fig. 1–3)**. Constituents of these granules are histamine, a small amount of heparin, and eosinophil chemotactic factor-A, all of which have an important function in inducing and maintaining immediate hypersensitivity reactions.[25,35] Histamine is a vasoactive amine that contracts smooth muscle, and heparin is an anticoagulant. IgE, the immunoglobulin formed in allergic reactions, binds readily to basophil cell membranes, and granules release their constituents when they contact an antigen. The granules lack hydrolytic enzymes, although peroxidase is present. Basophils exist for only a few hours in the bloodstream.

## Mast Cells

Tissue mast cells resemble basophils, but they are connective tissue cells of mesenchymal origin.[36] They are widely distributed throughout the body and are larger than basophils, with a small round nucleus and more granules **(Fig. 1–4)**. Unlike basophils, they have a long life span of between 9 and 18 months.[36] The enzyme content of the granules helps to distinguish them from basophils, as they

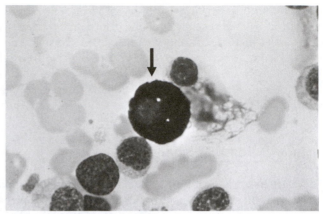

**FIGURE 1–4.** Photo of a mast cell. *(From Harmening, D. Clinical Hematology and Fundamentals of Hemostasis, ed 4. F. A. Davis, Philadelphia, 2002. Color Plate 42.) See Color Plate 4.*

contain acid phosphatase, alkaline phosphatase, and protease.[25] The mast cell, like the basophil, plays a role in hypersensitivity reactions by binding IgE.

## Monocytes

Monocytes, or mononuclear cells, are the largest cells in the peripheral blood, with a diameter that can vary from 12 to 22 μm; they have an average size of 18 μm. One distinguishing feature is an irregularly folded or horseshoe-shaped nucleus that occupies almost one-half of the entire cell's volume **(Fig. 1–5)**. The abundant cytoplasm stains a dull grayish blue and has a ground-glass appearance due to the presence of fine dustlike granules. These granules are actually of two types, one of which contains peroxidase, acid phosphatase, and arylsulfatase; this indicates that these granules are similar to the lysosomes of neutrophils.[25] The other type of granule may contain β-glucuronidase, lysozyme, and lipase, but no alkaline phosphatase. Digestive vacuoles may also be observed in the cytoplasm. These make up between 4 and 10 percent of total circulating white blood cells; however, they do not remain in the circulation for long. They stay in peripheral blood for up to 70 hours, and then they migrate to the tissues and become known as *macrophages*.

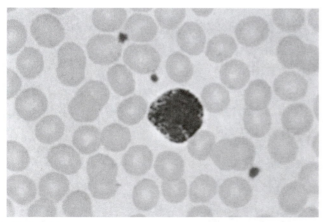

**FIGURE 1–3.** Photo of a basophil. *(From Harmening, D. Clinical Hematology and Fundamentals of Hemostasis, ed 4. F. A. Davis, Philadelphia, 2002. Color Plate 13.) See Color Plate 3.*

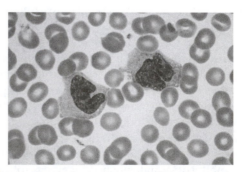

**FIGURE 1–5.** Photo of two monocytes. *(From Harmening, D. Clinical Hematology and Fundamentals of Hemostasis, ed 4. F. A. Davis, Philadelphia, 2002. Color Plate 17.) See Color Plate 5.*

## Tissue Macrophages

All tissue macrophages arise from monocytes, which can be thought of as macrophage precursors, because additional differentiation and cell division takes place in the tissues. The transition from monocyte to macrophage is characterized by progressive cellular enlargement to between 25 and 80 μm.[25] As the monocyte matures into a macrophage, there is an increase in endoplasmic reticulum, lysosomes, and mitochondria. Unlike monocytes, macrophages contain no peroxidase.[25,35] There are no conclusive data to indicate that monocytes are predestined for any particular tissue, so tissue distribution appears to be a random phenomenon.

Macrophages have specific names according to their particular tissue location. Some are immobile, while others progress through the tissues by means of amoeboid action. Macrophages in the lung are alveolar macrophages; in the liver, Kupffer cells; in the brain, microglial cells; and in connective tissue, histiocytes. Macrophages may not be as efficient as neutrophils in phagocytosis, because their motility is slow compared to that of the neutrophils. However, their life span appears to be in the range of months rather than days.

The monocyte–macrophage system plays an important role in initiating and regulating the immune response. Their functions include microbial killing, tumoricidal activity, intracellular parasite eradication, phagocytosis, secretion of cell mediators, and antigen presentation. Killing activity is enhanced when macrophages become "activated" by contact with microorganisms or with chemical messengers called *cytokines*, which are released by T lymphocytes during the immune response. (See Chapter 5 for a complete discussion of cytokines.)

## Dendritic Cells

Dendritic cells are so named because they are covered with long membranous extensions that make them resemble nerve cell dendrites. Their main function is to phagocytose antigen and present it to helper T lymphocytes. While their actual developmental lineage is not known, they are believed to be descendents of the myeloid line. They are classified according to their tissue location, in a similar manner to macrophages. Langerhans cells are found on skin and mucous membranes; interstitial dendritic cells populate the major organs such as the heart, lungs, liver, kidney, and the gastrointestinal tract; and interdigitating dendritic cells are present in the T lymphocyte areas of secondary lymphoid tissue and the thymus. After capturing antigen in the tissue by phagocytosis or endocytosis, they migrate to the blood and to lymphoid organs, where they present antigen to T lymphocytes to initiate the acquired immune response. They are the most potent phagocytic cell in the tissue.

## Toll–like Receptors

While each of the aforementioned cells has its own unique receptors to attach to microorganisms, an additional mechanism recently discovered on certain cells is Toll-like receptors. Toll is a protein originally discovered in the fruit fly *Drosophila*, where it plays an important role in antifungal immunity in the adult fly. Very similar molecules are found on human leukocytes and some nonleukocyte cell types, and these are called **Toll-like receptors (TLRs).** The highest concentration of these receptors occurs on monocytes, macrophages, and neutrophils.[37] There are 11 slightly different TLRs in humans.[37] Each of these receptors recognizes a different microbial product. For example, TLR2 recognizes teichoic acid and peptidoglycan found in gram-positive bacteria, while TLR4 recognizes lipopolysaccharide found in gram-negative bacteria **(Fig. 1–6)**. Once a receptor binds to its particular substance, or ligand, phagocytosis may be stimulated, or the cell produces cytokines that enhance inflammation and eventual destruction of the microorganism. Thus, they play an important role in enhancing natural immunity.

## Phagocytosis

The process of phagocytosis consists of four main steps: (1) physical contact between the white cell and the foreign particle, (2) formation of a phagosome, (3) fusion with cytoplasmic granules to form a phagolysosome, and (4) digestion and release of debris to the outside **(Fig. 1–7)**. Physical contact occurs as neutrophils roll along until they encounter the site of injury or infection.[33] They adhere to receptors on the endothelial cell wall of the blood vessels and penetrate through to the tissue by means of diapedesis. This process is aided by chemotaxis, whereby cells are attracted to the site of inflammation by chemical substances such as soluble bacterial factors, complement components, or C-reactive protein. Receptors on neutrophils or monocytes come into contact with the foreign particle surface,

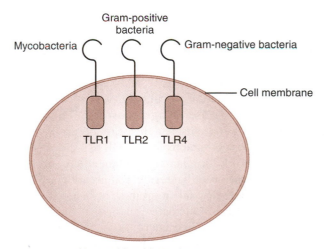

**FIGURE 1–6.** Toll-like receptors on a white cell membrane. Each of the 11 different Toll-like receptors recognizes a different pathogenic product. A few examples are shown here. TLR1 recognizes lipoprotein found in mycobacteria; TLR2 binds to peptidoglycan in gram-positive bacteria; TLR4 recognizes lipopolysaccharide in gram-negative bacteria.

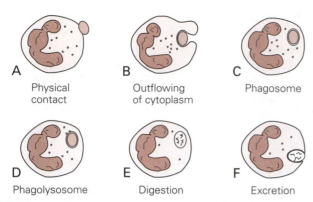

**FIGURE 1–7.** Steps involved in phagocytosis. *(A)* Adherence: physical contact between the phagocytic cell and the microorganism occurs, aided by opsonins. *(B)* Outflowing of cytoplasm to surround the microorganism. *(C)* Formation of phagosome: microorganism is completely surrounded by a part of the cell membrane. *(D)* Formation of the phagolysome: cytoplasmic granules fuse with membrane of phagosome, emptying contents into this membrane-bound space. *(E)* Digestion of the microorganism by hydrolytic enzymes. *(F)* Excretion of contents of phagolysosome to the outside by exocytosis.

enhanced by **opsonins,** a term derived from the Greek word meaning "to prepare for eating." Opsonins are serum proteins that attach to a foreign substance and help prepare it for phagocytosis. C-reactive protein, complement components, and antibodies are all important opsonins. Phagocytic cells have receptors for immunoglobulins and for complement components, which aid in contact and in initiating ingestion. Opsonins may act by neutralizing the surface charge on the foreign particle, making it easier for the cells to approach one another.

Once attachment has occurred, the cellular cytoplasm flows around the particle and eventually fuses with it. An increase in oxygen consumption, known as the **respiratory, or oxidative, burst,** occurs within the cell as the pseudopodia enclose the particle within a vacuole. The structure formed is known as a **phagosome.** The phagosome is gradually moved toward the center of the cell. Next, contact with cytoplasmic granules takes place, and fusion between granules and the phagosome occurs. At this point, the fused elements are known as a **phagolysosome.** The granules then release their contents, and digestion occurs. Any undigested material is excreted from the cells by exocytosis. The actual process of killing is oxygen-dependent and results from the generation of bactericidal metabolites. Heavily opsonized particles are taken up in as little as 20 seconds, and killing is almost immediate.[32]

Resting cells derive their energy from anaerobic glycolysis; however, when phagocytosis is triggered, the respiratory burst produces greater energy via oxidative metabolism. The hexose monophosphate shunt is used to change nicotinamide adenine dinucleotide phosphate (NADP) to its reduced form by adding a hydrogen. NADPH. NADPH then donates an electron to oxygen in the presence of NADPH oxidase, a membrane-bound enzyme, which is only activated through conformational change triggered by microbes themselves.[38] A radical known as $O_2^-$ (superoxide) is formed. Superoxide is highly toxic but can be rapidly converted to more lethal products. By adding hydrogen ions, the enzyme superoxide dismutase (SOD) converts superoxide to hydrogen peroxide or the hydroxyl radical OH. Hydrogen peroxide has long been considered an important bactericidal agent, and it is more stable than any of the free radicals. Its effect is potentiated by the formation of hypochlorite ions. This is accomplished through the action of the enzyme myeloperoxidase in the presence of chloride ions. Hypochlorite ions are powerful oxidizing agents. All of these substances contribute to killing within the phagocyte **(Fig. 1–8).**

However, new evidence indicates that an electron-transport system that alters the charge across the membrane of the phagolysosome is more important than actual formation of oxygen radicals themselves.[32] NADPH oxidase may depolarize the membrane, allowing hydrogen and potassium ions to enter the vacuole. When hydrogen combines with the superoxides, the pH increases, which in turn activates proteases that contribute to microbial killing. NADPH oxidase is known to be central to the killing of microbes, because its dysfunction causes chronic granulomatous disease. Patients with this disease suffer from recurring, severe bacterial infections.

## Inflammation

The overall reaction of the body to injury or invasion by an infectious agent is known as **inflammation.** Both cellular and humoral mechanisms are involved in this complex,

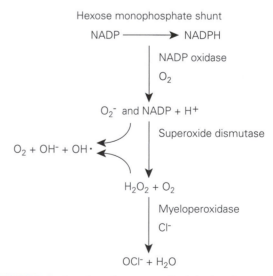

**FIGURE 1–8.** Creation of oxygen radicals in the phagocytic cell. The hexose monophosphate shunt is used to reduce NADP to NADPH. NADPH can reduce oxygen in the presence of NADPH oxidase to $O_2^-$, known as superoxide. Superoxide is converted to hydrogen peroxide through the action of the enzyme superoxide dismutase. Myeloperoxidase catalyzes formation of the hypochlorite radical, a very powerful oxidizing agent. Hydroxyl radicals, other powerful oxidizing agents, may also be formed.

highly orchestrated process. Each individual reactant plays a role in initiating, amplifying, or sustaining the reaction, and a delicate balance must be maintained for the process to be speedily resolved. The four cardinal signs or clinical symptoms are redness, swelling, heat, and pain. Major events associated with the process of inflammation are (1) increased blood supply to the infected area; (2) increased capillary permeability caused by retraction of endothelial cells lining the vessels; (3) migration of white blood cells, mainly neutrophils, from the capillaries to the surrounding tissue; and (4) migration of macrophages to the injured area[25] **(Fig. 1–9)**.

Chemical mediators such as histamine, which are released from injured mast cells, cause dilation of the blood vessels and bring additional blood flow to the affected area, resulting in redness and heat. The increased permeability of the vessels allows fluids in the plasma to leak to the tissues. This produces the swelling and pain associated with inflammation. Soluble mediators, including acute-phase reactants, initiate and control the response. Amplification occurs through formation of clots by the coagulation system and then the triggering of the fibrinolytic system.

As the endothelial cells of the vessels contract, neutrophils move through the endothelial cells of the vessel and out into the tissues. They are attracted to the site of injury or infection by the chemotaxins mentioned previously. Neutrophils, which are mobilized within 30 to 60 minutes after the injury, are the major type of cell present in *acute inflammation*. Neutrophil emigration may last 24 to 48 hours and is proportional to the level of chemotactic factors present in the area.

Migration of macrophages from surrounding tissue and from blood monocytes occurs several hours later and peaks at 16 to 48 hours. Macrophages attempt to clear the area through phagocytosis, and in most cases the healing process is completed with a return of normal tissue structure. However, when the inflammatory process becomes prolonged, it is said to be *chronic*, and tissue damage and loss of function may result. Specific immunity with infiltration of lymphocytes may contribute to the damage. Thus, a failure to remove microorganisms or injured tissue may result in continued tissue damage.

## SUMMARY

The study of immunology began as an interest in achieving immunity, or resistance to disease. Edward Jenner, an Englishman, performed the first successful vaccination against smallpox and ushered in the age of immunologic investigation. Another well-known name in the early history of immunology is Louis Pasteur, whose discovery of attenuated vaccines formed the basis of today's vaccination programs. The controversy over cellular versus humoral immunity was responsible for spawning much important research in the early years. Elie Metchnikoff identified phagocytic cells as a part of cellular immunity, and other researchers postulated that a humoral, or noncellular, factor in the blood was also involved in immunity. Both of these theories were brought together by Almuth Wright, an English physician who observed that both circulating and cellular factors are necessary to produce immunity.

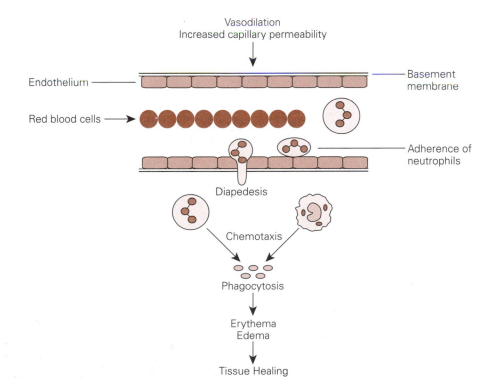

**FIGURE 1–9.** Events in the inflammatory response. Increased blood supply to the affected area is followed by increased capillary permeability and migration of neutrophils and macrophages to the tissues. Macrophages in the tissue are directed to the area. Acute-phase reactants stimulate phagocytosis of microorganisms. Clinical signs at the site of inflammation include edema and erythema. Tissue healing, with or without scarring, eventually results.

Natural, or innate, immunity encompasses all the body's defense mechanisms for resisting disease. These are always present, and the response is nonspecific, in that it is the same for any infectious agent encountered. External defenses are structural barriers such as skin, mucous membranes, and cilia that keep microorganisms from entering the body. Internal defenses are centered on the process of phagocytosis, which is the engulfment of cells or particulate matter by leukocytes, macrophages, and other cells. This process destroys most of the foreign cells that penetrate the external defenses.

Cells that are most active in phagocytosis include neutrophils, monocytes, and macrophages. Physical contact between the phagocytic cell and the foreign particle is aided by chemotaxis, whereby cells are attracted to the area, and opsonization, or coating of the foreign particle by serum proteins such as complement and antibody. Once contact occurs, cytoplasm flows around the foreign particle to form a phagosome. Fusion of the phagosome with lysosomal granules creates a phagolysosome. Inside this structure, enzymes are released, and the foreign particle is digested. The process is oxygen-dependent, and killing results from the creation of hypochlorite and hydroxyl ions, which damage protein irreversibly.

Acute-phase reactants are serum constituents that increase rapidly in response to infection or injury to the tissues. They enhance the process of phagocytosis by attracting leukocytes to the area of injury and by coating the foreign material so that it can be ingested more easily. Other functions of the acute-phase reactants include neutralization of mediators and proteolytic enzymes generated during the process of responding to pathogens. CRP is the most widely monitored of the acute-phase reactants and is the best indicator of acute inflammation.

Inflammation is the body's response to injury or invasion by a pathogen, and it is characterized by increased blood supply to the affected area, increased capillary permeability, migration of neutrophils to the surrounding tissue, and migration of macrophages to the injured area. Inflammation and the process of phagocytosis are considered natural immunity in that the response to any injury or pathogen is nonspecific. Phagocytosis, however, must occur before the specific immune response can be initiated, so this process is essential to both natural and acquired immunity.

# CASE STUDIES

1. A 45-year-old male named Rick went to his physician for an annual checkup. Although he was slightly overweight, his lab results indicated that both his total cholesterol and his HDL cholesterol were within normal limits. His fibrinogen level was 450 mg/dL, and his CRP level was 3.5 mg/dL. His physical examination was perfectly normal. The physician cautioned Rick that he might be at risk for a future heart attack, and he counseled him to be sure to exercise and eat a healthy, low-fat diet. Rick's wife told him that as long as his cholesterol level was normal, he didn't have anything to worry about. Who is correct? Explain your answer.

2. A 20-year-old female college student went to the infirmary with symptoms of malaise, fatigue, sore throat, and a slight fever. A complete blood count was performed, and both the red cell and white cell count were within normal limits. A rapid strep test was performed, and this was negative. A slide agglutination test for infectious mononucleosis was indeterminate, while a slide agglutination test for CRP was positive. Results of a semiquantitative CRP determination indicated an increased level of approximately 20 mg/dL. The student was advised to return in a few days for a repeat mono test. How does a test result showing an increase in CRP help in a presumptive diagnosis of infectious mononucleosis?

# EXERCISE

## IN VITRO PHAGOCYTOSIS

### Principle

A drop of whole blood is mixed with a drop of a bacterial culture and incubated at room temperature to demonstrate engulfment of bacteria by leukocytes.

### Materials

Test tubes, 12 × 75 mm

Broth culture of *Staphylococcus epidermidis*

Lancets for finger puncture

Heparinized microhematocrit tubes

Microscope slides

Wright stain

### Procedure

1. Take two 12 × 75 mm test tubes and label one 0 minutes and the other 5 minutes. If there is enough blood available, a 10-minute tube can also be set up.

2. Do a finger puncture and fill a heparinized microhematocrit tube about three-quarters full of blood. Note that blood drawn in an EDTA tube within the last 10 minutes can also be used.

3. Using a black rubber bulb, expel one drop of blood into each labeled test tube.

4. Add one drop of *Staphylococcus epidermidis* culture to each tube, using a disposable Pasteur pipette. The culture should be no more than a 0.5 McFarland standard in concentration. Dilute in an additional broth tube or in sterile saline if necessary.

5. Shake the tubes to mix, and make a blood film of the 0 tube immediately. Let the other tubes incubate for 5 minutes and 10 minutes, respectively, at room temperature before making blood films of them.

#### Method for Making Blood Smears

1. Obtain two clean glass slides, one of which will be used as a spreader slide.

2. With a Pasteur pipette, carefully place a small drop of blood at one end of a microscope slide.

3. Holding the spreader slide with the thumb and forefinger, place the spreader slide slightly in front of the drop of blood on the other slide, maintaining a 25-degree angle between the slides.

4. Move the spreader slide back toward the drop of blood. As soon as the slide comes in contact with the drop of blood, the blood will start to spread along the edge.

5. Keeping the spreader slide at a 25-degree angle, push it rapidly over the length of the slide. There should be a feathered edge on the end of the smear.

#### Wright Stain

1. Allow the blood smear to air dry.

2. Stain according to typical laboratory protocol for staining blood smears.

3. Blot the back of the slides to remove excess stain and let them air dry.

4. Use immersion oil and look for engulfment.

### Comments

These blood smears will be more watery than usual due to the addition of the broth culture with bacteria; therefore, it may be difficult to get a blood smear with a feathered edge. The feathered edge is not essential, as long as the blood cells are spread out on the slide. There should be a noticeable difference between the 0- and the 5-minute slide. The 0-minute slide will probably not show much engulfment, but bacteria may be seen in contact with leukocytes. The 5-minute slide should show bacteria within the cell as small purple dots. Neutrophils will be the predominant phagocytic cells, but an occasional monocyte may be seen. If lymphocytes are the only white blood cell seen, the bacterial suspension was too heavy, and the phagocytic cells destroyed themselves in attempting to engulf the bacteria present.

# EXERCISE

## LATEX AGGLUTINATION TEST FOR C-REACTIVE PROTEIN PRINCIPLE

Latex particles coated with antibody to CRP are reacted with patient serum. In this case, the CRP is acting as the antigen. If CRP is present above normal threshold levels, the antigen–antibody combination will result in a visible agglutination reaction. An elevated CRP level is a sensitive, although nonspecific, indicator of inflammation.

### Reagents

**(Kit from Wampole, Remel, or other manufacturers)**

CRP latex reagent, which contains a 1 percent suspension of polystyrene latex particles coated with anti–human CRP produced in goats or rabbits

Positive human serum control with a concentration of approximately 20 mg/dL of CRP

Negative human serum control

Disposable sampling pipettes

Disposable test slides

Not in kit but needed:

Timer; disposable stirrers; serological pipettes; test tubes, 12 × 75 mm

> **CAUTION:** The human serum used in the preparation of controls is tested by an FDA-approved method for the presence of antibodies to HIV as well as for hepatitis B surface antigen and HCV and found to be negative. However, because no test method can offer complete assurance that HIV, hepatitis B, hepatitis C, or other infectious agents are absent, the reagent should be handled with the same care as a clinical specimen.
>
> Reagents in the kit contain sodium azide as a preservative. Sodium azide may form lead or copper azide in laboratory plumbing. An explosion may occur upon percussion. Flush drains thoroughly with water after disposing of fluids containing sodium azide.

### Specimen Collection

Collect blood aseptically by venipuncture into a clean, dry, sterile tube and allow it to clot. Separate the serum without transferring any cellular elements. Do not use grossly hemolyzed, excessively lipemic, or bacterially contaminated specimens. Fresh nonheat inactivated serum is recommended for the test. However, if the test cannot be performed immediately, serum may be stored between 2°C and 8°C for up to 2 days. If there is any additional delay, freeze the serum at −20°C or below.

### Procedure*

#### Qualitative Slide Test

1. Be sure reagents and specimens are at room temperature.
2. Using one of the pipettes provided, fill it about two-thirds full with undiluted serum. While holding the pipette perpendicular to the slide, deliver one free-falling drop to the center of one oval on the slide. If a calibrated pipetter is used instead of the pipettes provided, adjust the pipetter to deliver 0.05 mL (50 mL).
3. Using the squeeze-dropper vials provided, add one drop of positive control and one drop of negative control to separate ovals on the slide. Note: A positive and a negative control should be run with each test.
4. Resuspend the latex reagent by gently mixing the vial until the suspension is homogeneous. Place one drop of CRP latex reagent next to each serum specimen and to each control.
5. Using separate stirrers, mix each specimen and control until the entire area of each oval is filled.
6. Tilt the slide back and forth, slowly and evenly, for 2 minutes. Place the slide on a flat surface and observe for agglutination using a direct light source.
7. The CRP positive control serum must show distinct agglutination, and the negative control must be nonreactive. If the reagent fails to agglutinate with the positive control, or does agglutinate with the negative control, it should be discarded.

#### Semiquantitative Slide Test

1. If a positive reaction is obtained, the specimen may be serially diluted with a glycine-saline buffer in order to obtain a semiquantitative estimate of the CRP level.
2. Begin with a 1:2 dilution of patient serum obtained by mixing equal parts specimen and glycine-saline buffer. Blend the tube contents thoroughly.
3. Add 0.1 mL of buffer to the desired number of test tubes. Add 0.1 mL of 1:2 dilution to the first tube; mix and transfer 0.1 mL to the next additional tube. Continue until all tubes are diluted.
4. Perform a slide agglutination test on each dilution by repeating the procedure (steps 3 through 7) as above, and look for agglutination.

## Results

1. A positive reaction is reported when the specimen shows agglutination, indicating the presence of CRP in the serum at a level equal to or greater than 0.6 mg/dL.

2. The titer is represented by the last dilution that shows a positive reaction.

3. A negative reaction is characterized by a lack of visible agglutination in the undiluted specimen.

## Comments

The latex agglutination test for CRP is a screening test for elevated levels of CRP in serum. A level of 0.6 mg/dL or higher gives a positive result with the undiluted specimen. Normal levels range from 0.1 mg/dL in newborns to 0.5 mg/dL in adults. Usually, with the onset of a substantial inflammatory stimulus, such as infection, myocardial infarction, or surgical procedures, the CRP level increases very significantly (>tenfold) above the value reported for healthy individuals. Following surgery, CRP levels rise sharply and usually peak between 48 and 72 hours. Levels decrease after the third postoperative day and should return to near normal between the fifth and seventh postoperative day. Thus, CRP levels can be used to monitor the outcome of surgery. CRP testing can also be used to monitor graft rejection, drug therapy with anti-inflammatory agents, and recurrence of malignancies. For patients with rheumatoid arthritis, elevated CRP can be used as an indicator of the active stage of the disease. In most situations, however, it is desirable to have more than one determination so that base levels can be established.

## Limitations of Procedures

1. Reagent, controls, and test specimens should be brought to room temperature and gently mixed before using.

2. Reagent and control should not be used after the expiration date indicated on the outside kit label.

3. Do not use the CRP reagent if there is evidence of freezing.

4. False-negative reactions may be due to high levels of CRP in undiluted specimens. A 1:5 dilution should always be run for this reason. False-positive reactions may occur with a reaction time longer than 2 minutes or with specimens that are lipemic, hemolyzed, or contaminated with bacteria. Therefore, any visibly contaminated, lipemic, or hemolyzed specimen should not be used.

5. Discard buffer if contaminated (evidence of cloudiness or particulate material in solution).

> **WARNING**  Latex reagent controls and buffer contain 0.1 percent sodium azide as a preservative. Sodium azide may react with lead and copper plumbing to form highly explosive metal azides. On disposal, flush with a large volume of water to prevent azide buildup.

* From Remel SeraTest CRP Latex, Package insert, Remel Incorporated, Lenexa, KS 66215

# REVIEW QUESTIONS

1. Enhancement of phagocytosis by coating of foreign particles with serum proteins is called
   a. opsonization.
   b. agglutination.
   c. solubilization.
   d. chemotaxis.

2. Jenner's work with cowpox, which provided immunity against smallpox, demonstrates which phenomenon?
   a. Natural immunity
   b. Attenuation of vaccines
   c. Phagocytosis
   d. Cross-immunity

3. Which of the following can be attributed to Pasteur?
   a. Discovery of opsonins
   b. Research on haptens
   c. First attenuated vaccines
   d. Discovery of the ABO blood groups

4. Which of the following peripheral blood cells plays a key role in killing of parasites?
   a. Neutrophils
   b. Monocytes
   c. Lymphocytes
   d. Eosinophils

5. Which of the following plays an important role as an external defense mechanism?
   a. Phagocytosis
   b. C-reactive protein
   c. Lysozyme
   d. Complement

6. The process of inflammation is characterized by all of the following except
   a. increased blood supply to the area.
   b. migration of white blood cells.
   c. decreased capillary permeability.
   d. appearance of acute-phase reactants.

7. Skin, lactic acid secretions, stomach acidity, and the motion of cilia represent which type of immunity?
   a. Natural
   b. Acquired
   c. Adaptive
   d. Auto

8. The structure formed by the fusion of engulfed material and enzymatic granules within the phagocytic cell is called a
   a. phagosome.
   b. lysosome.
   c. vacuole.
   d. phagolysosome.

9. Which of the following white blood cells is capable of further differentiation in the tissues?
   a. Neutrophil
   b. Eosinophil
   c. Basophil
   d. Monocyte

10. The presence of normal flora acts as a defense mechanism by which of the following means?
    a. Maintaining an acid environment
    b. Competing with pathogens for nutrients
    c. Keeping phagocytes in the area
    d. Coating mucosal surfaces

11. Measurement of CRP levels can be used for all of the following except
    a. monitoring drug therapy with anti-inflammatory agents.
    b. tracking the normal progress of surgery.
    c. diagnosis of a specific bacterial infection.
    d. determining active phases of rheumatoid arthritis.

12. Which of the following are characteristics of acute-phase reactants?
    a. Rapid increase following infection
    b. Enhancement of phagocytosis
    c. Nonspecific indicators of inflammation
    d. All of the above

13. A latex agglutination test for CRP is run on a 12-year-old girl who has been ill for the past 5 days with an undiagnosed disease. The results obtained are as follows: weakly reactive with the undiluted serum and negative for both the positive and negative controls. What should the technologist do next?
    a. Repeat the entire test
    b. Report the results as indeterminate
    c. Report the result as positive
    d. Obtain a new sample

14. Which is the most significant agent formed in the phagolysosome for the killing of microorganisms?
    a. Proteolytic enzymes
    b. Hydroxyl radicals
    c. Hydrogen peroxide
    d. Superoxides

15. The action of CRP can be distinguished from that of an antibody in which of the following ways?
    a. CRP acts before the antibody appears.
    b. Only the antibody triggers the complement cascade.
    c. Binding of the antibody is calcium-dependent.
    d. Only CRP acts as an opsonin.

# References

1. http://www.keratin.com/am/am003.shtml, accessed November 16, 2006.
2. Silverstein, AM: The history of immunology. In Paul, WE (ed): Fundamental Immunology, ed. 4. Lippincott Williams & Wilkins, Philadelphia, 1999, pp. 19–35.
3. Clark, WR. The Experimental Foundation of Modern Immunology, ed. 4. John Wiley & Sons, New York, 1991.
4. Fearon, DT. The instructive role of innate immunity in the acquired response. Science 272:50, 1996.
5. Gabay, C, and Kushner, I. Acute-phase proteins and other systemic responses to inflammation. N Engl J Med 340:448, 1999.
6. McPherson, RA: Specific proteins. In McPherson, RA, and Pincus, MR (eds.): Henry's Clinical Diagnosis and Management by Laboratory Methods, ed. 21. Saunders Elsevier, Philadelphia, 2007, pp. 231–244.
7. Yudkin, JS, Kumari, M, Humphries, SE, and Mohamed-Ali, V. Inflammation, obesity, stress and coronary heart disease: Is interleukin-6 the link? Atherosclerosis 148:209–14, 2000.
8. Weinberg, MD, Hooper, WC, and Dangas, G. Cardiac biomarkers for the prediction and diagnosis of atherosclerotic disease and its complications. Curr Mol Med 6:557–569, 2006.
9. Pepys, MB, and Hirschfield, GM. C-reactive protein: A critical update. J Clin Invest 111:1805–1812, 2003.
10. Woodhouse, S. C-reactive protein: From acute phase reactant to cardiovascular disease risk factor. MLO 12–20, March 2002.
11. Hutchinson, WL, et al. Immunoradiometric assay of circulating C-reactive protein: Age-related values in the adult general population. Clin Chem 46:934–938, 2000.
12. Ross, R, and Epstein, FH. Atherosclerosis—An inflammatory disease. New Engl J Med 340:115–26, 1999.
13. Pai, JK, Pischon, T, Ma, J, Manson, JE, et al. Inflammatory markers and the risk of coronary heart disease in men and women. N Engl J Med 321:2599–2610, 2004.
14. Cushman, M, Arnold, AM, Psaty, BM, et al. C-reactive protein and the 10-year incidence of coronary heart disease in older men and women: The cardiovascular health study. Circulation 112:25–31, 2005.
15. Boekholdt, SM, Hack, CE, Sandhu, et al. C-reactive protein levels and coronary artery disease incidence and mortality in apparently healthy men and women: The epic Norfolk prospective population study 1993–2003. Atherosclerosis 187:415–422, 2006.
16. Ridker, PM, Cannon, CP, Morrow, D, et al. C-reactive protein levels and outcomes after statin therapy. N Engl J Med 352:20–28, 2005.
17. Woloshin, S, and Schwartz, LM. Distribution of C-reactive protein values in the United States. N Engl J Med 352:1611–1613, 2005.
18. Lakoski, SG, Cushman, M, Criqui, M, Rundek, T, et al. Gender and C-reactive protein: Data from the multiethnic study of atherosclerosis (MESA) cohort. Am Heart 152:593–598, 2006.
19. Kisilevsky, R, and Tam, S-P. Acute phase serum amyloid A, cholesterol metabolism, and cardiovascular disease. Pediatr Path Mol Med 21:291–305, 2002.
20. Manley, PN, Ancsin JB, and Kisilevsky, R. Rapid recycling of cholesterol: The joint biologic role of C-reactive protein and serum amyloid A. Med Hypotheses 66:784–792, 2006.
21. Lannergard, A, Larsson, A, Kragsbjerg, P, and Friman, G. Correlations between serum amyloid A protein and C-reactive protein in infectious diseases. Scand J Clin Lab Invest 63:267–272, 2003.
22. Ezekowitz, RA. Role of the mannose-binding lectin in innate immunity. JID 187(Suppl 2) S335–S339, 2003.
23. Wulfsberg, EA, Hoffmann, DE, Cohen, MM. α1-antitrypsin deficiency: Impact of genetic discovery on medicine and society. JAMA 271:217–22, 1994.
24. Stoller, JK, and Aboussouan, LS. α1 antitrypsin deficiency. Lancet 365:2225–36, 2005.
25. McKenzie, SB. The Leukocyte. In Clinical Laboratory Hematology. Prentice Hall, Upper Saddle River, NJ, 2004, pp. 85–121.
26. Bamm, VV, Tsemakhovich, VA, Shaklai, M, and Shaklai, N. Haptoglobin types differ in their ability to inhibit heme transfer from hemoglobin to LDL. Biochemistry 43:3899–3906, 2004.
27. Yerbury, JJ, Rybehyn, MS, Esterbrook-Smith, SB, Henriques, C, et al. The acute phase protein haptoglobin is a mammalian extracellular chaperone with an action similar to clusterin. Biochemistry 44:10914–10925, 2005.
28. Ridker, PM, Hennekens, CH, Buring, JE, et al. C-reactive protein and other markers of inflammation in the prediction of cardiovascular disease in women. N Engl J Med 342:836, 2000.
29. Rose, VL, and Foody, JM. Elevated fibrinogen levels increase risk of heart disease in women. Am Fam Physician 59:3158, 1999.
30. Schilsky, MI. Diagnosis and treatment of Wilson's disease. Pediatr Transplantation 6:15–19, 2002.
31. Das, SK, and Ray, K. Wilson's disease: An update. Nat Clin Pract Neurol 2:482–93, 2006.
32. Segal, AW. How neutrophils kill microbes. Annu Rev Immunol 23:197–223, 2005.
33. Parsons, DD, Marty, J, and Strauss, RG: Cell biology, disorders of neutrophils, infectious mononucleosis, and related lymphocytosis. In Harmening, DM (ed.): Clinical Hematology and Fundamentals of Hemostasis, ed. 4. F. A. Davis, Philadelphia, 2002, pp. 251–271.
34. Simon, SI, and Green, CE. Molecular mechanics and dynamics of leukocyte recruitment during inflammation. Ann Rev Biomed Eng 7:151–185, 2005.
35. Lawrence, LW. The phagocytic leukocytes-morphology, kinetics, and function. In Steine-Martin EA, Lotspeich-Steininger, CA, and Koepke, JA: Clinical Hematology, ed. 2. Lippincott, Philadelphia, 1998.
36. Mathur, S, Schexneider, K, and Hutchison, RE. Hematopoiesis. In McPherson, RA, and Pincus, MR (eds): Henry's Clinical Diagnosis and Management by Laboratory Methods, ed. 21. Saunders Elsevier, Philadelphia, 2007, pp. 484–503.
37. Mak, TW, and Saunders, ME. The Immune Response: Basic and Clinical Principles. Elsevier, Burlington, MA, 2006, pp. 69–92.
38. Nauseef, WM. Assembly of the phagocyte NADPH oxidase. Histochem Cell Biol 122:277–291, 2004.

# The Lymphoid System

## LEARNING OBJECTIVES

*After finishing this chapter, the reader will be able to:*

1. Differentiate between primary and secondary lymphoid organs.
2. Describe the function and architecture of a lymph node.
3. Compare a primary and a secondary follicle.
4. Discuss the role of the thymus in T cell maturation.
5. Describe maturation of a B cell from the pro-B cell to a plasma cell.
6. Explain what constitutes a cluster of differentiation.
7. Identify and discuss the function of the following key antigens on T cells: CD2, CD3, CD4, and CD8.
8. Compare and contrast the CD3 receptor on a T cell and the surface immunoglobulin on a B cell.
9. Describe a cytokine.
10. Differentiate T cell subsets on the basis of antigenic structure and function.
11. Explain how natural killer (NK) cells recognize target cells.
12. Apply knowledge of T- and B-cell function to immunologically based disease states.

## KEY TERMS

____ Antibody-dependent cell cytotoxicity

____ Apoptosis

____ Bone marrow

____ Cell flow cytometry

____ Clusters of differentiation (CD)

____ Cytokine

____ Germinal center

____ Lymph node

____ Memory cell

____ Negative selection

____ Periarteriolar lymphoid sheath

____ Plasma cell

____ Positive selection

____ Primary follicle

____ Rosette technique

____ Secondary follicle

____ Spleen

____ Thymocyte

____ Thymus

# CHAPTER OUTLINE

The key cell involved in the immune response is the lymphocyte. Lymphocytes represent between 20 and 40 percent of the circulating white blood cells. The typical small lymphocyte is between 7 and 10 µm in diameter and has a large rounded nucleus that may be somewhat indented. The nuclear chromatin is dense and tends to stain a deep blue (**Fig. 2–1**, Color Plate 6).[1] Cytoplasm is sparse, containing few organelles and no specific granules, and consists of a narrow ring surrounding the nucleus.[2] The cytoplasm stains a lighter blue. These cells are unique, because they arise from a hematopoietic stem cell and then are further differentiated in the primary lymphoid organs. They can be separated into two main classes, depending on where this differentiation takes place. The primary lymphoid organs in humans are the bone marrow and the thymus.

Once lymphocytes mature in the primary organs, they are released and make their way to secondary organs, which include the spleen, lymph nodes, appendix, tonsils, and other mucosal-associated lymphoid tissue. It is in the secondary organs that the main contact with foreign antigens takes place. The spleen serves as a filtering mechanism for antigens in the bloodstream, and lymph nodes filter fluid from the tissues. Mucosal surfaces in the respiratory and alimentary tracts are backed with lymphoid tissue as an additional means of contacting foreign antigens as they enter the body. Lymphocyte circulation is complex and is regulated by different cell surface adhesion molecules and by chemical messengers called *cytokines*.

Lymphocytes are segregated within the secondary organs according to their particular functions. T lymphocytes are effector cells that serve a regulatory role, and B lymphocytes produce antibody. Both types of cells recirculate continuously from the bloodstream to the secondary lymphoid organs and back, in an attempt to increase contact with foreign antigens. A third type of lymphocyte, the NK cell, is large, granular, and plays a role in both the innate and adaptive immune response.

This chapter describes the primary lymphoid organs and examines their role in the maturation of lymphocytes. Secondary organs are presented in terms of the climate produced for development of the immune response. Specific characteristics of each of the three types of lymphocytes are discussed, as well as how these characteristics or markers can be used to identify them in the laboratory.

## PRIMARY LYMPHOID ORGANS

### Bone Marrow

All lymphocytes arise from pluripotential hematopoietic stem cells that appear initially in the yolk sac of the developing embryo and are later found in the fetal liver. **Bone marrow** assumes this role when the infant is born. It can be considered the largest tissue of the body, with a total weight of

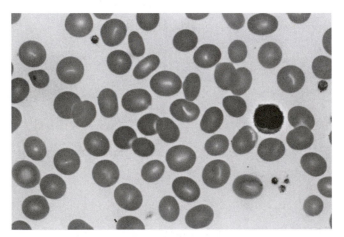

**FIGURE 2–1.** Typical lymphocyte found in peripheral blood. *(From Harr, R. Clinical Laboratory Science Review. F. A. Davis, Philadelphia, 2000, Color Plate 31.) See Color Plate 6.*

1300 to 1500 g in the adult.[2] Bone marrow fills the core of all long bones and is the main source of hematopoietic stem cells, which develop into erythrocytes, granulocytes, monocytes, platelets, and lymphocytes. Each of these lines has specific precursors that originate from the pluripotential stem cells. Most authorities agree that T, B, and NK cells arise from a common precursor known as the *common lymphoid precursor (CLP)* (see **Fig. 2–2**).[3] Lymphocyte precursors are further developed in the primary lymphoid organs.

The bone marrow functions as the center for antigen-independent lymphopoiesis. Lymphocyte stem cells are released from the marrow and travel to additional primary lymphoid organs where further maturation takes place. One subset goes to the thymus and develops into T cells. In humans, B-cell maturation takes place within the bone marrow itself. In peripheral blood, approximately 10 to 20 percent of all lymphocytes are B cells, 61 to 89 percent are T cells, and up to 22 percent are NK cells.[4]

## Thymus

T cells develop their identifying characteristics in the **thymus,** which is a small, flat, bilobed organ found in the thorax, or chest cavity, right below the thyroid gland and overlying the heart **(Fig. 2–3).** In humans, it weighs an

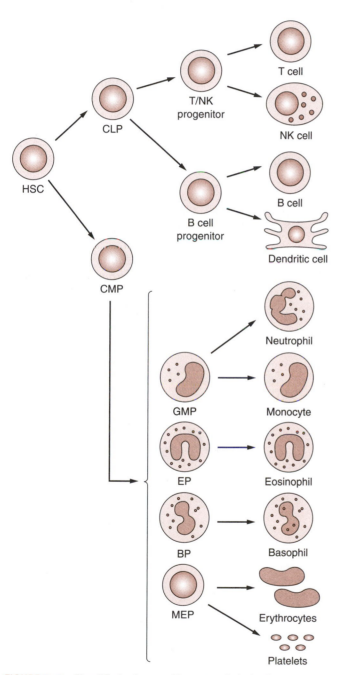

FIGURE 2–2.  Simplified scheme of hematopoiesis. In the marrow, hematopoietic stem cells (HSC) give rise to two different lines—a common lymphoid precursor (CLP) and a common myeloid precursor (CMP). CLPs give rise to T/NK progenitors, which differentiate into T and NK cells, and to B-cell progenitors, which become B cells and dendritic cells. The CMP differentiates into neutrophils, monocytes/macrophages, eosinophils, basophils, erythrocytes, and platelets.

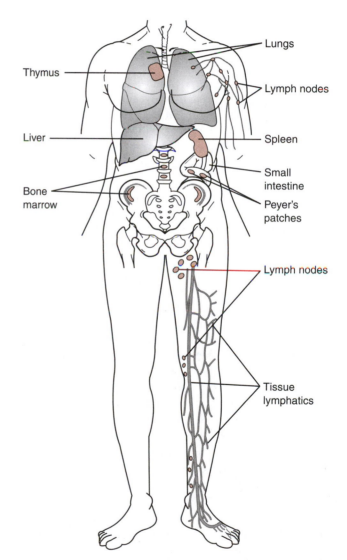

FIGURE 2–3.  Sites of lymphoreticular tissue. Primary organs include the bone marrow and the thymus. Secondary organs are distributed throughout the body and include the spleen, lymph nodes, and mucosal-associated lymphoid tissue. The spleen filters antigens in the blood, while the lymphatic system filters fluid from the tissues. *(From Widmann, FK. An Introduction to Clinical Immunology. F. A. Davis, Philadelphia, 1989, with permission.)*

average of 30 g at birth, reaches about 35 g at puberty, and then gradually atrophies.[5] It was first presumed that early in life, the thymus produces enough virgin T lymphocytes to seed the entire immune system, making it unnecessary later on. However, new evidence indicates that although the thymus diminishes in size, it is still capable of producing T lymphocytes until at least the fifth or sixth decade of life.[6]

Each lobe of the thymus is divided into lobules filled with epithelial cells that play a central role in this differentiation process. Surface antigens are acquired as the lymphocytes travel from the cortex to the medulla over a period of 2 to 3 weeks. Mature T lymphocytes are then released from the medulla.

Progenitors of T cells appear in the fetus as early as 8 weeks in the gestational period.[6] Thus, differentiation of lymphocytes appears to take place very early in fetal development and is essential to acquisition of immunocompetence by the time the infant is born.

## SECONDARY LYMPHOID ORGANS

Once differentiation occurs, mature T and B lymphocytes are released from the bone marrow and the thymus. They migrate to secondary lymphoid organs and become part of a recirculating pool. Each lymphocyte spends most of its life span in solid tissue, entering the circulation only periodically to go from one secondary organ to another. The *secondary lymphoid organs* include the spleen, lymph nodes, tonsils, appendix, Peyer's patches in the intestines, and other mucosal-associated lymphoid tissue (MALT; see Fig. 2–3). Lymphocytes in these organs travel through the tissue and return to the bloodstream by way of the thoracic duct. A specific lymphocyte may make the journey from blood to secondary lymphoid organs and back one to two times per day.[7] This continuous recirculation increases the likelihood of a lymphocyte coming into contact with its specific antigen.

Lymphopoiesis, or reproduction of lymphocytes, occurs in the secondary tissue, but this is strictly dependent on antigenic stimulation, while formation of lymphocytes in the bone marrow is antigen-independent. Most naïve or resting lymphocytes die within a few days after leaving the primary lymphoid organs unless activated by the presence of a foreign antigen. It is this second process that gives rise to long-lived memory cells and shorter-lived effector cells that are responsible for the generation of the immune response.

## Spleen

The **spleen** is the largest secondary lymphoid organ, having a length of approximately 12 cm and weighing 150 g in the adult. It is located in the upper-left quadrant of the abdomen, just below the diaphragm and surrounded by a thin connective tissue capsule. The organ can be characterized as a large discriminating filter, as it removes old and damaged cells and foreign antigens from the blood.

Splenic tissue can be divided into two main types: red pulp and white pulp. The red pulp makes up more than one-half of the total volume, and its function is to destroy old red blood cells. Blood flows from the arterioles into the red pulp and then exits by way of the splenic vein. The white pulp comprises approximately 20 percent of the total weight of the spleen and contains the lymphoid tissue, which is arranged around arterioles in a **periarteriolar lymphoid sheath (PALS; see Fig. 2–4)**. This sheath contains mainly T cells. Attached to the sheath are **primary follicles,** which contain B cells that are not yet stimulated by antigen. Surrounding the PALS is a marginal zone containing dendritic cells that trap antigen. Lymphocytes enter and leave this area by means of the many capillary branches that connect to the arterioles. Each day, an adult's blood volume passes through the spleen approximately four times, where lymphocytes and macrophages can constantly survey for infectious agents or other foreign matter.[7]

## Lymph Nodes

**Lymph nodes** are located along lymphatic ducts and serve as central collecting points for lymph fluid from adjacent tissues. Lymph fluid arises from passage of fluids and low-molecular-weight solutes out of blood vessel walls and into the interstitial spaces between cells. Some of this interstitial fluid returns to the bloodstream through venules, but a portion flows through the tissues and is eventually collected in thin-walled vessels known as *lymphatic vessels.*

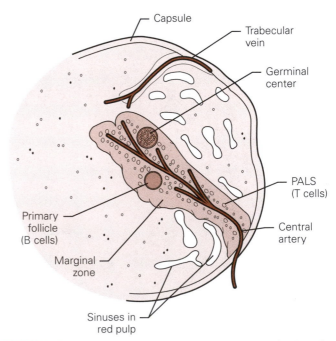

FIGURE 2–4. Cross-section of the spleen showing organization of the lymphoid tissue. T cells surround arterioles in the PALS. B cells are just beyond in follicles. When stimulated by antigen, the B cells form germinal centers. All of the lymphoid tissue is referred to as the *white pulp.*

Lymph nodes are especially numerous near joints and where the arms and legs join the body. Nodes range in size from 1 mm to about 25 mm in diameter. Filtration is a main function of these organs. The lymph fluid flows slowly through spaces called *sinuses,* which are lined with macrophages, creating an ideal location for phagocytosis to take place. The tissue is organized into an outer cortex, a paracortex, and an inner medulla **(Fig. 2–5).**

Lymphocytes and any foreign antigens present enter nodes via afferent lymphatic vessels. Numerous lymphocytes also enter the nodes from the bloodstream by means of specialized venules called *high endothelial venules,* located in paracortical areas.[5] The outermost layer, the cortex, contains macrophages and aggregations of B cells in primary follicles similar to those found in the spleen. These are the mature, resting B cells that have not yet been exposed to antigen. Specialized cells called *follicular dendritic cells* are also located here. They are found only in lymphoid follicles and have long cytoplasmic processes that radiate out like tentacles. These cells exhibit a large number of receptors for antibody and complement and help to capture antigen to present to T and B cells.

**Secondary follicles** consist of antigen-stimulated proliferating B cells. The interior of a secondary follicle is known as the **germinal center,** because it is here that blast transformation of the B cells takes place. **Plasma cells,** which actively secrete antibody, and **memory cells,** which are just a step away from forming plasma cells, are present. Generation of B-cell memory is a primary function of lymph nodes.[7]

T lymphocytes are mainly localized in the paracortex, the region between the follicles and the medulla. T lymphocytes are in close proximity to antigen-presenting cells called *interdigitating cells.* The medulla is less densely populated but contains some T cells (in addition to B cells), macrophages, and numerous plasma cells.

Particulate antigens are removed as the fluid travels across the node from cortex to medulla. The transit time through a lymph node is approximately 18 hours. Fluid and lymphocytes exit by way of the efferent lymph vessels. Such vessels form a larger duct that eventually connects with the thoracic duct and the venous system. In this manner, lymphocytes are able to recirculate continuously between lymph nodes and the peripheral blood.

If contact with antigen takes place, lymphocyte traffic shuts down due to the proliferation of activated cells.[7] Accumulation of lymphocytes and other cells causes the lymph nodes to become enlarged, a condition known as *lymphadenopathy.* Recirculation of expanded numbers of lymphocytes then occurs.

## Other Secondary Organs

Additional areas of lymphoid tissue include the MALT, tonsils, appendix, and cutaneous-associated lymphoid tissue. MALT, the mucosal associated lymphoid tissue, is found in the gastrointestinal, respiratory, and urogenital tracts. Here, macrophages and lymphocytes are localized at some of the main ports of entry for foreign organisms. Peyer's patches represent a specialized type of MALT and are located at the lower ileum of the intestinal tract.

The tonsils are another area of lymphoid tissue found in the mucous membrane lining of the oral and pharyngeal cavities. Their function is to respond to pathogens entering the respiratory and alimentary tracts. An additional location of lymphoid tissue is the appendix. All of these secondary organs function as potential sites for contact with foreign antigen, and they increase the probability of an immune response.

The epidermis contains a number of intraepidermal lymphocytes. Most of these are T cells, which are uniquely positioned to combat any antigens that enter through the skin. This association of lymphocytes is known as the *cutaneous-associated lymphoid tissue.*

Within each of these secondary organs, T and B cells are segregated and perform specialized functions. B cells

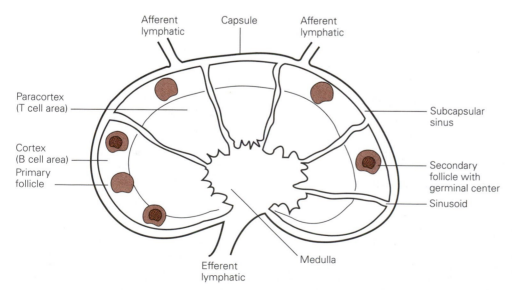

**FIGURE 2–5.** Structure of a lymph node. A lymph node is surrounded by a tough outer capsule. Right underneath is the subcapsular sinus, where lymph fluid drains from afferent lymphatic vessels. The outer cortex contains collections of B cells in primary follicles. When stimulated by antigen, secondary follicles are formed. T cells are found in the paracortical area. Fluid drains slowly through sinusoids to the medullary region and out the efferent lymphatic vessel to the thoracic duct.

differentiate into memory cells and plasma cells and are responsible for *humoral immunity* or antibody formation. T cells play a role in *cell-mediated immunity*, and as such, they produce sensitized lymphocytes that secrete cytokines. **Cytokines** are small polypeptides that regulate the functions of lymphocytes and other cells involved in the immune response. The characteristics and markers for each type of lymphocyte are considered separately.

## SURFACE MARKERS ON LYMPHOCYTES

Proteins that appear on cell surfaces can be used as markers to differentiate T cells and B cells. Proteins can also be used to distinguish the developmental stages of the two types of cells according to when these proteins appear. Such proteins, or antigens, have been detected by monoclonal antibodies, which are extremely specific antibodies made by cloning a single antibody-producing cell. (Refer to Chapter 4 for a discussion of preparation of monoclonal antibodies.)

Several laboratories have developed monoclonal antibodies, and each used its own nomenclature for the sets of antigens found. In an attempt to relate research findings and standardize the nomenclature, scientists set up the International Workshops on Human Leukocyte Antigens, beginning in 1982.[8] Panels of antibodies from different laboratories were used for analysis, and antibodies reacting similarly with standard cell lines were said to define **clusters of differentiation (CD).** As each antigen, or CD, was found, it was assigned a number.

The name *cluster of differentiation* came about because the exact nature of the proteins identified by the various antibodies was not known. This CD classification now acts as a reference in standardizing names of membrane proteins found on all human white blood cells. The most recent Workshop and Conference on Human Leukocyte Differentiation Antigens, now called Human Cell Differentiation Molecules, was held in December of 2004, and the list of CD designations currently numbers more than 350.[8] The antigens that are most important in characterizing T lymphocytes and B lymphocytes are shown in **Table 2–1** and are referred to in the following discussion of T-cell and B-cell development.

| Table 2–1. | Surface Markers on T and B Cells | | |
|---|---|---|---|
| **ANTIGEN** | **MOLECULAR WEIGHT (KD)** | **CELL TYPE** | **FUNCTION** |
| CD2 | 45–58 | Thymocytes, T cells, NK cells | Involved in T-cell activation |
| CD3 | 20–28 | Thymocytes, T cells | Associated with T-cell antigen receptor; role in TCR signal transduction |
| CD4 | 55 | Helper T cells, monocytes, macrophages | Coreceptor for MHC class II; receptor for HIV |
| CD5 | 58 | Mature T cells, thymocytes, subset of B cells (B1) | Positive or negative modulation of T and B cell receptor signaling |
| CD8 | 60–76 | Thymocyte subsets, cytotoxic T cells | Coreceptor for MHC class I |
| CD10 | 100 | B and T cell precursors, bone marrow stromal cells | Protease; marker for pre-B CALLA |
| CD16 | 50–80 | Macrophages, NK cells, neutrophils | Low affinity Fc receptor, mediates phagocytosis and ADCC |
| CD19 | >120 | B cells, follicular dendritic cells | Part of B cell coreceptor, signal transduction molecule that regulates B-cell development and activation |
| CD21 | 145 | B cells, follicular dendritic cells, subset of immature thymocytes | Receptor for complement component C3d; part of B-cell coreceptor with CD19 |
| CD23 | 45 | B cells, monocytes, follicular dendritic cells | Regulation of IgE synthesis; triggers release of Il-1, Il-6, and GM-CSF from monocytes |
| CD25 | 55 | Activated T, B cells, monocytes | Receptor for IL-2 |
| CD44 | 85 | Most leukocytes | Adhesion molecule mediating homing to peripheral lymphoid organs |
| CD45R | 180 | Different forms on all hematopoietic cells | Essential in T and B cell antigen-stimulated activation |
| CD 56 | 175–220 | NK cells, subsets of T cells | Not known |
| CD 94 | 70 | NK cells, subsets of T cells | Subunit of NKG2-A complex involved in inhibition of NK cell cytotoxicity |

NK = Natural killer; TCR = CD3-αβ receptor complex; MHC = major histocompatibility class; HIV = human immunodeficiency virus; CALLA = common acute lymphoblastic leukemia antigen; Fc = Fragment crystallizable; ADCC = antibody-dependent cell cytotoxicity; IgE = immunoglobulin E; GM-CSF = granulocyte-macrophage colony-stimulating factor

# STAGES IN B-CELL DIFFERENTIATION

## Pro-B Cells

B cells are derived from a multipotential progenitor cell (MMP), a lymphoid-myeloid precursor that differentiates to become either a common myeloid progenitor or an early lymphocyte progenitor.[9,10] Early lymphocyte progenitors become T cell, B cell, NK cell, or dendritic cell precursors, depending on exposure to different cytokines (see Fig. 2–2). B cells remain in the microenvironment provided by bone marrow stromal cells, and the earliest B-cell precursor can be recognized by the presence of a surface molecule called CD45R (B220 in mice).[9,11] B-cell precursors go through a developmental process that prepares them for their role in antibody production and, at the same time, restricts the types of antigens to which any one cell can respond. This part of B-cell development is known as the *antigen-independent phase*. Figure 2–6 depicts the changes that occur as B cells mature from the pro-B stage to become memory cells or plasma cells.

Several transcription, or growth, factors are necessary to differentiate common lymphoid precursors into pro-B cells. Some of these factors are E2A, EBF (early B-cell factor), and paired box protein 5 (PAX).[9,10] In addition, a cytokine called *interleukin-7* (IL-7) is also necessary at this early development stage. All of these factors are produced in the microenvironment of the bone marrow.

During this maturation process, the first step is the rearrangement of genes that code for the heavy and light chains of an antibody molecule. The end result is a B lymphocyte programmed to produce a unique antibody molecule, which consists of two identical light chains and two identical heavy chains (see Chapter 4 for details). Although portions of each chain are identical for every antibody molecule, it is the so-called variable regions that make each antibody molecule specific for a certain antigen or group of antigens. Heavy chains are coded for on chromosome 14, and light chains are coded for on chromosomes 2 and 22.

The pro-B cell has distinctive markers that include surface antigens CD19, CD45R, CD43, CD24, and c-Kit. Intracellular proteins found at this stage are terminal deoxyribonucleotide transferase (TdT) and recombination-activating genes RAG-1 and RAG-2, which code for enzymes involved in gene rearrangement **(Fig. 2–6A)**.[11,12,13] Gene rearrangement of the DNA that codes for antibody production occurs in a strict developmental sequence.[13] Rearrangement of genes on chromosome 14, which code for the heavy-chain part of the antibody molecule, takes place first in a random fashion (see Chapter 4 for details). C-Kit on the pro-B cell interacts with a cell surface molecule called *stem cell factor*, which is found on stromal cells. This interaction triggers the activation process. Recombinase enzymes RAG-1 and RAG-2 cleave the DNA at certain possible recombination sites, and TdT helps to join the pieces back together by incorporating additional nucleotides in the joining areas.[14] Successful

rearrangement commits a B cell to further development. CD19 acts as a coreceptor that helps to regulate further B-cell development and activation. CD45 is a membrane glycoprotein found on all hematopoietic cells, but the type found on B cells is the largest form, and it is designated CD45R. This is a tyrosine-specific phosphatase that is involved in signaling during B-cell activation. CD19, CD24, and CD45R remain on the cell surface throughout subsequent developmental stages.

Differentiation of pro-B cells into pre-B cells occurs upon successful rearrangement of heavy-chain genes. Stromal cells interact directly with pro-B cells, and they secrete cytokines, hormones, chemokines, and adhesion molecules, all of which are necessary for this developmental process.[14,15]

## Pre-B Cells

When synthesis of the heavy chain part of the antibody molecule occurs, the *pre-B stage* begins.[14,15] The first heavy chains synthesized are the μ chains, which belong to the class of immunoglobulins called IgM. The μ chains accumulate in the cytoplasm. Pre-B cells also lose the CD43 marker as well as c-Kit and TdT.[3] Pre-B cells may also express μ chains on the cell surface, accompanied by an unusual light chain molecule called a *surrogate light chain*.[14,15] Surrogate light chains consist of two short polypeptide chains that are noncovalently associated with each other **(Fig. 2–6B)**. They are not immunoglobulin proteins but are thought to be essential for regulating B-cell development. The combination of the two heavy chains with the surrogate light chains plus two very short chains, Ig-α/Ig-β form the pre-B cell receptor. This receptor adheres to bone marrow stromal cell membranes and transmits a signal to prevent rearrangement of any other heavy-chain genes.[9,10] It appears that only pre-B cells expressing the μ heavy chains in association with surrogate light chains survive and proceed to further differentiation.[15] Once the pre-B receptor (preBCR) is expressed, neighboring pre-B cells may send signals for further maturation.[15] This stimulates a burst of clonal expansion.[9]

## Immature B Cells

Immature B cells are distinguished by the appearance of complete IgM molecules on the cell surface[9,12] **(Fig. 2–6C)**. This indicates that rearrangement of the genetic sequence coding for light chains on either chromosome 2 or 22 has taken place by this time. Completion of light chain rearrangement commits a cell to produce an antibody molecule with specificity for a particular antigen or group of related antigens. *Variable regions*, which occur on both the light and heavy chains, determine this specificity. Once surface immunoglobulins appear, μ chains are no longer detectable in the cytoplasm.

Other surface proteins that appear on the immature B cell include CD21, CD 40, and major histocompatibility complex (MHC) class II molecules (see Chapter 3).[12] CD21 acts as a receptor for a breakdown product of the complement component C3, known as C3d (see Chapter 6 for details on complement). This enhances the likelihood of contact between B cells and antigen, because antigen frequently becomes coated with complement fragments during the immune response. CD40 and MHC class II are important for interaction of B cells with T cells.

At this stage, there is evidence that self-antigens give a negative signal to immature B cells, resulting in arrested maturation and cell death.[9,12] Immature B cells that tightly bind self-antigens through cross-linking of surface IgM molecules receive a signal to halt development, and they are eliminated or inactivated.[12] Thus, many B cells capable of producing antibody to self-antigens are deleted from the marrow by the process of programmed cell death, or **apoptosis.** It is estimated that more than 90 percent of B cells die in this manner without leaving the bone marrow.[14] Immature B cells leave the bone marrow and proceed to seed the spleen and other secondary lymphoid organs.

## Mature B Cells

In the spleen, immature B cells develop into mature cells known as *marginal zone B cells.*[9] These B cells remain in the spleen in order to respond quickly to any blood-borne pathogens they may come into contact with. Other immature B cells become follicular B cells, which are found in lymph nodes and other secondary organs. Unlike marginal B cells that remain in the spleen, follicular B cells are constantly recirculating throughout the secondary lymphoid organs.[9] In addition to IgM, all mature B cells exhibit IgD, another class of antibody molecule, on their surface **(Fig. 2–6D).** Both IgM and IgD have the same specificity for a particular antigen or group of antigens. These surface immunoglobulins provide the primary activating signal to B cells when contact with antigen takes place.[14] IgD is not required for B-cell function, but it may prolong the life span of mature B cells in the periphery.[12] Unless contact with antigen occurs, the life span of a mature B cell is

typically only a few days.[12,14] If, however, a B cell is stimulated by antigen, it undergoes transformation to a blast stage, which eventually forms memory cells and antibody-secreting plasma cells. This process is known as the *antigen-dependent phase* of B-cell development. These B cells have a half-life of more than 6 weeks.[12]

## Activated B Cells

Antigen-dependent activation of B cells takes place in the primary follicles of peripheral lymphoid tissue. This ocurs when antigens cross-link several surface immunoglobulins on select B cells **(Fig. 2–7).** Activated B cells exhibit identifying markers that include CD25, which is found on both activated T and B cells and acts as a receptor for interleukin-2 (IL-2), a growth factor produced by T cells. Additional receptors that appear at this time are specific for other growth factors produced by T cells. When B cells are activated in this manner, they transform into blasts that will give rise to both plasma cells and so-called memory cells.

## Plasma Cells

Plasma cells are spherical or ellipsoidal cells between 10 and 20 μm in size and are characterized by the presence of abundant cytoplasmic immunoglobulin and little to no surface immunoglobulin **(Fig. 2–8,** Color Plate 7).[1] The nucleus is eccentric or oval with heavily clumped chromatin that stains darkly. An abundant endoplasmic reticulum and a clear well-defined Golgi zone are present in the cytoplasm. This represents the most fully differentiated lymphocyte, and its main function is antibody production. Plasma cells are not normally found in the blood but are located in germinal centers in the peripheral lymphoid organs. Plasma cells are nondividing, and after several days of antibody production, they die without further proliferation.[9]

Memory cells (see Fig. 2-7) are also found in germinal centers and have a much longer life span than a resting

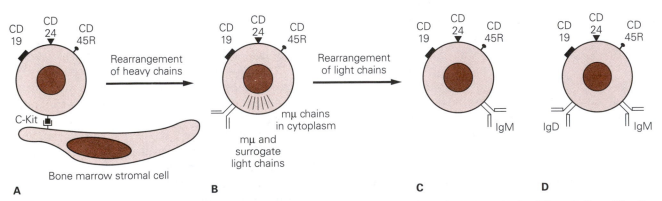

**FIGURE 2–6.** B-cell development in the bone marrow. Selected markers are shown for the various stages in the differentiation of B cells. Stages up to the formation of mature B cells occur in the bone marrow. (A) Pro-B cell. (B) Pre-B cell. (C) Immature B cell. (D) Mature B cell.

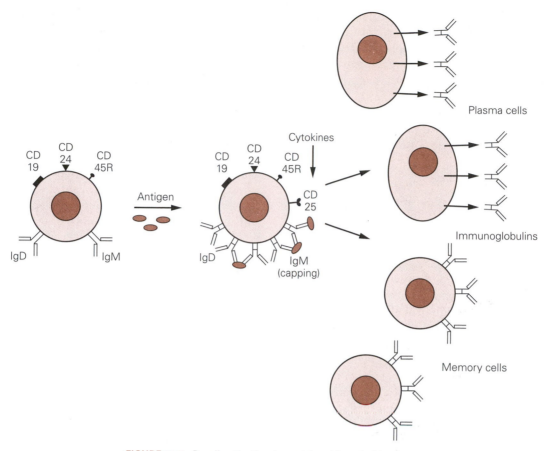

FIGURE 2–7. B-cell activation in peripheral lymphoid organs.

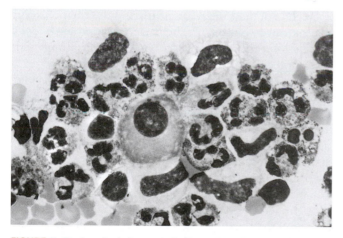

FIGURE 2–8. A typical plasma cell. *(From Harr, R. Clinical Laboratory Science Review. F. A. Davis, Philadelphia, 2000, Color Plate 28.) See Color Plate 7.*

B cell.[5] These represent progeny of antigen-stimulated B cells that are capable of responding to antigen with increased speed and intensity. They are similar in appearance to unstimulated B cells, but they remain in an activated state for months or years, ready to respond to the initial antigen.

## T-CELL DIFFERENTIATION

Sixty to 80 percent of circulating lymphocytes in the peripheral blood are T cells, and these become differentiated in the thymus. Lymphocyte precursors called **thymocytes** enter the thymus from the bone marrow. Within the lobules of the thymus are two main zones, the outer cortex and the inner medulla. Early precursors enter the thymus at the cortico-medullary junction and migrate to the outer cortex. Migration occurs in waves and is driven by chemical messengers called *chemokines*.[16–18] Early surface markers on thymocytes that are committed to becoming T cells include CD44 and CD25.[6,16–18]

As thymocytes travel through the thymus, they go through a process similar to that of B cells in the marrow: There is an orderly rearrangement of the genes coding for the antigen receptor. At the same time, distinct surface markers appear during specific stages of development. Maturation is an elaborate process that takes place over a 3-week period as cells filter through the cortex to the medulla. Thymic stromal cells include epithelial cells, macrophages, fibroblasts, and dendritic cells, all of which play a role in T-cell development. Interaction with stromal cells under the influence of cytokines, especially interleukin-7, is critical for growth and differentiation.[3,13] A significant selection process occurs as maturation takes place, because it is estimated that approximately 97 percent of the cortical cells die intrathymically before becoming mature T cells.[17]

## Double-Negative Stage

Early thymocytes lack CD4 and CD8 markers, which are important to their later function; hence they are known as *double-negative thymocytes* (DN) **(Fig. 2–9).** These large double-negative thymocytes actively proliferate in the outer cortex under the influence of interleukin-7.

Rearrangement of the genes that code for the antigen receptor known as TCR begins at this stage (Fig. 2–9).[14] CD3, the complex that serves as the main part of the T-cell antigen receptor, consists of eight noncovalently associated chains, six of which are common to all T cells.[4,20] However, two chains, the alpha (α) and beta (β) chains, contain variable regions that recognize specific antigens **(Fig. 2–10).** These are coded for by selecting gene segments and deleting others, as is the case with B cells. Rearrangement of the β chain occurs first.[16] The appearance of a functional β chain on the cell surface sends a signal to suppress any further

β chain gene rearrangements. The combination of the β chain with the rest of CD3 forms the pre-TRC receptor. Signaling by the β chain also triggers the thymocyte to become CD4-positive (CD4+) and CD8-positive (CD8+).[16,17]

Early on, some thymocytes, representing 10 percent or less of the total number, rearrange and express two other chains, gamma (γ) and delta (δ). It is not known how this process is controlled, but these cells proceed down a different developmental pathway. Cells expressing the γδ receptor typically remain negative for both CD4 and CD8. However, as mature T cells, they appear to represent the dominant T-cell population in the skin, intestinal epithelium, and pulmonary epithelium. New evidence indicates that they may act like natural killer (NK) cells, because they can bind to a broad range of cell surface molecules in their natural, unprocessed form.[19] They are capable of recognizing antigens without being presented by MHC proteins, so they may represent an important bridge between natural and adaptive immunity.

## Double-Positive Stage

At this second stage, when thymocytes express both CD4 and CD8 antigens, they are called *double-positive*. Double-positive thymocytes proliferate and then begin to rearrange the genes coding for the alpha chain.[17,18] When the CD3-αβ receptor complex (TCR) is expressed on the cell surface, a **positive selection** process takes place that allows only double-positive cells with functional TCR receptors to survive. T cells must recognize foreign antigen in association with class I or class II MHC molecules (Fig. 2–9). Any thymocytes that are unable to recognize self-MHC antigens die without leaving the thymus. This weeding out is important, because functioning T cells must be able to recognize foreign antigen along with MHC molecules.

Those cells expressing moderate levels of TCR receptor bind by means of the αβ chains to MHC antigens on cells within the thymus.[18,19] In fact, this recognition of MHC protein associated with small peptides has been found to be essential for positive selection.[18,21] TCR binding transmits a signal that results in activation of several enzymes called *kinases* that are necessary for further development and survival.[18] This process appears to take place in the cortex, although there are indications that interaction with epithelial cells in the medulla may be necessary to complete the process.[16]

A second selection process, known as **negative selection,** takes place among the surviving double-positive T cells. Strong reactions with self-peptides send a signal to delete the developing T cell by means of apoptosis, or programmed cell death. .[18,20] Most T cells that would be capable of an autoimmune response are eliminated in this manner. This selection process is very rigorous, because only 1 to 3 percent of the double-positive thymocytes in the cortex survive.[16]

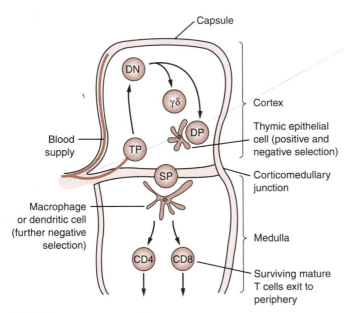

**FIGURE 2–9.** T-cell maturation in the thymus. T lymphocyte precursors (TP) enter the thymus at the cortico-medullary junction. They migrate upward in the cortex and begin development of the T-cell receptor. A small percent of precursors develop gamma-delta chains, while the majority develop alpha-beta chains and become double-positive (DP) (both CD4 and CD8 are present). Positive and negative selection take place through the CD3/T cell receptor for antigen. If positively selected, the T cell becomes single-positive (SP); that is, either CD4+ or CD8+. Further interaction with macrophages or dendritic cells take place to weed out any T cells able to respond to self-antigen. Surviving CD4+ and CD8+ cells exit the thymus to the peripheral blood.

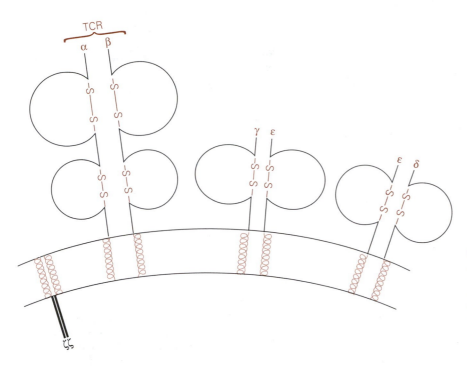

**FIGURE 2–10.** The CD3:T-cell receptor complex. The T-cell receptor that recognizes antigen consists of two chains, α and β, which have constant and variable regions. Four other types of chains are collectively known as CD3. These are ε, γ, δ, and ζ. They take part in signaling to the interior of the cell when antigen binding occurs.

## Mature T Cells

Survivors of selection exhibit only one type of marker, either CD4 or CD8, and they migrate to the medulla. It is not certain why one marker is down-regulated, but it may depend on which MHC protein the cell interacts with, and exposure to certain cytokines.[19] CD4+ T cells recognize antigen along with MHC class II protein, while CD8+ T cells interact with antigen and MHC class I proteins. The two separate mature T-cell populations created differ greatly in function. T cells bearing the CD4 receptor are termed *helper*, or *inducer*, *cells*, while the CD8-positive (CD8+) population consists of cytotoxic T cells. Approximately two-thirds of peripheral T cells express CD4 antigen, while the remaining one-third express CD8 antigen. These mature T cells are released from the thymus and seed peripheral lymphoid organs. Resting T cells have a life span of up to several years in these peripheral organs.[5]

T helper cells consist of two subsets, termed Th1 and Th2 cells. They each have a different role to play in the immune response. Th1 cells produce interferon gamma (IFN-γ) and tumor necrosis factor-beta (TNF-β), which protect cells against intracellular pathogens.[22] Th2 cells produce a variety of interleukins, including IL-4, IL-5, IL-10, and IL-13. The essential role of the Th2 cells is to help B cells produce antibody against extracellular pathogens.[22]

Recently, an additional T-cell subpopulation has been described. These are called T regulatory cells (T reg), and they possess the CD4 antigen and CD25.[5] These cells comprise approximately 5 to 10 percent of all CD4-positive T cells.[23,24] T regs play an important role in suppressing the immune response to self-antigens. They may do so by

producing interleukins such as IL-10 and transforming growth factor B, which switch off the immune response.[25]

Single positive T cells spend approximately 12 days in the medulla.[16] If any of the surviving cells are reactive to tissue antigens, a further deletion process takes place.[16] This ensures that most T cells leaving the thymus will not react to self-antigens. However, the process does not wipe out all self-reactivity, so the presence of T regulatory cells is necessary to prevent autoimmune responses.[16] Additional proliferation of these carefully screened T cells occurs, and then they leave the thymus to seed secondary lymphoid organs. They recirculate through the bloodstream and peripheral organs approximately once every 12 to 24 hours.[19] This is important for T cells to be able to make contact with antigen.[22] T cells remain metabolically active through continuous contact with self-peptide/MHC complexes on antigen-presenting cells and the action of interleukin-7 (IL-7).

## Antigen Activation

Antigen must be transported to the T-cell zones of the secondary lymphoid tissue.[22] When antigen recognition occurs, T lymphocytes are transformed into large activated cells that are characterized by polyribosome-filled cytoplasm. Activated T lymphocytes express receptors for IL-2, just as activated B cells do **(Fig. 2–11)**. T lymphoblasts differentiate into functionally active small lymphocytes that produce cytokines. Activities of specific cytokines include assisting B cells in commencing antibody production, killing tumor and other target cells, rejecting grafts, stimulating hematopoiesis in the bone marrow, and initiating delayed hypersensitivity allergic reactions. This type of immune

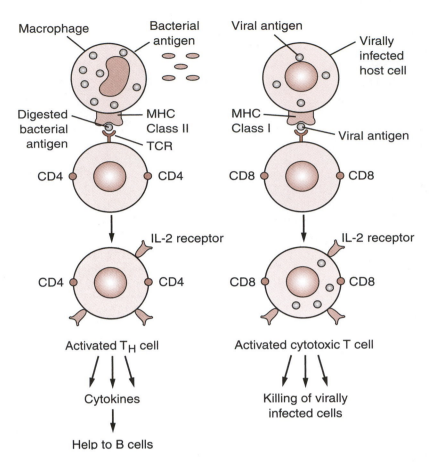

**FIGURE 2–11.** Activation of T cells—exposure to antigen causes production of CD25 receptors for interleukin-2 (IL-2). IL-2 causes sensitized CD4+ T cells to secrete cytokines that enhance antibody production by B cells. CD8+ T cells have increased cytotoxicity to recognize and kill virally infected cells.

response is known as *cell-mediated immunity* (see Chapter 5 for a full description of cell-mediated immunity). In addition to effector cells, T memory cells are also generated. They have a higher affinity for antigen than unstimulated T cells, and they may represent precursors in the later stage of the primary response.[22] In a similar manner to memory B cells, they are able to proliferate sooner than naïve T cells. They also express a broader array of cytokines and appear to persist for years.[26] **Table 2–2** summarizes the differences between T cells and B cells in structure and function.

## THIRD POPULATION OR NATURAL KILLER CELLS

A small percentage of lymphocytes do not express the markers of either T cells or B cells. These lymphocytes are generally larger than T cells and B cells at approximately 15 μm in diameter, and they contain kidney-shaped nuclei with condensed chromatin and prominent nucleoli. They have a higher cytoplasmic-nuclear ratio, and the cytoplasm contains a number of azurophilic granules.[27] These large granular lymphocytes make up 5 to 10 percent of the circulating lymphoid pool[5] and are found mainly in the spleen and peripheral blood. They have been named natural killer, or NK, cells because they have the

ability to mediate cytolytic reactions and kill target cells without prior exposure to them. They play an important role as a transitional cell bridging the innate and the acquired response to pathogens.[3,23] The fact that they lack specificity in their response is essential to their function as early defenders against pathogens.[28,29] This gives time for the acquired response of specific T and B cells to be activated.

NK cells arise from the common lymphocyte precursor (CLP) and differentiate into a T/NK cell that can become either a T cell or an NK cell.[28,29] Precursors that go to the thymus become T cells, while the influence of bone marrow stromal cells is necessary for NK cell differentiation.[13,28,32] Within the bone marrow, interleukin-15 plays a critical role in NK cell development.[3]

There are no surface antigens that are unique to NK cells, but they express a specific combination of antigens that can be used for identification. One such antigen is CD16, which is a receptor for the fragment crystallizable portion, or nonspecific end, of the immunoglobulin molecule IgG. This allows NK cells to attach to and lyse any cells that are coated with antibody.[30] The other main surface antigen is CD56. Two subsets of NK cells exist—those that have a high level of CD56 and low or no CD16, and those with some CD56 and high levels of CD16. The former produce more cytokines and help support antibody production, while the

| Table 2-2. | Comparison of T and B Cells |
|---|---|
| **T CELLS** | **B CELLS** |
| Develop in the thymus | Develop in the bone marrow |
| Found in blood (60%–80% of circulating lymphocytes), thoracic duct fluid, lymph nodes | Found in bone marrow, spleen, lymph nodes |
| Identified by rosette formation with SRBCs | Identified by surface immunoglobulin |
| End products of activation are cytokines | End product of activation is antibody |
| Antigens include CD2, CD3, CD4, CD8 | Antigens include CD19, CD20, CD21, CD40, MHC class II |
| Located in paracortical region of lymph nodes | Located in cortical region of lymph nodes |

SRBC = Sheep red blood cells

latter have a higher cytotoxic activity.[3,5, 31,32] The cytokines produced include interferon gamma and tumor necrosis factor-alpha, so NK cells may also play a role in amplifying the immune response in addition to their cytolytic activity.[3,32,33]

Due to the fact that NK cells are capable of recognizing any foreign cell and destroying it without regard to MHC restriction, they represent the first line of defense against virally infected and tumor cells.[13,31] They accumulate at the maternal-fetal interface, so they may also play an essential role in maintaining pregnancy.[28,32] Mature NK cells have a half-life of 7 to 10 days, and in addition to the uterus, they are mainly found in peripheral blood, the spleen, and the liver.[28,32]

NK cell activity is stimulated by exposure to cytokines such as interleukin-12, interferon gamma, and interferon beta.[31] Since these rise rapidly during a viral infection, NK cells are able to respond early on during an infection, and their activity peaks in about 3 days, well before antibody production or a cytotoxic T cell response.

## Mechanism of Cytotoxicity

For years it had been a mystery how NK cells tell the difference between normal and abnormal cells. However, the mechanism is now beginning to be understood. It appears that there is a balance between activating and inhibitory signals that enables NK cells to distinguish healthy cells from infected or cancerous ones.[31] There are two main classes of receptors on NK cells that govern this response: inhibitory receptors, which deliver inhibitory signals, and activatory receptors, which deliver signals to activate the cytotoxic mechanisms.[31] The inhibitory signal is based on recognition of MHC class I protein, which is expressed on all healthy cells. If NK cells react with MHC class I proteins, then inhibition of natural killing occurs. One specific type of receptor on NK cells responsible for

this binding include killer cell immunoglobulin-like receptors (KIRs).[28,33] Other inhibitory receptors include ILT/LIR and CD94/NKG2A receptors, which also bind MHC class I molecules. All three receptors can be found on NK cells at the same time.[29]

Diseased and cancerous cells tend to lose their ability to produce MHC proteins. NK cells are thus triggered by a lack of MHC antigens, sometimes referred to as recognition of "missing self."[31,33,34] This lack of inhibition appears to be combined with an activating signal switched on by the presence of proteins produced by cells under stress, namely those cells that are infected or cancerous. These proteins are named MICA and MICB. Receptors called CD94/NKG2C and CD94/NKG2D on NK cells bind MICA or MICB and send a signal to destroy the cell.[29,32,34] If an inhibitory signal is not received at the same time, then NK cells release substances called *perforins* and *granzymes* (**Fig. 2–12**). Perforins are pore-forming proteins that polymerize in the presence of Ca2+ and form channels in the target cell membrane.[29] Granzymes are packets of serine esterase enzymes that may enter through the channels and mediate cell lysis. Thus, NK cells are constantly monitoring potential target cells through binding to either activating or inhibitory receptors, and the NK cell either detaches and moves on or binds and activates cell destruction.

## Antibody-Dependent Cell Cytotoxicity

A second method of destroying target cells is also available to NK cells. They recognize and lyse antibody-coated cells through a process called **antibody-dependent cell cytotoxicity.** Binding occurs through the CD16 receptor for IgG. Any target cell coated with IgG can be bound

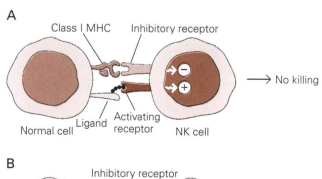

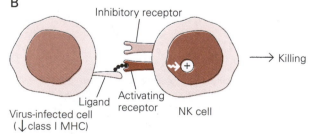

**FIGURE 2–12.** Mechanism of NK cell cytotoxicity. *(From Kindt, TJ, Goldsby, RA, and Osborne, BA. Kuby Immunology, ed. 6. WH Freeman, New York, 2007, p. 363, with permission.)*

and destroyed. This method is not unique to NK cells, as monocytes, macrophages, and neutrophils also exhibit such a receptor and act in a similar manner. Nonetheless, the overall importance of NK cells as a defense mechanism is demonstrated by the fact that patients who lack these cells have recurring, serious viral infections.[28]

## LABORATORY IDENTIFICATION OF LYMPHOCYTES

Identification of lymphocytes as either T cells or B cells may be useful in diagnosis of any of the following states: lymphoproliferative malignancies, immunodeficiency diseases, unexplained infectious diseases, monitoring of transplants, and acquired immunologic abnormalities such as AIDS. Most methods are based on separation of mononuclear cells from whole blood and detection of specific cell surface markers.

One of the most frequently used methods for obtaining lymphocytes is density gradient centrifugation with Ficoll-Hypaque.[35] Ficoll-Hypaque is available commercially and has a specific gravity that varies between 1.077 and 1.114, depending on the manufacturer. Diluted defibrinated or heparinized blood is carefully layered on top of the solution, and the tube is centrifuged. Centrifugation produces three distinct layers: plasma at the top of the tube, a mononuclear layer banding on top of the density gradient solution, and erythrocytes and granulocytes at the bottom of the tube **(Fig. 2–13).**

Once a lymphocyte population has been obtained, segregation into subsets is accomplished via flow cytometry. This technique relies on the use of labeled monoclonal antibodies against specific surface antigens. Some of the more common antigens tested for include CD2, CD3, CD4, CD7, and CD8 on T cells and CD19, CD20, CD22, and surface immunoglobulin on B cells. **Cell flow cytometry** is an automated system for identifying cells based on the scattering of light as cells flow in single file through a laser beam. Fluorescent antibodies are used to screen for subpopulations, such as B cells, T helper cells, and T cytotoxic cells. The antibodies used are monoclonal, and each has a different fluorescent tag. The principles of flow cytometry are discussed more fully in in Chapter 12.

### Manual Method

The **rosette technique** using red blood cells from sheep has been a historical method for enumeration of T lymphocytes. Lymphocytes are separated from whole blood and then mixed with a suspension of sheep red blood cells. If three or more red blood cells are attached to a lymphocyte, it is considered a rosette **(Fig. 2–14).** Sheep cells attach to the CD2 antigen, found only on T cells. Using a counting chamber, 200 cells are counted and the percent forming rosettes is calculated. This represents the percentage of T cells, and the percent of B cells is calculated by subtracting this number from 100. There should be approximately twice as many T cells as B cells. This technique is not as precise as those mentioned previously, because rosetting can be influenced by cold-reacting anti-lymphocyte antibodies that are formed in diseases such as rheumatoid arthritis and infectious mononucleosis. Therefore, this method is no longer used in clinical laboratories.

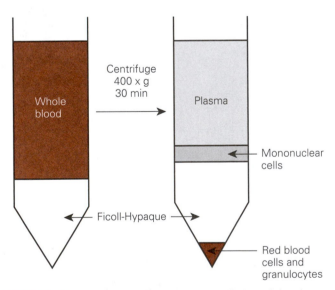

**FIGURE 2–13.** Ficoll-Hypaque separation of cells in peripheral blood. Whole blood diluted with buffer is layered onto Ficoll-Hypaque medium in a plastic centrifuge tube. Tubes are spun at 4003 g for 30 minutes. Red blood cells and granulocytes settle to the bottom of the tube, while mononuclear cells (monocytes and lymphocytes) form a band at the interface of the Ficoll-Hypaque and plasma.

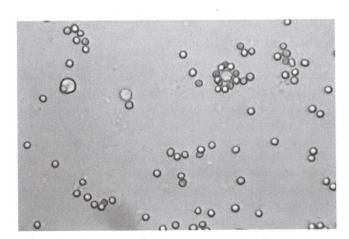

**FIGURE 2–14.** T-cell rosette. T cell surrounded by sheep red blood cells that attach to CD2 receptors on T cell.

## SUMMARY

All undifferentiated lymphocytes arise in the bone marrow from hematopoietic stem cells. They mature in the primary lymphoid organs. For B cells, this takes place in the bone marrow, while T cells acquire their specificity in the thymus. B and T cells can be recognized by the presence of surface antigens, or CDs, that are detected by monoclonal antibodies. B cell markers include CD19, MHC class II proteins, and surface immunoglobulins. The surface immunoglobulins act as receptors for antigen. MHC class II proteins allow B cells to interact with T helper cells in the production of antibody. When contact with specific antigen occurs, B cells differentiate into plasma cells, which produce antibody. In the process, memory cells are also created. These can rapidly respond the next time that same antigen is seen. Production of antibody is known as humoral immunity

T cells are distinguished by the presence of CD3, CD2, and either CD4 or CD8. CD2 is the receptor that interacts with sheep red blood cells to form rosettes, a simple test for the enumeration of T cells. Cells that express CD4 belong to a T-cell subset that includes helper/inducer cells, while CD8-carrying T cells are cytotoxic/suppressor cells. The CD3 marker serves as the receptor for antigen. The major portion of it is common to all T cells, but two chains—alpha and beta—contain variable regions that can bind to only certain antigens. T cells go through a positive and then a negative selection process, whereby the surviving cells recognize MHC determinants along with foreign antigen. The T cells are responsible for cell-mediated immunity, which involves production of cytokines that serve as regulatory factors for the immune response.

A third class of lymphocytes, known as NK cells, are found in the peripheral blood and represent 5 to 15 percent of the total lymphocyte population. These are larger and contain more cytoplasm and granules than T or B cells. They are responsible for killing target cells, including those that are virally infected or cancerous, without previous exposure or sensitization to them. They do this by recognizing missing self-MHC antigens, in addition to detecting the presence of stress proteins on infected and cancerous cells. This is an important first line of defense against invasion by such cells.

Laboratory determination of individual lymphocyte populations is essential in diagnosis of such conditions as lymphomas, immunodeficiency diseases, unexplained infections, or acquired immune diseases such as AIDS. Lymphocytes are identified using monoclonal antibodies directed against specific surface antigens. They are enumerated through the use of cell flow cytometry, which categorizes cells on the basis of light scattering. Automated methods eliminate subjectivity and are more precise, although more costly.

# CASE STUDY

A 2-year-old boy is sent for immunologic testing because of recurring respiratory infections, including several bouts of pneumonia. The results show decreased immunoglobulin levels, especially of IgG. Although his white blood cell count was within the normal range, the lymphocyte count was low. Flow cytometry was performed to determine if a particular subset of lymphocytes was low or missing. It was determined that he had a low number of CD3+lymphocytes, although the CD19+ lymphocyte population was normal. How can this be interpreted? How can this account for his recurring infections?

# EXERCISE

## ENUMERATION OF T CELLS

### Principle

Lymphocytes are separated from whole blood by using a ficoll density gradient, which causes erythrocytes and granulocytes to settle at the bottom of a conical centrifuge tube while mononuclear cells form a layer at the gradient's top. Red blood cells from sheep are used to identify the T-cell population of lymphocytes, because these spontaneously complex with T cells through the CD2 receptor. If three or more sheep cells surround a T cell, this is known as a *rosette*. Quantitation of T cells provides information about cell-mediated immunity, which plays an important role in regulation of the immune response and defense against virally infected or cancerous cells.

### Specimen Collection

Collect blood by venipuncture using sterile technique. A freshly drawn heparinized blood specimen is needed for this procedure, because use of ethylenediaminetetraacetic acid (EDTA) will result in poor recovery of mononuclear cells. An additional EDTA tube may be drawn for a complete blood cell count and a differential.

### Reagents Materials, and Equipment

Centrifuge

Microscope slides

Coverslips, 22 × 22 mm

Pasteur pipettes

Disposable serologic pipettes: 1 mL, 5 mL, 10 mL

Conical plastic centrifuge tubes

Glass test tubes, 12 × 75 mm

Histopaque-1077 (Sigma Diagnostics, St. Louis, Missouri) or other Ficoll-Hypaque solution

Sheep red blood cells (Becton-Dickinson)

Sterile phosphate buffered saline (PBS)

### Procedure

1. Add 3 mL of Histopaque-1077 to a 15 mL plastic conical centrifuge tube.

2. Dilute 3 mL of heparinized blood with an equal amount of sterile phosphate buffered saline (PBS). Mix and carefully layer on top of the Histopaque-1077.

3. Centrifuge at $400 \times g$ at room temperature for 30 minutes. Allow the centrifuge to coast to a stop. Do not use the brake. The opaque interface that develops is the mononuclear layer.

4. Aspirate and discard the upper layer to within 0.5 cm of the mononuclear layer.

5. Carefully remove the opaque interface with a capillary pipette and dispense into a 15 mL centrifuge tube. Do not exceed 1.5 mL total volume in the transfer. Add 10 mL of PBS, mix well, and centrifuge at $400 \times g$ for 10 minutes.

6. Decant the supernatant, and drain the last drops by inverting the tube on top of a paper towel.

7. Add 1 mL of PBS, and resuspend the cells by aspirating carefully with a Pasteur pipette.

8. Obtain a final cell count of $6 \times 10^6$ cells/mL with a hemacytometer. Fill the counting chamber, and count the cells in the four corner squares of the chamber. Multiply by 20 to obtain the total number of mononuclear cells harvested. Add more buffer if further dilution is necessary.

> NOTE: The instructor can prepare the cell suspension before the laboratory begins if time is short.

9. Prepare sheep red blood cell suspension by placing about 3 mL of sheep red blood cells in a 15 mL centrifuge tube and filling with buffer. Centrifuge for 10 minutes at $400 \times g$. Resuspend 0.1 mL of packed cells in 19.9 mL buffer to achieve a concentration of 0.5 percent.

10. Pipette 0.5 mL of the lymphocyte suspension into a 12 × 75 mm test tube. Pipette 0.5 mL of sheep red blood cell suspension into the same tube, and mix well.

11. Centrifuge mix at $250 \times g$ for 5 minutes. Remove the centrifuge tube carefully so the cells are not disturbed. Incubate at room temperature for 1.5 to 2 hours. Cells can also be incubated overnight at 4°C, if preferred.

12. After incubation, carefully resuspend the cells by holding the tube almost horizontal and carefully twisting around the long axis.

13. With a capillary pipette and no bulb, gently transfer the rosettes to a clean microscope slide and add a cover slip. Place the cover slip carefully so that no air bubbles are formed. Observe the rosettes using a 40× objective.

14. Count only those lymphocytes that are surrounded by three or more sheep red cells. Count a total of 200 lymphocytes, including those that do not form rosettes. The percent of T lymphocytes can be obtained by dividing the number of lymphocytes in rosettes by the total number of lymphocytes counted.

## Interpretation of Results

In a normal adult, T lymphocytes compose 52 to 81 percent of the total number of lymphocytes. A low percent of T lymphocytes may indicate a T-cell disorder. Some of these conditions include AIDS, Hodgkin's disease, chronic lymphocytic leukemia, and immunodeficiency diseases.

Care must be taken when performing this procedure. Rosettes can be disrupted, so resuspension after centrifugation must be done very gently; otherwise the percent of T lymphocytes will be falsely lowered. In addition, lymphocytes must be distinguished from sheep red blood cells, because both cells are about the same size. Lymphocytes, however, are more refractile because of the presence of a nucleus.

The mononuclear layer also contains monocytes. These should not be counted as nonrosetting lymphocytes, because this, too, will falsely lower the percent of T cells found. Monocytes are considerably larger than lymphocytes, and they contain more cytoplasm, which has a granular appearance.

This technique is not as accurate a detection of specific antigens with monoclonal antibody because of the fragile nature of the rosettes formed. It is, however, less expensive to perform and is of historic significance, because this represents the first means of T-cell identification.

# REVIEW QUESTIONS

1. Which of the following is a primary lymphoid organ?

   a. Lymph node
   b. Spleen
   c. Thymus
   d. MALT

2. What type of cells would be found in a primary follicle?

   a. Unstimulated B cells
   b. Germinal centers
   c. Plasma cells
   d. Memory cells

3. Which of the following is true of NK cells?

   a. They rely on memory for antigen recognition.
   b. They share antigens with B cells.
   c. They are found mainly in lymph nodes.
   d. They recognize a lack of MHC proteins.

4. Where are all undifferentiated lymphocytes made?

   a. Bone marrow
   b. Thymus
   c. Spleen
   d. Lymph nodes

5. In the thymus, positive selection of immature T cells is based upon recognition of which of the following?

   a. Self-antigens
   b. Stress proteins
   c. MHC antigens
   d. μ chains

6. Which of these are found on a mature B cell?

   a. IgG and IgD
   b. IgM and IgD
   c. Alpha and beta chains
   d. CD3

7. Which receptor on T cells is responsible for rosetting with sheep red blood cells?

   a. CD2
   b. CD3
   c. CD4
   d. CD8

8. Which of the following can be attributed to antigen-stimulated T cells?

   a. Humoral response
   b. Plasma cells
   c. Cytokines
   d. Antibody

9. Which is a distinguishing feature of a pre-B cell?

   a. μ chains in the cytoplasm
   b. Complete IgM on the surface
   c. Presence of CD21 antigen
   d. Presence of CD25 antigen

10. When does genetic rearrangement for coding of light chains take place?

    a. Before the pre-B cell stage
    b. As the cell becomes an immature B cell
    c. Not until the cell becomes a mature B cell
    d. When the B cell becomes a plasma cell

11. Which of the following antigens are found on the T cell subset known as helper/inducers?

    a. CD3
    b  CD4
    c. CD8
    d. CD11

12. Where does the major portion of antibody production occur?

    a. Peripheral blood
    b. Bone marrow
    c. Thymus
    d. Lymph nodes

13. Which of the following would represent a double-negative thymocyte?

    a. CD2–CD3+CD4–CD8+
    b. CD2+CD3–CD4–CD8–
    c. CD2–CD3+CD4+CD8–
    d. CD2+CD3+CD4+CD8–

14. Which of the following best describes the T-cell receptor for antigen?

    a. It consists of IgM and IgD molecules.
    b. It is the same for all T cells.
    c. It is present in the double-negative stage.
    d. Alpha and beta chains are unique for each antigen.

# References

1. Bell, A. Morphology of human blood and marrow cells. In Harmening, DM: Clinical Hematology and Fundamentals of Hemostasis, ed. 4. F. A. Davis, Philadelphia, 2002, pp. 1–38.

2. Vajpayee, N, Graham, SS, and Bern, S. Basic examination of blood and bone marrow. In McPherson, RA, and Pincus, MR (eds): Henry's Clinical Diagnosis and Management by Laboratory Methods, ed. 21. WB Saunders, Philadelphia, 2007, pp. 457–483.

3. Blom, B, and Spits, H. Development of human lymphoid cells. Annu Rev Immunol 24:287–320, 2006.

4. Holmer, LD, Hamoudi, W, and Bueso-Ramos, CE. Chronic leukemia and related lymphoproliferative disorders. In Harmening, DM: Clinical Hematology and Fundamentals of Hemostasis, ed. 4. F. A. Davis, Philadelphia, 2002, pp. 301–330.

5. Kindt, TJ, Goldsby, RA, and Osborne, BA. Kuby Immunology, ed. 6. WH Freeman and Co, New York, 2007, pp. 23–75.

6. Robertson, P, and Poznansky, MC. T-lymphocyte development and models of thymopoietic reconstitution. Transpl Infect Dis 5:38–42, 2003.

7. Mak, TW, and Saunders, ME. The Immune Response: Basic and Clinical Principles. Elsevier Inc, Burlington, MA, 2006, pp. 35–67.

8. http://bloodjournal.hematologylibrary.org/cgi/content/full/106/9/3123. Zola, H, Swart, B, Nicholson, I, Aasted, B. et al. CD molecules 2005: Human cell differentiation molecules. Accessed May 29, 2007.

9. Matthias, P, and Rolink, AG. Transcriptional networks in developing and mature B cells. Nat Rev/Immunol 5:497–508, 2005.

10. Allman, D, and Miller, JP. The aging of early B-cell precursors. Immunol Rev 205:18–29, 2005.

11. Nagasawa, T. Miroenvironmental niches in the bone marrow required for B-cell development. Nat Rev/Immunol 6:107–116, 2006.

12. Mak, TW, and Saunders, ME. The Immune Response: Basic and Clinical Principles. Elsevier, Burlington, MA, 2006, pp. 209–245.

13. Mathur, S, Schexneider, K, and Hutchison, RE. Hematopoiesis. In McPherson, RA, and Pincus, MR (eds): Henry's Clinical Diagnosis and Management by Laboratory Method, ed. 21. WB Saunders, Philadelphia, 2007, pp. 484–503.

14. Kindt, TJ, Goldsby, RA, and Osborne, BA. Kuby Immunology, ed. 6. WH Freeman and Co, New York, 2007, pp. 271–301.

15. Milne, CD, Fleming, HE, Zhang, Y, and Paige, CJ. Mechanisms of selection mediated by interleukin-7, the preBCR, and hemokinin-1 during B-cell development. Immunol Rev 197:75–88, 2004.

16. Takahama, Y. Journey through the thymus: Stromal guides for T-cell development and selection. Nat Rev/Immunol 6:127–135, 2006.

17. Kindt, TJ, Goldsby, RA, and Osborne, BA. Kuby Immunology, ed. 6. WH Freeman and Co, New York, 2007, pp. 245–270.

18. Starr, TK, Jameson, SC, and Hogquist, KA. Positive and negative selection of T cells. Annu Rev Immunol 21:139–176, 2003.

19. Mak, TW, and Saunders, ME. The Immune Response: Basic and Clinical Principles. Elsevier, Burlington, MA, 2006, pp. 311–337.

20. Sprent, J, and Kishimoto, H. The thymus and negative selection. Immunol Rev 185:126–135, 2002.

21. Barton, GM, and Rudensky, AY: Requirements for diverse, low-abundance peptides in positive selection of T cells. Science 283:67, 1999.

22. Sprent, J, and Surh, CD. T cell memory. Annu Rev Immunol 20:551–579, 2002.

23. O'Garra, A, and Viera, P. Regulatory T cells and mechanisms of immune system control. Nat Med 10: 801–805, 2004.

24. Becker, C, Stoll, S, Bopp, T, Schmitt, E, et al. Regulatory T cells: Present and future hopes. Med Microbiol Immunol 195:113–124, 2006.

25. Franzke, A, Hunger, JK, Dittmar, KEJ, Ganser, A, et al. Regulatory T-cells in the control of immunological diseases. Ann Hematol 85:747–758, 2006.

26. Hagmann, M. How the immune system walks memory lane. Science Now July 12:4, 2000.

27. Yokoyama, WM. Natural killer cells. In Paul, WE (ed): Fundamental Immunology, ed. 6 Lippincott Williams & Wilkins, Philadelphia, 2008, pp. 483–517.

28. Yokoyama, WM, Kim, S, and French, AR. The dynamic life of natural killer cells. Annu Rev Immunol 22:405–29, 2004.

29. Mak, TW, and Saunders, ME. The Immune Response: Basic and Clinical Principles. Elsevier, Burlington, MA, 2006, pp. 518–552.

30. McPherson, RA, and Massey, D. Overview of the Immune System and Immunologic Disorders. In McPherson, RA, and Pincus, MR (eds): Henry's Clinical Diagnosis and Management by Laboratory Method, ed. 21. WB Saunders, Philadelphia, 2007, pp. 789–792.

31. Kindt, TJ, Goldsby, RA, and Osborne, BA. Kuby Immunology, ed. 6. WH Freeman and Co, New York, 2007, pp. 351–370.

32. Di Santo, JP. Natural killer cell developmental pathways: A question of balance. Annu Rev Imminol 24:257–286, 2006.

33. Lanier, L. NK cell recognition. Annu Rev Immunol 23:225–274, 2005.

34. Bauer, S, Groh, V, and Wu, J, et al. Activation of NK cells and T cells by NKG2D, a receptor for stress-inducible MICA. Science 285:727, 1999.

35. Stevens, RA, Lempicki, RA, Natarajan, V, Higgins, J, et al. General immunologic evaluation of patients with human immunodeficiency virus infection. In Detrick, B, Hamilton, RG, and Folds, JD (eds): Manual of Molecular and Clinical Laboratory Immunology, ed. 7. ASM Press, Washington, DC, 2006, pp. 847–861.

# Nature of Antigens and the Major Histocompatibility Complex

## LEARNING OBJECTIVES

*After finishing this chapter, the reader will be able to:*

1. Define and characterize the nature of immunogens.
2. Differentiate an immunogen from an antigen.
3. Identify the characteristics of a hapten.
4. Describe how an epitope relates to an immunogen.
5. Discuss the role of adjuvants.
6. Differentiate heterophile antigens from alloantigens and autoantigens.
7. Explain what a haplotype is in regard to inheritance of major histocompatibility complex (MHC) antigens.
8. Describe differences in structure of class I and class II proteins.
9. Compare the transport of antigen to cellular surfaces by class I and class II proteins.
10. Describe the role of transporters associated with antigen processing (TAP) in selecting peptides for binding to class I molecules.
11. Discuss the differences in the source and types of antigen processed by class I and class II molecules.
12. Explain the clinical significance of the class I and class II molecules.

## KEY TERMS

____ Adjuvant
____ Allele
____ Alloantigen
____ Autoantigen
____ Class I MHC (HLA) molecule
____ Class II MHC (HLA) molecule
____ Conformational epitope
____ Epitope
____ Haplotype
____ Hapten
____ Heteroantigen
____ Heterophile antigen
____ Major histocompatibility complex (MHC)
____ Immunogen
____ Invariant chain (Ii)
____ Linear epitope
____ Transporters associated with antigen processing (TAP)

## CHAPTER OUTLINE

The immune response of lymphocytes is triggered by materials called **immunogens,** macromolecules capable of triggering an adaptive immune response by inducing the formation of antibodies or sensitized T cells in an immunocompetent host. Immunogens can then specifically react with such antibodies or sensitized T cells. The term *antigen* refers to a substance that reacts with antibody or sensitized T cells but may not be able to evoke an immune response in the first place. Thus, all immunogens are antigens, but the converse is not true. However, many times the terms are used synonymously, and the distinction between them is not made. In discussing serological reactions or particular names of substances such as blood groups, the term *antigen* is still more commonly used; hence both terms are used in this chapter.

One of the most exciting areas of research focuses on how and why we respond to particular immunogens. This response is actually caused by a combination of factors: the nature of the immunogen itself, genetic coding of MHC molecules that must combine with an immunogen before T cells are able to respond, and immunogen processing and presentation. This chapter focuses on all three areas and discusses future clinical implications of some recent findings.

## FACTORS INFLUENCING THE IMMUNE RESPONSE

Several factors such as age, overall health, dose, route of inoculation, and genetic capacity influence the nature of this response. In general, older individuals are more likely to have a decreased response to antigenic stimulation. At the other end of the age scale, neonates do not fully respond to immunogens, because their immune systems are not completely developed. Overall health plays a role, as individuals who are malnourished, fatigued, or stressed are less likely to mount a successful immune response.

There appears to be a threshold dose for each individual immunogen. This allows the innate immune response to take care of small amounts of pathogens and leave the adaptive response for pathogens that are present in large numbers. Generally, the larger the dose of an immungen one is exposed to, the greater the immune response is. However, very large doses can result in T- and B-cell tolerance, a phenomenon that is not well understood. It is possible that memory cells become overwhelmed and therefore nonresponsive.[1] The actual amount of immunogen needed to generate an immune response differs with the route of inoculation. Such routes include intravenous (into a vein), intradermal (into the skin), subcutaneous (beneath the skin), and oral administration. Where the immunogen enters the body determines which cell populations will be involved in the response and how much is needed to trigger a response.

Lastly, a genetic predisposition may be involved that allows individuals to respond to particular immunogens. This predisposition is linked to the MHC (discussed in the section on the clinical significance of the MHC molecules) and to the receptors generated during T and B lymphocyte development.

## TRAITS OF IMMUNOGENS

In general, the ability of an immunogen to stimulate a host response depends on the following characteristics: (1) macromolecular size, (2) chemical composition and molecular complexity, (3) foreignness, and (4) the ability to be processed and presented with MHC molecules.[1,2] Usually an immunogen must have a molecular weight of at least 10,000 to be recognized by the immune system, and the best immunogens typically have a molecular weight of over 100,000 daltons.[1,2] However, there are exceptions, because a few substances with a molecular weight of less than 1000 have been known to induce an immune response. For the most part, the rule of thumb is that the greater the molecular weight, the more potent the molecule is as an immunogen.

Immunogenicity is also determined by a substance's chemical composition and molecular complexity. Proteins and polysaccharides are the best immunogens. Proteins are powerful immunogens, because they are made up of a variety of units known as *amino acids*. The particular sequential arrangement of amino acids, the primary structure, determines the secondary structure, which is the relative orientation of amino acids within the chain. The tertiary structure embodies the spatial or three-dimensional orientation of the entire molecule; and the quaternary structure is based on the association of two or more chains into a single polymeric unit. Because of the variations in subunits, proteins may have an enormous variety of three-dimensional shapes. B cells recognize structures that project from the external surfaces of macromolecules, and the more complexity or branching there is, the easier it is for B cells to respond. Proteins have epitopes that also stimulate T cells, which is essential to generating T-cell help in antibody production.[1] In contrast, synthetic polymers such as nylon or Teflon are made up of a few simple repeating units with no bending or folding within the molecule, and these materials are nonimmunogenic. For this reason, they are used in making artificial heart valves, elbow replacements, and other medical appliances.

Carbohydrates are somewhat less immunogenic than protein, because the units of sugars are more limited than the number of amino acids in protein. As immunogens, carbohydrates most often occur in the form of glycolipids or glycoproteins. Many of the blood group antigens are comprised of such carbohydrate complexes. For example, the A, B, and H blood group antigens are glycolipids, and the Rh and Lewis antigens are glycoproteins.[3] Pure nucleic acids and lipids are not immunogenic by themselves, although a response can be generated when they are attached to a suitable carrier molecule.[4] This is the case for autoantibodies to DNA that are formed in systemic lupus erythematosus. These autoantibodies are actually stimulated by a DNA-protein complex rather than by DNA itself.

Another characteristic that all immunogens share is foreignness. The immune system is normally able to distinguish between self and nonself, and those substances recognized as nonself are immunogenic. This ability is acquired as lymphocytes mature in the primary lymphoid organs. Any lymphocyte capable of reacting with self-antigen is normally eliminated. Typically, the more distant taxonomically the source of the immunogen is from the host, the better it is as a stimulus. For example, plant protein is a better immunogen for an animal than is material from a related animal. Occasionally, however, autoantibodies, or antibodies to self-antigens, exist. This is the exception rather than the rule, and this phenomenon is discussed in Chapter 14.

Furthermore, for a substance to elicit an immune response, it must be subject to antigen processing, which involes enzymatic digestion to create small peptides or pieces that can be complexed to MHC molecules to present to responsive lymphocytes. If a macromolecule can't be degraded and presented with MHC molecules, then it would be a poor immunogen. The particular MHC molecules produced also determine responsiveness to individual antigens. Each individual inherits the ability to produce a certain limited repertoire of MHC molecules, discussed in the section on the genes coding for MHC molecules.

## NATURE OF EPITOPES

Although an immunogen must have a molecular weight of at least 10,000, only a small part of the immunogen is actually recognized in the immune response. This key portion of the immunogen is known as the *determinant site* or **epitope.** Epitopes are molecular shapes or configurations that are recognized by B or T cells, and there is evidence that for proteins, epitopes recognized by B cells may consist of as few as 6 to 15 amino acids.[1,2] Large molecules may have numerous epitopes, and each one may be capable of triggering specific antibody production or a T-cell response. Epitopes may be repeating copies, or they may have differing specificities. They may also be sequential or **linear** (i.e., amino acids following one another on a single chain), or they may be conformational. A **conformational epitope** results from the folding of one chain or multiple chains, bringing certain amino acids from different segments of a linear sequence or sequences into close proximity with each other so they can be recognized together **(Fig. 3–1).**

Epitopes recognized by B cells may differ from those recognized by T cells.[1,2] Surface antibody on B cells may react with both linear and conformational epitopes present on the surface of an immunogen. Anything that is capable of cross-linking surface immunoglobulin molecules is able to trigger B-cell activation. The immunogen does not necessarily have to be degraded first. If the immunogen is a protein, B cells may recognize the primary, secondary, tertiary, or even the quaternary structure. For polysaccharides, the branch points of branched chains may contribute most to recognition.[2] T cells, on the other hand, recognize an epitope only as a part of a complex formed with MHC proteins on the surface of an antigen-presenting cell. The antigen-presenting

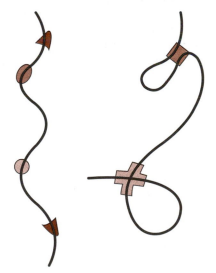

**A** Linear epitopes          **B** Conformational epitopes

**FIGURE 3–1.** Linear versus conformational epitopes. (A) Linear epitopes consist of sequential amino acids on a single polypeptide chain. There may be several different types on one chain. (B) Conformational epitopes result from the folding of a polypeptide chain or chains, and nonsequential amino acids are brought into close proximity.

cell must process an immunogen first and degrade it into small peptides for it to be recognized by T cells (see the section on antigen processing). Thus, T-cell epitopes are linear but may be molecules found anywhere in the cell, rather than strictly surface molecules.

## HAPTENS

Some substances are too small to be recognized by themselves, but if they are complexed to larger molecules, they are then able to stimulate a response. **Haptens** are nonimmunogenic materials that, when combined with a carrier, create new antigenic determinants. Once antibody production is initiated, the hapten is capable of reaction with antibody even when the hapten is not complexed to a carrier molecule; however, precipitation or agglutination reactions will not occur, because a hapten has a single determinant site and cannot form the cross-links with more than one antibody molecule that are necessary for precipitation or agglutination **(Fig. 3–2)**.

Haptens may be complexed artificially with carrier molecules in a laboratory setting, or this may occur naturally within a host and set off an immune response. An example of the latter is an allergic reaction to poison ivy. Poison ivy (*Rhus radicans*) contains chemical substances called *catechols*, which are haptens. Once in contact with the skin, these can couple with tissue proteins to form the immunogens that give rise to contact dermatitis. Another example of haptens coupling with normal proteins in the body to provoke an immune response occurs with certain drug-protein conjugates that can result in a life-threatening allergic response. The best known example of this occurs with penicillin.

The most famous study of haptens was conducted by Karl Landsteiner, a German scientist who was known for his discovery of the ABO blood groups. In his book *The Specificity of Serological Reactions*, published in 1917, he detailed the results of an exhaustive study of haptens that has contributed greatly to our knowledge of antigen–antibody reactions. He discovered that antibodies recognize not only chemical features such as polarity, hydrophobicity, and ionic charge, but the overall three-dimensional configuration is also important.[1,2] The spatial orientation and the chemical complementarity are responsible for the lock-and-key relationship that allows for tight binding between antibody and epitope **(Fig. 3–3)**. Today it is known that many therapeutic drugs and hormones can function as haptens.[2]

## RELATIONSHIP OF ANTIGENS TO THE HOST

Antigens can be placed in broad categories according to their relationship to the host. **Autoantigens** are those antigens that belong to the host. These do not evoke an immune response under normal circumstances. **Alloantigens** are from other members of the host's species, and these are capable of eliciting an immune response. They are important to consider in tissue transplantation and in blood transfusions. **Heteroantigens** are from other species, such as other animals, plants, or microorganisms.

**Heterophile antigens** are heteroantigens that exist in unrelated plants or animals but are either identical or closely related in structure so that antibody to one will cross-react with antigen of the other. An example of this is the human blood group A and B antigens, which are related to bacterial polysaccharides.[4] It is believed that anti-A antibody, which is normally found in individuals with blood types other than A (e.g., type B and type O), is originally formed after exposure to pneumococci or other similar bacteria. Naturally occurring anti-B antibody is formed after exposure to a similar bacterial cell wall product.

Normally in serological reactions, the ideal is to use a reaction that is completely specific, but the fact that cross-reactivity exists can be helpful for certain diagnostic purposes. Indeed, the first test for infectious mononucleosis (IM) was based on a heterophile antibody reaction. During the early states of IM, a heterophile antibody is formed, stimulated by an unknown antigen. This antibody was found

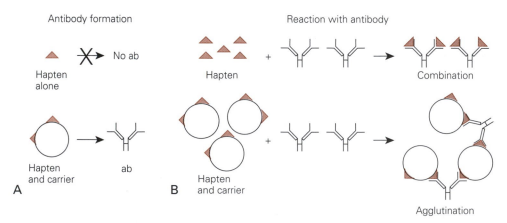

FIGURE 3–2. Characteristics of hapten. (A) Hapten alone cannot stimulate antibody formation. It can react with antibody, but it is monovalent, so no complexes form. (B) When complexed to a carrier, the hapten can stimulate antibody formation. If hapten is complexed to a carrier at multiple sites, then agglutination can take place.

Reactivity with

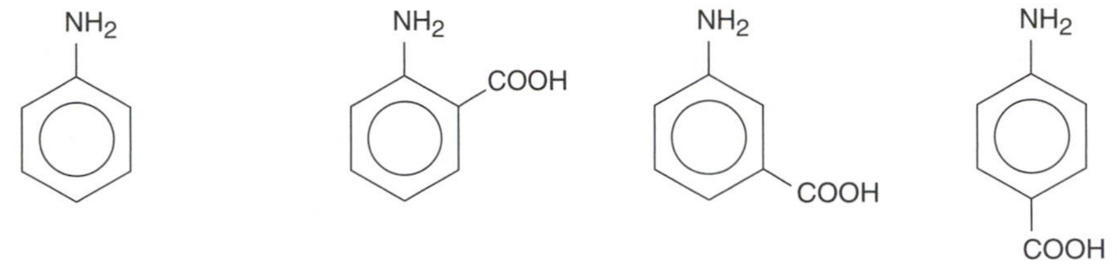

| Antiserum against | Aminobenzene (aniline) | o-Aminobenzoic acid | m-Aminobenzoic acid | p-Aminobenzoic acid |
|---|---|---|---|---|
| Aminobenzene | +++ | 0 | 0 | 0 |
| o-Aminobenzoic acid | 0 | +++ | 0 | 0 |
| m-Aminobenzoic acid | 0 | 0 | ++++ | 0 |
| p-Aminobenzoic acid | 0 | 0 | 0 | +++/++++ |

FIGURE 3–3. Landsteiner's study of the specificity of haptens. Spatial orientation of small groups is recognized, because antibodies made against aminobenzene coupled to a carrier will not react with other similar haptens. The same is true for antiserum to o-aminobenzoic acid, m-aminobenzoic acid, and p-aminobenzoic acid. Antibody to a carboxyl group in one location would not react with a hapten, which has the carboxyl group in a different location. *(From Landsteiner, K. The specificity of serological reactions, revised edition. Dover Press, New York, 1962.)*

to react with sheep red blood cells, and this formed the basis of the Paul-Bunnell screening test for mononucleosis (see Chapter 22). This procedure was a useful screening test when the causative agent of IM had not been identified. Current rapid screening tests for IM are based on the principle of detection of heterophile antibody.

## ADJUVANTS

The power of immunogens to generate an immune response can be increased through the use of adjuvants. An **adjuvant** is a substance administered with an immunogen that increases the immune response. It acts by producing a local inflammatory response that attracts a large number of immune system cells to the injection site.[1] Aluminum salts are the only ones approved for clinical use in the United States, and these are used to complex with the immunogen to increase its size and to prevent a rapid escape from the tissues.[5] It must be injected into the muscle to work. The hepatitis B vaccination is an example of using this type of adjuvant.

Another common adjuvant is Freund's complete adjuvant, which consists of mineral oil, emulsifier, and killed mycobacteria (0.5 mg/mL). Antigen is mixed with adjuvant and then injected. It is released slowly from the injection site. Freund's adjuvant produces granulomas, or large areas of scar tissue, and thus is not used in humans. Adjuvants are thought to enhance the immune response by prolonging the existence of immunogen in the area, increasing the effective size of the immunogen, and increasing the number of macrophages involved in antigen processing.[1,2]

## MAJOR HISTOCOMPATIBILITY COMPLEX

For years, scientists searched to identify postulated immune response genes that would account for differences in how individuals respond to particular immunogens. Evidence now indicates that the genetic capability to mount an immune response is linked to a group of molecules originally referred to as *human leukocyte antigens* (HLA). The French scientist Dausset gave them this name, because they were first defined by discovering an antibody response to circulating white blood cells.[4,6] These antigens are also known as *MHC molecules*, because they determine whether transplanted tissue is histocompatible and thus accepted or recognized as foreign and rejected. MHC molecules are actually found on all nucleated cells in the body, and they play a pivotal role in the development of both humoral and cellular immunity. Their main function is to bring antigen to the cell surface for recognition by T cells, because T-cell activation will occur only when antigen is combined with MHC molecules. Clinically, they are relevant, because they may be involved in transfusion reactions, graft rejection, and autoimmune diseases. Genes controlling expression of these molecules are actually a system of genes known as the **major histocompatibility complex (MHC)**.

### Genes Coding for MHC Molecules (HLA Antigens)

The MHC system is the most polymorphic system found in humans.[6,7] It is thought that this polymorphism is essential to our survival, because MHC molecules play a pivotal role in triggering the immune response to diverse immunogens.[8] Genes coding for the MHC molecules in humans are found on the short arm of chromosome 6 and are divided into three categories or classes. Class I molecules are coded for at three different locations or loci, termed A, B, and C. Class II genes are situated in the D region, and there are several different loci, known as DR, DQ, and DP. For the class II molecules, there is a gene that codes for the alpha chain and one or more genes that code for the beta chain. Between the class I and class II regions on chromosome 6 is the area of class III genes, which code for complement proteins and cytokines such as tumor necrosis factor (Fig. 3–4). Class III proteins are secreted proteins that have an immune function, but they are not expressed on cell surfaces. Class I and II gene products are involved in antigen recognition and influence the repertoire of antigens to which T cells can respond.

At each of these loci, or locations, there is the possibility of multiple alleles. **Alleles** are alternate forms of a gene that code for slightly different varieties of the same product. The MHC system is described as polymorphic, because there are so many possible alleles at each location. For example, at least 580 different alleles of HLA-A, 921 alleles of HLA-B, and 312 alleles of HLA-C have been identified at this time.[9]

The probability that any two individuals will express the same MHC molecules is very low. An individual inherits two copies of chromosome 6, and thus there is a possibility of two different alleles for each gene on the chromosome, unless that person is homozygous (has the same alleles) at a given location. These genes are described as *codominant*, meaning that all alleles that an individual inherits code for products that are expressed on cells. Since the MHC genes are closely linked, they are inherited together as a package called a **haplotype.** Thus, each inherited chromosomal region consists of a package of genes for A, B, C, DR, DP, and DQ. The full genotype would consist of two of each gene at a particular locus. Because there are numerous alleles or varient forms at each locus, an individual's MHC type is about as unique as a fingerprint.

Traditionally, HLA nomenclature had been defined serologically through the use of a battery of antibodies.

Currently, however, advances in DNA analysis have made identification of actual genes possible. The nomenclature has become correspondingly more complex. For instance, the notation HLA DRB1*1301 indicates the actual gene involved in coding for an HLA DR1 antigen, with the B standing for the beta chain, which is a part of the antigen, and the 1301 indicating a specific allele. The uniqueness of the HLA antigens creates a major problem in matching organ donors to recipients, because these antigens are highly immunogenic. However, in cases of disputed paternity, polymorphisms can be used as a helpful identification tool.

## Structure of Class I Molecules

Each of the MHC genes codes for a protein product that appears on cell surfaces. All the proteins of a particular class share structural similarities and are found on the same types of cells. **Class I MHC molecules** are expressed on all nucleated cells, although they differ in the level of expression. They are highest on lymphocytes and low or undetected on liver hepatocytes, neural cells, muscle cells, and sperm.[6,10] This may explain why HLA matching is not done in the case of liver transplants. Additionally, HLA-C antigens are expressed at a lower level than HLA-A and HLA-B antigens, so the latter two are the most important to match for transplantation.[10]

Each class I antigen is a glycoprotein dimer, made up of two noncovalently linked polypeptide chains. The α chain has a molecular weight of 45,000. A lighter chain associated with it, called a β₂–microglobulin, has a molecular weight of 12,000 and is encoded by a single gene on chromosome 15 that is not polymorphic.[6] The α chain is folded into three domains, α1, α2, and α3, and it is inserted into the cell membrane via a transmembrane segment that is hydrophobic.[10] The three external domains consist of about 90 amino acids each, the transmembrane domain has about 25 hydrophobic amino acids along with a short stretch of about 5 hydrophilic amino acids, and an anchor of 30 amino acids (Fig. 3–5). β₂–microglobulin does not penetrate the cell membrane, but it is essential for proper folding of the α chain. X-ray crystallographic studies indicate that the α1 and α2 domains each form an alpha helix and that these

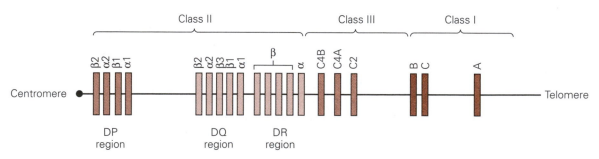

FIGURE 3–4. The major histocompatibility complex. Location of the class I, II, and III genes on chromosome 6. Class I consists of loci A, B, and C, while class II has at least three loci, DR, DQ, and DP.

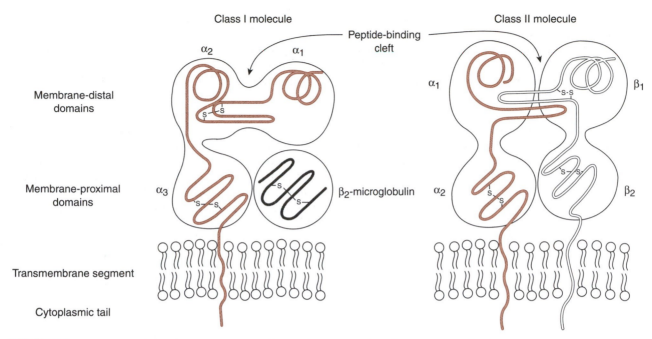

**FIGURE 3–5.** Structure of class I and II MHC products. *(From Goldsby, RA, Kindt, TJ, and Osborne, BA. Immunology, ed. 4. WH Freeman, New York, 2000, p. 178, with permission.)*

serve as the walls of a deep groove at the top of the molecule that functions as the peptide-binding site in antigen recognition.[6,7] This binding site is able to hold peptides that are between 8 and 10 amino acids long. Most of the polymorphism resides in the α1 and α2 regions, while the α3 and β2 regions are similar to the constant regions found in immunoglobulin molecules.[6,10] The α3 region reacts with CD8 on cytotoxic T cells.

Another group of molecules called the nonclassical class I antigens are designated E, F, and G. This group of molecules, except for G, are not expressed on cell surfaces and do not function in antigen recognition but may play other roles in the immune response. G antigens are expressed on trophoblast cells during the first trimester of pregnancy and are thought to help ensure tolerance for the fetus by protecting placental tissue from the action of NK cells.[6]

## Structure of Class II Molecules

The occurrence of **class II MHC molecules** is much more restricted than that of class I, because they are found primarily on antigen-presenting cells, which include B lymphocytes, monocytes, macrophages, and dendritic cells. The major class II molecules—DP, DQ, and DR—consist of two noncovalently bound polypeptide chains that are both encoded by genes in the MHC complex. DR is expressed at the highest level, as it accounts for about one-half of all the class II molecules on a particular cell.[6] The DR β gene is the most highly polymorphic, as 18 different alleles are known at this time.[6]

Both the α chain, with a molecular weight of 33,000, and the β chain, with a molecular weight of 27,000, are anchored to the cell membrane.[11] Each has two domains, and it is the

α1 and the β1 domains that come together to form the peptide-binding site, similar to the one found on class I molecules[7,10] (see Fig. 3–5). However, both ends of the peptide-binding cleft are open, and this allows for capture of longer peptides than is the case for class I molecules. At least three other class II genes have been described—DM, DN, and DO, the so-called nonclassical class II genes. Products of these genes play a regulatory role in antigen processing.[7]

The main role of the class I and class II MHC molecules is to bind peptides within cells and transport them to the plasma membrane, where T cells can recognize them in the phenomemon known as *antigen presentation.* T cells can only "see" and respond to antigens when they are combined with MHC molecules. While one individual can express only a small number of MHC molecules, each molecule can present a large number of different antigenic peptides to T cells.[12] It is thought that the two main classes of these molecules have evolved to deal with two types of infectious agents: those that attack cells from the outside (such as bacteria) and those that attack from the inside (viruses and other intracellular pathogens).Class I molecules mainly present peptides that have been synthesized within the cell to CD8 (cytotoxic) T cells, while class II molecules present antigen to CD4 (helper) T cells. Class II molecules mainly bind exogenous proteins—those taken into the cell from the outside and degraded.[13,14] Class I molecules are thus the watchdogs of viral, tumor, and certain parasitic antigens that are synthesized within the cell, while class II molecules stimulate CD4 T cells in the case of bacterial infections or the presence of other material that is endocytosed by the cell.[13,15] In either case, for a T-cell response to be triggered, peptides must be available in adequate supply for MHC molecules to bind, they must be able to be bound effectively, and they must be recognized by a T-cell receptor.[16] Some viruses, such as herpes simplex and adenovirus, have managed to block the immune response by interfering with one or more processes involved in antigen presentation.[8,17] These viruses are able to maintain a lifelong presence in the host (see Chapter 22 for details).

The difference in functioning of the two molecules is tied to the mechanisms by which processed antigen is transported to the surface. Both types of molecules, however, must be capable of presenting an enormous array of different antigenic peptides to T cells. The chemistry of the MHC antigens controls what sorts of peptides fit in the binding pockets. These two pathways are discussed here.

## Role of Class I Molecules

Both class I and class II molecules are synthesized in the rough endoplasmic reticulum, and for a time they remain anchored in the endoplasmic reticulum membrane. Class I molecules, however, actually bind peptides while still in the endoplasmic reticulum.[7] In fact, binding helps to stabilize the association of the α chain of class I with the $\beta_2$–microglobulin.[16] However, before binding with antigen occurs, newly synthesized α chains freely bind a molecule called *calnexin*. This 88-kd molecule is membrane-bound in the endoplasmic reticulum, and it keeps the α chain in a partially folded state while it awaits binding to $\beta_2$–microglobulin.[13,18] When $\beta_2$–microglobulin binds, calnexin is released, and three other chaperone molecules—calreticulin, tapasin, and ERp57—are associated with the complex and help to stabilize it for peptide binding[17,18] **(Fig. 3–6).**

Peptides that associate with the class I molecules are approximately eight to ten amino acids in length and are derived from partial digestion of proteins synthesized in the cytoplasm. These intracellular peptides may include viral,

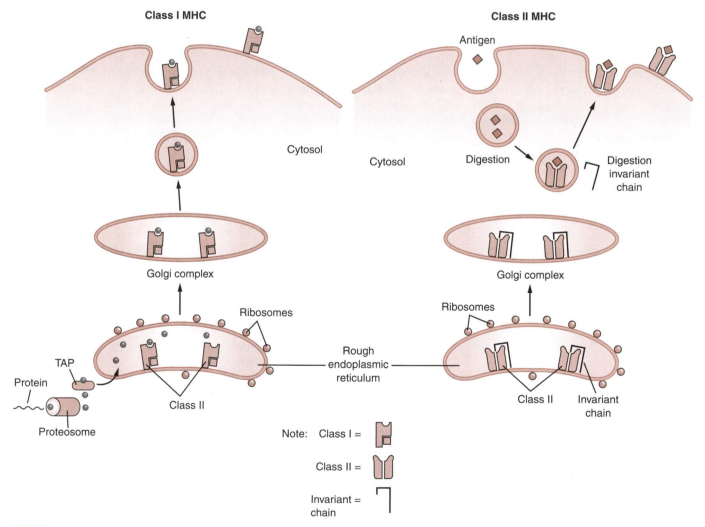

**FIGURE 3–6.** Separate antigen processing pathways for endogenous and exogenous antigens. Class I MHC molecules are made in the rough endoplasmic reticulum (ER), where small peptides made within the cell are transported to the ER. Upon combining with MHC class I, the peptide-MHC complex is transported through the Golgi complex to the cell surface. The binding site of MHC class II molecules are first occupied by an invariant chain (Ii). This is degraded and exchanged for short exogenous peptides in an endosomal compartment. The exogenous peptide-MHC class II complex is then transported to the cell surface.

tumor, or even bacterial antigens.[12] Such peptides may be newly made proteins that fail to fold correctly and hence are defective. These are called *defective ribosomal products* (DRiPs).[12] Twenty to 70 percent of all proteins synthesized in a cell may fall into this category.[8,19] Digestion of these defective or early proteins is carried out by proteases that reside in large cylindrical cytoplasmic complexes called *proteasomes*.[13] Proteasomes are a packet of enzymes that play a major role in antigen presentation.[13] Peptides must be unfolded before entering the cylindrical chamber of the proteosome, and then they are cleaved into the proper size for delivery to class I molecules. Once cleaved, the peptides must then be pumped into the lumen of the endoplasmic reticulum by specialized transporter proteins.[7,15] These two proteins, **transporters associated with antigen processing (TAP1 and TAP2)**, are responsible for the adenosine triphosphate–dependent transport, from the cytoplasm to the lumen of the endoplasmic reticulum, of peptides suitable for binding to class I molecules.[8,17,18] TAP1 and TAP2 are most efficient at transporting peptides that have 12 amino acids or less.[15,17] Tapasin brings the TAP transporters into close proximity to the newly formed MHC molecules and mediates interaction with them so that peptides can be loaded onto the class I molecules.[13,15] Once the α chain has bound the peptide, the MHC I-peptide complex is rapidly transported to the cell surface (see Fig. 3–6).[6]

Of the thousands of peptides that may be processed in this manner, only a small fraction of them (1 percent or less) actually induce a T-cell response.[15] Binding is based on interaction of only two or three amino acid residues with the class I binding groove. Different class I molecules will have slightly different binding affinities, and it is these small differences that determine to which particular antigens one individual will respond.

It is estimated that a single cell may express about $10^5$ copies of each class I molecule, so many different peptides can be captured and expressed in this manner.[10] As few as 10 to 100 identical antigen-MHC I complexes can induce a cytotoxic response.[15] In healthy cells, most of these MHC I complexes contain self-peptides that are ignored by the T cells, while in diseased cells, peptides are derived from viral proteins or proteins associated with cancerous states. Display of hundreds of class I molecules complexed to antigen allows CD8+ T cells to continuously check cell surfaces for the presence of nonself-antigen. If it recognizes an antigen as being foreign, the CD8+ T cell produces cytokines that cause lysis of the entire cell **(Fig. 3–7)**.

## Role of Class II Molecules

Unlike class I molecules, class II molecules must be transported from the endoplasmic reticulum (ER) to an endosomal compartment before they can bind peptides.[7] Dendritic cells are the most potent activators of T cells, and they are excellent at capturing and digesting exogenous antigens such as bacteria. Class II molecules in the endoplasmic

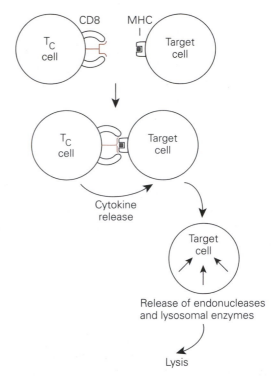

**FIGURE 3–7.** The CD8+ T cell recognizes antigen in asociation with MHC class I. If the antigen is recognized as being foreign, cytokines are released, causing destruction of the target cell.

reticulum associate with a protein called the **invariant chain (Ii),** which prevents interaction of the binding site with any endogenous peptides in the endoplasmic reticulum.[7,13] The invariant chain is a 31-kd protein that is made in excess so that enough is available to bind with all class II molecules shortly after they are synthesized. Ii may be responsible for helping to bring α and β chains together in the ER lumen and then moving them out through the Golgi complex to the endocytic vesicles, where digested antigen is found.[16] Because the open structure of class II molecules would permit binding of segments of intact proteins within the ER, Ii serves to protect the binding site.[20]

Once bound to the invariant chain, the class II molecule is transported to an endosomal compartment, where it encounters peptides derived from endocytosed, exogenous proteins. Antigen processing may help to unfold molecules and uncover functional sites that are buried deep within the native protein structure.[3] The invariant chain is degraded by a protease, leaving just a small fragment called *class II invariant chain peptide* (CLIP) attached to the peptide-binding cleft.[14,21] CLIP is then exchanged for exogenous peptides. Selective binding of peptides is favored by the low pH of the endosomal compartment.[16] HLA-DM molecules help to mediate the reaction by removing the CLIP fragment.[6,10,21] Generally, peptides of approximately 13 to 18 amino acid residues can bind, because the groove is open on both ends, unlike class I molecules, which have a closed end.[10,14,22,23] Within a central core of 13 amino acids, 7 to 10 residues provide the major contact points.[10]

Hydrogen bonding takes place along the length of the captured peptide, in contrast to class I molecules, which only bond at the amino and carboxy terminal ends.[23,24] There are also several pockets in the class II proteins that easily accommodate amino acid side chains. This gives class II proteins more flexibility in the types of peptides that can be bound.[23,24] Once binding has occurred, the class II protein-peptide complex is stabilized and is transported to the cell surface (see Fig. 3–6). On the cell surface, class II molecules are responsible for forming a trimolecular complex that occurs between antigen, class II molecule, and an appropriate T-cell receptor. If binding occurs with a T-cell receptor on a CD4+ T cell, the T helper cell recruits and triggers a B-cell response, resulting in antibody formation **(Fig. 3–8).**

## Clinical Significance of MHC

Testing for MHC antigens has typically been done, because both class I and class II molecules can induce a response that leads to graft rejection. Testing methodology has changed from serological principles to molecular methods, which are much more accurate. The role of the laboratory in transplantation is presented in Chapter 17. MHC antigens also appear to play a role in development of autoimmune

diseases. The link between MHC antigens and autoimmune diseases is discussed more fully in Chapter 14.

However, the evidence that both class I and class II molecules play a major role in antigen presentation has more far-reaching consequences. They essentially determine the types of peptides to which an individual can mount an immune response. Although the MHC molecules typically have a broad binding capacity, small biochemical differences in these proteins are responsible for differences seen in the ability to react to a specific antigen.[12] It is possible that nonresponders to a particular vaccine such as hepatitis B do not have the genetic capacity to respond. On the other hand, presence of a particular MHC protein may confer additional protection, as the example of HLA B8 and increased resistance to HIV infection shows.[8] Therefore, it will be important to know an individual's MHC type for numerous reasons.

Much of the recent research has focused on the types of peptides that can be bound by particular MHC molecules.[23–25] Future developments may include tailoring vaccines to certain groups of such molecules. As more is learned about antigen processing, vaccines containing certain amino acid sequences that serve as immunodominant epitopes can be specifically developed. This might avoid the risk associated with using live organisms. Additionally, if an individual suffers from allergies, knowing a person's MHC type might also help predict the types of allergens to which they may be allergic, because research in this area is attempting to group allergens according to amino acid structure.[25] It is likely that knowledge of the MHC molecules will affect many areas of patient care in the future.

## SUMMARY

To fully comprehend the specificity of antigen–antibody combination, it is essential to understand the principal characteristics of antigens. Antigens are macromolecules that elicit formation of immunoglobulins or sensitized cells in an immunocompetent host. Immunogen is a term that is often used synonymously with antigen. The term immunogen emphasizes the fact that a host response is triggered, while the term antigen is sometimes used to denote a substance that does not elicit a host response but reacts with antibody once it has been formed.

Although immunogenicity is influenced by factors such as age, health, route of inoculation, and genetic capacity, there are certain specific characteristics that are shared by most immunogens: a molecular weight of at least 100,000, molecular complexity, and foreignness to the host. While Immunogens are fairly large molecules, the immune response is keyed to only small portions of these molecules, or epitopes, and very small differences in these epitopes can be detected by the immune system.

Adjuvants are substances that can be mixed with antigen to enhance the immune response. Most adjuvants work by

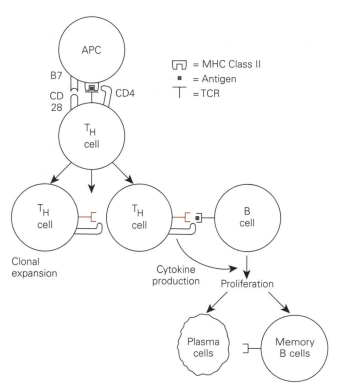

**FIGURE 3–8.** CD4+ T cells recognize exogenous antigen on phagocytic antigen presenting cells along with MHC class II. T cells are stimulated by contact with antigen, and clonal expansion takes place. These CD4+ helper T cells secrete cytokines that cause an antigen activated B cell to proliferate and produce plasma cells, which make antibody.

keeping the antigen in the area and by increasing the number of cells involved in the immune response.

The genetic capability to mount an immune response is linked to a group of molecules known as the MHC antigens. The two main classes of these molecules, sometimes referred to as HLA antigens, have evolved to deal with infectious agents that attack cells from the outside (such as bacteria) and those that attack from the inside (viruses and other intracellular pathogens). Class I and class II molecules bind peptides within cells and transport them to the plasma membrane, where they can be recognized by T cells. Class I MHC molecules are found on all nucleated cells, and these molecules associate with foreign antigens, such as viral proteins, synthesized within a host cell. Class I molecules are stabilized by the binding of antigen, and the complex is readily transported to the cellular surface. Class II molecules, on the other hand, have a more limited distribution, and these associate with foreign antigens taken into the cell from the outside. Binding of antigen to the class II molecules occurs in endosomal compartments, and then this complex is moved to the outside of the cell. The binding sites on both types of molecules may limit the size and the nature of the antigen bound. Thus, these molecules play a key role in antigen processing and recognition.

# CASE STUDY

A 15-year-old boy needs to have a kidney transplant due to the effects of severe diabetes. His family members consist of his father, mother, and two sisters. All of them are willing to donate a kidney so that he can come off dialysis. He is also on a list for a cadaver kidney. His physician suggests that the family be tested first for the best HLA match.

## Questions

a. How many alleles would be shared by mother and son? Father and son?

b. What are the chances that one of the sisters would be an exact match?

c. Is there a possibility that a cadaver kidney might be a better match than any of the family members?

# EXERCISE

## SPECIFICITY OF ANTIGEN–ANTIBODY REACTIONS

### Principle

Typing serum is an antibody that will react only with the specific red blood cell antigen against which it is directed. Agglutination indicates the presence of that particular antigen.

### Reagents, Materials, and Equipment

Anti-A typing serum

Anti-B typing serum

Group A, group B, and group O reagent red blood cells

Microscope slides

Disposable stirrers

### Procedure

1. Divide each microscope slide in half, using a wax marking pencil. Label the left side "A" and the right side "B" for the two antisera that will be used.
2. Place one drop of anti-A on the left side of slide and one drop of anti-B on the right side.
3. Add one drop of reagent red blood cell suspension to each side.
4. Mix each side thoroughly with a separate disposable stirrer.
5. Rock slide gently back and forth for 2 minutes.
6. Observe for agglutination.
7. Repeat this procedure for each type of reagent red blood cell.

### Results

1. Report any cells that agglutinate with anti-A serum as type A cells and any cells that agglutinate with anti-B serum as type B cells.
2. Agglutination with both types of antisera indicates that both A and B antigens are present, and this is type AB.
3. No agglutination indicates cells have neither antigen, and these belong to group O.

### Interpretation of Results

Red blood cell antigens consist of a lipid–sugar complex that is inserted into the cell's membrane. The H antigen serves as the building block for both A and B antigens. As can be seen in **Figure 3–9**, all three antigens differ only by the presence or absence of one sugar. If only H antigen is present, then these cells are typed as O cells. Specific antibody is able to detect the one sugar difference in each of the antigens, and an agglutination reaction will occur only with the antigen against which the antibody is directed.

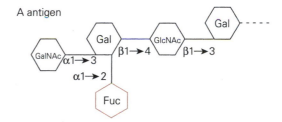

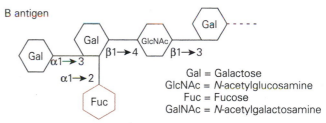

FIGURE 3–9. Structure of H, A, and B red cell antigens. *(From Cooling, L. ABO, H, and Lewis blood groups and structurally related antigens. In Roback, J, Combs, MR, Grossman B, Hillyer, C (eds.): Technical Manual, ed. 16. American Association of Blood Banks, Bethesda, MD, 2008, pp. 361–85 with permission.)*

# REVIEW QUESTIONS

1. All of the following are characteristic of a good immunogen except
   a. internal complexity.
   b. large molecular weight.
   c. the presence of numerous epitopes.
   d. found on host cells.

2. Which of the following best describes a hapten?
   a. Not able to react with antibody
   b. Antigenic only when coupled to a carrier
   c. Has multiple determinant sites
   d. A large chemically complex molecule

3. Which would be the best immunogen?
   a. Protein with a molecular weight of 200,000
   b. Nylon
   c. Polysaccharide with a molecular weight of 250,000
   d. Protein with a molecular weight of 175,000

4. All of the following describe an epitope except
   a. same as an antigenic determinant site.
   b. area of an immunogen recognized by T cells.
   c. consists of sequential amino acids only.
   d. key portion of the immunogen.

5. Adjuvents act by which of the following methods?
   a. Complex to antigen to increase its size
   b. Prevent rapid escape from the tissues
   c. Increase processing of antigen
   d. All of the above

6. A heterophile antigen is one that
   a. is a self-antigen.
   b. exists in unrelated plants or animals.
   c. has been used previously to stimulate antibody response.
   d. is from the same species but is different from the host.

7. Which of the following is true of MHC (HLA) class II antigens?
   a. They are found on all nucleated cells.
   b. They are found on B cells and macrophages.
   c. They all originate at one locus.
   d. They are coded for on chromosome 9.

8. MHC molecules are associated with which of the following?
   a. Graft rejection
   b. Autoimmune diseases
   c. Determining to which antigens an individual responds
   d. All of the above

9. Which of the following best describes the role of TAP?
   a. They bind to class II molecules to help block the antigen-binding site.
   b. They bind to class I proteins in proteosomes.
   c. They transport peptides into the lumen of the endoplasmic reticulum.
   d. They help cleave peptides for transport to endosomes.

10. An individual is recovering from a bacterial infection and tests positive for antibodies to a protein normally found in the cytoplasm of this bacterium. Which of the following statements is true of this situation?
    a. Class I molecules have presented bacterial antigen to CD8+ T cells.
    b. Class I molecules have presented bacterial antigen to CD4+ T cells.
    c. Class II molecules have presented bacterial antigen to CD4+ T cells.
    d. B cells have recognized bacterial antigen without help from T cells.

# References

1. Mak, TW, and Saunders, ME. The Immune Response: Basic and Clinical Principles. Elsevier, Burlington, MA, 2006, pp. 121–146.

2. Kindt, TJ, Goldsby, RA, and Osborne, BA. Kuby Immunology, ed. 6. WH Freeman and Co., New York, 2007, pp. 76–110.

3. Berzofsky, JA, and Berkower, IJ. Immunogenicity and antigen structure. In Paul, WE (ed): Fundamental Immunology, ed. 4. Lippincott Williams & Wilkins, Philadelphia, 1999, pp. 651–698.

4. Beadling, WV, and Cooling, L. Immunohematology. In Henry's Clinical Diagnosis and Management by Laboratory Methods, ed. 21. Saunders, Philadelphia, 2007, pp. 617–668.

5. Mak, TW, and Saunders, ME. The Immune Response: Basic and Clinical Principles. Elsevier, Burlington, MA, 2006, pp. 695–749.

6. Massey, HD, and McPherson, RA. Human Leukocyte Antigen: The Major Histocompatibility Complex of Man. In Henry's Clinical Diagnosis and Management by Laboratory Methods, ed. 21. Saunders, Philadelphia, 2007, pp. 876–893.

7. Mak, TW, and Saunders, ME. The Immune Response: Basic and Clinical Principles. Elsevier, Burlington, MA, 2006, pp. 247–277.

8. Groothuis, TAM, Griekspoor, AC, Neijssen, JJ, Herberts, CA, et al. MHC class I alleles and their exploration of the antigen-processing machinery. Immunol Rev. 207:60–76, 2005.

9. HLA Informatics Group, The Anthony Nolan Trust. The HLA Sequence Database. Accessed July 23, 2007, at http://www.anthonynolan.org.uk/HIG/lists/class1list.html.

10. Kindt, TJ, Goldsby, RA, and Osborne, BA. Kuby Immunology, ed. 6. WH Freeman and Co., New York, 2007, pp. 189–222.

11. Pieters, J. MHC class II-restricted antigen processing and presentation. Adv Immunol 75:159–208, 2000.

12. Shastri, N, Cardinaud, S, Schwab, SR, Serwold, T, et al. All the peptides that fit: The beginning, the middle, and the end of the MHC class I antigen-processing pathway. Immunol Rev 207:31–41, 2005.

13. Loureiro, J, and Ploegh, HL. Antigen presentation and the ubiquitin-proteosome system in host-pathogen interactions. Adv Immunol 92:226–306, 2006.

14. Li, P, Gregg, JL, Wang, N, Zhou, D, et al. Compartmentalization of class II antigen presentation: Contribution of cytoplasmic and endosomal processing. Immunol Rev 207:206–217, 2005.

15. Koch, J, and Tampe, R. The macromolecular peptide-loading complex in MHC class I-dependent antigen presentation. Cell Mol Life Sci 63:653–662, 2006.

16. Germain, RN. Antigen processing and presentation. In Paul, WE (ed): Fundamental Immunology, ed. 4. Lippincott Williams & Wilkins, Philadelphia, 1999, pp 287–336.

17. Scholz, C, and Tampe, R. The intracellular antigen transport machinery TAP in adaptive immunity and virus escape mechanisms. J Bioenerg and Biomembr 37:509–515, 2005.

18. Cresswell, P, Ackerman, AL, Giodini, A, Peaper, DR, et al. Mechanisms of MHC class-I restricted antigen processing and cross-presentation. Immunol Rev 207:147–157, 2005.

19. Yewdell, JW. The seven dirty little secrets of major histocompatibility complex class I antigen processing. Immunol Rev 207:8–18, 2005.

20. Mak, TW, and Saunders, ME. Antigen processing and presentation. In The Immune Response: Basic and Clinical Principles. Elsevier, Burlington, MA, 2006, pp. 279–309.

21. Ghosh, P, Amaya, M, and Mellins, E, et al. The structure of an intermediate in class II MHC maturation: CLIP bound to HLA-DR3. Nature 378:457–462, 1995.

22. Brown, JH, Jardetzky, TS, and Gorga, JC, et al. Three-dimensional structure of the human class II histocompatibility antigen HLA-DR1. Nature 364:33, 1993.

23. Jardetzky, TS, Brown, JH, and Gorga, JC, et al. Crystallographic analysis of endogenous peptides associated with HLA-DR1 suggests a common, polyproline II-like conformation for bound peptides. Proc Natl Acad Sci USA 93:734–738, 1996.

24. Stern, LJ, Brown, JH, and Jardetzky, TS, et al. Crystal structure of the human class II MHC protein HLA-DR1 complexed with an influenza virus peptide. Nature 368:215–21, 1994.

# 4 Antibody Structure and Function

# CHAPTER OUTLINE

When B lymphocytes are stimulated by antigen and undergo differentiation, the end product is antibody or immunoglobulin. **Immunoglobulins** are glycoproteins found in the serum portion of the blood. They are composed of 82 to 96 percent polypeptide and 2 to 14 percent carbohydrate.[1] When subjected to electrophoresis at pH 8.6, immunoglobulins appear primarily in the gamma ($\gamma$) band **(Fig. 4–1)**. Each

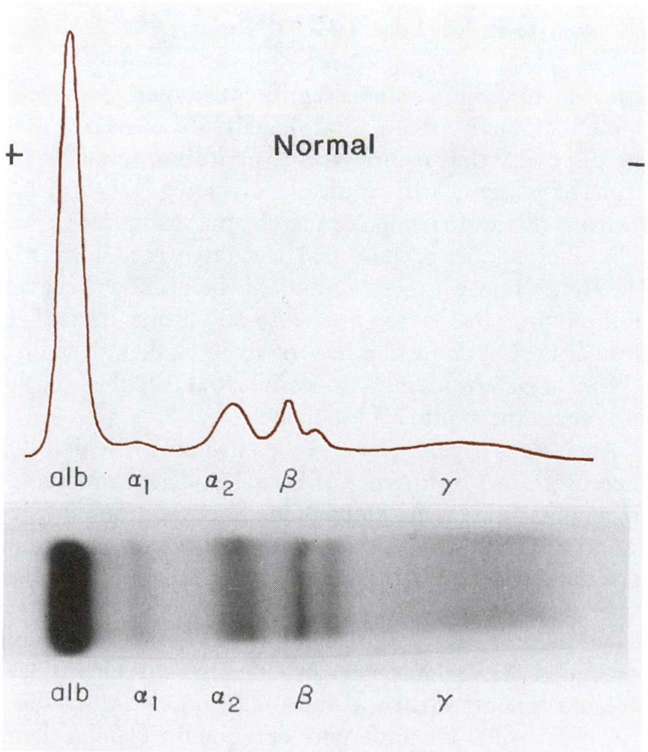

FIGURE 4–1. Serum electrophoresis. (From Widmann, FK. An Introduction to Clinical Immunology. FA Davis, Philadelphia, 1989, with permission.)

of the five major classes has slightly different electrophoretic properties. These classes are designated IgG, IgM, IgA, IgD, and IgE (*Ig* is an abbreviation for "immunoglobulin").

Immunoglobulins are considered to be the humoral branch of the immune response. They play an essential role in antigen recognition and in biological activities related to the immune response such as opsonization and complement activation. Although each class has unique properties, all immunoglobulin molecules share many common features. This chapter presents the nature of this generalized structure and discusses the characteristics of each immunoglobulin type. Specific functions for each of the classes are examined in relation to structural differences.

## TETRAPEPTIDE STRUCTURE OF IMMUNOGLOBULINS

All immunoglobulin molecules are made up of a basic four-chain polypeptide unit that consists of two large chains called **heavy** or **H chains** and two smaller chains called **light** or **L chains.** These chains are held together by noncovalent forces and disulfide interchain bridges. The basic structure of immunoglobulins was elucidated in the 1950s and 1960s by the efforts of two men: Gerald Edelman, working at the Rockefeller Institute in the United States, and Rodney Porter at Oxford University in England. For their contributions, these men shared the Nobel Prize in physiology and medicine in 1972. They chose to work with immunoglobulin G.

Edelman's work centered on using the analytic ultracentrifuge to separate out immunoglobulins on the basis of molecular weight.[2] He found that intact IgG molecules had a sedimentation coefficient of 7 S (the Svedberg unit [S] indicates the sedimentation rate in an analytical ultracentrifuge).

Larger molecules will travel farther and thus have a larger sedimentation coefficient. On obtaining a purified preparation of IgG, Edelman used 7 M urea to unfold the molecule. Once unfolded, the exposed sulfhydryl bonds could be cleaved by a reducing agent such as mercaptoethanol. After such treatment, the material was subjected again to ultracentrifugation, and two separate fractions, one at 3.5 S and one at 2.2 S, were obtained.

The 3.5 S fraction, with a molecular weight of approximately 50,000, was designated the H chain; the 2.2 S fraction, with a molecular weight of 22,000, was named the L chain.[3] These two pieces occurred in equal amounts, indicating that the formula for IgG had to be $H_2L_2$. This is the generalized formula for all immunoglobulins.

## Cleavage with Papain

Porter's work was based on the use of the proteolytic enzyme papain, which was used to cleave IgG into three pieces of about equal size, each having a sedimentation coefficient of 3.5 S and representing a molecular weight of approximately 45,000 to 50,000 d.[3,4] Carboxymethyl cellulose ion exchange chromatography separated this material into two types of fragments, one of which spontaneously crystallized at 4°C. This fragment, known as the **Fc fragment** (for "fragment crystallizable"), had no antigen-binding ability and is now known to represent the carboxy-terminal halves of two H chains that are held together by S–S bonding.[3] The Fc fragment is important in effector functions of immunoglobulin molecules, which include opsonization and complement fixation.

The remaining two identical fragments were found to have antigen-binding capacity and were named **Fab fragments** (fragment antigen-binding). Because precipitation would not occur if Fab fragments were allowed to react with antigen, it was guessed that each fragment represented one antigen-binding site and that two such fragments were present in an intact antibody molecule; such a molecule would be able to form a cross-linked complex with antigen, and the complex would precipitate. Each Fab fragment thus consists of one L chain and one-half of an H chain, held together by disulfide bonding.[4]

## Pepsin Digestion

Alfred Nisonoff used pepsin to obtain additional evidence for the structure of immunoglobulins.[3] This proteolytic enzyme was found to cleave IgG at the carboxy-terminal side of the interchain disulfide bonds, yielding one single fragment with a molecular weight of 100,000 d and all the antigen-binding ability, known as F(ab)$_2$. An additional fragment called Fc' was similar to Fc except that it disintegrated into several smaller pieces. Thus, a basic picture of the four-chain unit of the immunoglobulin molecule was obtained, which indicated that each L chain was bonded to an H chain by means of an S–S bond, and the H chains were joined to each other by one or more S–S bonds **(Fig. 4–2)**. The exact

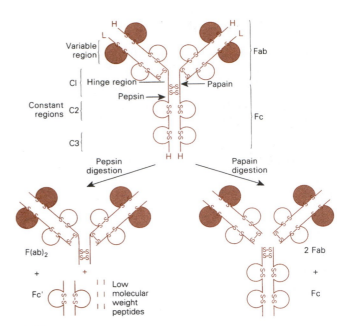

**FIGURE 4–2.** Generalized structure of an immunoglobulin molecule. The basic structure of an immunoglobulin is a tetrapeptide, consisting of two H and two L chains linked by disulfide bonds. Intrachain disulfide bonds create flooded regions or domains. The amino-terminal end of each chain is a variable region, while the carboxy-terminal end is one or more constant regions. Pepsin digestion yields an F(ab)$_2$ fragment, with all the antibody activity, and an Fc$_1$ fragment. Papain digestion yields two F(ab) fragments and an Fc portion.

number of disulfide bonds differs among antibody classes and subclasses.

## THE NATURE OF LIGHT CHAINS

The difficulty in obtaining a significant amount of a specific immunoglobulin for amino acid analysis was overcome by the discovery that **Bence-Jones proteins,** found in the urine of patients with multiple myeloma, were in fact L chains that were being secreted by the malignant plasma cells.[3] Bence-Jones proteins had been discovered in 1845 by Dr. Henry Bence-Jones, who noted the peculiar behavior of these proteins: When heated to 60°C, they precipitate from urine, but on further heating to 80°C, they redissolve. These characteristics made it possible to isolate the L chains and obtain the amino acid sequence.

Analysis of several Bence-Jones proteins revealed that there were two main types of L chains, designated **kappa (ε)** and **lambda (λ).** Each contained between 200 and 220 amino acids, and from position number 111 on (the amino terminus is position number 1), it was discovered that each type had essentially the same sequence. This region was called the **constant region,** and the amino-terminal end was called the **variable region.** Thus, all κ L chains have an almost identical carboxy-terminal end, and the same is true of λ chains. The difference between the κ and λ chains lies in the amino acid substitutions at a few locations along the chain. There are no functional differences between the two types. Both κ and λ L chains are found in all five classes of immunoglobulins, but only one type is present in a given molecule.

## HEAVY CHAIN SEQUENCING

H chain sequencing demonstrated the presence of domains similar to those in the L chains—that is, variable and constant regions. The first approximately 110 amino acids at the amino-terminal end constitute the variable domain, and the remaining amino acids can typically be divided up into three or more constant regions with very similar sequences, designated $C_H1$, $C_H2$, and $C_H3$. Constant regions of the H chain are unique to each class and give each immunoglobulin type its name. Hence, IgG has an γ H chain, IgM a μ chain, IgA an α chain, IgD a δ chain, and IgE an ε chain. Each of these represents an **isotype,** a unique amino acid sequence that is common to all immunoglobulin molecules of a given class in a given species. Minor variations of these sequences that are present in some individuals but not others are known as **allotypes (Fig. 4–3).** Allotypes occur in the four IgG subclasses, in one IgA subclass, and in the kappa light chain.[3] These genetic markers are found in the constant region and are inherited in simple Mendelian fashion. Some of the best-known examples of allotypes are variations of the γ chain known as G1m3 and G1m17.

The variable portions of each chain are unique to a specific antibody molecule, and they constitute what is known as the **idiotype** of the molecule. The amino-terminal ends of both L and H chains contain these regions, which are essential to the formation of the antigen-binding site. Together they serve as the antigen-recognition unit.

## HINGE REGION

The segment of H chain located between the $C_H1$ and $C_H2$ regions is known as the **hinge region.** It has a high content of proline and hydrophobic residues; the high proline content allows for flexibility.[3,5] This ability to bend lets the two antigen-binding sites operate independently. The flexibility also assists in effector functions such as initiation of the complement cascade (see Chapter 6 for details). Gamma, delta, and alpha chains all have a hinge region, but mu and epsilon chains do not. However, the $C_H2$ domains of these latter two chains are paired in such a way as to confer flexibility to the Fab arms.[1]

In addition to the four polypeptide chains, all types of immunoglobulins contain a carbohydrate portion, which is localized between the $C_H2$ domains of the two H chains. Functions of the carbohydrate include (1) increasing the solubility of immunoglobulin, (2) providing protection against degradation, and (3) enhancing functional activity of the Fc domains. This latter function may be the most important, because recognition by Fc receptors correlates with the presence of the carbohydrate moiety.[5]

## THREE-DIMENSIONAL STRUCTURE OF ANTIBODIES

The basic four-chain structure of all immunoglobulin molecules does not actually exist as a straight γ shape, but in fact it is folded into compact globular subunits, based on the formation of balloon-shaped loops at each of the domains.[6] Intrachain disulfide bonds stabilize these globular regions. Within each of these regions or domains, the polypeptide chain is folded back and forth on itself to form what is called a β-pleated sheet. The folded domains of the H chains line up with those of the L chains to produce a cylindrical structure called an *immunoglobulin fold* or *barrel* (**Fig. 4–4**).[1,3] Antigen is captured within the barrel by binding to a small number of amino acids at strategic locations on each chain known as *hypervariable regions.*

Three small hypervariable regions consisting of approximately 30 amino acid residues are found within the

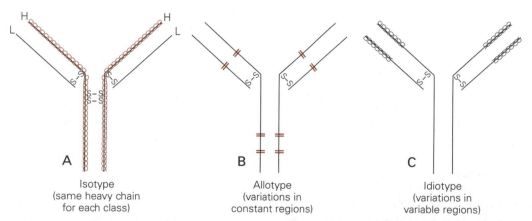

**FIGURE 4–3.** Antibody variations. *(A)* Isotype—the H chain that is unique to each immunoglobulin class. *(B)* Allotype—genetic variations in the constant regions. *(C)* Idiotype—variations in variable regions that give individual antibody molecules specificity.

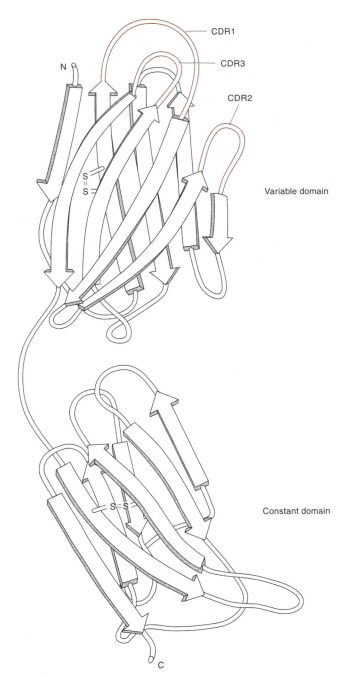

FIGURE 4–4. Three-dimensional structure of an L chain. In this ribbon diagram tracing the polypeptide backbone, B strands are shown as wide ribbons, other regions as narrow strings. Each of the two globular domains consists of a barrel-shaped assembly of seven to nine antiparallel B strands. The three hypervariable regions (CDR1, CDR2, and CDR3) are flexible loops that project outward from the amino-terminal end of the $V_L$ domain. *(From Parslow, TG, et al. Medical Immunology, ed. 10. McGraw-Hill/Appleton & Lange, 2001, with permission.)*

variable regions of both H and L chains. Each of these regions, called *complementarity-determining regions* (CDRs), is between 9 and 12 residues long.[3] They occur as loops in the folds of the variable regions of both L and H chains, and the antigen-binding site is actually determined by the apposition of the six hypervariable loops, three from each

chain (see Fig. 4–4). Antigen binds in the middle of the CDRs, with at least four of the CDRs involved in the binding.[1,3,6,7] Thus, a small number of amino acids can create an immense diversity of antigen-binding sites. Properties of individual antibody classes are considered in the following sections.

## IgG

IgG is the predominant immunoglobulin in humans, comprising approximately 75 to 80 percent of the total serum immunoglobulins. As seen in **Table 4–1**, IgG has the longest half-life of any immunoglobulin class, approximately 23 to 25 days, which may help to account for its predominance in serum. There are four major subclasses, with the following distribution: IgG1, 67 percent; IgG2, 22 percent; IgG3, 7 percent; and IgG4, 4 percent.[1,3] These subclasses differ mainly in the number and position of the disulfide bridges between the γ chains, as seen in Figure 4–5. Variability in the hinge region affects the ability to reach for antigen and the ability to initiate important biological functions such as complement activation.[8] IgG3 has the largest hinge region and the largest number of interchain disulfide bonds; therefore, it is the most efficient at binding complement, followed by IgG1.[1,3] IgG2 and IgG4 have shorter hinge segments, which tend to make them poor mediators of complement activation.[5]

Major functions of IgG include the following: (1) providing immunity for the newborn because IgG can cross the placenta; (2) fixing complement; (3) coating antigen for enhanced phagocytosis (opsonization); (4) neutralizing toxins and viruses; and (5) participating in agglutination and precipitation reactions. All subclasses of IgG appear to be able to cross the placenta, although IgG2 is the least efficient.[3]

Macrophages, monocytes, and neutrophils have receptors on their surfaces that are specific for the Fc region of IgG. This enhances contact between antigen and phagocytic cells and generally increases the efficiency of phagocytosis. IgG1 and IgG3 are particularly good at initiating phagocytosis, because they bind most strongly to Fc receptors.[1,9]

IgG has a high diffusion coefficient that allows it to enter extravascular spaces more readily than other immunoglobulin types. In fact, it is distributed almost equally between the intravascular and extravascular spaces.[1] Thus, it plays a major role in neutralizing toxins and viruses.

Agglutination and precipitation reactions take place in vitro, although it is not known how significant a role these play in vivo. IgG is better at precipitation reactions than at agglutination, because precipitation involves small soluble particles, which are more easily brought together by the relatively small IgG molecule. Agglutination is the clumping together of larger particles such as red blood cells, and being a larger molecule, IgM is much more efficient at this than IgG.

## Table 4–1.    Properties of Immunoglobulins

|  | IgG | IgM | IgA | IgD | IgE |
|---|---|---|---|---|---|
| Molecular weight | 150,000 | 900,000 | 160,000– | 180,000 | 190,000 |
| Sedimentation coefficient | 7 S | 19 S | 7 S | 7 S | 8 S |
| H chain | γ | μ | α | δ | ε |
| H chain subclasses | γ1, γ2, γ3, γ4 | None | α1, α2 | None | None |
| H chain molecular weight | 50,000–60,000 | 70,000 | 55,000–60,000 | 62,000 | 70,000–75,000 |
| Constant domains (H chain) | 3 | 4 | 3 | 3 | 4 |
| Percent of total immunoglobulin | 70–75 | 10 | 10–15 | <1 | 0.002 |
| Serum concentration (mg/dL) | 800–1600 | 120–150 | 70–350 | 1–3 | 0.005 |
| Serum half-life (days) | 23 | 6 | 5 | 1–3 | 2–3 |
| Carbohydrate content (weight percent) | 2–3 | 12 | 7–11 | 9–14 | 12 |
| Electrophoretic migration | γ2–α1 | γ1–β12 | γ2–β2 | γ1 | γ1 |
| Complement fixation | Yes | Yes | No | No | No |
| Crosses placenta | Yes | No | No | No | No |

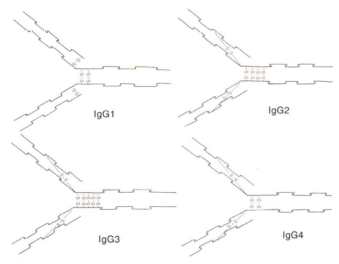

FIGURE 4–5. IgG subclasses. There are four subclasses of IgG: IgG1, IgG2, IgG3, and IgG4. These differ in the number and linkages of the disulfide bonds. *(From Bryant, NJ. Laboratory Immunology and Serology, ed. 3. WB Saunders, Philadelphia, 1992, p. 29, with permission.)*

## IgM

IgM is known as a *macroglobulin*, because it has a sedimentation rate of 19 S, which represents a molecular weight of approximately 970,000.[1] As seen in Table 4–1, the half-life of IgM is about 10 days—much shorter than that of IgG. It accounts for between 5 and 10 percent of all serum immunoglobulins.

If IgM is treated with mercaptoethanol, it dissociates into five 7 S units, each having a molecular weight of 190,000 and a four-chain structure that resembles IgG. The molecular weight of the H or μ chain is approximately 70,000. It consists of about 576 amino acids and includes one more constant domain than is found on the γ chain. The pentamer form is found in secretions, while the monomer form occurs on the surface of B cells.[5,10]

The five monomeric units are held together by a **J** or **joining chain,** which is a glycoprotein with several cysteine residues. These serve as linkage points for disulfide bonds between two adjacent monomers. Linkage occurs at the carboxy-terminal end of two of the μ chains, and it appears that the J chain may initiate polymerization by stabilizing Fc sulfhydryl groups so that cross-linking can occur.[3] The molecular weight of the J chain is approximately 15,000. One J chain is present per pentamer.

IgM thus configured assumes a starlike shape (**Fig. 4–6**) with 10 functional binding sites; only about five of these are used unless the antigen is extremely small.[1] The high valency of IgM antibodies contravenes the fact that they tend to have a low affinity for antigen.

Because of its large size, IgM is found mainly in the intravascular pool and not in other body fluids or tissues. It cannot cross the placenta. IgM is known as the primary response antibody, because it is the first to appear after antigenic stimulation, and it is the first to appear in the maturing infant. It is synthesized only as long as antigen remains present, because there are no memory cells for IgM. **Figure 4–7** depicts the difference between the primary response, which is predominantly IgM, and the secondary response, which is mainly IgG. The primary response is characterized by a long lag phase, while the secondary response has a shortened lag period and a much more rapid increase in antibody titer.

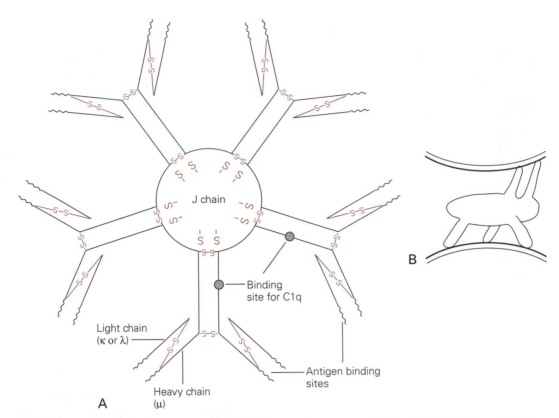

FIGURE 4–6. Structure of immunoglobulin M. (A) Pentameric structure of IgM, which is linked by a J chain. (B) Spacial configuration of IgM. Monomers can extend in different directions. (From Bryant, NJ. Laboratory Immunology and Serology, ed. 3. WB Saunders, Philadelphia, 1992, p. 31, with permission.)

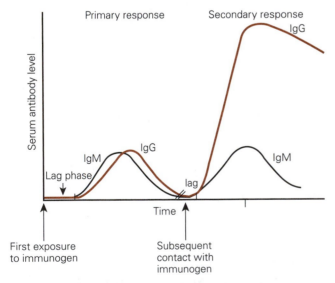

FIGURE 4–7. A comparison of the primary and secondary response to immunogen. The primary response is characterized by a long lag phase, slow exponential increase in antibody, and short-lived response. The secondary or anamnestic response has a shortened lag period, antibody rise is much more rapid, and serum levels remain higher for longer periods. This is caused by the large number of antigen-specific memory T and B cells generated during the primary response.

The functions of IgM include (1) complement fixation, (2) agglutination, (3) opsonization, and (4) toxin neutralization. IgM is the most efficient of all immunoglobulins at triggering the classical complement pathway (see Chapter 6), because a single molecule can initiate the reaction as a result of its multiple binding sites. This probably represents the most important function of IgM. The larger number of binding sites also makes IgM more efficient at agglutination reactions, especially with multivalent antigens. Thus, IgM forms a potent defense against many bacterial diseases. Because IgM has a J chain, it can ocasionally acquire a secretory component like IgA does, and this allows it to traverse epithelial cells and patrol mucous membranes.[1]

IgM also serves as a surface receptor for antigen. In the cytoplasm of the pre-B cell, μ chains first appear. When they associate with the early surrogate L chains, a signal is sent to exclude rearrangement of the other H chain locus and to begin rearrangement of the genes controlling L chain synthesis.[5] Later, as L chains are synthesized, IgM monomers are formed and become inserted into the plasma membrane. The presence of membrane IgM classifies lymphocytes as mature B cells. (See Chapter 2 for a complete discussion of B-cell development.)

## IgA

In the serum, IgA represents 10 to 15 percent of all circulating immunoglobulin, and it appears as a monomer with a molecular weight of approximately 160,000. It has a sedimentation coefficient of 7 S and migrates between the μ and β regions on electrophoresis. The H chain, called the α chain, has a molecular weight between 55,000 and 60,000 and consists of about 472 amino acids. There are two subclasses, designated IgA1 and IgA2. They differ in content by 22 amino acids, 13 of which are located in the hinge region and are deleted in IgA2.[11] The lack of this region appears to make IgA2 more resistant to some bacterial proteinases that are able to cleave IgA1.[11] Hence IgA2 is the predominant form in secretions at mucosal surfaces, while IgA1 is mainly found in serum.

IgA2, is found as a dimer along the respiratory, urogenital, and intestinal mucosa, and it also appears in milk, saliva, tears, and sweat.[11,12] Since mucosal surfaces are a major point of entry for pathogens, IgA2 serves to keep antigens from penetrating further into the body. The dimer consists of two monomers held together by a J chain that has a molecular weight of about 15,000. Secretory IgA is synthesized in plasma cells found mainly in mucosal-associated lymphoid tissue, and it is released in dimeric form. IgA is synthesized at a much greater rate than that of IgG—approximately 3 grams per day in the average adult—but because it is mainly in secretory form, the serum concentration is much lower.[11]

A **secretory component (SC),** which has a molecular weight of about 70,000, is later attached to the FC region around the hinge portion of the α chains.[3,11,13] This protein, consisting of five immunoglobulin-like domains, is derived from epithelial cells found in close proximity to the plasma cells.[3] As **Figure 4-8** indicates, SC precursor, with a molecular weight of 100,000, is actually found on the surface of epithelial cells and serves as a specific receptor for IgA. Plasma cells that secrete IgA actually home to subepithelial tissue, where IgA can bind as soon as it is released from the plasma cells.[3] This homing of activated lymphocytes depends upon a high level of certain adhesion molecules that allow binding to epithelial cells.[11] Once binding takes place, IgA and SC precursor are taken inside the cell and then released to the opposite surface by a process known as *transcytosis.* The vesicle carrying IgA and the SC receptor fuses with the membrane on the cell's opposite side, and a small fragment of SC is cleaved to liberate the IgA dimer with the remaining SC.[11] The SC may thus act to facilitate transport of IgA to mucosal surfaces.[12] It also makes the dimer more resistant to enzymatic digestion by masking sites that would be susceptible to protease cleavage.[3]

The main function of secretory IgA is to patrol mucosal surfaces and act as a first line of defense. It plays an important role in neutralizing toxins produced by microorganisms, and it helps to prevent bacterial adherence to mucosal surfaces.[13] Complexes of IgA and antigen are easily trapped in mucus and then eliminated by the ciliated epithelial cells of the respiratory or intestinal tract. This prevents pathogens from colonizing the mucosal epithelium.[12] Since IgA is found in breast milk, breastfeeding helps to maintain the health of newborns.

It appears that IgA is not capable of fixing complement by the classical pathway, although aggregation of immune complexes may trigger the alternate complement pathway.[11] (Refer to Chapter 6 for a complete discussion of the complement pathways.) Lack of complement activation may actually assist in clearing antigen without triggering an inflammatory response, thus minimizing tissue damage.[11–13]

Additionally, neutrophils, monocytes, and macrophages possess specific receptors for IgA. Binding to these sites triggers a respiratory burst and degranulation.[12] This occurs for both serum and secretory IgA, indicating that they are capable of acting as opsonins. The success of oral immunizations such as the Sabin vaccine, which induces IgA almost exclusively, demonstrates the effectiveness of IgA's protective role on mucosal surfaces.

## IgD

IgD was not discovered until 1965, when it was found in a patient with multiple myeloma. It is extremely scarce in the serum, representing less than 0.001 percent of total immunoglobulins. It is synthesized at a low level and has a half-life of only 2 to 3 days. The molecule has a molecular weight of approximately 180,000, and it migrates as a fast γ protein. The δ H chain has a molecular weight of 62,000 and appears to have an extended hinge region consisting of 58 amino acids.[10]

Most of the IgD present is found on the surface of immunocompetent but unstimulated B lymphocytes. It is the second type of immunoglobulin to appear (IgM being the first), and it may play a role in B-cell activation. The high level of surface expression and its intrinsic flexibility make it an ideal early responder to antigen.[5] Those cells bearing only IgM receptors appear incapable of an IgG

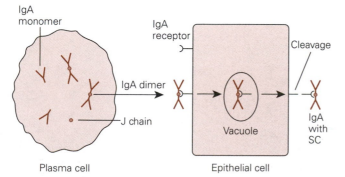

**FIGURE 4-8.** Formation of secretory IgA. IgA is secreted as a dimer from plasma cells and is captured by specific receptors on epithelial cells. The receptor is actually an SC, which binds to IgA and exits the cell along with it.

response, while those with both IgM and IgD receptors are capable of responding to T-cell help and switching to synthesis of IgG, IgA, or IgE.[5] Thus, IgD may play a role in regulating B-cell maturation and differentiation.[1,10]

Because of its unusually long hinge region, IgD is more susceptible to proteolysis than other immunoglobulins. This may be the main reason for its short half-life. In the secreted form in the serum, IgD does not appear to serve a protective function, because it does not bind complement, it does not bind to neutrophils or macrophages, and it does not cross the placenta.[1]

## IgE

IgE is the least abundant immunoglobulin in the serum, accounting for only 0.0005 percent of total serum immunoglobulins.[1] It is an 8 S molecule with a molecular weight of approximately 190,000. The $\kappa$ or H chain is composed of around 550 amino acids that are distributed over one variable and four constant domains. A single disulfide bond joins each $\kappa$ chain to an L chain, and two disulfide bonds link the H chains to one another.

IgE is the most heat-labile of all immunoglobulins; heating to 56°C for between 30 minutes and 3 hours results in conformational changes and loss of ability to bind to target cells. IgE does not participate in typical immunoglobulin reactions such as complement fixation, agglutination, or opsonization. Additionally, it is incapable of crossing the placenta. Instead, shortly after synthesis, it attaches to basophils and tissue mast cells by means of specific surface proteins, termed *high-affinity FC ε RI receptors*, which are found exclusively on these cells.[3,5] The molecule binds at the $C_H3$ domain on the FC region.[9] This leaves the antigen-binding sites free to interact with specific antigen **(Fig. 4–9)**. Plasma cells that produce IgE are located primarily in the lung and in the skin.[5]

Mast cells are also found mainly in the skin and in the lining of the respiratory and alimentary tracts. One such cell may have several hundred thousand receptors, each capable of binding an IgE molecule. When two adjacent IgE molecules on a mast cell bind specific antigen, a cascade of cellular events is initiated that results in degranulation of the mast cells with release of vasoactive amines such as histamine and heparin. Release of these mediators induces what is known as a type I immediate hypersensitivity or allergic reaction (see Chapter 13). Typical reactions include hay fever, asthma, vomiting and diarrhea, hives, and life-threatening anaphylactic shock.

While IgE appears to be a nuisance antibody, it may serve a protective role by triggering an acute inflammatory reaction that recruits neutrophils and eosinophils to the area to help destroy invading antigens that have penetrated IgA defenses.[1] Eosinophils, especially, play a major part in the destruction of large antigens such as parasitic worms that cannot be easily phagocytized (see Chapter 20 for details).

## ANTIBODY DIVERSITY

Attempts to explain the specificity of antibody for a particular antigen began long before the actual structure of immunoglobulins was discovered. The central issue was whether an antigen selected lymphocytes with the inherent capability of producing specific antibody to it or whether the presence of antigen added a new specificity to a generalized type of antibody.

### Ehrlich's Side-Chain Theory

One of the first theories to be formulated was that of Paul Ehrlich in the early 1900s, termed the *side-chain theory*. Ehrlich postulated that certain cells had specific surface receptors for antigen that were present before contact with antigen occurred. Once antigen was introduced, it would select the cell with the proper receptors, combination would take place, and then receptors would break off and enter the circulation as antibody molecules. New receptors would form in place of those broken off, and this process could be repeated. Although this represented a rather simplistic explanation for antibody synthesis, two key premises emerged: (1) the lock-and-key concept of the fit of antibody for antigen and (2) the idea that an antigen selected cells with the built-in capacity to respond to it. Although this theory did not explain the kinetics of the immune response or the idea of immunologic memory, it laid the foundation for further hypotheses.

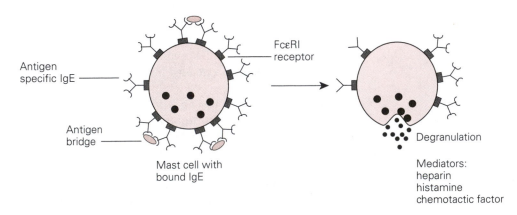

Antigen specific IgE

Antigen bridge

Mast cell with bound IgE

FcεRI receptor

Degranulation

Mediators:
heparin
histamine
chemotactic factor

FIGURE 4–9. Action of IgE on mast cells. IgE binds to specific ε receptors on mast cells. When antigen bridges two nearby IgE molecules, the membrane is disturbed and degranulation results. Chemical mediators are released.

## Clonal Selection

In the 1950s, Niels Jerne and Macfarlane Burnet independently supported the idea of a clonal selection process for antibody formation.[14–16] The key premise is that individual lymphocytes are genetically preprogrammed to produce one type of immunoglobulin and that a specific antigen finds or selects those particular cells capable of responding to it, causing them to proliferate. The receptors Ehrlich originally postulated are the surface immunoglobulins IgM and IgD, found on unstimulated B lymphocytes. Repeated contact with antigen would continually increase a specific lymphocyte pool. Such a model provides an explanation for the kinetics of the immune response.

The main drawback to the **clonal selection theory** was consideration of the genetic basis for the diversity of antibody molecules. If separate genes were present to code for antibody to every possible antigen, an overwhelming amount of DNA would be needed. In 1965, Dryer and Bennett proposed a solution to this dilemma by suggesting that the constant and variable portions of immunoglobulin chains are actually coded for by separate genes.[17] There could be a small number coding for the constant region and a larger number coding for the variable region. This would considerably simplify the task of coding for such variability. This notion implied that although all lymphocytes start out with identical genetic germ-line DNA, diversity is created by a series of recombination events that occur as the B cell matures. Scientific evidence now indicates that this is exactly what happens, as explained in the following discussion.

## GENES CODING FOR IMMUNOGLOBULINS

Tonegawa did some pioneering experiments with DNA and discovered that chromosomes contain no intact immunoglobulin genes, only building blocks from which genes can be assembled. This confirmed the hypothesis of Dryer and Bennett.[18] Tonegawa was awarded the Nobel Prize in 1987 for this monumental discovery. Human immunoglobulin genes are found in three unlinked clusters: H chain genes are located on chromosome 14, κ chain genes are on chromosome 2, and λ chain genes are on chromosome 22. Within each of these clusters, a selection process occurs. The genes cannot be transcribed and translated into functional antibody molecules until this rearrangement, assisted by special recombinase enzymes, takes place. Once this rearrangement does occur, it permanently changes the DNA of the particular lymphocyte.

## Rearrangement of Heavy Chain Genes

The selection process begins with rearrangement of the genes for the heavy chains. All H chains are derived from a single region on chromosome 14. The genes that code for the variable region are divided into three groups—$V_H$, D, and J. There are at least 39 $V_H$ (variable) genes, approximately

23 functional D (diversity) genes, and 6 J (joining) genes.[19–21] In addition, there is a set of genes (C) that codes for the constant region. This includes one gene for each H chain isotype. They are located in the following order: Cμ, Cδ, Cγ3, Cγ1, Cα1, Cγ2, Cγ4, Cε, and Cα2. Only one of these constant regions is selected at any one time. For synthesis of the entire H chain, a choice is made from each of the sections so as to include one $V_H$ gene, one D gene, one J gene, and one constant region. During the process of B-cell maturation, the pieces are spliced together to commit that B lymphocyte to making antibody of a single specificity.

Joining of these segments occurs in two steps: First, at the DNA level, one D and one J are randomly chosen and are joined with deletion of the intervening DNA **(Fig. 4–10)**. Next, a V gene is joined to the DJ complex, resulting in a rearranged V(D)J gene. The VJD combination codes for the entire variable region of the heavy chain. This rearrangement occurs early in B-cell development in pro-B cells.[21,22] (See Chapter 2 for additional details.) The recombinase enzymes RAG-1 and RAG-2, which are distinctive markers of this stage, are essential for initiating this process. The recombinase enzymes recognize specific target sequences called *recombination signal sequences* that flank all immunoglobulin gene segments.[21] However, joining of the V, J, and D segments doesn't always occur at a fixed position, so each sequence can vary by a small number of nucleotides. This contributes additional diversity.[20] If a successful rearrangement of DNA on one chromosome 14 occurs, then the genes on the second chromosome are not rearranged; this phenomenon is known as **allelic exclusion.** If the first rearrangement is nonproductive, then rearrangement of the second set of genes on the other chromosome 14 occurs.

The variable and constant regions are joined at the ribonucleic acid (RNA) level, thus conserving the DNA of the constant regions and allowing for a later phenomenon called **class switching,** whereby daughter plasma cells can produce antibody of another type. During transcription and synthesis of messenger ribonucleic acid (mRNA), a constant region is spliced to the V(D)J complex.[23] Because C μ is the region closest to the J region, μ H chains are the first to be synthesized, and these are the markers of the pre-B lymphocytes. The C δ region, which lies closest to the C μ region, is often transcribed along with C μ. The presence of DNA for both the C μ and C δ regions allows for RNA for IgD and IgM to be transcribed at the same time. Thus, a B cell could express IgD and IgM with the same variable domain on its surface at the same time. The process of switching to other immunoglobulin classes occurs later, resulting from a looping out and deletion of other constant regions. This allows the same VJD region to be coupled with a different C region to produce antibody of a different class (i.e., IgA, IgG, or IgE) but with the identical specificity for antigen. Contact with T cells and with cytokines provides the signal for switching to take place.[23]

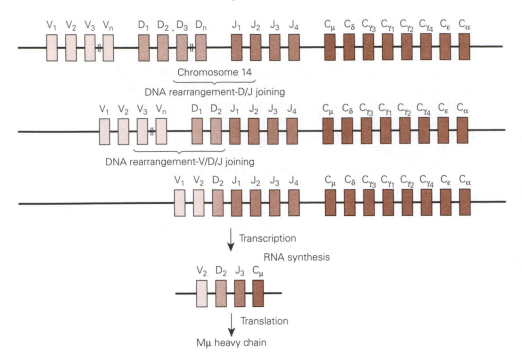

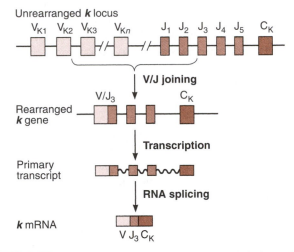

**FIGURE 4–10.** Coding for immunoglobulin H chains. Four separate regions on chromosome 14 code for H chains. DJ regions are spliced first, and then this segment is joined to a variable region. When RNA synthesis occurs, one constant region is attached to the VDJ combination. μ H chains are made first, but the cell retains its capacity to produce immunoglobulin of another class.

## Light Chain Rearrangement

Because L chain rearrangement occurs only after μ chains appear, μ-chain synthesis represents a pivotal step in the process. L chains exhibit a similar genetic rearrangement, except they lack a D region. Recombination of segments on chromosome 2, coding for κ chains, occurs prior to that on chromosome 22, which codes for λ chains. Chromosome 2 contains approximately 40 functional $V_\kappa$ regions, 5 J regions, and one $C_\kappa$ region.[21] The process of VJ joining is accomplished by an excision of intervening DNA. This results in $V_\kappa$ and $J_\kappa$ segments becoming permanently joined to one another on the rearranged chromosome. Transcription begins at one end of the $V_\kappa$ segment and proceeds through the $J_\kappa$ and $C_\kappa$ segments. Unrearranged J segments are removed during RNA splicing, which occurs in the translation **(Fig. 4–11).**

A productive rearrangement of the κ genes with subsequent protein production keeps the other chromosome 2 from rearranging, and it shuts down any recombination of the λ-chain locus on chromosome 22.[18] Only if a nonfunctioning gene product arises from κ rearrangement does λ chain synthesis occur. The lambda locus contains $30V_\lambda$, $4J_\lambda$, and four functional $C_\lambda$ segments.[20] If functional heavy and light chains are not produced by these rearrangements, then the particular B cell dies by apoptosis.

L chains are then joined with μ chains to form a complete IgM antibody, which first appears in immature B cells. Once IgM and IgD are present on the surface membrane, the B lymphocyte is fully mature and capable of responding to antigen (see Chapter 2). The large variety of V, J, D, and C combinations for each type of chain, plus the different possibilities for L and H chain combination, make for

**FIGURE 4–11.** Assembly and expression of the κ L chain locus. A DNA rearrangement fuses one V segment to one J segment. The VJ segment is then transcribed along with a unique C region to form mature κ mRNA. Unarranged J segments are removed during RNA splicing. (*From Parslow, TG, et al. Medical Immunology, ed. 10. McGraw-Hill/Appleton & Lange, 2001, with permission.*)

more than enough configurations to allow us to respond to any antigen in the environment.

## MONOCLONAL ANTIBODY

The knowledge that B cells are genetically preprogrammed to synthesize very specific antibody has been used in developing antibodies for diagnostic testing known as **monoclonal antibodies.** Normally, the response to an antigen is heterogeneous, because even a purified antigen has multiple epitopes that stimulate a variety of B-cell clones. In 1975, Georges Kohler and Cesar Milstein discovered a technique to produce antibody arising from a single B cell, which has revolutionized serological testing. For their pioneering research, they were awarded the Nobel Prize in 1984.

Kohler and Milstein's technique fuses an activated B cell with a myeloma cell that can be grown indefinitely in the laboratory. Myeloma cells are cancerous plasma cells. Normally, plasma cells produce antibody, so a particular cell line that is not capable of producing antibody is chosen. In addition, this cell line has a deficiency of the enzyme hypoxanthine guanine phosphoribosyl transferase (HGPRT) that renders it incapable of synthesizing nucleotides from hypoxanthine and thymidine, which are needed for DNA synthesis.

## Hybridoma Production

A mouse is immunized with a certain antigen, and after a time, spleen cells are harvested. Spleen cells are combined with myeloma cells in the presence of polyethylene glycol (PEG), a surfactant. The PEG brings about fusion of plasma cells with myeloma cells, producing a **hybridoma.** Only a small percentage of cells actually fuse, and some of these are like cells—that is, two myeloma cells or two spleen cells. After fusion, cells are placed in culture using a selective medium containing hypoxanthine, aminopterin, and thymidine (HAT). Culture in this medium is used to separate the hybridoma cells by allowing them to grow selectively. Myeloma cells are normally able to grow indefinitely in tissue culture, but in this case they cannot, because both pathways for the synthesis of nucleotides are blocked. One pathway, which builds DNA from degradation of old nucleic acids, is blocked, because the myeloma cell line employed is deficient in the required enzymes HGPRT and thymidine kinase.[24] The other pathway, which makes DNA from new nucleotides, is blocked by the presence of aminopterin. Consequently, the myeloma cells die out. Normal B cells cannot be maintained continuously in cell culture, so these die out as well. This leaves only the fused hybridoma cells, which have the ability (acquired from the myeloma cell) to reproduce indefinitely in culture and the ability (acquired from the normal B cell) to synthesize nucleotides by the HGPRT and thymidine kinase pathway **(Fig. 4–12).**

## Selection of Specific Antibody-Producing Clones

The remaining hybridoma cells are diluted out and placed in microtiter wells, where they are allowed to grow. Each well, containing one clone, is then screened for the presence of the desired antibody by removing the supernatant. Once identified, a hybridoma is capable of being maintained in cell culture indefinitely, and it produces a permanent and uniform supply of monoclonal antibody that reacts with a single epitope.[24]

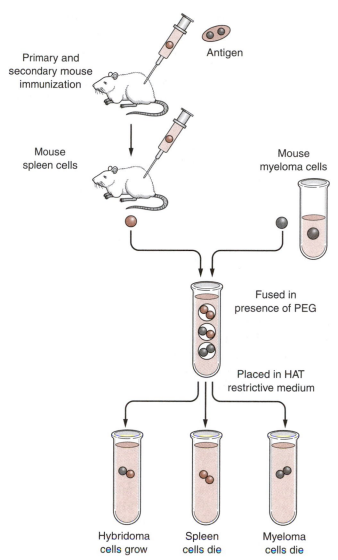

**FIGURE 4–12.** Formation of a hybridoma in monoclonal antibody production. A mouse is immunized, and spleen cells are removed. These cells are fused with nonsecreting myeloma cells and then plated in a restrictive medium. Only the hybridoma cells will grow in this medium, where they synthesize and secrete a monoclonal immunoglobulin specific for a single determinant on an antigen. *(From Barrett, JT. Textbook of Immunology, ed. 5. Mosby, St. Louis, 1988, with permission.)*

## Clinical Applications

Monoclonal antibodies were initially used for in vitro diagnostic testing. A familiar example is pregnancy testing, which uses antibody specific for the β chain of human chorionic gonadotropin, thereby eliminating many false-positive reactions. Other examples include detection of tumor antigens and measurement of hormone levels.

Recently, however, there has been an emphasis on the use of monoclonal antibodies as therapeutic agents. One of the biggest success stories is in the treatment of two autoimmune diseases: rheumatoid arthritis and Crohn's disease (a progressive inflammatory colitis). Both of these diseases have been treated with a monoclonal antibody called inflixmab that blocks the action of tumor necrosis factor-alpha.[25–29] Another tumor necrosis factor blocker, adalimumab (Humira), has also proven effective in decreasing symptoms of these two diseases.[30–32]

Monoclonal antibodies have also been used to treat various types of cancers. In the case of metastatic breast cancer, trastuzumab (Herceptin), an antibody directed against HER-2/neu protein, which is present in large numbers on tumor cells, has been helpful in slowing the disease's progress.[33,34] Another example is rituximab (Rituxan), used to treat non-Hodgkin lymphoma. Other monoclonal antibodies approved by the FDA include cetuximab (Erbitux) to treat colorectal cancer and head and neck cancers and bevacizumab (Avastin) to treat colorectal, non-small lung, and breast cancers.[33] Additionally, some monoclonal antibodies are conjugated with radioactive substances that are delivered directly to cancerous cells. Drugs in this category include ibritumomab tiuxetan (Zevalin), for cancerous B lymphocytes, and tositumomab (Bexxar) to treat some non- Hodgkin lymphomas that no longer respond to rituximab.[33] The fact that monoclonal antibodies can now be humanized by recombinant technology has cut down on reactions to the reagents themselves, which used to be of mouse origin. This area of research in pharmacology is rapidly expanding and is likely to continue to grow in the future.

## SUMMARY

The basic structural unit for all immunoglobulins is a tetrapeptide composed of two L and two H chains joined together by disulfide bonds. While $\mu$ and $\lambda$ L chains are found in all types of immunoglobulins, the H chains differ for each immunoglobulin class. The five classes are IgM, IgG, IgA, IgD, and IgE. IgG, IgD, and IgE exist as monomers, IgA has a dimeric form, and IgM is a pentamer whose subunits are held together by a J chain.

Each immunoglobulin molecule has constant and variable regions. The variable region is at the amino-terminal end, called the Fab fragment and this determines the specificity of that molecule for a particular antigen. The constant region, located at the carboxy-terminal end of the molecule and named the Fc fragment, is responsible for binding to effector cells such as neutrophils, basophils, eosinophils, and mast cells to amplify the inflammatory process and speed up antigen removal.

Structural differences determine specific functions for each of the immunoglobulin types. For instance, IgG is relatively small and easily penetrates into tissues, while IgM is much larger and excels at complement fixation. IgA has an SC that protects it from enzymatic digestion while it patrols mucosal surfaces. An extended hinge region gives IgD an advantage as a surface receptor for antigen. IgE binds to mast cells to initiate a local inflammatory reaction.

Ehrlich's side-chain theory was the first attempt to account for antibody diversity, and it is based on the antigen selecting the correctly programmed B lymphocyte. The clonal selection theory took this a step further and postulated that lymphocytes are generally pre-endowed to respond to one antigen or a group of antigens, with IgM and IgD acting as surface receptors that interact with specific antigen to trigger proliferation of a clone of identical cells.

Genetic preprogramming of lymphocytes can best be explained by the concept of gene recombination. More than one gene controls synthesis of a particular immunoglobulin, and through a random selection process, these individual segments are joined to commit that lymphocyte to making antibody of a single specificity.

A working example of the clonal selection theory is the production of monoclonal antibodies. A cancerous cell or myeloma is fused with an antibody-producing cell to form a hybridoma. Hybridomas formed by fusion of one of each cell type (e.g., myeloma and B cell) are identified by using HAT, a selective medium. Then hybridomas are diluted out and placed in microtiter wells. The clone producing the desired antibody is located by testing the supernatant in each well. Monoclonal antibodies are used both in diagnosis and treatment of disease.

# CASE STUDIES

1. A 15-year-old male exhibited symptoms of fever, fatigue, nausea, and sore throat. He went to his primary care physician, and a rapid strep test and a test for infectious mononucleosis were performed in the office. The rapid strep test result was negative, but the test result for infectious mononucleosis was faintly positive. The patient mentioned that he thought he had previously had mononucleosis, but it was never officially diagnosed. His serum was sent to a reference laboratory to test with specific Epstein-Barr viral antigens. The results indicated the presence of IgM only.

## Question

a. Is this a reactivated case of mononucleosis? Explain your answer.

2. A 10-year-old female experienced one cold after another in the springtime. She had missed several days of school, and her mother was greatly concerned. The mother took her daughter to the pediatrician, worried that she might be immunocompromised because she couldn't seem to fight off infections. A blood sample was obtained and sent to a reference laboratory for a determination of antibody levels, including an IgE level. The patient's IgM, IgG, and IgA levels were all normal for her age, but the IgE level was greatly increased.

## Question

a. What does this indicate about the patient's state of health?

# EXERCISE

## SERUM PROTEIN ELECTROPHORESIS

### Principle

Electrophoresis is the migration of charged particles in an electrical field through an electrolyte solution toward the electrode of the opposite charge. At a pH of 8.6, all serum proteins are negatively charged, and when placed in an electrical field, they migrate toward the anode at a rate that depends on the net negative charge. Five distinct bands are obtained: albumin, alpha₁, alpha₂, beta, and gamma. Immunoglobulins are located in the gamma band. The relative proportions of these fractions is useful in the diagnosis of immunodeficiency diseases and immunoproliferative disorders.

### Sample Preparation

Obtain serum from whole blood by using a sterile clot tube. Centrifuge and remove the supernatant. Discard any samples that appear to be hemolyzed. Serum is stable for up to 5 days if the specimen is refrigerated. Avoid freezing samples because this tends to denature protein. Urine and cerebrospinal fluid can also be used. They may be stored covered at 2 to 8°C for up to 72 hours.

### Reagents, Materials, and Equipment

Agarose gel electrophoresis system

Agarose film

Buffer kit

Stain

Microliter pipette

Stir-stain dishes

5 percent acetic acid

Sample cups

Other equipment, depending upon the kit used

### Procedure

Refer to the procedure for the specific gel eletrophoresis system used.

### Interpretation of Results

All serum proteins should migrate toward the anode. The rate of migration is influenced by the net charge on the molecule, the molecule's size, the buffer's pH, the buffer's ionic strength, and the gel concentration. Albumin has the greatest negative charge at pH 8.6, and hence it will travel the farthest in a given time. Because it is present in the greatest concentration, a dark compact band should be seen. Next, a more faint alpha₁ band will be seen, followed by an alpha₂ band and the beta band. Immunoglobulins will migrate within the gamma region, but as these are the least charged, they will remain in a diffuse band near the origin.

Protein bands are not visible until after staining with amido black or acid blue. Once the film is dried and then rinsed in 5 percent acetic acid, the stain will remain localized only on protein bands. If normal controls are run along with patient serum, bands can be visually compared to determine any possible abnormalities in immunoglobulin production. Infection may be indicated by an overall increase in intensity of color within the gamma region. A sharp band within the region would indicate monoclonal gammopathies with specific antibody production. Lack of immunocompetence would be demonstrated by an overall decrease in color in the gamma region.

If a densitometer is available, a more quantitative approach is possible. The following represents a normal distribution for serum proteins: albumin, 58 to 70 percent; alpha₁, 2 to 5 percent; alpha₂, 6 to 11 percent; beta, 8 to 14 percent; and gamma, 9 to 18 percent. If a total serum protein determination has been made, these percentages can then be turned into actual mg/dL amounts. To determine abnormalities of specific immunoglobulin classes, immunoelectrophoresis must be performed.

# REVIEW QUESTIONS

1. Which is characteristic of variable domains of immunoglobulins?
   a. They occur on both the H and L chains.
   b. They represent the complement binding site.
   c. They are at the carboxy-terminal ends of the molecules.
   d. All of the above

2. All of the following are true of IgM *except* that it
   a. can cross the placenta.
   b. fixes complement.
   c. has a J chain.
   d. is a primary response antibody.

3. How many antigen binding sites does a typical IgM molecule have?
   a. 2
   b. 4
   c. 6
   d. 10

4. Bence-Jones proteins are identical to which of the following?
   a. H chains
   b. L chains
   c. IgM molecules
   d. IgG molecules

5. An Fab fragment consists of
   a. two H chains.
   b. two L chains.
   c. one L chain and one-half of an H chain.
   d. one L chain and an entire H chain.

6. Which of the following pairs represents two different immunoglobulin allotypes?
   a. IgM and IgG
   b. IgM1 and IgM2
   c. Antihuman IgM and antihuman IgG
   d. IgG1m3 and IgG1m17

7. Which of the following are L chains of antibody molecules?
   a. κ
   b. γ
   c. μ
   d. α

8. If the results of serum protein electrophoresis show a significant decrease in the gamma band, which of the following is a likely possibility?
   a. Normal response to active infection
   b. Muliple myeloma
   c. Immunodeficiency disorder
   d. Monoclonal gammopathy

9. The subclasses of IgG differ mainly in
   a. the type of L chain.
   b. the arrangement of disulfide bonds.
   c. the ability to act as opsonins.
   d. molecular weight.

10. Which best describes the role of the SC of IgA?
    a. A transport mechanism across endothelial cells
    b. A means of joining two IgA monomers together
    c. An aid to trapping antigen
    d. Enhancement of complement fixation by the classical pathway

11. Which represents the main function of IgD?
    a. Protection of the mucous membranes
    b. Removal of antigens by complement fixation
    c. Enhancing proliferation of B cells
    d. Destruction of parasitic worms

12. Which antibody is best at agglutination and complement fixation?
    a. IgA
    b. IgG
    c. IgD
    d. IgM

13. Which of the following can be attributed to the clonal selection theory of antibody formation?
    a. Plasma cells make generalized antibody.
    b. B cells are preprogrammed for specific antibody synthesis.
    c. Proteins can alter their shape to conform to antigen.
    d. Cell receptors break off and become circulating antibody.

14. All of the following are true of IgE *except* that it
    a. fails to fix complement.
    b. is heat stable.
    c. attaches to tissue mast cells.
    d. is found in the serum of allergic persons.

**15.** Which best describes coding for immunoglobulin molecules?

   a. All genes are located on the same chromosome.
   b. L chain rearrangement occurs before H chain rearrangement.
   c. Four different regions are involved in coding of H chains.
   d. λ rearrangement occurs before κ rearrangement.

**16.** What is the purpose of HAT medium in the preparation of monoclonal antibody?

   a. Fusion of the two cell types
   b. Restricting the growth of unfused myeloma cells
   c. Restricting the growth of unfused spleen cells
   d. Restricting antibody production to the IgM class

## References

1. Mak, TW, and Saunders, ME. B cell receptor structure and function. In Mak, TW, and Saunders, ME: The Immune Response: Basic and Clinical Principles. Elsevier, Burlington, MA, 2006, pp. 93–120.
2. Edelman, GM. The structure and function of antibodies. Sci Am 223:34, 1970.
3. Kindt, TJ, Goldsby, RA, and Osborne, BA. Antigens and antibodies. In Kindt, TJ, Goldsby, RA, and Osborne, BA: Kuby Immunology, ed. 6. WH Freeman, New York, 2007, pp. 76–110.
4. Porter, RR. The structure of antibodies. Sci Am 217:81, 1967.
5. Frazer, JK, and Capra, JD. Immunoglobulins: Structure and function. In Paul, WE (ed): Fundamental Immunology, ed. 4. Lippincott Williams & Wilkins, Philadelphia, 1999, pp. 37–74.
6. Davies, DR, and Cohen, GH. Interactions of protein antigens with antibodies. Proc Natl Acad Sci USA 93:7–12, 1996.
7. Wedemayer, GJ, Patten, PA, and Wang, LH, et al. Structural insights into the evolution of an antibody combining site. Science 276:1665–1669, 1997.
8. Harris, LJ, Larson, SB, and McPherson, A. Comparison of intact antibody structures and the implications for effector function. Adv Immunol 72:191–208, 1999.
9. Nezlin, R, and Ghetie, V. Interactions of immunoglobulins outside the antigen-combining site. Adv Immunol 82:155–215, 2004.
10. McPherson, RA, and Massey, HD. Laboratory evaluation of immunoglobulin function and humoral immunity. In McPherson, RA, and Pincus, MR (ed): Henry's Clinical Diagnosis and Management by Laboratory Methods, ed. 21. Saunders Elsevier, Philadelphia, 2007, pp. 835–848.
11. Brandtzaeg, P, and Johansen, F. Mucosal B cells: Phenptypic characteristics, transcriptional regulation, and homing properties. Immunol Rev 206:32–63, 2005.
12. Wines, B, and Hogarth, P. IgA receptors in health and disease. Tissue Antigens 68: 103–114, 2006.
13. Woof, JM, and Mestecky, J. Mucosal immunoglobulins. Immunol Rev 206:64–82, 2005.
14. MacKay, IR. History of immunology in Australia: Events and identities. Int Med J 36:394–398, 2006.
15. Jerne, NK. The natural selection theory of antibody production. Proc Natl Acad Sci USA 41:849–857, 1955.
16. Burnet, FM. A modification of Jerne's theory of antibody production using the concept of clonal selection. Aust J Sci 20:67–69, 1957.
17. Dreyer, WJ, and Bennett, JC. The molecular basis of antibody formation: A paradox. Proc Natl Acad Sci USA 54:864, 1965.
18. Mak, TW, and Saunders, ME. The immunoglobulin genes. In Mak, TW, and Saunders, ME. The Immune Response: Basic and Clinical Principles. Elsevier, Burlington, MA, 2006, pp. 179–208.
19. Delves, PJ, and Roitt, IM. The immune system. First of two parts. N Engl J Med 343:37–49, 2000.
20. Kindt, TJ, Goldsby, RA, and Osborne, BA. Organization and expression of immunoglobulin genes. In Kindt, TJ, Goldsby, RA, and Osborne, BA: Kuby Immunology, ed. 6. WH Freeman, New York, 2007, pp. 111–144.
21. Dudley, DD, Chaudhuri, J, Bassing, CH, and Alt, FW. Mechanism and control of V(d)J recombination versus classswitch recombination: Similarities and differences. Adv Immunol 86:43–112, 2005.
22. Cobb, RM, Oestreich, KJ, Osipovich, OA, Oltz, EM. Accessibility control of V(D)J recombination. Adv Immunol 91:45–110, 2006.
23. Chaudhuri, J, Basu, U, Zarrin, A, Yan, C, et al. Evolution of the immunoglobulin heavy chain class switch recombination mechanism. Adv Immunol 94:157–214, 2007.
24. Mak, TW, and Saunders, ME. Exploring antigen-antibody interaction. In Mak, TW, and Saunders, ME. The Immune Response: Basic and Clinical Principles. Elsevier, Burlington, MA, 2006, pp. 147–176.
25. Maini, R, St. Clair, EW, and Breedveld, F, et al. Infliximab (chimeric anti-tumour necrosis factor-alpha monoclonal antibody) versus placebo in rheumatoid arthritis patients receiving concomitant methotrexate: A randomised phase III trial. ATTRACT Study Group. Lancet 354:1932–1939, 1999.
26. Nikas, S, Temekonidis, T, Zikou, A, Argyropoulou, M, et al. Treatment of resistant rheumatoid arthritis by intra-articular infliximab injections: A pilot study. Ann Rheum Dis 63(1):102–103, 2004.
27. Kristensen, LE, Saxne, T, Nilsson, J, and Geborek, P. Impact of concomitant DMARD therapy on adherence to treatment with etanercept and infliximab in rheumatoid arthritis. Results from a six-year observational study in southern Sweden. Arthritis Res Ther 8(6):R174, 2006.
28. Abe T, Takeuchi T, Miyasaka N, Hashimoto H, Kondo H, et al. A multicenter, double-blind, randomized, placebo controlled trial of infliximab combined with low dose methotrexate in Japanese patients with rheumatoid arthritis. J Rheumatol 33(1):37–44, 2006.
29. Present, DH, Rutgeerts, P, and Targan, S, et al. Infliximab for the treatment of fistulas in patients with Crohn's disease. N Engl J Med 340:1398–1405, 1999.
30. Hochberg, M, Tracy, J, Hawkins-Holt, M, and Flores, R. Comparison of the efficacy of the tumour necrosis factor α blocking agents adalimumab, etanercept, and infliximab when

added to methotrexate in patients with active rheumatoid arthritis. Ann Rheum Dis 62(Suppl 2): ii13–ii16. 2003.

31. FDA approves new therapy for rheumatoid arthritis. www.fda.gov/bbs/topics/ANSWERS/2002/ANS01186.html. Accessed September 14, 2007.

32. FDA approves new treatment for Crohn's disease. www.fda.gov/ bbs/topics/NEWS/2007/NEW01572.html. Accessed September 14, 2007.

33. Monoclonal antibodies. http://www.cancer.org/docroot/ETO/ content/ETO_1_4X_Monoclonal_Antibody_Therapy. Accessed September 10, 2007.

34. Biological therapies for cancer: Q and A. http:// cancernet.nci.nih.gov/cancertopics/factsheet/Therapy/ biological. Accessed September 1, 2007.

# 5

# Cytokines

*Timothy Stegall, PhD.*

## LEARNING OBJECTIVES

*After finishing this chapter, the reader will be able to:*

1. Define cytokine.
2. Define pleiotropy as it relates to cytokine activities.
3. Distinguish between autocrine, paracrine, and endocrine effects of cytokines.
4. Explain the functions of interleukin-1 (IL-1) in mediating the immune response.
5. Explain the effects of tumor necrosis factor (TNF).
6. Compare the functions of type 1 and type 2 interferons (IFN).
7. Describe the actions of interleukin-2 (IL-2) on target cells.
8. Discuss the biological roles of the hematopoietic growth factors.
9. Describe the biological role of colony stimulating factors.
10. Describe the current types of anticytokine therapies.
11. Describe clinical assays for cytokines.

## KEY TERMS

____ Acute phase response
____ Adaptive immune response
____ Adaptive T regulatory 1 cells (TR1)
____ Antagonist
____ Autocrine
____ Chemokine
____ Colony stimulating factor (CSF)
____ Cytokines
____ Endocrine
____ Endogenous pyrogen
____ Erythropoietin (EPO)
____ Granulocyte-CSF (G-CSF)
____ Granulocyte-macrophage-CSF (GM-CSF)
____ Innate immune response
____ Integrins
____ Interferons (IFN)
____ Interleukins (IL)
____ Macrophage-CSF (M-CSF)
____ Paracrine
____ Pleiotropic
____ Redundancy
____ Transforming growth factor beta (TGF-β)
____ T regulatory (Treg) cells
____ Tumor necrosis factor (TNF)

# CHAPTER OUTLINE

## INTRODUCTION TO CYTOKINES

**Cytokines** are small soluble proteins that regulate the immune system, orchestrating both innate immunity and the adaptive response to infection. These chemical messengers, produced by several different types of cells, have activity-modulating effects on the hematopoietic and immune systems through activation of cell-bound receptor proteins.[1] Cytokines are induced in response to specific stimuli—such as bacterial lipopolysaccharides, flagellin, or other bacterial products—through the ligation of cell-adhesion molecules or through the recognition of foreign antigens by host lymphocytes. The effects of cytokines in vivo include regulation of growth, differentiation, and gene expression by many different cell types, including leukocytes. These effects are achieved through both **autocrine stimulation** (i.e., affecting the same cell that secreted it) and **paracrine** (i.e., affecting a target cell in close proximity) activities. Occasionally, cytokines will also exert systemic or **endocrine** activities. Individual cytokines do not act alone but in conjunction with many other cytokines that are induced during the process of immune activation. The resulting network of cytokine expression regulates leukocyte activity and leads to the elimination of the infection.

The cytokine cascade produces a spectrum of activities that lead to the rapid generation of innate and adaptive immune responses. In fact, the ability or inability to generate certain cytokine patterns often determines the outcome and the clinical course of infection. In extreme circumstances, massive overproduction and dysregulation produces a "cytokine storm" that leads to shock, multiorgan failure, or even death, thus contributing to pathogenesis.[2,3]

Initially, cytokines were named based on their activities and the types of cells from which they were first isolated. The major cytokine families include tumor necrosis factors (TNF), interferons (IFN), chemokines, transforming growth factors (TGF), and colony stimulating factors (CSF). There are also the interleukins (IL), which currently number from IL-1 to IL-32.[4] The **interleukins** are unrelated cytokines that must satisfy three criteria in order to be classified as interleukins: they must have had their genes cloned, they must be inducible in leukocytes, and their biological activities in inflammatory processes must be catalogued.

Cytokines were originally thought to act solely on cells of the immune system, but it soon became apparent that many also act on cells outside the immune system. The **pleiotropic** (i.e., having many different effects) nature of cytokine activity relates to the widespread distribution of cytokine receptors on many cell types and the ability of cytokines to alter expression of numerous genes. Many different cytokines may share properties—that is, they activate some of the same pathways and genes. This **redundancy** may be explained by the fact that many cytokines share receptor subunits. For instance, IL-6, IL-11, leukemia inhibitory factor, oncostatin M, ciliary neurotrophic factor, and cardiotrophin all utilize the gp130 subunit as part of their receptors.[5] The specificity for each cytokine is contained in the other subunits in the respective receptors, but much of the signal transmitted through the receptors is generated by the gp130 subunit. Thus, some cytokines may have overlapping effects and may alter the activity of many of the same genes. However, redundancy of cytokine activities cannot be explained entirely by shared receptor subunits. TNF-α, IL-1, and IL-6 exert many of the same biological activities, but each utilizes a distinct receptor. Here, the cytokines are activating similar immune response pathways through different signaling pathways. **Figure 5–1** illustrates some of the different actions of cytokines.

The increasing clinical usage of cytokines, cytokine antagonists, and cytokine receptor antagonists in conditions such as rheumatoid arthritis, psoriasis, asthma, Crohn's disease, transplantation, and cancer treatments will drive demand for cytokine assays in the clinical laboratory. The pattern of cytokine expression can also determine whether the host will be able to mount an effective defense against and survive certain infections. In addition, numerous

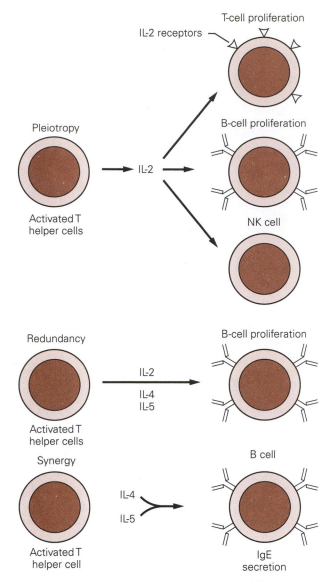

**FIGURE 5–1.** Cytokine characteristics of pleiotropy, redundancy, and antagonism. *(Adapted from Kindt, TJ, Goldsby, RA, and Osborne, BA. Kuby Immunology, ed. 6. WH Freeman, New York, 2007, with permission.)*

immunodeficiency syndromes and leukemias are caused by defects in cytokines or their receptors/signal transduction circuits.[6] Genetic and proteomic analyses of these defects will occur within the clinical laboratory in order to assess treatment modalities, effectiveness, and potential gene-replacement therapies.

## CYTOKINES IN THE INNATE IMMUNE RESPONSE

Cytokines involved in the innate immune response are responsible for many of the physical symptoms attributed to inflammation, such as fever, swelling, pain, and cellular infiltrates into damaged tissues. The **innate immune response** is nonspecific but occurs within hours of first contact with microorganisms (see Chapter 1). It may play a

crucial part in recovery from infection. The main function of the innate immune response is to recruit effector cells to the area. Cytokines involved in triggering this response are interleukin-1, tumor necrosis factor-alpha, interleukin-6, chemokines, transforming growth factor-beta, and interferons-alpha and beta. The function of each is discussed here.

## Interleukin-1 (IL-1)

The IL-1 family consists of IL-1α, IL-1β, and IL-1RA (IL-1 receptor antagonist).[7] IL-1α and IL-1β are proinflammatory cytokines produced by monocytes and macrophages. IL-1 production may be induced by the presence of microbial pathogens, bacterial lipopolysaccharides, or other cytokines. IL-1α and IL-1β exhibit the same activities in many test systems and share about 25 percent sequence homology.[7] However, IL-1α remains intracellular within monocytes and macrophages and is rarely found outside these cells. IL-1α can be released after cell death and can help attract inflammatory cells to areas where cells and tissues are being killed or damaged.

IL-1β is responsible for most of the systemic activity attributed to IL-1, including fever, activation of phagocytes, and production of acute phase proteins. It is cleaved intracellularly to an active form that is then secreted by monocytes.

IL-1 acts as an **endogenous pyrogen** and induces fever in the **acute phase response** through its actions on the hypothalamus.[8] The hypothalamus acts as the thermostat for the human body, and IL-1 sets the thermostat at a higher level. Elevated body temperatures may serve to inhibit the growth of pathogenic bacteria and viruses and also increases lymphocyte activity. Additionally, IL-1 induces the production of vascular cell-adhesion molecules as well as chemokines and IL-6. These chemokines and cell-adhesion molecules attract and assist leukocytes to enter the inflamed area by a process known as *diapedesis* (see Chapter 1). IL-1 also induces the production of colony stimulating factors in the bone marrow, thereby increasing the available number of phagocytic cells that can respond to the damaged tissues.[9]

IL-1RA is also produced by monocytes and macrophages. It acts as an antagonist to IL-1 by blocking the IL-1 receptor and limiting the availability of the receptor for IL-1. This helps to regulate the physiological response to IL-1 and turn off the response when no longer needed.

## Tumor Necrosis Factor-α (TNF-α)

**Tumor necrosis factors (TNF)** were first isolated from tumor cells and were so named because they induced lysis in these cells. TNF-α is the most prominent member of the TNF superfamily, which consists of at least 19 different peptides that have diverse biological functions.[10] TNF-α exists in both membrane-bound and soluble forms and causes vasodilation and increased vasopermeability. The soluble form is derived from the membrane-bound form by proteolytic cleavage with TNF-α-converting enzyme. However, the soluble form is unstable and has a short half-life. Membrane-bound TNF-α can mediate all the cytotoxic and inflammatory effects of TNF through cell-to-cell contact. The main trigger for TNF-α production is the presence of lipopolysaccharide, found in gram-negative bacteria.

TNF-α secreted by activated monocytes and macrophages can activate T cells through its ability to induce expression of MHC class II molecules, vascular adhesion molecules, and chemokines, in a similar manner to IL-1. These actions enhance antigen presentation and activate T cells to respond to the pathogen that triggered the initial inflammatory response. However, when secreted at higher levels, TNF can have deleterious systemic effects, leading to septic shock. This condition results from large amounts of TNF secreted in response to gram-negative bacterial infections, causing a decrease in blood pressure, reduced tissue perfusion, and disseminated intravascular coagulation. The latter may lead to uncontrolled bleeding.

TNF-α and IL-1 are both present in rheumatoid synovial fluids and synovial membranes of patients with rheumatoid arthritis (RA). Studies with anti-TNF-α and anti-IL-1 demonstrate that TNF-α is the central mediator of pathological processes in RA and other inflammatory illnesses such as Crohn's disease.[11]

TNFR1 (TNF receptor 1) is constitutively expressed on most tissues, binds soluble TNF-α, and is the primary mediator of TNF-α signal transduction in most cell types. TNFR2 is usually expressed in epithelial cells and cells of the immune system and is activated by the membrane-bound form of TNF-α. Overall, TNF-α activity is at least partially regulated by soluble forms of both TNF receptors. These act to bind excess TNF-α and, combined with the short half-life of the soluble form, serve to limit the cytokine's signaling activity.

## IL-6

IL-6 is a single protein produced by both lymphoid and nonlymphoid cell types. It is part of the cytokine cascade released in response to lipopolysaccharide and plays an important role in acute phase reactions and the adaptive immune response. IL-6 is expressed by a variety of normal and transformed cells, including T cells, B cells, monocytes and macrophages, fibroblasts, hepatocytes, keratinocytes,

astrocytes, vascular endothelial cells, and various tumor cells. IL-1 primarily triggers its secretion.

This pleiotropic cytokine affects inflammation, acute phase reactions, immunoglobulin synthesis, and the activation states of B cells and T cells. IL-6 stimulates B cells to proliferate and differentiate into plasma cells and induces CD4+ T cells to produce greater quantities of both pro- and anti-inflammatory cytokines.[5]

Only one IL-6 receptor has been identified, and it consists of IL-6Rα (the IL-6-specific receptor) and gp130 (the common signal-transducing receptor subunit utilized by several cytokines). Binding of IL-6 to the IL-6Rα induces dimerization of gp130 with the α-subunit **(Fig. 5–2)**. Homodimerization following IL-6 binding causes conformational changes in gp130 that expose tyrosine residues in the intracellular portion of the molecule. Through a series of phosphorylation reactions, genes for acute phase proteins such as CRP, C3, and fibrinogen are activated, as is interferon regulatory factor-1 (IRF-1). B- and T-cell genes are turned on in the same manner.

## Chemokines

**Chemokines** are a family of cytokines that enhance motility and promote migration of many types of white blood cells toward the source of the chemokine (chemotaxis).[12] Most of the chemotactic activity of leukocytes is regulated by the activities of chemokines, including the response to infectious diseases, autoimmune inflammation, cancer, and the homing of lymphocytes to all the lymphoid tissues. The chemokines are classified into four families based on the position of N-terminal cysteine residues. The first group—the alpha, or CXC, chemokines—contains a single amino acid between the first and second cysteines. The second group—the beta, or CC, chemokines—has adjacent cysteine residues. The third group—the C chemokines—lacks one of the cysteines. CX3C, the last major group, has three amino acids between the cysteines. Chemokines play key roles in the initiation and development of inflammatory responses in numerous disease processes. Currently, over 40 chemokines and 20 chemokine receptors have been identified **(Table 5–1).**

Both TNF-α and IL-6 are among the many cytokines that induce chemokine production in the inflammatory response. Combined with cell adhesion molecules, the

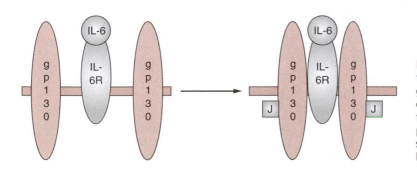

FIGURE 5–2. IL-6 binding to the IL-6R subunit recruits two gp130 subunits to the receptor complex. Signal transduction takes place through tyrosine phosphorylation of the gp130 subunits by one of the Janus kinases (J).

| Table 5–1. | Select Chemokines and Their Receptors | |
|---|---|---|
| CHEMOKINE GROUP | CHEMOKINE NAMES | CHEMOKINE RECEPTORS |
| CC Chemokines | MCP-1, MCAF, JE | CCR2 |
| | MIP-1α | CCR1, CCR5 |
| | MIP-1β | CCR5 |
| | RANTES | CCR1, CCR3, CCR5 |
| | Eotaxin | CCR3 |
| CXC Chemokines | GROα, MGSA, MIP-2, KC | CXCR2 |
| | IL-8 | CXCR1, CXCR2 |
| | IP-10, CRG-2 | CXCR3 |
| | SDF-1 | CXCR4 |

chemokines facilitate the extravasation of leukocytes into the tissues. Leukocytes rolling on capillary endothelial cells activate their chemokine receptors in the presence of chemokines. This, in turn, activates **integrins,** or cell adhesion molecules, on leukocytes and leads to firm adhesion to the endothelial cells. Shared expression of chemokine receptors among different types of leukocytes allows for the co-localization of multiple cell types to the damaged tissue and helps to broaden the response to tissue damage. The gradient of chemokine concentration enables the leukocytes to migrate between the endothelial cells into the tissue in the direction of increasing chemokine concentration.

The spectrum of chemokines and cytokines expressed in the inflammatory response determines the types of cells that respond and the genes that are turned on in response to the stimuli. The types of cell surface receptors expressed by leukocytes are often developmentally regulated—for example, immature T cells possess only the chemokine receptors related to lymphoid tissue homing. Only mature T cells express the receptors that allow them to participate in an ongoing immune reaction.

The chemokine receptors CXCR4 and CCR5 are utilized by HIV as co-receptors for infection of CD4$^+$ T lymphocytes and macrophages.[13] Individuals with certain polymorphisms in these chemokine receptors are long-term nonprogressors. They remain asymptomatic, have normal CD4$^+$ T-cell counts and normal immune function, and have low or undetectable viral loads. The altered protein sequences of the receptors block or diminish the virus's ability to enter the cells and thereby increase the infected individual's chances of survival. The CCR5-Δ32 polymorphism is a 32 bp deletion in the CCR5 gene and is the most important of the host resistance factors. Homozygous individuals are protected from HIV infection while heterozygous persons exhibit longer periods from infection to AIDS development. In addition, certain polymorphisms in SDF1 (the ligand for CXCR4) and RANTES (the ligand for CCR5) can block the virus's ability to bind to and enter T cells and can delay the progression to full-blown AIDS.

## TGF-β

The **transforming growth factor beta (TGF-β)** superfamily is composed of three isoforms: TGF-β1, β2, and β3. TGF-β was originally characterized as a factor that induced growth arrest in tumor cells. Later, it was identified as a factor that induces antiproliferative activity in a wide variety of cell types. Active TGF-β is primarily a regulator of cell growth, differentiation, apoptosis, migration, and the inflammatory response. Thus, it acts as a control to help down-regulate the inflammatory response when no longer needed.

In the immune response, TGF-β functions as both an activator and an inhibitor of proliferation, depending on the developmental stage of the affected cells.[14] TGF-β regulates the expression of CD8 in CD4$^-$CD8$^-$ thymocytes and acts as an autocrine inhibitory factor for immature thymocytes. It inhibits the activation of macrophages and the growth of many different somatic cell types and functions as an anti-inflammatory factor for mature T cells. TGF-β blocks the production of IL-12 and strongly inhibits the induction of IFN-γ. In addition, the production of TGF-β by T helper 2 cells is now recognized as an important factor in the establishment of oral tolerance to bacteria normally found in the mouth. In activated B cells, TGF-β typically inhibits proliferation and may function as an autocrine regulator to limit the expansion of activated cells.

## IFN-α and IFN-β

**Interferons** were originally so named because they interfere with viral replication. However, it is the type I interferons consisting of IFN-α and IFN-β that function primarily in this manner. These interferons are produced by dendritic cells and induce production of proteins and pathways that directly interfere with viral replication and cell division.[15] In most cases, this helps limit the infection to one relatively small area of the body. Type I IFN activates natural killer cells and enhances the expression of MHC class I proteins, thus increasing the recognition and killing of virus-infected cells.

The type I interferons are also active against certain malignancies and other inflammatory processes. For instance, IFN-β is efficacious in treating multiple sclerosis, although the exact mechanism of action remains unclear.[16] IFN-α has been used to treat hepatitis C and Kaposi's sarcoma, as well as certain leukemias and lymphomas.[17]

## CYTOKINES IN THE ADAPTIVE IMMUNE RESPONSE

Cytokines involved in the innate immune response are produced by many different cell types and function mainly to increase acute phase reactants and to recruit white cells to the area of infection. In contrast, cytokines involved in the

**adaptive immune response** are mainly secreted by T cells, especially T helper (Th) cells, and affect T- and B-cell function more directly. There are three main subclasses of Th cells, Th1, Th2, and Treg (T regulatory cells). Each has a specific function and produces a different set of cytokines. Once the T-cell receptor (TCR) captures antigen, clonal expansion of those particular CD4$^+$ T helper cells occurs.[18] Differentiation into Th1, Th2, or Treg cell lineages is influenced by the spectrum of cytokines expressed in the initial response.[19] The Th1 lineage is driven by the expression of IL-12 by dendritic cells and is primarily responsible for cell-mediated immunity, while Th2 cells drive antibody-mediated immunity and are developmentally regulated by IL-4. Treg cells are derived from IL-10-responsive naïve T cells and help to regulate the activities of Th1 and Th2 cells **(Figs. 5–3 and 5–4).**

## Th1 Cytokines

Dendritic cells in damaged tissues produce IL-12 in response to certain stimuli such as mycobacteria, intracellular bacteria, and viruses. It is also produced by macrophages and B cells and has multiple effects on both T cells and natural killer (NK) cells. IL-12 binds to its receptor on naïve T cells and causes the expression of a new set of genes, including those that determine maturation into the Th1 lineage. Activation of Th1 cells induces high-level expression of IFN-γ.[20] IL-12 also increases the cytolytic ability of natural killer (NK) cells; therefore, it serves as an important link between the innate and adaptive immune responses by enhancing defenses against intracellular pathogens.

### IFN-γ

IFN-γ is the principal molecule produced by Th1 cells, and it affects the RNA expression levels of more than 200 genes.[21,22] Genes involved in regulation and activation of CD4$^+$ Th1 cells, CD8$^+$ cytotoxic lymphocytes, NK cells, bactericidal activities, IL-12R and IL-18R are all regulated

by IFN-γ. In addition, IFN-γ stimulates antigen presentation by MHC I and MHC II molecules. The increased expression of MHC class I and II molecules on antigen-presenting cells increases the likelihood of antigen capture and the involvement of additional lymphocytes.

In addition to the above listed actions, IFN-γ is a strong stimulator of macrophages and boosts their tumoricidal activity. Thus, IFN-γ enhances the immune response in a number of key ways.

IFN-γ production can be stimulated in mature Th1 cells by two means: (1) ligation of the T-cell receptor (TCR) by MHC-peptide antigen presentation or (2) cytokine stimulation by IL-12 and IL-18. IL-12 and IL-18 act synergistically to stimulate IFN-γ production, even in the absence of TCR ligation. In addition, IL-12 and IL-18 can activate IFN-γ secretion by CD8$^+$ lymphocytes.

### IL-2

Th1 cells also secrete IL-2 in addition to IFN-γ. IL-2 is also known as the *T-cell growth factor.* It drives the growth and differentiation of both T and B cells and induces lytic activity in NK cells. IL-2 and IFN-γ induce the development of Th1 cells, which, in turn, induces macrophage activation and delayed type hypersensitivity. Th1 cells stimulate the production of IgG1 and IgG3 opsonizing and complement fixing antibodies by antigen-activated B cells. These isotypes assist in the kinds of cell-mediated immune responses that are driven by Th1 cells.

IL-2 alone can activate proliferation of Th2 cells and helps to generate IgG1 and IgE producing cells. The clonal expansion of activated T helper cells is a necessary part of mounting an adequate immune response to any immunologic challenge. The cytokine network that develops will continue to regulate T-cell growth and differentiation until the challenge is gone and the response must subside.

Transcription of the gene for IL-2 and IL-2R begins within 1 hour of TCR ligation. The functional IL-2R consists of α, β, and γ or β and γ subunits. The β and γ subunits increase the affinity of the receptor for IL-2 and are responsible for most of the signal transduction through the receptor. The γ chain is also shared by the receptors for IL-4, IL-7, IL-9, IL-15, and IL-21.[23] The importance of the γ chain is demonstrated in individuals who have mutations in this chain. These persons have X-linked severe combined immunodeficiency syndrome and lack functional T and B cells.[24]

## Th2 Cytokines

### IL-4

As mentioned previously, Th2 cells are primarily responsible for antibody-mediated immunity. IL-4 is one of the key cytokines regulating Th2 immune activities and helps drive antibody responses in a variety of diseases.[24] The IL-4 receptor is expressed on lymphocytes and on numerous

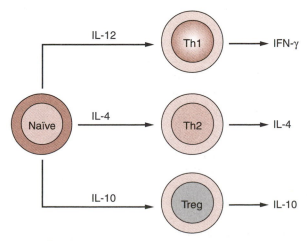

**FIGURE 5–3.** Development of T helper and T regulatory cells.

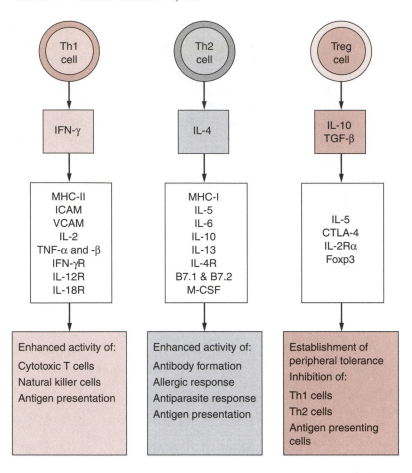

FIGURE 5-4. Individual T cell classes produce different products that determine the range of activities for the class.

nonhematopoietic cell types. IL-4 activity on naïve T cells turns on the genes that generate Th2 cells and turns off the genes that promote Th1 cells, such as IFN-γ and IFN-γ R subunits. The chemokine MCP-1 enhances IL-4 production by naïve T cells and could play a role in moving naïve T cells toward the Th2 pathway.

Th2 cells are responsible for regulating many aspects of the immune response, including those related to allergies, autoimmune diseases, and fighting off parasites. Among the many genes induced by IL-4 are MHC-I, IL-5, IL-13, and the co-stimulatory molecules B7.1 and B7.2. IL-4 promotes the production of IgG2a and IgE and, along with IL-5, drives the differentiation and activation of eosinophils in both allergic immune responses and the response to parasitic infections.[24] IL-13 is a cytokine with many of the same properties as IL-4, and both cytokines induce worm expulsion and favor IgE-class switching.

## IL-10

IL-10 has anti-inflammatory and suppressive effects on Th1 cells. It is produced by monocytes, macrophages, CD8+ T cells, and Th2 CD4+ T cells. It inhibits antigen presentation by macrophages and dendritic cells and stimulates CD8+ T cells. It also induces the production of MHC-II on B cells. However, one of the major effects of IL-10 is the inhibition of IFN-γ production via the suppression of IL-12 synthesis by accessory cells and the promotion of a Th2 cytokine

pattern.[25] Thus, in contrast to most other cytokines, IL-10 serves as an **antagonist** to IFN-γ—it is a down-regulator of the immune response.

## Cytokines Associated with T Regulatory Cells

The third major subclass of CD4+ T cells are the **T regulatory (Treg) cells.** Tregs are CD4+ CD25+ T cells that are selected in the thymus.[26] They play a key role in establishing peripheral tolerance to a wide variety of self-antigens, allergens, tumor antigens, transplant antigens, and infectious agents. CD4+ CD25+ Tregs affect T cell activity primarily through the actions of TGF-β. TGF-β induces expression of Foxp3, a transcription factor that causes Treg cells to suppress the activity of other T cells.[27] Tregs may be found in transplanted tissue and help to establish tolerance to the graft by the host immune system through the alteration of antigen presentation.

Tregs are also responsible for inducing IL-10 and TGF-β expression in **adaptive T regulatory 1 (Tr1) cells** in the peripheral circulation. Tr1 cells are CD4+ T cells that are induced from antigen-activated naïve T cells in the presence of IL-10. They exert their suppressive activities on both Th1 and Th2 cells by producing more IL-10, TGF-β, or IL-5. T-cell suppression occurs through IL-10 inhibition of proinflammatory cytokines and inhibition of costimulatory molecule expression on antigen presenting cells (APCs), while TGF-β down-regulates the function of APCs and blocks proliferation and cytokine production by CD4+ T cells. All of these activities lead to down-regulation of the immune response and the prevention of chronic inflammation.

These two types of regulatory T cells operate through a network of cytokines to establish peripheral tolerance to certain antigens; therefore, they play a key role in limiting autoimmunity. The relative importance of each phenotype depends largely on the antigen involved, the context of antigen presentation, and the biology of the tissue.

## ERYTHROPOIETIN AND COLONY STIMULATING FACTORS

The **colony stimulating factors (CSFs)** include IL-3, **erythropoietin (EPO)** and **granulocyte, macrophage,** and **granulocyte-macrophage colony stimulating factors (G-CSF, M-CSF,** and **GM-CSF,** respectively).[18,28-30] In response to inflammatory cytokines such as IL-1, the different colony stimulating factors act on bone marrow cells at different developmental stages and promote specific colony formation for the various cell lineages. IL-3 is a multilineage colony stimulating factor that induces CD34+ bone marrow stem cells to form T and B cells. In conjunction with IL-3, the CSFs direct immature bone marrow stem cells to develop into red blood cells (RBCs), platelets, and the various types of white blood cells **(Fig. 5–5).** IL-3 acts

on bone marrow stem cells to begin the differentiation cycle, and the activity of IL-3 alone drives the stem cells into the lymphocyte differentiation pathway.

GM-CSF acts to drive differentiation toward other white cell types. If M-CSF is activated, the cells become macrophages. M-CSF also increases phagocytosis, chemotaxis, and additional cytokine production in monocytes and macrophages. If G-CSF is activated, the cells become neutrophils. G-CSF enhances the function of mature neutrophils and affects the survival, proliferation, and differentiation of all cell types in the neutrophil lineage. It decreases IFN-γ production and increases IL-4 production in T cells, and it mobilizes multipotential stem cells from the bone marrow. These stem cells are utilized to repair damaged tissues and create new vasculature in these areas. These activities are necessary to reconstruct tissues following an infection. However, IL-3 in conjunction with GM-CSF drives the development of basophils and mast cells, while the addition of IL-5 to IL-3 and GM-CSF drives the cells to develop into eosinophils. The net effect is an increase in white blood cells to respond to the ongoing inflammatory processes.

EPO regulates RBC production in the bone marrow but is primarily produced in the kidneys. The protein in its physiological form is a 34 kD monomer with a high carbohydrate content. Glycosylation of the protein is required for activity and accounts for the structural differences between recombinant EPO-α and EPO-β. Both proteins have the same amino acid sequence and similar activities as endogenous EPO, but EPO-α is the form licensed for clinical use by the FDA. EPO-α is often prescribed to improve the red cells counts for individuals with anemia and for those with cancer who have undergone radiation and chemotherapy.

RBC proliferation induced by EPO improves oxygenation of the tissues and eventually switches off EPO production. The normal serum EPO values range from 5 to 28 U/L but must be interpreted in relation to the hematocrit, as levels can increase by up to a thousandfold during anemia.

## CYTOKINES AND ANTICYTOKINE THERAPIES

Cytokine-inhibiting biologics disrupt the interaction between cytokines and their cognate receptors.[31] Initial studies used murine monoclonal antibodies that were able to function only for short periods of time before the host mounted an immune response against them. Recombinant DNA techniques have allowed for the production of humanized monoclonal antibodies that are much less immunogenic and that function as cytokine antagonists. An example is infliximab (Remicade), a chimeric antibody containing human constant regions and murine antigen-specific arms that bind human TNF-α. Remicade blocks the activity of TNF-α in rheumatoid arthritis (RA) and Crohn's disease. A single dose alleviates symptoms and reduces swollen joints

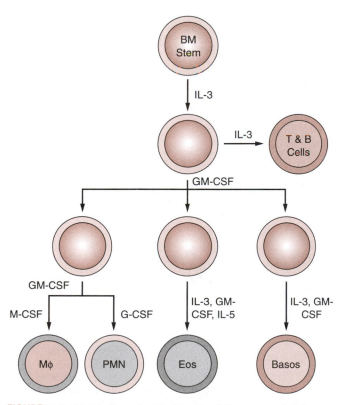

**FIGURE 5–5.** Maturation of white blood cell lineages under the influence of colony stimulating factors.

in RA patients for up to 4 weeks. Multiple infusions achieve 60 to 70 percent improvement in symptoms in these individuals.

Monoclonal antibodies can be further humanized so that the complementarity-determining regions are the only murine components remaining (e.g., Zenapax, which is directed at human IL-2Rα). These antibodies generally have lower affinity and extended half-life, but reduced immunogenicity. As an alternative, transgenic mice that have human immunoglobulin genes are able to produce fully human monoclonal antibodies from mouse hybridoma cells following immunization. These antibodies have high affinities and long half-lives and are not immunogenic.

Another approach to anti-cytokine therapy is the development of hybrid proteins containing cytokine receptor binding sites attached to immunoglobulin constant regions. The only member of this class that has been approved for human use is etanercept (Enbrel). Enbrel consists of the extracellular domains of the type 2 TNF receptor fused to the heavy chain constant region of IgG1. This fusion protein can bind TNF-α, block its activity, and has a 4.8-day half-life in serum. However, about 16 percent of treated individuals develop antibodies to the TNFR2 moiety. Some of these antibodies may be able to bind to native receptors and activate signaling pathways, thus mimicking TNF-α activity and negating the protein's therapeutic effects.[32]

## CLINICAL ASSAYS FOR CYTOKINES

Activation of the immune system is a significant component of autoimmune diseases such as rheumatoid arthritis,[11] psoriasis,[33] and inflammatory bowel disease.[34,35] In addition, the role of cytokines in developing an effective immune response to certain infectious diseases has been well studied.[2] For example, tuberculosis is controlled by cell-mediated immunity, not humoral immunity, and immunity is therefore driven by Th1 cytokines. Clinical evaluation of the cytokine profile in the patient could be of prognostic and diagnostic value to the physician.[36,37]

Although there are several cytokine assay formats available in Europe, none have been approved for clinical use by the FDA at this time. The most basic test is the ELISpot assay, which employs the enzyme-linked immunosorbent assay (ELISA; see **Fig. 5–6**) technique on in vitro activated peripheral white blood cells. In this process, either a monoclonal or polyclonal antibody specific for the chosen cytokine is precoated onto a microplate. Antigen-stimulated, mitogen-stimulated (positive control), or saline-stimulated (negative control) white blood cells are pipetted into the wells, and the microplate is placed into a humidified $CO_2$ incubator at 37°C for a specified period of time. During the incubation period, the immobilized antibody, in the immediate vicinity of the secreting cells, binds the secreted cytokine. After any cells and unbound substances are washed away, a biotinylated polyclonal antibody specific for the

chosen cytokine is added to the wells. Following a wash to remove any unbound biotinylated antibody, alkaline-phosphatase conjugated to streptavidin is added. Unbound enzyme is subsequently washed away, and a substrate solution is added. A colored precipitate forms and appears as spots at the sites of cytokine localization, with each spot representing an individual cytokine-secreting cell. The spots can be counted with a stereomicroscope or with an automated ELISpot reader.

Multiplexed ELISAs utilize several detector antibodies bound to individual microwells or antibody microarrays and allow for simultaneous detection of several cytokines from serum.[38] Current formulations allow for the detection of 12 to 25 pro- and anti-inflammatory cytokines in one reaction. In the microarray format, each well on the slide contains a microarray of spotted antibodies, with four "spots" for each of the 12 cytokines plus additional spots for positive and negative controls. The replicate spots allow for acquisition of reliable quantitative data from a single sample.

New microbead assays allow for the simultaneous detection of multiple cytokines in a single tube. Each bead type has its own fluorescent wavelength, which, when combined with the fluorescent secondary antibody bound to a specific cytokine, allows for the detection of up to 100 different analytes in one tube. The use of a multiplexed bead array enabled simultaneous measurement of representative proinflammatory cytokines such as IL-1β, IL-1RA, IL-6, IL-8, and TNF-α; Th1/Th2 distinguishing cytokines IFN-γ,

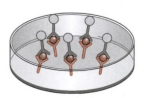
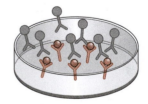
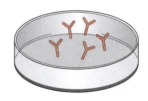
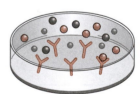

1. Capture antibody attached to well.

2. Cell culture supernatant containing cytokines is added. Wash off unbound material.

3. Enzyme-labeled secondary antibody is added. Wash off unbound antibody.

4. Substrate changes color in the presence of the enzyme-labeled antibody bound to the cytokine.

**FIGURE 5–6.** A standard ELISA assay.

IL-2, IL-4, IL-5, and IL-10; nonspecific acting cytokines IFN-α, IL-13, IL-15, and IL-17; and chemokines IP-10, MCP-1, MIP-1α, and RANTES.

One drawback of protein-based technologies is the short half-life of certain cytokines. This can be overcome by looking at RNA expression in cells using reverse transcription polymerase chain reaction (PCR). The PCR product is made using a fluorescent-labeled primer and can be hybridized to either solid-phase or liquid microarrays. Solid-phase arrays have up to 40,000 spots containing specific ssDNA oligonucleotides representing individual genes. Clinically useful arrays generally have substantially fewer genes represented. Fluorescence of a spot indicates that the gene was expressed in the cell and that the cell was producing the cytokine.

The liquid arrays utilize the same beads as the antibody microbead arrays discussed earlier. However, instead of antibodies, these beads have oligonucleotides on their surfaces and allow up to 100 different cDNAs to be identified. The combination of the bead fluorescence and the fluorescence of the labeled cDNA produces an emission spectrum that identifies the cytokine gene that was expressed in the cells.

## SUMMARY

Cytokines are the functional regulatory proteins for the immune system and are secreted by white blood cells and a variety of other cells. They exert activity-modulating effects on cells of the hematopoietic and immune systems through the activation of cell-bound receptor proteins. Cytokines are induced in response to specific stimuli such as bacterial lipopolysaccharides, flagellin, or other bacterial products through the ligation of cell-adhesion molecules or through the recognition of foreign antigens by host lymphocytes. The effects of cytokines in vivo include regulation of growth, differentiation, and gene expression by many different cell types, including leukocytes, through both autocrine and paracrine activities. Occasionally, cytokines will also exert systemic or endocrine activities.

Individual cytokines do not act alone but in conjunction with many other cytokines that are induced during the process of immune activation. The resulting network of cytokine expression regulates the activities of leukocytes by modulating cytokine activities; this leads to the elimination of the infection. The combined cytokines produce a spectrum of activities that lead to the rapid generation of innate and adaptive immune responses. In fact, the ability or inability to generate certain cytokine patterns often determines the outcome and clinical course of infection. In certain circumstances, massive overproduction produces a "cytokine storm" that leads to shock, multiorgan failure, or even death, thus contributing to pathogenesis.

The cytokines were originally thought to act solely on cells of the immune system, but we now know that many cytokines also act on cells outside the immune system. Vascular endothelial cells, astrocytes, liver cells, muscle cells, and many other cell types respond to cytokines. The pleiotropic nature of cytokine activity relates to the widespread distribution of cytokine receptors on many cell types and the ability of cytokines to alter expression of many genes. Several different cytokines may share properties (i.e., they activate some of the same pathways and genes). This redundancy may be explained by the sharing of cytokine receptor subunits by many cytokines. However, redundancy of cytokine activities cannot be explained entirely by shared receptor subunits. TNF-α, IL-1, and IL-6 exert many of the same biological activities, but each utilizes a distinct receptor. Here, the cytokines are activating similar immune response pathways through different signaling pathways.

The major cytokines involved in the initial stages of the inflammatory response are IL-1, IL-6, TNF-α, and the chemokines. These cytokines are responsible for many of the physical symptoms attributed to inflammation such as fever, swelling, pain, and cellular infiltrates into damaged tissues.

Engagement of the TCR by the appropriate peptide-MHC complex triggers clonal expansion of $CD4^+$ T helper cells. Naïve T cells can differentiate into Th1, Th2, or Treg cell lineages, with the spectrum of cytokines expressed in the initial response determining the lineage. The Th1 lineage is driven by the expression of IL-12 by dendritic cells and is primarily responsible for cell-mediated immunity, while Th2 cells drive antibody-mediated immunity and are developmentally regulated by IL-4. Treg cells are derived from IL-10-responsive naïve T cells and help to regulate the activities of Th1 and Th2 cells through the activities of IL-10 and TGF-β.

The colony stimulating factors (CSFs) include IL-3; erythropoietin (EPO); and granulocyte, macrophage, and granulocyte-macrophage colony stimulating factors (G-CSF, M-CSF, and GM-CSF, respectively). The CSFs are responsible for inducing differentiation and growth of all white cell classes and help to drive the immune response by ensuring that the numbers and types of cells available are adequate.

Anticytokine therapies continue to be developed for many pathological conditions such as Crohn's disease and rheumatoid arthritis. These therapies will drive the need for laboratory assays for cytokines and other markers of immune activation.

# CASE STUDY

A 55-year-old woman being treated for acute lymphocytic leukemia (ALL) was found to be severely neutropenic (477 neutrophils/mL). Her physicians felt that increasing the dosage of her chemotherapy drugs was necessary to eliminate the cancer, but they could not risk further lowering of the neutrophil count due to the increased risk of infection. Since timely full-dose chemotherapy greatly improves survival, it was considered necessary to continue with treatment. However, in order to continue with chemotherapy, treatment for the neutropenia was also necessary.

While undergoing treatment, the patient was also enrolled in a research study designed to look at cytokine expression in ALL patients with neutropenia. The study utilized a liquid bead array that included the colony stimulating factors and the cytokines typically seen in the innate immune response and in Th1 and Th2 responses.

## Questions

a. What colony stimulating factor should the physicians prescribe to overcome the neutropenia?

b. What are some of the cytokines that might be detected in a Th1 type response?

c. What are some of the cytokines that might be detected in a Th2 type response?

# REVIEW QUESTIONS

1. The ability of a single cytokine to alter the expression of several genes is called
   a. redundancy.
   b. pleiotropy.
   c. autocrine stimulation.
   d. endocrine effect.

2. Which of the following can be attributed to IL-1?
   a. Mediator of the innate immune response
   b. Differentiation of stem cells
   c. Halts growth of virally infected cells
   d. Stimulation of mast cells

3. Which of the following are target cells for IL-3?
   a. Myeloid precursors
   b. Lymphoid precursors
   c. Erythroid precursors
   d. All of the above

4. A lack of IL-4 might result in which of the following?
   a. Inability to fight off viral infections
   b. Increased risk of tumors
   c. Lack of IgE
   d. Decreased eosinophil count

5. Which of the following is also known as the T-cell growth factor?
   a. IFN-$\gamma$
   b. IL-12
   c. IL-2
   d. IL-10

6. Which chemokine receptor does HIV need for cell-specific binding?
   a. CCR1
   b. CCR3
   c. CCR4
   d. CCR5

7. IFN-$\alpha$ and IFN-$\beta$ differ in which way from IFN-$\gamma$?
   a. IFN-$\alpha$ and IFN-$\beta$ are called immune interferons, and IFN-$\gamma$ is not.
   b. IFN-$\alpha$ and IFN-$\beta$ primarily activate macrophages, while IFN-$\gamma$ halts viral activity.
   c. They are made primarily by activated T cells, while IFN-$\gamma$ is made by fibroblasts.
   d. IFN-$\alpha$ and IFN-$\beta$ inhibit cell proliferation, while IFN-$\gamma$ stimulates antigen presentation by class II MHC molecules.

8. A patient in septic shock caused by a gram-negative bacterial infection exhibits the following symptoms: high fever, very low blood pressure, and disseminated intravascular coagulation. Which cytokine is the most likely contributor to these symptoms?
   a. IL-2
   b. TNF
   c. IL-12
   d. IL-7

9. IL-10 acts as an antagonist to what cytokine?
   a. IL-4
   b. TNF-$\alpha$
   c. IFN-$\gamma$
   d. TGF-$\beta$

10. Which would be the best assay to measure a specific cytokine?
    a. Blast formation
    b. T-cell proliferation
    c. Measurement of leukocyte chemotaxis
    d. ELISA testing

# References

1. Thomson, A. The Cytokine Handbook. Academic Press, London, 1991.

2. Lucey, DR, Clerici, M, and Shearer, GM. Type 1 and type 2 cytokine dysregulation in human infectious, neoplastic, and inflammatory diseases. Clin Microbiol Rev 9:532–562, 1996.

3. Glickstein, LJ, and Huber, BT. Karoushi—death by overwork in the immune system. J Immunol 155:522–524, 1995.

4. http://www.genenames.org/genefamily/il.php. Accessed March 11, 2008.

5. Heinrich, PC, Behrmann, I, Muller-Newen, G, Schaper, F, and Graeve, L. Interleukin-6-type cytokine signaling through the gp130/Jak/STAT pathway. Biochem J 334:297–314, 1998.

6. Lim, MS, and Elenitoba-Johnson, KSJ. The molecular pathology of primary immunodeficiencies. J Mol Diag 6:59–83, 2004.

7. Dinarello, CA. Interleukin-1 and interleukin-1 antagonism. Blood 77:1627–1652, 1991.

8. Turnbull, AV, and Rivier, CL. Regulation of the hypothalamic-pituitary-adrenal axis by cytokines: Actions and mechanisms of action. Physiol Rev 79:1–71, 1999.

9. Metcalf, D. The molecular control of cell division, differentiation commitment, and maturation in hematopoietic cells. Nature 339:27–30, 1989.

10. Lockesley, RM, Killeen, N, and Lenardo, MJ. The TNF and TNF receptor superfamilies: Integrating mammalian biology. Cell 104:487–501, 2001.

11. Feldmann, M, Brennan, FM, and Maini, RN. Role of cytokines in rheumatoid arthritis. Ann Rev Immunol 14:397–440, 1996.

12. Kim, CH. Chemokine-chemokine receptor network in immune cell trafficking. Curr Drug Targets—Immune, Endocrine, Metab Disord 4:343–361, 2004.

13. Reiche, EMV, Bonametti, AM, Voltarelli, JC, Morimoto, HK, and Watanabe, MAE. Genetic polymorphisms in the chemokine and chemokine receptors: Impact on clinical course and therapy of the Human Immunodeficiency Virus type 1 infection (HIV-1). Curr Medicin Chem 14:1325–1334, 2007.

14. Rahimi, RA, and Leof, EB. TGF-β signaling: A tale of two responses. J Cell Biochem 102:593–608, 2007.

15. Liu, Y-J. IPC: Professional type I interferon-producing cells and plasmacytoid dendritic cell precursors. Ann Rev Immunol 23:275–306, 2005.

16. Van Weyenbergh, J, Weitzerbin, J, Rouillard, D, Barral-Netto, M, and Liblau, R. Treatment of multiple sclerosis patients with interferon-beta primes monocyte-derived macrophages for apoptotic cell death. J Leukoc Biol 70:745–748, 2001.

17. Melian, EB, and Plosker, GL. Interferon alfacon-1: A review of its pharmacology and therapeutic efficacy in the treatment of chronic hepatitis C. Drugs 61:1661–1691, 2001.

18. Currier, JR. T-lymphocyte activation and cell signalling. In Detrick, B, Hamilton, RG, and Folds, JD (eds): Manual of Molecular and Clinical Laboratory Immunology, ed. 7. ASM Press, Washington, DC, 2006.

19. Tsugi, NM. Antigen-specific CD4+T cells in the intestine. Inflamm Aller Drug Targets 5:191–201, 2006.

20. Szabo, SJ., Costa, GL, Zhang, X, and Glimcher, LH. A novel transcription factor, T-bet, directs Th1 lineage commitment. Cell 100:655–669, 2000.

21. Boehm, U, Klamp, T, Groot, M, and Howard, JC. Cellular responses to interferon gamma. Ann Rev Immunol 15:749–795, 1997.

22. Murphy, KM, and Reiner, SL. The lineage decisions of helper T cells. Nature Rev Immunol 2:933–944, 2002.

23. Sugamura, K, Asao, H, Kondo, M, Tanaka, N, Isii, N, Ohbo, K, Nakamura, M, and Takeshita, T. The interleukin-2 receptor γ chain: Its role in multiple cytokine receptor complexes and T cell development in XSCID. Annu Rev Immunol 14:179–205, 1996.

24. Abbas, AK, Murphy, KM, and Sher, A. Functional diversity of helper T lymphocytes. Nature 383:787–793, 1996.

25. Assadullah, K, Sterry, W, and Volk, HD. Interleukin-10 therapy—review of a new approach. Pharmacol Rev 55:241–269, 2003.

26. Wan, YY, and Flavell, RA. The roles for cytokines in the generation and maintenance of regulatory T cells. Immunolog Rev 212:114–130, 2006.

27. Fonenot, JD, and Rudensky, AY. A well adapted regulatory contrivance: Regulatory T cell development and the forkhead family transcription factor Foxp3. Nature Immunol 6:331–337, 2005.

28. Parissis, J, Filippatos, G, Adamopoulos, S, Li, X, Kremastinos, DT, and Uhal, BD. Hematopoietic colony stimulating factors in cardiovascular and pulmonary remodeling: Promoters or inhibitors. Curr Pharmaceu Design 12:2689–2699, 2006.

29. Sloand, EM, Kim, S, Maciejewski, JP, Van Rhee, F, Chauduri, A, Barrett, J, and Young, NS. Pharmacologic doses of granulocyte colony stimulating factor affect cytokine production by lymphocytes in vitro and in vivo. Blood 95:2269–2274, 2000.

30. Varlet-Marie, E, Gaudard, A, Audran, M, and Bressolle, F. Pharmacokinetics/pharmacodynamics of recombinant human erythropoietins in doping control. Sports Med 33:301–315, 2003.

31. Song, XR, Torphy, TJ, Griswold, DE, and Shealy, D. Coming of age: Anti-cytokine therapies. Molecu Interven 2:36–46, 2002.

32. Engelmann, H, Holtmann, H, Nophar, Y, Hadas, E, Leitner, O, and Wallach, D. Antibodies to a soluble form of tumor necrosis factor (TNF) receptor have TNF-like activity. J Biol Chem 265:14497–14504, 1990.

33. Jacob, SE, Nassiri, M, Kerdel, FA, and Vincek, V. Simultaneous measurement of multiple Th1 and Th2 serum cytokines in psoriasis and correlation with disease severity. Mediat Inflam 12:309–313, 2003.

34. Propst, A, Propst, T, Herold, M, Vogel, W, and Judmaier, G. Interleukin-1 receptor antagonist in differential diagnosis of inflammatory bowel diseases. Eur J Gastroenterol Hepatol 7:1031–1036, 1995.

35. Desai, D, Faubion, WA, and Sandborn, WJ. Review article: Biological activity markers in inflammatory bowel disease. Aliment Pharmacol Therapeut 25:247–255, 2007.

36. Madariaga, MG, Jalali, Z, and Swindells, S. Clinical utility of interferon gamma assay in the diagnosis of tuberculosis. J Am Board Fam Med 20:540–547, 2007.

37. Dosanjh, DPS, Hinks, TSC, Innes, JA, Deeks, JJ, Pasvol, G, Hackforth, S, Varia, H, Millington, KA, Gunatheesan, R, Guyot-Revol, V, and Lalvani, A. Improved diagnostic evaluation of suspected tuberculosis. Ann Int Med 148:325–336, 2008.

38. Remick, DG. Multiplex cytokine assays. In Detrick, B, Hamilton, RG, and Folds, JD (eds): Manual of Molecular and Clinical Laboratory Immunology, ed. 7. ASM Press, Washington, DC, 2006.

# Complement System

## LEARNING OBJECTIVES

*After finishing this chapter, the reader will be able to:*

1. Describe the nature of the complement components.
2. Differentiate between the classical and the alternative pathways, including proteins and activators involved in each.
3. Discuss formation of the three principal units of the classical pathway: recognition, activation, and membrane attack units.
4. Describe how initiation of the mannose-binding lectin (MBL) pathway occurs.
5. Explain how C3 plays a key role in all pathways.
6. Describe regulators of the complement system.
7. Discuss the role of the following cell membrane receptors: CR1, DAF, MCP, CR2, CR3, CR4, CD59, and MCP.
8. Relate biological manifestations of complement activation to generation of specific complement products.
9. Describe the complement deficiency associated with the following conditions: hereditary angioedema and paroxysmal nocturnal hemoglobinuria.
10. Differentiate tests for functional activity of complement from measurement of individual complement components.
11. Analyze laboratory findings and indicate disease implications in relation to complement abnormalities.

## KEY TERMS

____ Activation unit
____ Alternative pathway
____ Anaphylatoxin
____ Bystander lysis
____ C1 inhibitor (C1INH)
____ C4-binding protein (C4BP)
____ Classical pathway
____ Complement receptor type 1 (CR1)
____ Decay-accelerating factor (DAF)
____ Factor H
____ Factor I
____ Hemolytic titration (CH$_{50}$) assay
____ Hereditary angioedema
____ Immune adherence
____ Lectin pathway
____ Mannose-binding lectin (MBL)
____ Membrane attack complex
____ Membrane cofactor protein (MCP)
____ Paroxysmal nocturnal hemoglobinuria (PNH)
____ Properdin
____ Recognition unit
____ S protein

# CHAPTER OUTLINE

As described in Chapter 1, complement is a complex series of more than 30 soluble and cell-bound proteins that interact in a very specific way to enhance host defense mechanisms against foreign cells. Originally recognized in the 1890s as a heat-labile substance present in normal nonimmune serum, *complement* was so coined by Paul Ehrlich because it complements the action of antibody in destroying microorganisms.[1] Jules Bordet was awarded the Nobel Prize in 1919 for his role in elucidating the nature of complement.

While complement promotes opsonization and lysis of foreign cells and immune complexes, chronic activation can lead to inflammation and tissue damage. It is the latter that occurs in autoimmune diseases; therefore, complement activation needs to be carefully regulated in order to minimize tissue damage. In addition to the major proteins involved in activation, there are numerous proteins that act as controls or regulators of the system. The three pathways for activation of complement will be discussed along with major system controls.

Most plasma complement proteins are synthesized in the liver, with the exception of C1 components, which are mainly produced by intestinal epithelial cells, and factor D, which is made in adipose tissue.[1,2] Other cells, such as monocytes and macrophages, are additional sources of early complement components, including C1, C2, C3, and C4.[3,4] Most of these proteins are inactive precursors, or zymogens, which are converted to active enzymes in a very precise order. **Table 6–1** lists the characteristics of the main complement proteins.

| Table 6–1. | Proteins of the Complement System | | |
|---|---|---|---|
| **SERUM PROTEIN** | **MOLECULAR WEIGHT, kD** | **CONCENTRATION (μg/mL)** | **FUNCTION** |
| **Classical Pathway** | | | |
| C1q | 410 | 150 | Binds to Fc region of IgM and IgG |
| C1r | 85 | 50 | Activates C1s |
| C1s | 85 | 50 | Cleaves C4 and C2 |
| C4 | 205 | 300–600 | Part of C3 convertase (C4b) |
| C2 | 102 | 25 | Binds to C4b—forms C3 convertase |
| C3 | 190 | 1200 | Key intermediate in all pathways |
| C5 | 190 | 80 | Initiates membrane attack complex |
| C6 | 110 | 45 | Binds to C5b in MAC |
| C7 | 100 | 90 | Binds to C5bC6 in MAC |
| C8 | 150 | 55 | Starts pore formation on membrane |
| C9 | 70 | 60 | Polymerizes to cause cell lysis |

## Table 6-1. Proteins of the Complement System—Cont'd

| SERUM PROTEIN | MOLECULAR WEIGHT, kD | CONCENTRATION (µg/mL) | FUNCTION |
|---|---|---|---|
| **Alternative Pathway** | | | |
| Factor B | 93 | 200 | Binds to C3b to form C3 convertase |
| Factor D | 24 | 2 | Cleaves factor B |
| Properdin | 55 | 15–25 | Stabilizes C3bBb–C3 convertase |
| **MBL Pathway** | | | |
| MBL | 200–600 | 0.0002–10 | Binds to mannose |
| MASP-1 | 93 | 1.5–12 | Unknown |
| MASP-2 | 76 | Unknown | Cleaves C4 and C2 |

Fc = Fragment crystallizable; Ig = immunoglobulin; MAC = membrane attack complex; MBL = mannose-binding lectin; MASP = MBL-associated serine protease.

The complement system can be activated in three different ways. The first is the **classical pathway,** which involves nine proteins that are triggered by antigen–antibody combination. Pillemer and colleagues later discovered an antibody-independent pathway in the 1950s, and this plays a major role as a natural defense system.[5] The second pathway, the **alternative pathway,** was originally called the *properdin system,* because the the protein properdin was thought to initiate this pathway. Now, however, it is known that properdin's major function is to stabilize a key enzyme complex formed along the pathway. The third pathway, the **lectin pathway,** is another antibody-independent means of activating complement proteins. Its major constituent, **mannose-** (or mannan-) **binding lectin (MBL),** adheres to mannose found mainly in the cell walls or outer coating of bacteria, viruses, yeast, and protozoa. While each of these pathways will be considered separately, activation seldom involves only one pathway.

The complement system plays a major part in the inflammatory response directed against foreign antigens. Although the end product of complement activation is lysis of the invading cell, many other important events take place along the way. Complement fragments acting as opsonins, for which specific receptors are present on phagocytic cells, enhance metabolism and clear immune complexes. In fact, uptake of immune complexes in the spleen appears to be complement-dependent.[1] Complement components are also able to increase vascular permeability, recruit monocytes and neutrophils to the area of antigen concentration, and trigger secretion of immunoregulatory molecules that amplify the immune response.[4] Any deficiencies in the complement system can result in an increased susceptibility to infection or in the accumulation of immune complexes with possible autoimmune manifestations. Thus, these proteins play a significant role as a host defense mechanism.

## THE CLASSICAL PATHWAY

The classical pathway or cascade is the main antibody-directed mechanism for triggering complement activation.

However, not all immunoglobulins are able to activate this pathway. Those classes that can include IgM, IgG1, IgG2, and IgG3. IgM is the most efficient, because it has multiple binding sites; thus, it takes only one molecule attached to two adjacent antigenic determinants to initiate the cascade. Two IgG molecules must attach to antigen within 30 to 40 nm of each other before complement can bind, and it may take at least 1000 IgG molecules to ensure that two are close enough to initiate such binding.[1,6] Some epitopes, notably the Rh group, are too far apart on the cell for this to occur, so they are unable to fix complement. Within the IgG group, IgG3 is the most effective, followed by IgG1 and then IgG2.[6]

In addition to antibody, there are a few substances that can bind complement directly to initiate the classical cascade. These include C-reactive protein, several viruses, mycoplasmas, some protozoa, and certain gram-negative bacteria such as *Escherichia coli.*[6] However, most infectious agents can directly activate only the alternative pathway.

Complement activation can be divided into three main stages, each of which is dependent on the grouping of certain reactants as a unit. The first stage involves C1, which is known as the **recognition unit.** Once C1 is fixed, the next components activated are C4, C2, and C3, known collectively as the **activation unit.** C5 through C9 comprise the **membrane attack complex,** and it is this last unit that completes lysis of the foreign particle. Each of these is discussed in detail in the following sections. **Figure 6–1** depicts a simplified scheme of the entire pathway.

## The Recognition Unit

The first complement component to bind is C1, a molecular complex of 740,000 d. It consists of three subunits: C1q, C1r, and C1s, which are stabilized by calcium.[1,6] The complex is made up of one C1q subunit and two each of the C1r and C1s subunits. Although the C1q unit is the part that binds to antibody molecules, the C1r and C1s subunits generate enzyme activity to begin the cascade. The $(C1r, C1s)_2$ complex is an S-shaped structure with several domains of

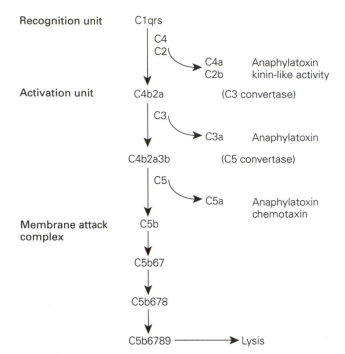

Recognition unit    C1qrs

Activation unit    C4b2a

Membrane attack complex    C5b

**FIGURE 6–1.** The classical complement cascade. C1qrs is the recognition unit that binds to the Fc portion of two antibody molecules. C1s is activated and cleaves C4 and C2 to form C4b2a, which is known as *C3 convertase*. C3 convertase cleaves C3 to form C4b2a3b, known as *C5 convertase*. The combination of C4b2a3b is the activation unit. C5 convertase cleaves C5. C5b attracts C6, C7, C8, and C9, which bind together, forming the membrane attack complex. C9 polymerizes to cause lysis of the target cell.

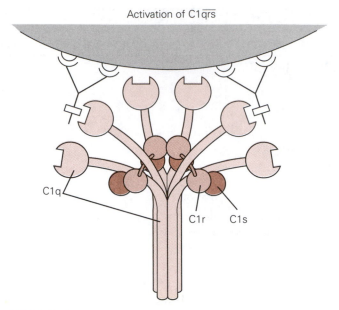

**FIGURE 6–2.** Structure of C1qrs. When two or more globular heads of C1q attach to bound immunoglobulin molecules, the collagen-like stalks change their configuration. The resulting shape change causes C1r to become a serine protease. This cleaves a small fragment off C1s, uncovering the C1s protease, whose only targets are C4 and C2.

C1s has a limited specificity, with its only substrates being C4 and C2. Once C1s is activated, the recognition stage ends.

## The Activation Unit

Phase two, the formation of the activation unit, results in the production of an enzyme known as *C5 convertase*. C4 is the second-most-abundant complement protein, with a serum concentration of approximately 600 µg/mL.[6] It consists of three polypeptide chains and has a molecular weight of approximately 198,000. C1s cleaves C4 to split off a 77-amino acid fragment called C4a. In the process, it opens a thioester-containing active site on the remaining part, C4b. C4b must bind to protein or carbohydrate within a few seconds, or it will react with water molecules to form iC4b, which is rapidly degraded. Thus, C4b binds mainly to antigen in clusters that are within a 40 nm radius of C1. This represents the first amplification step in the cascade, because for every one C1 attached, approximately 30 molecules of C4 are split and attached.[2]

C2 is the next component to be activated. Complement proteins were named as they were isolated, before the sequence of activation was known—hence the irregularity in the numbering system. C2 is a single-chain glycoprotein with a molecular weight of 102,000.[2] The C2 gene is closely associated with the gene for *factor B* (alternative pathway) on chromosome 6 in the major histocompatability complex, and each serves a similar purpose in its particular pathway.[8]

When combined with C4b in the presence of magnesium ions, C2 is cleaved by C1s to form C2a (which has a

unequal size. The sequence of binding is C1s-C1r-C1r-C1s.[1] It is hypothesized that this structure assumes the shape of a distorted figure eight, and it wraps itself around the arms of C1q **(Fig. 6–2)**.

C1q has a molecular weight of 410,000 and is composed of six strands that form six globular heads with a collagen-like tail portion. This structure has been likened to a bouquet with six blossoms extending outward (see Fig. 6–2). Each of the six stalks is composed of three homologous polypeptide chains—A, B, and C—that form a triple helix.[1] Alanine residues, which interrupt the triple helix, make a semiflexible joint that allows the "stems" to bend. As long as calcium is present in the serum, C1r and C1s remain associated with C1q.

C1q "recognizes" the fragment crystallizable (Fc) region of two adjacent antibody molecules, and at least two of the globular heads of C1q must be bound to initiate the classical pathway. This binding occurs at the $C_H2$ region for IgG and at the $C_H3$ region for IgM. C1r and C1s are both serine protease proenzymes or zymogens. As binding of C1q occurs, both are converted into active enzymes. Autoactivation of C1r results from a conformational change that takes place as C1q is bound. Mechanical stress transmitted from the stems as binding occurs opens up the active site on C1r.[7] Once activated, C1r cleaves a thioester bond on C1s, which activates it. Activated C1r is extremely specific, because its only known substrate is C1s. Likewise,

molecular weight of 70,000) and C2b (which has a molecular weight of 34,000) **(Fig. 6–3A)**. This is the only case for the designation *a* to be given to the cleavage piece with enzyme activity. C2 must be within a 60 nm radius of bound C1s for cleavage to occur. Binding of C2 to C4b can occur in the fluid phase, but C4b attached to antigen is much more efficient in accepting C2. This serves to keep the reaction localized.

The combination of C4b and C2a is known as *C3 convertase* **(Fig. 6–3B)**. This is written as C4b2a to indicate that the complex is an active enzyme. This complex is not very stable. The half-life is estimated to be between 15 seconds and 3 minutes, so C3 must be bound quickly. If binding does occur, C3 is cleaved into two parts, C3a and C3b.

C3 is the major constituent of the complement system and is present in the plasma at a concentration of 1200 µg/mL.[6] It serves as the pivotal point for all three pathways, and cleavage of C3 to C3b represents the most significant step in the entire process of complement activation.[9] The molecule has a molecular weight of 190,000, and it consists of two polypeptide chains, alpha and beta. The alpha chain contains a highly reactive thioester group, and when C3a is removed by cleavage of a single bond in the αchain, the thioester is exposed; the remaining piece, C3b, is then capable of binding to hydroxyl groups on carbohydrates and proteins in the immediate vicinity.[6,7,9] Only a small percentage of cleaved C3 molecules bind to antigen; most are hydrolyzed by water molecules and decay in the fluid phase.[6,10] C3b is estimated to have a half-life of 60 microseconds if not bound to antigen.

The cleavage of C3 represents a second and major amplification process, because about 200 molecules are split for every molecule of C4b2a.[1] In addition to being required for the formation of the membrane attack complex, C3b also serves as a powerful opsonin. Macrophages have specific receptors for it (discussed later in the chapter), and this contributes greatly to the process of phagocytosis. However, a large number of molecules are needed for this to occur; hence the need for amplification.

If C3b is bound within 40 nm of the C4b2a, then this creates a new enzyme known as *C5 convertase*. **Figure 6–3C** depicts this last step in the formation of the activation unit. The cleaving of C5 with deposition of C5b at another site on the cell membrane constitutes the beginning of the membrane attack complex (MAC).

## The Membrane Attack Complex

C5 consists of two polypeptide chains, α and β, which are linked by disulfide bonds to form a molecule with a molecular weight of about 190,000. C5 convertase, consisting of C4b2b3b, splits off a 74-amino-acid piece known as C5a, and C5b attaches to the cell membrane, forming the beginning of the MAC. The splitting of C5 and the cleavage of C3 represents the most significant biological consequences of the complement system, as explained in the "Biological Manifestations of Complement Activation" section. However,

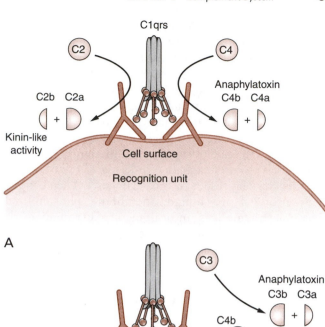

A

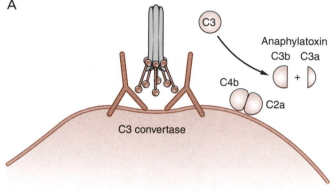

B

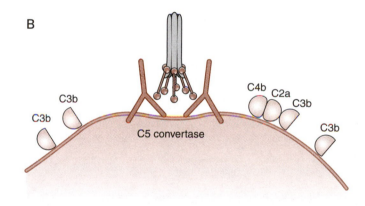

C

**FIGURE 6–3.** Formation of the activation unit. *(A)* C1qrs is able to cleave C4 and C2. *(B)* The larger pieces, C4b and C2a, bind to the target cell surface and form the enzyme C3 convertase. This cleaves C3 into C3a and C3b. *(C)* C3b is a powerful opsonin, and it binds to the target in many places. If some remains associated with C4bC2a, the enzyme C5 convertase is formed. The association of C4bC2aC3b is known as the *activation unit.*

C5b is extremely labile, and it is rapidly inactivated unless binding to C6 occurs.[1]

Subsequent binding involves C6, C7, C8, and C9. None of these proteins have enzymatic activity, and they are all present in much smaller amounts in serum than the preceding components. C6 and C7 each have molecular weights of approximately 110,000, and both have similar physical and chemical properties. C8 is made up of three dissimilar chains joined by disulfide bonds and has a total molecular weight of about 150,000.[2] C9 is a single polypeptide chain with a molecular weight of 70,000. The carboxy-terminal end is hydrophobic, while the amino-terminal end is hydrophilic. The hydrophobic part serves to anchor the MAC within the target membrane. Formation of the membrane attack unit is pictured in **Figure 6–4.**

Membrane damage is caused by at least two different mechanisms: channel formation and the binding of phospholipids. The latter causes a reordering and reorientation of molecules that results in leaky patches.[6] When complement proteins are bound, membrane phospholipids rearrange themselves into domains surrounding the C5b6789 complex, and the integrity of the membrane is destroyed. Ions then are able to pass freely out of the cell.

The membrane attack unit begins when C6 binds to C5b, thereby stabilizing it. Then this complex attaches to the cell surface. C7 binds next, forming a trimolecular complex that

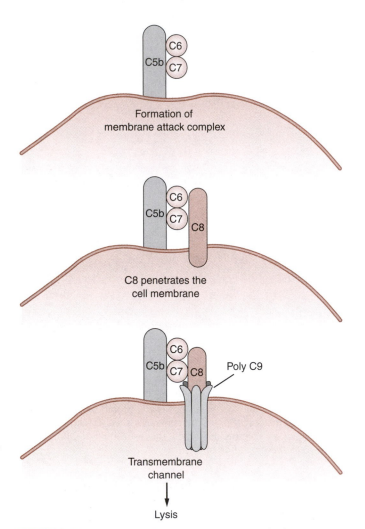

**FIGURE 6–4.** Formation of the membrane attack unit. C5 convertase cleaves C5 into C5a and C5b. C5b binds to the target cell, and C6 and C7 become attached to it. C8 binds to these associated molecules and begins to penetrate the cell membrane. C9 binds to the complex and polymerizes to form the transmembrane channel, which causes lysis of the cell.

has a high affinity for lipid constituents of the cell membrane. This allows for insertion of the C7 part of the C5b67 complex into the membrane of the target cell.[3]

Next, C8 binds to C7 and exposes a hydrophobic region that interacts with the cell membrane to form a small hole in the membrane as C8 is inserted into the lipid bilayer.[3] Lysis can be observed at this stage, but the addition of C9 accelerates the process. Binding of C8 causes a loss of potassium from the cell, which is followed by leakage of amino acids and ribonucleotides. The pore formed by the binding of C5b678 is small, capable of lysing erythrocytes but not nucleated cells.[1] For lysis of nucleated cells to be achieved, C9 must bind to the complex.

When C9 binds to the C5–C8 complex, it unfolds, becomes inserted into the lipid bilayer, and polymerizes. Anywhere from 1 to 18 molecules of C9 can bind to one C8 molecule.[3] C9 polymerizes only when bound, and it is believed that the C5–C8 complex acts as a catalyst to enhance the rate of reaction.[2] Polymerized C9 forms a hollow, thin-walled cylinder, which can be seen on electron microscopy and constitutes the transmembrane channel. The completed MAC unit has a functional pore size of 70 to 100Å.[1,3] One such unit can lyse erythrocytes, but lysis of nucleated cells is a multihit phenomenon; it was originally believed that lysis of all cells was a single-hit phenomenon. Destruction of target cells actually occurs through an influx of water and a corresponding loss of electrolytes.

## THE ALTERNATIVE PATHWAY

Pathogens can be destroyed in the absence of antibody by means of the alternative pathway, which acts as part of innate or natural immunity. This pathway is important as an early defense against pathogens. Phylogenetically, this represents the oldest of the C3 activating pathways. First described by Pillemer and his associates in the early 1950s, the pathway was originally named for the protein **properdin,** a constituent of normal serum with a concentration of approximately 5 to 15 μg/mL.[11] Now it is known that properdin does not initiate this pathway but rather stabilizes the C3 convertase formed from activation of other factors. In addition to properdin, the serum proteins that are unique to this pathway include factor B and factor D. C1, C2, and C4, found in the classical pathway, are not used at all in this system. C3, however, is a key component of both pathways. The alternative pathway is summarized in **Figure 6–5.**

Triggering substances for the alternative pathway include bacterial cell walls, especially those containing lipopolysaccharide; fungal cell walls; yeast; viruses; virally infected cells; tumor cell lines; and some parasites, especially trypanosomes.[1] All of these can serve as sites for binding the complex C3bBb, one of the end products of this pathway. The conversion of C3 is the first step in this pathway.

In plasma, native C3 is not stable. Water is able to hydrolyze a thioester bond and thus spontaneously activates a small number of these molecules.[12] Once activated, it can

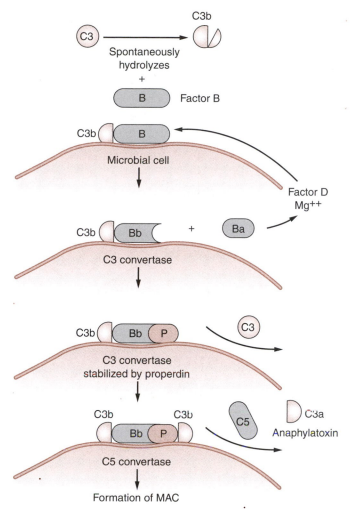

FIGURE 6-5. The alternative pathway. C3 is hydrolyzed by water to produce a C3b sometimes called iC3. This molecule can bind factor B. When factor B is bound to C3b, B is cleaved to form C3Bb, an enzyme with C3 convertase activity. More C3 is cleaved to form more C3bBb. This enzyme is stabilized by properdin, and it continues to cleave additional C3. If a molecule of C3 remains attached to the C3bBbP enzyme, the convertase now has the capability to cleave C5. The C5 convertase thus consists of C3bBb3bP. After C5 is cleaved, the pathway is exactly the same as the classical pathway.

bind to factor B, which has a molecular weight of 93,000 and is fairly abundant in the serum, at a level of 200 µg/mL.[6,8] Binding of C3b (sometimes called *iC3*) to B causes a conformational change that makes B more susceptible to cleavage by serine proteases. Thus, only bound factor B can be cleaved by factor D. The role of factor B is thus analogous to that of C2 in the classical pathway, because it forms an integral part of a C3 convertase.

Factor D is a plasma protein that goes through a conformational change when it binds to factor B.[7,8] It is a serine protease with a molecular weight of 24,000, and its only substrate is bound factor B. When bound to factor B, the catalytic site on factor D opens, making it an active enzyme. The concentration of factor D in the plasma is the lowest of all the complement proteins, approximately 2 µg/mL.[6] It cleaves factor B into two pieces: Ba (with a molecular weight

of 33,000) and Bb (with a molecular weight of approximately 60,000). Bb remains attached to C3b, forming the initial C3 convertase of the alternative pathway. Bb is rapidly inactivated unless it becomes bound to a site on one of the triggering cellular antigens.

As the alternative pathway convertase, *C3bBb* is then capable of cleaving additional C3 into C3a and C3b. Some C3b attaches to cellular surfaces and acts as a binding site for more factor B. This results in an amplification loop that feeds C3b into the classical and alternative pathways. All C3 present in plasma would be rapidly converted by this method were it not for the fact that the enzyme C3bBb is extremely unstable unless properdin binds to the complex. Binding of properdin increases the half-life of C3bBb from 90 seconds to several minutes.[6,8] In this manner, optimal rates of alternative pathway activation are achieved.[11]

C3bBb can also cleave C5, but it is much more efficient at cleaving C3.[13] If, however, some of the C3b produced remains bound to the C3 convertase, the enzyme is altered to form C3bBb3bP, which has a high affinity for C5 and exhibits C5 convertase activity.[12,13] C5 is cleaved to produce C5b, the first part of the membrane attack unit. From this point on, both the alternative and classical pathways are identical.

## THE LECTIN PATHWAY

The lectin pathway represents another means of activating complement without antibody being present. Lectins are proteins that bind to carbohydrates. This pathway provides an additional link between the innate and acquired immune response, because it involves nonspecific recognition of carbohydrates that are common constituents of microbial cell walls and that are distinct from those found on human cell surfaces.[14,15] One key lectin, called *mannose-binding, or mannan-binding, lectin (MBL)*, binds to mannose or related sugars in a calcium-dependent manner to initiate this pathway.[16] These sugars are found in glycoproteins or carbohydrates of a wide variety of microorganisms such as bacteria, yeasts, viruses, and some parasites. MBL is considered an acute phase protein, because it is produced in the liver and is normally present in the serum but increases during an initial inflammatory response.[15] It plays an important role as a defense mechanism in infancy, during the interval between the loss of maternal antibody and the acquisition of a full-fledged antibody response to pathogens.[17] In fact, deficiencies of MBL have been associated with serious infections such as neonatal pneumonia and sepsis.[15,18]

The structure of MBL is similar to that of C1q, and it is associated with three MBL-serine proteases (MASPs): MASP-1, MASP-2, and MASP-3. Once MBL binds to a cellular surface, MASP-2, which is homologous to C1s, autoactivates.[19] MASP-2 thus takes the active role in cleaving C4 and C2, while the functions of MASP-1 and MASP-3 are unclear at this time.[16,19] Once C4 and C2 are cleaved, the rest of the pathway is identical to the classical pathway. **Figure 6-6** shows the convergence of all three pathways.

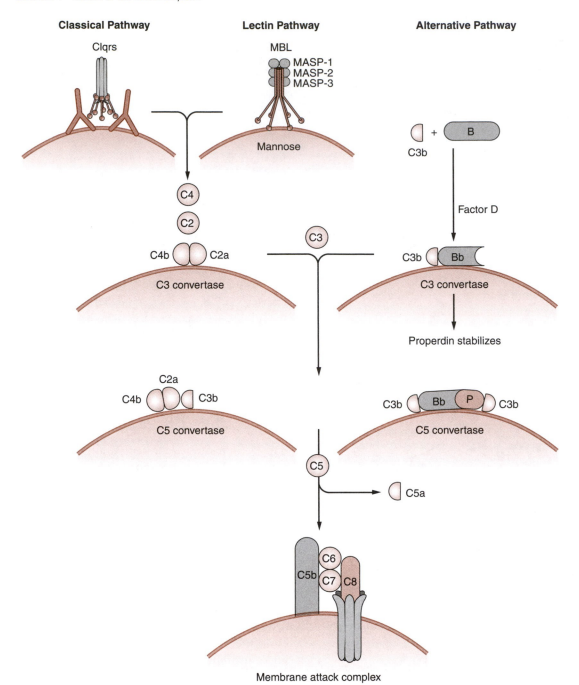

**FIGURE 6–6.** Convergence of the classical, alternative, and lectin pathways. The binding of C1qrs to two antibody molecules activates the classical pathway, while the alternative pathway is started by hydrolysis of C3. The lectin pathway is triggered by binding of MBP to mannose on bacterial cell walls. MASP-1, MASP-2, and MASP-3 bind to form an activated C1-like complex. MASP-2 cleaves C2 and C4 and proceeds like the classical pathway. Factor B and factor D operate in the alternative pathway. While C3 convertase is formed differently in each pathway, C3 is a key component in each one. The C5 convertase in the alternative pathway consists of C3bBb3bP. In the classical pathway, C5 convertase is made up of C4b2a3b. After C5 is cleaved, the pathway is common to all.

## SYSTEM CONTROLS

Activation of complement could cause tissue damage and have devastating systemic effects if it was allowed to proceed uncontrolled. To ensure that infectious agents and not self-antigens are destroyed and that the reaction remains localized, several plasma proteins act as system regulators. In addition, there are specific receptors on certain cells that also exert a controlling influence on the activation process. In fact, approximately one-half of the complement components serve as controls for critical steps in the activation process. Because activation of C3 is the pivotal step in all pathways, the majority of the control proteins are aimed at halting accumulation of C3b. However, there are controls at all crucial steps along the way. Regulators will be discussed according to their order of appearance in each of the three pathways. A brief summary of these is found in **Table 6–2.**

## Regulation of the Classical and Lectin Pathways

**C1 inhibitor,** or C1INH, is a glycoprotein with a molecular weight of 105,000 that inhibits activation at the first stages of both the classical and lectin pathways. Like most of the other complement proteins, it is mainly synthesized in the liver, but monocytes also may be involved to some extent in its manufacture. Its main role is to inactivate C1 by binding to the active sites of C1r and C1s. C1r and C1s become instantly and irreversibly dissociated from C1q.[2,6] C1q remains bound to antibody, but all enzymatic activity ceases. C1INH also inactivates MASP-2 binding to the MBL-MASP complex, thus halting the lectin pathway.[12,19]

Further formation of C3 convertase in the classical and lectin pathways is inhibited by four main regulators: soluble **C4b-binding protein (C4BP)** and three cell-bound receptors, **complement receptor type 1 (CR1), membrane cofactor protein (MCP),** and **decay accelerating factor (DAF).**[1,7] All of these act in concert with **factor I,** a serine protease that inactivates C3b and C4b when bound to one of these regulators. C4BP is abundant in the plasma and has a molecular weight of about 520,000. It is capable of combining with either fluid-phase or bound C4b, so C4b cannot bind C2 and is made available for degradation by factor I.[1] If C4BP attaches to cell-bound C4b, it can dissociate it from C4b2a complexes, thus causing the cessation of the classical pathway.

CR1, also known as CD35, is a large polymorphic glycoprotein with a molecular weight between 165,000 and 280,000.[3] It is found mainly on peripheral blood cells, including neutrophils, monocytes, macrophages, erythrocytes, eosinophils, B lymphocytes, some T lymphocytes, and follicular dendritic cells.[2] It binds C3b and C4b but has the greatest affinity for C3b.[2,20] Once bound to CR1, both C4b and C3b can then be degraded by factor I

Perhaps one of the main functions of CR1, however, is to act as a receptor on platelets and red blood cells and to mediate transport of C3b-coated immune complexes to the liver and spleen.[3,20] It is there that fixed tissue macrophages strip the immune complexes from the red blood cells, process the complexes, and return the red blood cells intact

to circulation. The ability of cells to bind complement-coated particles is referred to as **immune adherence.**

Membrane cofactor protein (MCP), or CD46, has a molecular weight between 50,000 and 70,000 and is found on virtually all epithelial and endothelial cells except erythrocytes.[3] MCP is the most efficient cofactor for factor I–mediated cleavage of C3b. It also serves as a cofactor for cleavage of C4b, but it is not as effective as C4BP. MCP also helps to control the alternative pathway, since binding of factor B to C3b is inhibited.

Decay-accelerating factor (DAF), or CD55, a 70,000 d membrane glycoprotein, is the third main receptor, and it has a wide tissue distribution. It is found on peripheral blood cells, on endothelial cells and fibroblasts, and on numerous types of epithelial cells.[3,6,21,22] DAF is capable of dissociating both classical and alternative pathway C3 convertases. It can bind to both C3b and C4b in a similar manner to CR1.[3] It does not prevent initial binding of either C2 or factor B to the cell but can rapidly dissociate both from their binding sites, thus preventing the assembly of an active C3 convertase.

The carboxy-terminal portion of DAF is covalently attached to a glycophospholipid anchor that is inserted into the outer layer of the membrane lipid bilayer. This arrangement allows DAF mobility within the membrane so it can reach C3 convertase sites that are not immediately adjacent to it **(Fig. 6–7).**[21] The presence of DAF on host cells protects them from **bystander lysis** and is one of the main mechanisms used in discrimination of self from nonself, because foreign cells do not possess this substance. However, it does not permanently modify C3b or C4b; thus, they are capable of re-forming elsewhere as active convertases.

## Regulation of the Alternative Pathway

The principal soluble regulator of the alternative pathway is **factor H,** which has a molecular weight of 160,000.[7,12] It acts by binding to C3b, thus preventing the binding of factor B. C3b in the fluid phase has a hundredfold greater affinity for factor H than for factor B, but on cell surfaces, C3b preferentially binds factor B. However, factor H also accelerates the dissociation of the C3bBb complex on cell surfaces. When factor H binds to C3bBb, Bb becomes

| SERUM PROTEIN | MOLECULAR WEIGHT (KD) | CONCENTRATION (mg/mL) | FUNCTION |
|---|---|---|---|
| C1 inhibitor (C1INH) | 105 | 240 | Dissociates C1r and C1s from C1q |
| Factor I | 88 | 35 | Cleaves C3b and C4b |
| Factor H | 150 | 300–450 | Cofactor with I to inactivate C3b; prevents binding of B to C3b |
| C4-binding protein | 520 | 250 | Acts as a cofactor with I to inactivate C4b (C4bp) |
| S protein (vitronectin) | 84 | 500 | Prevents attachment of the C5b67 complex to cell membranes |

**Table 6–2. Plasma Complement Regulators**

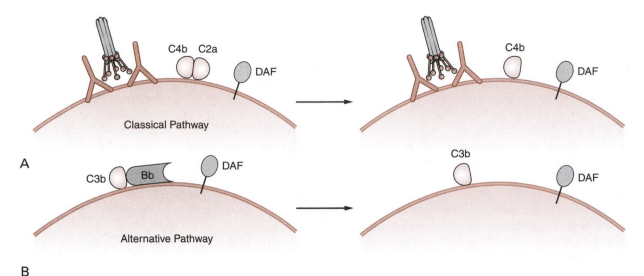

A

B

FIGURE 6–7. Inhibitory effects of DAF. DAF acts in both the classical and alternative pathways to dissociate C3b. When C3b binds to cell surfaces that have DAF present, DAF helps dissociate Bb from binding to C3b in the alternative pathway. In the classical pathway, DAF dissociates C2a from C4b.

displaced. In this manner, C3 convertase activity is curtailed in plasma and on cell surfaces.

Additionally, factor H acts as a cofactor that allows factor I to break down C3b. It appears that only those molecules with tightly bound factor H acquire high-affinity binding sites for factor I.[23] When factor I binds, a conformational change takes place and allows it to cleave C3b.[23] On cellular surfaces, C3b is cleaved to C3f, a small piece that is released into the plasma, and to iC3b, which remains attached but is no longer an active enzyme. iC3b is further broken down to C3c and C3dg by factor I in conjunction with another cofactor, the CR1 receptor (Fig. 6–8).[1]

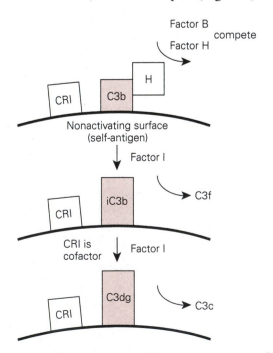

FIGURE 6–8. Complement controls. CR1 receptor acts as a cofactor in the inactivation of C3b. Factor I cleaves C3b to form C3dg and C3c. C3dg is not an effective opsonin, and it is not capable of further participation in the complement cascade.

## Regulation of Terminal Components

S protein is a soluble control protein that acts at a deeper level of complement activation. Also known as *vitronectin*, S protein interacts with the C5b67 complex as it forms in the fluid phase and prevents it from binding to cell membranes.[6] Binding of C8 and C9 still proceeds, but polymerization of C9 does not occur, and the complex is unable to insert itself into the cell membrane or to produce lysis.[3]

A receptor known by various terms, including *membrane inhibitor of reactive lysis (MIRL)*, or *CD59*, also acts to block formation of the membrane attack complex. MIRL is widely distributed on the cell membranes of all circulating blood cells, including red blood cells, and on endothelial, epithelial, and many other types of cells.[2,3] Its main function is to bind to C8 and prevent insertion of C9 into host cell membranes.[6,11] Table 6–3 lists the receptors and indicates the type of cell on which they are found.

## COMPLEMENT RECEPTORS AND THEIR BIOLOGICAL ROLES

Some complement receptors found on host cells amplify and enhance the immune response by augmenting phagocytosis and stimulating accessory cells, rather than acting as regulators. Table 6–3 summarizes the main characteristics of each and describes the cell types on which they are found. CR1 has been discussed in the previous section. A second receptor, CR2 or CD21, is found mainly on B lymphocytes and follicular dendritic cells.[2,4] Ligands for CR2 include degradation products of C3b, such as C3dg, C3d, and iC3b. In addition, the Epstein-Barr virus gains entry to B cells by binding to this receptor. CR2 is present only on mature B cells, and it is lost when conversion to plasma cells occurs.

| Table 6-3. | Receptors on Cell Membranes for Complement Components | | |
|---|---|---|---|
| **RECEPTOR** | **LIGAND** | **CELL TYPE** | **FUNCTION** |
| CR1 (CD35) | C3b, iC3b, C4b | RBCs, neutrophils, monocytes, macrophages, eosinophils, B and T cells, follicular dendritic cells | Cofactor for factor I; mediates transport of immune complexes |
| CR2 (CD21) | C3dg, C3d, iC3b | B cells, follicular dendritic cells, epithelial cells | B-cell coreceptor for antigen with CD19 |
| CR3 (CD11b/CD18) | iC3b, C3d, C3b | Monocytes, macrophages, neutrophils, NK cells | Adhesion and increased activity of phagocytic cells |
| CR4 (CD11c/CD18) | iC3b, C3b | Monocytes, macrophages, neutrophils, NK cells, activated T and B cells, dendritic cells | Adhesion and increased activity of phagocytic cells |
| DAF (CD55) | C3b, C4b | RBCs, neutrophils, platelets, monocytes, endothelial cells, fibroblasts, T cells, B cells, epithelial cells | Dissociates C2b or Bb from binding sites, thus preventing formation of C3 convertase |
| MIRL (CD59) | C8 | RBCs, neutrophils, platelets, monocytes, endothelial cells, epithelial cells | Prevents insertion of C9 into cell membrane |
| MCP (CD46) | C3b, C4b | Neutrophils, monocytes, macrophages, platelets, T cells, B cells, endothelial cells | Cofactor for factor I cleavage of C3b and C4b |

RBC = red blood cell; NK = natural killer

CR2 plays an important role as part of the B-cell coreceptor for antigen. Acting in concert with CD19, it binds complement-coated antigen and cross-links it to membrane immunoglobulin to activate B cells. In this manner, immune complexes are more effective at enhancing B-cell differentiation and production of memory cells than is antigen by itself.[3,4,21]

Another receptor, CR3 (CD11b/CD18), found on monocytes, macrophages, neutrophils, and natural killer cells, specifically binds particles opsonized with iC3b, a C3b degradation product.[3] It does this in a calcium-dependent manner. The CR3 receptor plays a key role in mediating phagocytosis of particles coated with these complement fragments **(Fig. 6–9)**. It consists of an α and a β chain, with molecular weights of 165,000 and 95,000, respectively.[24] These proteins trigger surface adhesion and increased activity of phagocytic cells.[6] Patients whose white blood cells lack these receptors fail to exhibit functions such as chemotaxis, surface adherence, and aggregation. Deficiencies in phagocytosis are also noted. These individuals have an impaired capacity to bind iC3b-coated particles and are subject to recurrent infections.

The CR4 (CD11c/CD18) receptor is very similar to CR3 in that it also binds iC3b fragments in a calcium-dependent fashion. CR4 proteins are found on neutrophils, monocytes, tissue macrophages, activated T cells, dendritic cells, NK cells, and activated B cells.[3] Neutrophils and monocytes,

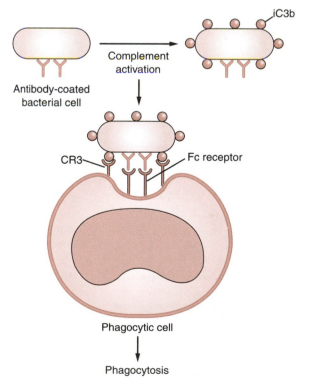

**FIGURE 6–9.** Role of C3b in opsonization. C3b-coated antigens are destroyed more easily due to interaction with the CR1 receptors found on phagocytic cells.

however, possess smaller amounts of CR4 than of CR3. Their function appears to be similar to that of CR3, and they may assist neutrophil adhesion to the endothelium during inflammation.

Receptors specific for Clq are found on neutrophils, monocytes, macrophages, B cells, platelets, and endothelial cells.[3,23] These receptors, known as *collectin receptors*, bind the collagen portion of Clq and generally enhance the binding of Clq to Fc receptors. Interacting only with bound Clq, the receptors appear to increase phagocytic cells' uptake of immune complexes opsonized with Clq. Additionally, on neutrophils, they may act to enhance the respiratory burst triggered by IgG binding to Fc receptors.

## BIOLOGICAL MANIFESTATIONS OF COMPLEMENT ACTIVATION

Activation of complement is a very effective means of amplifying the inflammatory response to destroy and clear foreign antigens. The cycle does not always have to proceed to lysis for this to be accomplished; hence, some of the initiating proteins are much more plentiful than proteins that form the membrane attack complex. Complement proteins also serve as a means of linking innate and natural immunity. They act as opsonins to facilitate destruction by phagocytic cells, and they play a major role in uptake and presentation of antigens so a specific immune response can occur. They also facilitate B-cell activation and may, in fact, be necessary for maintaining immunological memory. Effector molecules generated earlier in the cascade play a major role in all these areas. Such molecules can be classified into three main categories: anaphylatoxins, chemotaxins, and opsonins.

An **anaphylatoxin** is a small peptide that causes increased vascular permeability, contraction of smooth muscle, and release of histamine from basophils and mast cells. Proteins that play such a part are C3a, C4a, and C5a. All of these have a molecular weight between 9,000 and 11,000, and they are formed as cleavage products from larger complement components. Of these molecules, C5a is the most potent, at least 200 times more powerful than C3a, while C4a is the least effective.[6]

C3a, C4a, and C5a attach to specific receptors on neutrophils, basophils, mast cells, eosinophils, smooth muscle cells, and vascular endothelium.[4] C3a and C4a attach to the C3a receptor (C3aR), and C5a attaches to the C5a receptor (C5aR). When binding occurs on basophils and mast cells, histamine is released, thereby increasing vascular permeability and causing contraction of smooth muscles. C5a causes neutrophils to release hydrolytic enzymes, oxygen radicals, and prostaglandins, aiding in destruction of foreign antigens.[4,6]

C5a also serves as a chemotaxin for neutrophils, basophils, eosinophils, mast cells, monocytes, and dendritic cells. In this manner, these cells are directed to the source of antigen concentration. Because of increased vascular permeability, neutrophils migrate from blood vessels to the tissues and tend to aggregate.

Binding of C5a to monocytes causes them to undergo an oxidative burst that includes increased production of hydrolytic enzymes, neutrophil chemotactic factor, platelet activating factors, interleukin-1, and toxic oxygen metabolites.[13] Interleukin-1 is a protein that enhances T-cell activation. This may produce fever and an increase in acute phase reactants, both of which are characteristic of an inflammatory response.

As a means of localizing and controlling the effects of C3a, C4a, and C5a, these substances are rapidly inactivated by an enzyme in the plasma called *carboxypeptidase N*. C3a and C4a are cleaved in seconds, while conversion of C5a occurs more slowly.

The last major effect of complement-derived peptides is opsonization. C4b, C3b, and iC3b, which accumulate on cell membranes as complement activation proceeds, bind to specific receptors on erythrocytes, neutrophils, monocytes, and macrophages, as discussed earlier. This facilitates phagocytosis and clearance of foreign substances, and it is one of the key functions of the complement system. In addition, attachment of C3 products to an antigen has been found to enhance the B-cell response.

## COMPLEMENT AND DISEASE STATES

Although complement acts as a powerful weapon to combat infection by amplifying phagocytosis, in some cases it can actually contribute to tissue damage or death. Complement can be harmful if (1) activated systemically on a large scale as in gram-negative septicemia, (2) it is activated by tissue necrosis such as myocardial infarction, or (3) lysis of red cells occurs. In the case of septicemia due to a gram-negative organism, large quantities of C3a and C5a are generated, leading to neutrophil aggregation and clotting. Damage to the tiny pulmonary capillaries and interstitial pulmonary edema may result.[6]

Tissue injury following obstruction of the blood supply, such as occurs in myocardial infarction, or heart attack, can cause complement activation and deposition of membrane attack complexes on cell surfaces. Receptors for C3a and C5a have been found in coronary plaques, indicating that complement components may increase the damage to heart tissue.[26,27]

Lysis may be another end result of complement activation. Hemolytic diseases such as cold autoimmune hemolytic anemia are characterized by the presence of an autoantibody that binds at low temperatures. When these cells warm up, complement fixation results in lysis (see Chapter 14 for a more complete discussion of complement-mediated autoimmune diseases).

# COMPLEMENT DEFICIENCIES

## Major Pathway Components

Although excess activation of the complement system can result in disease states, lack of individual components also has a deleterious effect. Hereditary deficiency of any complement protein, with the exception of C9, usually manifests itself in increased susceptibility to infection and delayed clearance of immune complexes. Most of these conditions are inherited on an autosomal recessive gene, and they are quite rare, occurring in 0.03 percent of the general population.[26] The deficiency that occurs most often is that of C2, which is found in 1 in 20,000 individuals.[28–30] Recent evidence indicates that atherosclerosis may be related to a C2 deficiency.[28] Additionally, C2-deficient individuals may be more prone to recurrent streptococcal and staphylococcal infections.[28] The factor B locus is nearby, and often C2-deficient persons are reported to have decreases in factor B. Other types of complement deficiencies are less common.

A second deficiency that occurs with some frequency is that of mannose-binding lectin, found in 3 to 5 percent of the population. MBL is important during the interval between the loss of passively acquired maternal antibodies and the ability of infants to produce their own antibody.[10] Lack of MBL has been associated with pneumonia, sepsis, and meningococcal disease in infants.[15,17,18]

The most serious deficiency, however, is that of C3, because it is the key mediator in all pathways. Individuals with a C3 deficiency are prone to developing severe, recurrent life-threatening infections with encapsulated bacteria such as *Streptococcus pneumoniae* and may also be subject to immune complex diseases.[17] Such complexes can be lodged in the kidney and result in glomerulonephritis.[26,31]

It appears that a deficiency of any of the terminal components of the complement cascade (C5–C8) causes increased susceptibility to systemic *Neisseria* infections, including meningococcal meningitis and disseminated gonorrheal disease.[10,28] **Table 6–4** lists the complement components and the disease states associated with the absence of each individual factor.

## Regulatory Factor Components

A prime example of a disease due to a missing or defective regulatory component is **paroxysmal nocturnal hemoglobinuria (PNH).** Individuals with this disease have red blood cells that are deficient in DAF; hence, the cells are subject to lysis by means of the bystander effect once the complement system has been triggered. These individuals appear to have a deficiency in the glycophospholipid anchor of the DAF molecule that prevents its insertion into the cell membrane.[10,21] When C3b is deposited on erythrocytes because of activation of either pathway, the result is complement-mediated intravascular and extravascular hemolysis resulting in a chronic hemolytic anemia.

| Table 6-4. | Deficiencies of Complement Components |
|---|---|
| **DEFICIENT COMPONENT** | **ASSOCIATED DISEASE** |
| C1 (q, r, or s) | Lupuslike syndrome; recurrent infections |
| C2 | Lupuslike syndrome; recurrent infections; atherosclerosis |
| C3 | Severe recurrent infections; glomerlonephritis |
| C4 | Lupuslike syndrome |
| C5-C8 | *Neisseria* infections |
| C9 | No known disease association |
| C1INH | Hereditary angioedema |
| DAF | Paroxysmal nocturnal hemoglobinuria |
| MIRL | Paroxysmal nocturnal hemoglobinuria |
| Factor H or factor I | Recurrent pyogenic infections |
| MBL | Pneumococcal diseases, sepsis, *Neisseria* infections |
| Properdin | *Neisseria* infections |
| MASP-2 | Pneumococcal diseases |

C1INH – C1 inhibitor; DAF – decay accelerating factor; MIRL = membrane inhibitor of reactive lysis; MBL = mannose-binding lectin; MASP-2 = mannose-asociated serine protease.

Some studies indicate that a DAF deficiency is associated with a lack of CD59 (MIRL), and both are implicated in PNH.[17,32] CD59 has the same glycophospholipid anchor found in DAF, so the gene deficiency affects both molecules. As mentioned previously, CD59 prevents insertion of C9 into the cell membrane by binding to the C5b678 complex, thus inhibiting formation of transmembrane channels.[26] Therefore, the presence of both DAF and CD59 is important in protecting red blood cells against bystander lysis.

Recurrent attacks of angioedema that affect the extremities, the skin, the gastrointestinal tract, and other mucosal surfaces are characteristic of **hereditary angioedema.** This disease is caused by a deficiency or lack of C1INH, which occurs with a population frequency of 2 in 10,000.[17] Lack of C1INH results in excess cleavage of C4 and C2, keeping the classical pathway going and creating kinin-related proteins that increase vascular permeability. Thus, the response to a localized antigen is continued swelling or edema. The edema can be subcutaneous or within the bowel or upper-respiratory tract. Normally, this spontaneously subsides in 48 to72 hours, but if this occurs in the area of the oropharynx, life-threatening upper-airway obstruction may develop.[26]

The condition may be either hereditary or acquired. It is inherited as an autosomal dominant gene that codes for either a dysfunctional or an inactive protein. One normal gene does not produce enough inhibitor to keep up with the demand, and the condition is apparent in the heterozygous state. If the condition is hereditary, laboratory results indicate normal levels of C1q and C3 but reduced levels of C4 and C2.[30]

In contrast, individuals with an acquired C1INH deficiency show reduced levels of C1q because of excess activation of the classical cascade by antibody. This may result from a B-cell malignancy; presence of an autoimmune disease; or, in some rare instances, appearance of an autoantibody that binds to the active site of the C1 inhibitor.[14] In each instance, C1INH is present but quickly becomes depleted.

Other inhibitors for which there are genetic deficiencies include factors H and I. Lack of either component produces a constant turnover of C3 to the point of depletion. Recurrent bacterial infections may ensue.

## LABORATORY DETECTION OF COMPLEMENT ABNORMALITIES

Determining the levels of complement components can be a useful adjunct in diagnosing disease. Hereditary deficiencies can be identified, and much can be learned about inflammatory or autoimmune states by following the consumption of complement proteins. Techniques to determine complement abnormalities generally fall into two categories: (1) measurement of components as antigens in serum and (2) measurement of functional activity.[6] Many assays are not available in routine clinical laboratories and are restricted to research laboratories. Some of the more common assays will be discussed here.

### Immunologic Assays of Individual Components

The methods most frequently used to assay individual components include radial immunodiffusion (RID) and nephelometry.[17,26] Components that are usually measured and for which there are standardized reagents include C1q, C4, C3, C5, factor B, factor H, factor I, and C1 inhibitor. Kits are available for C3a, C4a, and C5a. Radial immunodiffusion uses agarose gel into which specific antibody is incorporated. Serum serves as the antigen and is placed in wells that are cut in the gel. Diffusion of the antigen from the well occurs in a circular pattern. The radius of the resulting circle can be related to antigen concentration (see Chapter 8 for further details on RID). This is a sensitive technique when performed correctly, but it takes at least 24 hours before test results are available.

Nephelometry measures concentration according to the amount of light scattered by a solution containing a reagent antibody and a measured patient sample (refer to Chapter 8 for more details on nephelometry). Generally, the more antigen–antibody complexes that are present, the more a beam of light will scatter as it passes through the solution. Such systems have a high degree of accuracy, results are available

quickly, and processing is easy because of the use of automation. However, it is necessary to purchase expensive equipment. Nephelometry and RID are both sensitive tests.[33]

None of the assays for individual components are able to distinguish whether the molecules are functionally active. Thus, although the preceding techniques give quantitative results and are relatively easy to perform, test results must be interpreted carefully.

### Assays for the Classical Pathway

Assays that measure lysis, the end point of complement activation, are functional tests that are frequently run in conjunction with testing of individual components. The **hemolytic titration (CH$_{50}$) assay** is most commonly used for this purpose.[17,26] This measures the amount of patient serum required to lyse 50 percent of a standardized concentration of antibody-sensitized sheep erythrocytes. Because all proteins from C1 to C9 are necessary for this to occur, absence of any one component will result in an abnormal CH$_{50}$, essentially reducing this number to zero.

The titer is expressed in CH$_{50}$ units, which is the reciprocal of the dilution that is able to lyse 50 percent of the sensitized cells.[6,17] The 50 percent point is used because this is when the change in lytic activity per unit change in complement is a maximum. Most labs need to establish their own normal values.

An additional CH$_{50}$ test has also been developed based on lysis of liposomes that release an enzyme when lysed. This can be read on an analyzer and is more accurate than traditional CH$_{50}$ testing.[26] However, lytic assays in general are complicated to perform and lack sensitivity. Individual labs must establish their own normal values. When the results are abnormal, the reasons cannot be determined. Such procedures are useful in establishing functional activity or lack thereof. Additional testing for individual components should be performed to follow up on any abnormality.

Lytic activity can also be measured by radial hemolysis in agarose plates. Rabbit red blood cells that have been sensitized with antibody are implanted in agarose, and patient serum is added to wells punched in the gel. Lysis appears as a clear zone around each well, and if complement standards are run, the size of the zone can be related to complement concentration.

ELISAs have been designed as another means of measuring activation of the classical pathway.[17,26,34] Solid-phase IgM attached to the walls of microtiter plates is used to initiate complement activation. Antihuman antibody to C9 conjugated to alkaline phosphatase is the indicator of complement activation. When a substrate is added, if any C9 is present and the antibody conjugate has attached, a color change will be evident. (Refer to Chapter 10 for a complete discussion of the principle of ELISA techniques.) This type of testing, which is very sensitive, is probably the best screen for complement abnormalities.[26] Additionally, split products that result from complement activation can also be detected by this same method. These products include C4a, C4d, C3a, and C5a, which are generated only if complement activation has occurred.

## Alternative Pathway Assays

Alternative pathway activation can be measured by several different means. An $AH_{50}$ can be performed in the same manner as the $CH_{50}$, except magnesium chloride and ethylene glycol tetraacetic acid are added to the buffer, and calcium is left out.[33] This buffer chelates calcium, which blocks classical pathway activation. Rabbit red cells are used as the indicator, because these provide an ideal surface for alternative pathway activation.

An additional means of testing for alternative pathway function is via ELISA. One such test can detect C3bBbP or C3bP complexes in very small quantities. Microtiter wells are typically coated with bacterial polysaccharide to trigger activation of the alternative pathway.

One test system has been developed that can determine the activity of all three pathways: the classical pathway, the alternative pathway, and the mannose-binding lectin pathway.[17,34] In this test system, strips used for the classical pathway are coated with IgM, strips for the alternative pathway are coated with lipopolysaccharide, and strips for the mannose-binding lectin pathway are coated with mannose. Such testing is easy to perform and is not dependent upon the use of animal erythrocytes, which may be hard to obtain. Deficiencies can be detected using the combined test results.

## Interpretation of Laboratory Findings

Decreased levels of complement components or activity may be due to any of the following: (1) decreased production, (2) consumption, or (3) in vitro consumption. The third condition must be ruled out before either of the other two is considered. Specimen handling is extremely important. Blood should be collected in a clot tube with no serum separator.[34] The tube should be spun down, and the serum should be frozen or placed on dry ice if it is not tested within 1 to 2 hours. If a specimen has been inadequately refrigerated, been subjected to multiple freeze–thaws, or been in prolonged storage, the results may be invalid, and the test needs to be repeated with a fresh specimen. Control serum should also be included with each batch of test sera.

A typical screening test for complement abnormalities usually includes determination of the following: C3, C4, and factor B levels, as well as hemolytic content.[17] Testing for products of complement activation such as C3a, C4a, C5a, and Ba as well as breakdown products, including C3dg, iC3b, and C4d, can also be performed as a means of monitoring inflammatory processes such as rheumatoid arthritis and systemic lupus erythematosus. **Table 6–5** presents some of the possible screening results from ELISA testing and correlates these with deficiencies of individual factors. An understanding of these patterns may be helpful in differentiating hereditary deficiencies from activational states

| Table 6–5. | Diagnosis of Complement Abnormalities | | |
|---|---|---|---|
| IMPAIRED FUNCTION/ DEFICIENCY | CLASSICAL PATHWAY | LECTIN PATHWAY | ALTERNATIVE PATHWAY |
| C1q, C1r, C1s | Low | Normal | Normal |
| C4, C2 | Low | Low | Normal |
| MBL, MASP2 | Normal | Low | Normal |
| B, D, P | Normal | Normal | Low |
| C3, C5, C6, C7, C8, C9 | Low | Low | Low |
| C1INH | Low | Low | Low |
| Factor H and I | Low | Low | Low |
| Improperly handled sera | Low | Low | Low |

Adapted from Seelen, MA, et al. An enzyme-linked immunosorbent assay-based method for functional analysis of the three pathways of the complement system. In Detrick, B, Hamilton, RG, and Folds, JD (eds): Manual of Molecular and Clinical Laboratory Immunology, ed. 7. ASM Press, Washington, D.C., 2006, p. 124.

that consume available complement components. Additional testing would be necessary, however, to actually pinpoint hereditary deficiencies.

## Complement Fixation Testing

Complement itself can actually be used as a reagent in the test known as *complement fixation*. Because complement fixation occurs after the binding of antigen and antibody, uptake of complement can be used as an indicator of the presence of either specific antigen or antibody. This technique has been used in the detection of viral, fungal, and rickettsial antibodies. The test involves a two-stage process: (1) a test system with antigen and antibody, one of which is unknown, and (2) an indicator system consisting of sheep red blood cells coated with hemolysin, which will lyse in the presence of complement.

To destroy any complement present, patient serum must be heated to 56°C for 30 minutes prior to testing. Then dilutions of the serum are combined with known antigen and a measured amount of guinea pig complement. Guinea pig complement can be used for testing, because complement is not species-specific. If patient antibody is present, it will combine with the reagent antigen, and complement will be bound. The test can also be performed with reagent antibody to detect the presence of antigen in the sample.

The second step involves adding sheep red blood cells that are coated with hemolysin. After an additional incubation, the tubes are centrifuged and then read for hemolysis. If hemolysis is present, this means that no patient antibody was present, and the test is negative. Lack of hemolysis is a positive test **(Fig. 6–10)**. Results are expressed as the highest dilution showing no hemolysis.

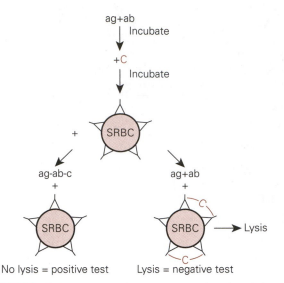

FIGURE 6–10. Patient serum and antigen are incubated, and then a measured amount of complement is added. After a second incubation, sheep red blood cells, which are coated with antibody, are added to the reaction tube. If patient antibody to the specific antigen is present, no hemolysis occurs. Lack of patient antibody allows the complement to combine with coated sheep red blood cells and lysis occurs.

The use of controls is extremely important to ensure the accuracy of test results. These include running known positive and negative sera, an antigen control, a patient serum control, a cell control, and a complement control. The antigen and patient serum controls test for the ability of complement to bind in the absence of antibody. These controls should show lysis with the sheep red blood cells. The cell control is a check on spontaneous lysis. Lysis should be absent or extremely low. The complement control tube should show lysis to indicate that the complement is working correctly. Due to the amount of manipulation required and the need for standardization and numerous controls, the use of complement fixation in the clinical laboratory is limited.

## SUMMARY

The complement system is a series of more than 30 proteins normally found in serum that play a major role in phagocytosis and clearance of foreign antigens from the body. While the end product of complement activation is lysis, other important events, such as opsonization, increase in vascular permeability, and chemotaxis of monocytes and neutrophils take place along the way to enhance host defense mechanisms. Most of the proteins of the complement system are inactive enzyme precursors, or zymogens, that are converted to active enzymes in a very precise order. One such means of activation is the classical pathway, which is triggered by antigen–antibody combination and involves nine of the proteins.

The alternative pathway acts as a natural means of defense against infection; it is triggered not by antigen–antibody combination but by the presence of microorganisms. The lectin pathway also involves nonspecific recognition of microorganisms by means of sugars such as mannose that are common constituents of microbial cell walls but that are distinct from those found on human cell surfaces. Although initial activation of these pathways involves proteins that are unique to each, C3 serves a major role in linking all three pathways. Cleavage of C3 to C3a and C3b represents one of the most significant steps in all pathways, because C3b is a powerful opsonin that greatly enhances phagocytosis. C3a is an anaphylatoxin that causes release of reactants from mast cells that amplify the inflammatory response. The end result is lysis of cells due to production of a membrane attack complex that drills holes in the cell membrane.

If activation of the complement system was to proceed uncontrolled, tissue damage and life-threatening systemic effects might result. Therefore, several proteins act as regulators to keep the reaction localized and ensure that infectious agents and not self-antigens are destroyed. Some of these are free-floating in the plasma, while others are found on cell surfaces as specific receptors.

One class of membrane receptors on host cells acts in conjunction with complement components to amplify the immune response. These receptors bind antigen–antibody complexes and facilitate phagocytosis. Other functions may include enhancing activity of phagocytes and production of increased memory B cells.

Complement plays a major role in several disease states. Decreased complement levels or a decline in lytic activity can indicate either hereditary deficiencies or extreme activation of the system. Paroxysmal nocturnal hemoglobinuria and hereditary angioedema are two conditions that result from missing or very low production of certain regulators. Deficiencies of some components, especially that of C3, may cause an increased risk of life-threatening infection or glomerulonephritis due to a lack of clearance of immune complexes.

Several laboratory assays have been devised to detect abnormal complement levels. One of these, the $CH_{50}$ hemolytic assay, uses 50 percent lysis of a standard concentration of antibody-sensitized sheep erythrocytes as an end point. This measures the presence of all proteins involved in the classical pathway. A similar assay, the $AH_{50}$ assay, measures the functioning of the alternative pathway. Other assays using RID or ELISA techniques measure levels of individual components. Proper handling of specimens is essential to ensure correct interpretation of laboratory testing.

Complement fixation tests use complement as a reagent to detect the presence of antigen or antibody. Antigen and antibody are allowed to combine with a measured amount of complement. Then indicator sheep red blood cells are added. These are coated with hemolysin (antisheep cell antibody), and if complement has not been tied up in the first reaction, then lysis of the cells occurs. Thus, lysis is a negative test, indicating that either antigen or antibody was not present. As in all complement testing, the use of standards and control is necessary for accurate results.

# CASE STUDIES

1. A 3-year-old child has a history of serious infections and is currently hospitalized with meningitis. The doctor suspects that he may have a complement deficiency and orders testing. The following results are obtained: decreased $CH_{50}$, normal C4 and C3 levels, and decreased radial hemolysis in agarose plates using a buffer that chelates calcium.

   Questions

   a. What do the results indicate about possible pathway(s) affected?

   b. Which component(s) are likely to be lacking?

   c. What sort of additional follow-up would be recommended?

2. A 25-year-old female appeared at the emergency room with symptoms of abdominal pain with severe vomiting and swelling of the legs and hands. She stated that she has had these symptoms on several previous occasions. After appendicitis was ruled out, a battery of tests, including some for abnormalities of complement components, was performed. The following results were obtained: red and white blood cell count normal, total serum protein normal, $CH_{50}$ decreased, alternative pathway function normal, C3 level normal, and C4 and C2 levels decreased.

   Questions

   a. What symptoms led physicians to consider a possible complement abnormality?

   b. What are possible reasons for a decrease in both C4 and C2?

   c. What other testing would confirm your suspicions?

# EXERCISE

## EZ COMPLEMENT CH$_{50}$ ASSAY

### Principle

Total hemolytic complement activity is measured by calculating the dilution of patient serum that is needed to lyse 50 percent of a standard concentration of optimally sensitized sheep red blood cells. Sheep erythrocytes have been previously sensitized with specific antibody. The value obtained is compared with those reported for a normal control. The degree of hemolysis is directly proportional to the total complement activity.

### Sample Preparation

Collect at least 2 mL of blood by venipuncture using sterile technique. Do not use any anticoagulants. Allow the blood to clot at room temperature. Separate the serum from the clot. If not used within a few hours, the serum can be aliquoted in 0.5 mL portions and quick-frozen at –70°C. Do not use plasma.

### Reagents, Materials, and Equipment

Sheep erythrocytes sensitized with antisheep antibody and preserved with sodium azide (Diamedix Corp., Miami, FL). These should be stored upright at 2°C to 8°C.

Complement reference serum (Diamedix or in-house controls)

High and low controls (Diamedix)

Pipette and disposable tips to dispense 5 μL

Centrifuge

Photometer that will read absorbance at 415 nm

> **CAUTION** The sensitized cells contain sodium azide. Azides are reported to react with lead and copper in plumbing to form compounds that may detonate on percussion. When disposing of solutions containing sodium azide, flush with large volumes of water to minimize the buildup of metal azide compounds.

### Procedure*

1. Reconstitute the standard with cold (2°C to 8°C) distilled water for immediate use. Discard any unused portion.

2. Reconstitute high and low controls with cold distilled water for immediate use. Discard the unused portion.

3. Place test tubes with sensitized cells in a rack and allow them to warm to room temperature. Set up one tube for each specimen, one for the reference serum, one each for the high and low controls, and one for the spontaneous lysis control. It is recommended that no more than 12 tubes be run at once.

4. Vortex tubes or shake vigorously for 10 seconds to resuspend cells.

5. Remove the stopper and transfer 5 μL of sample or standard into a tube. Replace the stopper and mix immediately by inverting the tube three to four times. The spontaneous lysis tube receives no sample but should also be mixed.

6. Allow tubes to stand at room temperature for 60 minutes.

7. Mix contents of all tubes again by inverting three to four times or by vortexing.

8. Centrifuge the tubes at approximately 1000 rpm for at least 5 minutes.

9. Read the absorbance of the supernatants at 415 nm within 15 minutes. If possible, read directly through the original tube, or use a photometer with a sipping device that can withdraw the supernatant without disturbing the sedimented cells.

   a. To read the absorbance, zero the photometer with a water blank.

   b. Read and record the absorbance of the spontaneous lysis control. If the absorbance value is greater than 0.1, the results of the assay will not be valid, and the test must be repeated with a new lot of sensitized cells.

   c. Zero the photometer again with the spontaneous lysis control. This will correct for any spontaneous lysis in test specimens.

   d. Read and record the absorbance value of the reference serum.

   e. Read and record the absorbance value of each test sample.

> **Note:** The volume of individual tubes is at the lowest limit of detection on Spectrometer 20 instruments used in many clinical laboratory science programs. An EZ Reader photometer designed specifically to read these tubes is available from Diamedix.

10. Calculate test results as follows: Divide the absorbance value of the supernate by the absorbance value of the reference serum and multiply by 100 to give the percent of reference.

---

* From the package insert for the EZ Complement CH$_{50}$ Assay by Diamedix Corporation, Miami, FL.

## Results

| Percent of Reference | Standard Complement Level |
|---|---|
| 0–50 | Absent or low |
| 51–150 | Normal |
| ≥150 | High |

## Interpretation of Results

This test will provide a quantitative value for the functional activity of total complement. It cannot identify the individual component or components that are abnormal. Abnormal specimens should be assayed for levels of each of the individual components of complement (C1–C9).

Depressed complement levels may be due to any of the following: genetic deficiencies; decreased complement synthesis accompanying liver disease; or fixation of complement due to chronic glomerulonephritis, rheumatoid arthritis, hemolytic anemias, graft rejection, SLE, or other autoimmune phenomena. Elevated levels are found in acute inflammatory conditions, leukemia, Hodgkin's disease, sarcoma, and Behçet's disease.

# REVIEW QUESTIONS

1. The classical complement pathway is activated by
   a. most viruses.
   b. antigen–antibody complexes.
   c. fungal cell walls.
   d. All of the above

2. All of the following are characteristic of complement components *except*
   a. normally present in serum.
   b. mainly synthesized in the liver.
   c. present as active enzymes.
   d. heat-labile.

3. All of the following are true of the recognition unit *except*
   a. it consists of C1q, C1r, and C1s.
   b. the subunits require calcium for binding together.
   c. binding occurs at the Fc region of antibody molecules.
   d. C1q becomes an active esterase.

4. Which is referred to as C3 convertase?
   a. C4b2a
   b. C3bBb
   c. iC3Bb
   d. All of the above

5. Mannose-binding protein in the lectin pathway is most similar to which classical pathway component?
   a. C3
   b. C1rs
   c. C1q
   d. C4

6. Which of the following describes the role of properdin in the alternative pathway?
   a. Stabilization of C3/C5 convertase
   b. Conversion of B to Bb
   c. Inhibition of C3 convertase formation
   d. Binding to the initiating antigen

7. Which best characterizes the membrane attack complex?
   a. Each pathway utilizes different factors to form it.
   b. C5 through C9 are not added in any particular order.
   c. One MAC unit is sufficient to lyse any type of cell.
   d. C9 polymerizes to form the transmembrane channel.

8. All of the following represent functions of the complement system *except*
   a. decreased clearance of antigen–antibody complexes.
   b. lysis of foreign cells.
   c. increase in vascular permeability.
   d. migration of neutrophils to the tissues.

9. Which of the following is true of the amplification loop in complement activation?
   a. It is found in the alternative pathway.
   b. iC3 binds factor B to generate amplification.
   c. C3b is the product that is increased.
   d. All of the above

10. Factor H acts by competing with which of the following for the same binding site?
    a. Factor B
    b. Factor D
    c. C3B
    d. Factor I

11. A lack of CR1 receptors on red blood cells would result in which of the following?
    a. Decreased binding of C3b to red blood cells
    b. Lack of clearance of immune complexes by the spleen
    c. Increased breakdown of C3b to C3d and C3dg
    d. All of the above

12. A lack of CR2 on cell membranes would result in which of the following?
    a. Decrease in hemolysis
    b. Increased susceptibility to infection
    c. Decreased antibody production
    d. Increase in antibody of the IgG class

13. Why is complement not activated with anti-Rh (D) antibodies?
    a. Rh antigens stimulate little antibody production.
    b. Rh antigens are too far apart on red blood cells.
    c. Rh antibodies are not capable of fixing complement.
    d. DAF protects red blood cells from buildup of antibody.

14. The $CH_{50}$ test measures which of the following?
    a. The dilution of patient serum required to lyse 50 percent of a standard concentration of sensitized sheep red blood cells
    b. Functioning of both the classical and alternative pathways
    c. Genetic deficiencies of any of the complement components
    d. All of the above

15. Which of the following would be most effective in preventing bystander lysis of red blood cells?
    a. C1INH
    b. Factor B
    c. DAF
    d. Factor H

**16.** Decreased $CH_{50}$ levels may be caused by

  a. inadequate refrigeration of specimen.
  b. coagulation-associated complement consumption.
  c. autoimmune disease process.
  d. All of the above

# References

1. Kindt, TJ, Goldsby, RA, and Osborne, BA. Kuby Immunology, ed. 6. WH Freeman and Co., New York, 2007, pp. 168–188.
2. Prodinger, WM, et al. Complement. In Paul, WE (ed): Fundamental Immunology, ed. 4. Lippincott-Raven, Philadelphia, 1999, pp. 967–995.
3. Mak, T, and Saunders, M. The Immune Response: Basic and Clinical Principles. Elsevier, Burlington, MA, 2004, pp. 553–581.
4. Carroll, MC. The complement system in regulation of adaptive immunity. Nat Immunol 5:981–986, 2004.
5. Pillemer, L, et al. The properdin system and immunity: Demonstration and isolation of a new serum protein, properdin, and its role in immune phenomena. Science 120:279, 1954.
6. Massey, HD, and Mcpherson, RA. Mediators of inflammation: Complement, cytokines, and adhesion molecules. In McPherson, RA, and Pincus, MR (ed): Henry's Clinical Diagnosis and Management by Laboratory Methods, ed. 21. Saunders Elsevier, Philadelphia, 2007, pp. 850–875.
7. Arlaud, GJ, Barlow, PN, Gaboriaud, C, Gross, P, et al. Deciphering complement mechanisms: The contributions of structural biology. Mol Immunol 44:3809–3822, 2007.
8. Xu, Y, Narayana, SVL, and Volanakis, JE. Structural biology of the alternative pathway convertase. Immunol Rev 180:123–135, 2001.
9. Janssen, BJC, Christodoulidou, A, McCarthy, A, Lambris, JD, et al. Structure of C3b reveals conformational changes that underlie complement activity. Nature 444:213–216, 2006.
10. Walport, MJ. Complement. Part I. New Engl J Med 344:1058–1066, 2001.
11. Mollnes, TE, Song, WC, and Lambris, JD. Complement in inflammatory tissue damage and disease. Trends Immunol 23:61–64, 2002.
12. Schwaeble, WJ, and Reid, KBM. Does properdin crosslink the cellular and the humoral response? Immunol Today 20:17–21, 1999.
13. Rawal, N, and Pangburn, MK. Structure/function of C5 convertases of complement. Int Immunopharmacol 1:415–422, 2001.
14. Medzhitov, R, and Janeway, C. Innate immunity. New Engl J Med 343:338–43, 2000.
15. Eisen, DP, and Minchinton, RM. Impact of mannose-binding lection on susceptibility to infectious diseases. CID 37:1496–1505, 2003.
16. Arnold, JN, Dwek, RA, Rudd, PM, and Sim, RB. Mannan binding lectin and its interaction with immunoglobulins in health and in disease. Immunol Lett 106:103–110, 2006.
17. Mollnes, TE, Jokiranta, TS, Truedsson, L, Nilsson, B, et al. Complement analysis in the 21st century. Mol Immunol 44:3838–3849, 2007.
18. Frakking, FNJ, Brouwer, N, van Eijkelenburg, NKA, Merkus, MP, et al. Low mannose-binding lectin (MBL) levels in neonates with pneumonia and sepsis. Clin Exp Immunol 150:255–262, 2007.
19. Kerr, FK, Thomas, AR, Wijeyewickrema, LC, Whisstock, JC, et al. Elucidation of the substrate specificity of the MASP-2 protease of the lectin complement pathway and identification of the enzyme as a major physiological target of the serpin, C1-inhibitor. Mol Immunol 45:670–677, 2008.
20. Smith, BO, Mallin, RL, Krych-HGoldberg, M, Wang, X, et al. Structure of the C3b binding site of CR1 (CD35), the immune adherence receptor. Cell 108:769–780, 2002.
21. Carroll, MC, and Fischer, MB. Complement and the immune response. Curr Opin Immunol 9:64–69, 1997.
22. Lubin, DM, and Atkinson, J. Decay-accelerating factor: Biochemistry, molecular biology, and function. Adv Immunol 7:35, 1989.
23. DiScipio, RG. Ultrastructures and interactions of complement factors H and I. J Immunol 149:2592, 1993.
24. Sun, X, et al. Role of decay-accelerating factor in regulating complement activation on the erythrocyte surface as revealed by gene targeting. Proc Natl Acad Sci, USA 96:628–633, 1999.
25. Kozono, Y, et al. Cross-linking CD21/CD35 or CD19 increases both B7–1 and B7–2 expression on murine splenic B cells. J Immunol 160:1565–1572, 1998.
26. Wen, L, Atkinson, JP, and Giclas, PC. Clinical and laboratory evaluation of complement deficiency. J Allergy Clin Immunol 113:585–593, 2004.
27. Oksjoki, R, Laine, P, Helske, S, Vehmaan-Kreula, P, et al. Receptors for the anaphylatoxins C3a and C5a are expressed in human atherosclerotic coronary plaques. Atherosclerosis 195:90–99, 2007.
28. Sjoholm, AG, Jonsson, G, Braconier, JH, Sturfelt, G, et al. Complement deficiency and disease: An update. Mol Immunol 43:78–85, 2006.
29. Pickering, MC, Botto, M, Taylor, PR, Lachmann, et al. Systemic lupus erythematosus, complement deficiency, and apoptosis. Adv Immunol 76:227–324, 2000.
30. Lewis, MJ, and Botto, M. Complement deficiencies in humans and animals: Links to autoimmunity. Autoimmunity 39:367–378, 2006.
31. Hughes, J, et al. C5-C9 membrane attack complex mediates endothelial cell apoptosis in experimental glomerulonephritis. Am J Physiol Renal Physiol 278:F747–57, 2000.
32. Song, WC. Complement regulatory proteins and autoimmunity. Autoimmunity 39:403–410, 2006.
33. Giclas, PC. Analysis of complement in the clinical laboratory. In Detrick, B, Hamilton, RG, and Folds, JD (eds): Manual of Molecular and Clinical Laboratory Immunology, ed. 7. ASM Press, Washington, D.C., 2006, pp. 115–117.
34. Seelen, MA, Roos, A, Wieslander, J, and Daha, MR. An enzyme-linked immunosorbent assay-based method for functional analysis of the three pathways of the complement system. In Detrick, B, Hamilton, RG, and Folds, JD (eds): Manual of Molecular and Clinical Laboratory Immunology, ed. 7. ASM Press, Washington, D.C., 2006, pp. 124–127.

# Basic Immunological Procedures

# 7 Safety and Specimen Preparation

*Susan K. Strasinger, DA, MT (ASCP) and Christine Stevens*

## LEARNING OBJECTIVES

*After finishing this chapter, the reader will be able to:*

1. List the components of the chain of infection and the safety precautions that will break the chain.
2. Correctly perform routine handwashing.
3. Describe the types of personal protective equipment used by laboratory personnel.
4. Differentiate between universal precautions, body substance isolation, and standard precautions.
5. Describe the acceptable methods for disposal of biological waste in the laboratory.
6. Following federal regulations and guidelines, prepare patient specimens for transport.
7. Safely dispose of sharp objects.
8. Describe the components of the Occupational Exposure to Bloodborne Pathogens Standard.
9. Describe safety precautions utilized when handling chemicals.
10. Discuss the components of chemical hygiene plans.
11. Identify the symbol for radiation.
12. Describe the following: serial dilution, solute, diluent, compound dilution.
13. Explain how an antibody titer is determined.
14. Calculate the amount of diluent needed to prepare a specific dilution of a serum specimen.

## KEY TERMS

___ Biohazardous
___ Body substance isolation
___ Chain of infection
___ Chemical Hygiene Plan
___ Diluent
___ Material safety data sheets
___ Occupational Safety and Health Administration (OSHA)
___ Personal protective equipment
___ Postexposure prophylaxis
___ Serial dilution
___ Solute
___ Standard precautions
___ Titer
___ Universal precautions

# CHAPTER OUTLINE

The clinical laboratory contains a wide variety of safety hazards, many capable of producing serious injury or life-threatening disease. To work safely in this environment, clinical laboratorians must learn what hazards exist and the basic safety precautions associated with them, and they must apply the basic rules of common sense required for everyday safety. Some hazards are unique to the health-care environment, and others are encountered routinely throughout life **(Table 7–1)**.

## BIOLOGICAL HAZARDS

In the immunology laboratory, the most significant hazard exists in obtaining and testing patient specimens. An understanding of the transmission—the **chain of infection**—of microorganisms is necessary to prevent infection. The chain of infection requires a continuous link between three elements: a source, a method of transmission, and a susceptible host. The most likely source of infection in serological testing is through contact with patient specimens, and the main concern is exposure to viruses such as the hepatitis viruses and human immunodeficiency virus (HIV). Therefore, safety precautions are designed to protect health-care workers from exposure to potentially harmful infectious agents. The ultimate goal of biological safety is to prevent completion of the chain by preventing transmission. **Figure 7–1** contains the universal symbol for **biohazardous** material and illustrates the chain of infection and how it can be broken by following safety practices.

Preventing the transmission of microorganisms from infected sources to susceptible hosts is critical in controlling the spread of infection. Procedures used to prevent microorganism transmission include handwashing, wearing **personal protective equipment (PPE),** isolating highly infective or highly susceptible patients, and properly disposing contaminated materials. Strict adherence to guidelines published by the Centers for Disease Control and Prevention (CDC) and the **Occupational Safety and Health Administration (OSHA)** is essential.

| Table 7–1. | Types of Safety Hazards | |
|---|---|---|
| **TYPE** | **SOURCE** | **POSSIBLE INJURY** |
| Biologic | Infectious agents | Bacterial, fungal, viral, or parasitic infections |
| Sharp | Needles, lancets, and broken glass | Cuts, punctures, or bloodborne pathogen exposure |
| Chemical | Preservatives and reagents | Exposure to toxic, carcinogenic, or caustic agents |
| Radioactive | Equipment and radioisotopes | Radiation exposure |
| Electrical | Ungrounded or wet equipment and frayed cords | Burns or shock |
| Fire/explosive | Bunsen burners and organic chemicals | Burns or dismemberment |
| Physical | Wet floors, heavy boxes, and patients | Falls, sprains, or strains |

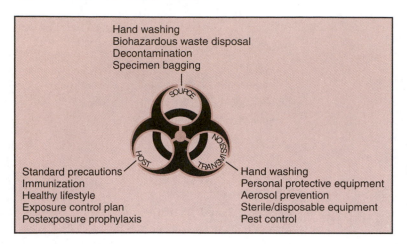

FIGURE 7-1. Chain of infection and safety practices related to the biohazard symbol. *(From Strasinger, SK, and DiLorenzo, MS. Urinalysis and Body Fluids, ed. 5. FA Davis, Philadelphia, 2008, with permission.)*

## Handwashing

Hand contact represents the number-one method of infection transmission. Hands should always be washed at the following times: before patient contact, when gloves are removed, prior to leaving the work area, whenever the hands have been knowingly contaminated, before going to designated break areas, and before and after using bathroom facilities. Correct routine handwashing technique includes the following:[1]

1. Wet hands with warm water.
2. Apply soap, preferably antimicrobial.
3. Rub to form a lather, create friction, and loosen debris.
4. Clean thoroughly between fingers, thumbs, and under fingernails and rings for at least 15 seconds and up to the wrist.
5. Rinse hands in a downward position.
6. Dry hands with a paper towel.
7. Turn off faucets with a clean paper towel to prevent recontamination.

## Personal Protective Equipment

Personal protective equipment encountered by laboratorians includes gloves, gowns or laboratory coats, masks, goggles, face shields, and Plexiglas countertop shields. Gloves are worn to protect the health-care worker's hands from contamination by patient body substances and to protect the patient from possible microorganisms on the health-care worker's hands. Wearing gloves is not a substitute for handwashing. Hands must always be washed when gloves are removed. A variety of gloves are available, including sterile and nonsterile, powdered and unpowdered, and latex and nonlatex.

Allergy to latex is increasing among health-care workers. Laboratorians should be alert for symptoms of reactions associated with latex contact, including irritant contact dermatitis that produces patches of dry, itchy irritation on the hands; delayed hypersensitivity reactions resembling poison ivy that appear 24 to 48 hours following exposure; and true immediate hypersensitivity reactions often characterized by facial flushing and respiratory difficulty (see Chapter 14). Handwashing immediately after removal of gloves and avoiding powdered gloves may aid in preventing the development of latex allergy. Replacing latex gloves with nitrile or vinyl gloves provides an acceptable alternative. Any signs of a latex reaction should be reported to a supervisor, as true latex allergy can be life-threatening.[2]

In the immunology laboratory, fluid-resistant laboratory coats with wrist cuffs are worn to protect skin and clothing from contamination by patient specimens. Coats are worn at all times when working with patient specimens. They must be completely buttoned with gloves pulled over the cuffs. Both gloves and laboratory coats should be changed as soon as possible if they become visibly soiled, and they must be removed when leaving the laboratory.

The mucous membranes of the eyes, nose, and mouth must be protected from specimen splashes and aerosols. A variety of protective equipment is available, including goggles, full-face plastic shields, and Plexiglas countertop shields (**Fig. 7–2**). Particular care should be taken to avoid splashes and aerosols when removing container tops and when transferring and centrifuging specimens. Never centrifuge specimens in uncapped tubes or in uncovered centrifuges. When specimens are received in containers with contaminated exteriors, the exterior of the container must be disinfected or, if necessary, a new specimen may be requested.

## Procedure Precautions

**Universal precautions (UP)** were instituted by the CDC in 1985 to protect health-care workers from exposure to bloodborne pathogens, primarily hepatitis B virus (HBV) and HIV. Under universal precautions, all patients are assumed to be possible carriers of bloodborne pathogens. Transmission may occur by skin puncture from a contaminated sharp object or by passive contact through open skin

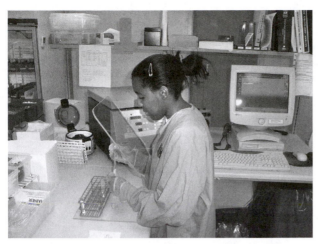

FIGURE 7–2. *Personal protective equipment. (From Strasinger, SK, and DiLorenzo, MA. Phlebotomy Workbook for the Multiskilled Healthcare Professional, ed. 2. FA Davis, Philadelphia, 2003, with permission.)*

lesions or mucous membranes. The guideline recommends wearing gloves when collecting or handling blood and body fluids contaminated with blood, wearing face shields when there is danger of blood splashing on mucous membranes, and disposing of all needles and sharp objects in puncture-resistant containers without recapping.

A modification of universal precautions, **body substance isolation (BSI)** is not limited to bloodborne pathogens and considers all body fluids and moist body substances to be potentially infectious. Personnel should wear gloves at all times when encountering moist body substances. A disadvantage of the BSI guideline is that it does not recommend handwashing after removing gloves unless visual contamination is present.

The major features of UP and BSI have now been combined and are called **standard precautions.** Standard precautions should be used for the care of all patients and include the following:[3]

**Handwashing.** Wash hands after touching blood, body fluids, secretions, excretions, and contaminated items, whether or not gloves are worn. Wash hands immediately after gloves are removed, between patient contacts, and when otherwise indicated to avoid transfer of microorganisms to other patients or environments. It may be necessary to wash hands between tasks and procedures on the same patient to prevent cross-contamination of different body sites.

**Gloves.** Wear gloves (clean, nonsterile gloves are adequate) when touching blood, body fluids, secretions, excretions, and contaminated items. Change gloves between tasks and procedures on the same patient after contact with material that may contain a high concentration of microorganisms. Remove gloves promptly after use, before touching noncontaminated items and environmental surfaces, and before going to another patient. Wash hands immediately to avoid transfer of microorganisms to other patients or environments.

**Mask, Eye Protection, and Face Shield.** Wear a mask and eye protection or a face shield to protect mucous membranes of the eyes, nose, and mouth during procedures and patient-care activities that are likely to generate splashes or sprays of blood, body fluids, secretions, and excretions.

**Gown.** Wear a gown (a clean, nonsterile gown is adequate) to protect skin and to prevent soiling of clothing during procedures and patient-care activities that are likely to generate splashes of blood, body fluids, secretions, or excretions. Select a gown that is appropriate for the activity and amount of fluid likely to be encountered. Remove a soiled gown as promptly as possible, and wash hands to avoid transfer of microorganisms to other patients or environments.

**Patient-Care Equipment.** Handle used patient-care equipment soiled with blood, body fluids, secretions, and excretions in a manner that prevents skin and mucous membrane exposures, contamination of clothing, and transfer of microorganisms to other patients and environments. Ensure that reusable equipment is not used for the care of another patient until it has been cleaned and reprocessed appropriately. Ensure that single-use items are discarded properly.

**Environmental Control.** Ensure that the hospital has adequate procedures for the routine care, cleaning, and disinfection of environmental surfaces, beds, bed rails, bedside equipment, and other frequently touched surfaces, and ensure that these procedures are being followed.

**Linen.** Handle, transport, and process used linen soiled with blood, body fluids, secretions, and excretions in a manner that prevents skin and mucous membrane exposure and contamination of clothing and that avoids transfer of microorganisms to other patients and environments.

**Occupational Health and Bloodborne Pathogens.** Take care to prevent injuries when using needles, scalpels, and other sharp instruments or when handling sharp instruments after procedures; when cleaning used instruments; and when disposing of used needles. Never recap used needles or otherwise manipulate them using both hands, and never use any technique that involves directing the point of a needle toward any part of the body; rather, use either a one-handed "scoop" technique or a mechanical device designed for holding the needle sheath. Do not remove used needles from disposable syringes by hand, and do not bend, break, or otherwise manipulate used needles by hand. Place used disposable syringes and needles, scalpel blades, and other sharp items in appropriate puncture-resistant containers, which are located as close as practical to the area in which the items were used. Place reusable syringes and needles in a puncture-resistant container for transport to the reprocessing area.

**Patient Placement.** Place a patient who contaminates the environment or who does not (or cannot be expected to) assist in maintaining appropriate hygiene or environmental control in a private room. If a private room is not available, consult with infection-control professionals regarding patient placement or other alternatives.

## Biological Waste Disposal

All biological waste, except urine, must be placed in appropriate containers labeled with the biohazard symbol. This includes not only specimens, but also the materials with which the specimens come in contact. Any supplies contaminated with blood and body fluids must also be disposed of in containers clearly marked with the biohazard symbol or with red or yellow color-coding. This includes alcohol pads, gauze, bandages, disposable tourniquets, gloves, masks, gowns, and plastic tubes and pipettes. Disposal of needles and other sharp objects is discussed in the next section.

Contaminated nondisposable equipment, blood spills, and blood and body fluid processing areas must be disinfected. The most commonly used disinfectant is a 1:10 dilution of sodium hypochlorite (household bleach) prepared weekly and stored in a plastic, not a glass, bottle. The bleach should be allowed to air-dry on the contaminated area prior to removal. The National Committee for Clinical Laboratory Standards (NCCLS) states that a 1:100 dilution can be used for routine cleaning.[4]

## Transporting Patient Specimens

Depending on the scope of testing performed in an immunology laboratory, transporting and receiving patient specimens must be considered. Therefore, regulations for packaging and labeling developed by the U.S. Department of Transportation (DOT), the International Air Transport Association (IATA), and the United Nations must be followed.

### Courier-Delivered Specimen Transport

Specimens transported by a hospital courier among clinics, physicians' offices, and the hospital laboratory are exempt from most DOT rules unless they are suspected of containing an infectious substance. The transport vehicle should be used exclusively for transport of these materials and should be equipped to secure the transport containers.[5] Minimum shipping standards for this type of transportation include[6]

1. Leak-proof, water-tight specimen containers.
2. Tightly capped tubes placed in a rack to maintain an upright position.
3. Leak-proof inner packaging surrounded by enough absorbent material to completely absorb all the liquid present.
4. A leak-proof plastic or metal transport box with a secure, tight-fitting cover.
5. Properly labeled transport boxes accompanied by specimen data and identification forms.

Specimens picked up by a courier that are to be shipped to an out-of-the-area laboratory, such as a reference laboratory, must follow DOT regulations. Many of these laboratories supply shipping containers to their clients.

### DOT and IATA Specimen Transport

Under DOT and IATA regulations, all diagnostic specimens require triple packaging (**Fig. 7–3**). This includes the following:

1. Watertight primary containers made of glass, metal, or plastic with a positive (screw-on) cap.
2. The primary container must be wrapped with enough absorbent material to be capable of absorbing all of its contents. Multiple specimens must be wrapped individually prior to placing them in the leak-proof secondary container.
3. The secondary container is placed in a sturdy outer container made of corrugated fiberboard, wood, metal, or rigid plastic. An itemized list of contents in a sealed plastic bag is also placed in the outer container. Ice packs are placed between the secondary and the outer container. Additional measures must be taken when using ice and dry ice.

In January 2007, labeling of the outer container changed. The terms *clinical specimen* and *diagnostic specimen* have been replaced with *biological substances, Category B*. This wording is placed next to the label UN 3373.[7,8]

## SHARPS HAZARDS

Sharp objects in the laboratory, including needles, lancets, and broken glassware, present a serious biological hazard for possible exposure to bloodborne pathogens caused by accidental puncture. Although bloodborne pathogens are also transmitted through contact with mucous membranes and nonintact skin, a needle or lancet used to collect blood has the capability to produce a very significant exposure to bloodborne pathogens. It is essential that safety precautions be followed at all times when sharp hazards are present.

The number-one personal safety rule when handling needles is to *never* manually recap one. Many safety devices are available for needle disposal, and they provide a variety of safeguards. These include needle holders that become a sheath, needles that automatically resheath or become blunt, and needles with attached sheathes. All sharps must be disposed of in puncture-resistant, leak-proof containers labeled with the biohazard symbol (**Fig. 7–4**). Containers should be located in close proximity to the work area and must always be replaced when the safe capacity mark is reached.

### Government Regulations

The federal government has enacted regulations to protect health-care workers from exposure to bloodborne pathogens. These regulations are monitored and enforced by OSHA. The Occupational Exposure to Bloodborne Pathogens Standard became law in 1991.[9] It requires all employers to have a written Bloodborne Pathogen Exposure Control Plan and to provide necessary protection, free of

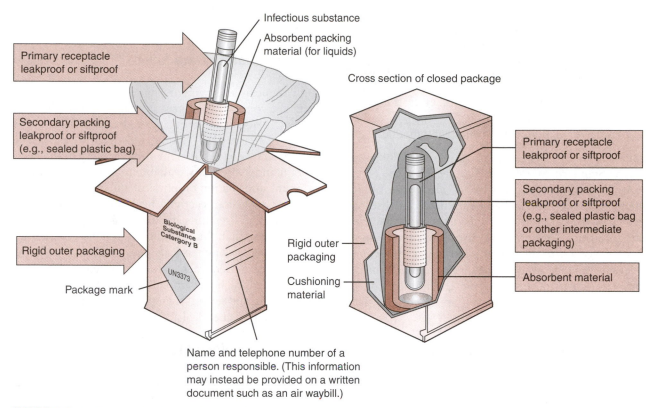

**FIGURE 7–3.** Packing and labeling of Category B infectious substances.

†If multiple fragile primary receptacles are placed in a single secondary package, they must be either individually wrapped or separated to prevent contact. *(From Pipeline and Hazardous Materials Safety Administration, U.S. Department of Transportation.)*

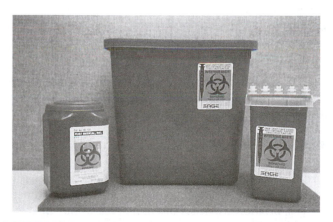

**FIGURE 7–4.** Examples of puncture-resistant containers. *(From Strasinger, SK, and DiLorenzo, MA. Phlebotomy Workbook for the Multiskilled Healthcare Professional, ed. 2. FA Davis, Philadelphia, 2003, with permission.)*

charge, for employees. Specifics of the OSHA standard include the following:

1. Requiring all employees to practice universal (standard) precautions.
2. Providing lab coats, gowns, face shields, and gloves to employees and providing laundry facilities for non disposable protective clothing.
3. Providing sharps disposal containers and prohibiting recapping of needles.
4. Prohibiting eating, drinking, smoking, and applying cosmetics in the work area.
5. Labeling all biohazardous materials and containers.
6. Providing immunization for the hepatitis B virus free of charge.
7. Establishing a daily work surface disinfection protocol. The disinfectant of choice for bloodborne pathogens is sodium hypochlorite (household bleach freshly diluted 1:10).
8. Providing medical follow-up to employees who have been accidentally exposed to bloodborne pathogens.
9. Documenting regular training of employees in safety standards.

The exposure control plan must be available to employees. It must be updated annually and must identify procedures and individuals at risk of exposure to bloodborne pathogens. The plan must also identify the engineering controls (i.e., sharps containers) and the procedures in place to prevent exposure incidents.

In 1999, OSHA issued a new compliance directive called Enforcement Procedures for the Occupational Exposure to Bloodborne Pathogens Standard.[10] The new directive placed more emphasis on using engineering controls to prevent accidental exposure to bloodborne pathogens. Additional changes to the directive were mandated by passage of the Needlestick Safety and Prevention Act, signed into law in 2001.[11] Under this law, employers must

1. Document their evaluations and implementation of safer needle devices.
2. Involve employees in the selection and evaluation of new devices.
3. Maintain a log of all injuries from contaminated sharps.

In June 2002, OSHA issued a revision to the Bloodborne Pathogens Standard compliance directive.[12] In the revised directive, the agency requires that all blood holders (adapters) with needles attached be immediately discarded into a sharps container after the device's safety feature is activated. Rationale for the new directive is based on the exposure of workers to the unprotected stopper-puncturing end of evacuated tube needles, the increased needle manipulation required to remove it from the holder, and the possible worker exposure from the use of contaminated holders.

## Occupational Exposure to Bloodborne Pathogens

Any accidental exposure to blood through needlestick, mucous membranes, or nonintact skin must be reported to a supervisor, and a confidential medical examination must be immediately started. Evaluation of the incident must begin right away to ensure appropriate **postexposure prophylaxis (PEP)**. Needlesticks are the most frequently encountered exposure and place the laboratorian in danger of contracting HIV, HBV, and hepatitis C virus (HCV). Each health-care institution is responsible for designing and implementing its own exposure control plan.[13]

## CHEMICAL HAZARDS

### General Precautions

Serological testing may involve use of chemical reagents that must be handled in a safe manner to avoid injury. General rules for safe handling of chemicals include taking precautions to avoid getting chemicals on your body, clothes, and work area; wearing PPE such as safety goggles when pouring chemicals; observing strict labeling practices; and following instructions carefully. Preparing reagents under a fume hood is also a recommended safety precaution. Chemicals should never be mixed together, unless specific instructions are followed, and they must be added in the order specified. This is particularly important when combining acid and water, as acid should always be added to water to avoid the possibility of sudden splashing.

When skin or eye contact occurs, the best first aid is to immediately flush the area with water for at least 15 minutes and then seek medical attention. Laboratorians must know the location of the emergency shower and eyewash station in the laboratory. Do not try to neutralize chemicals spilled on the skin.

## Material Safety Data Sheets

All chemicals and reagents containing hazardous ingredients in a concentration greater than 1 percent are required to have a **material safety data sheet (MSDS)** on file in the work area. By law, vendors must provide these sheets to purchasers; however, it is the responsibility of the facility to obtain and keep them available to employees. An MSDS contains information on physical and chemical characteristics, fire, explosion reactivity, health hazards, primary routes of entry, exposure limits and carcinogenic potential, precautions for safe handling, spill cleanup, and emergency first aid. Containers of chemicals that pose a high risk must be labeled with a chemical hazard symbol representing the possible hazard, such as flammable, poisonous, corrosive, and so on. State and federal regulations should be consulted for the disposal of chemicals.

## Chemical Hygiene Plan

OSHA requires that all facilities that use hazardous chemicals have a written **Chemical Hygiene Plan** available to employees.[14] The purpose of the plan is to detail the following:

1. Appropriate work practices
2. Standard operating procedures
3. Personal protective equipment
4. Engineering controls, such as fume hoods and flammables safety cabinets
5. Employee training requirements
6. Medical consultation guidelines

Each facility must appoint a chemical hygiene officer, who is responsible for implementing and documenting compliance with the plan. Examples of chemical safety equipment and information are shown in **Figure 7–5**.

## Chemical Waste Disposal

Hazardous chemical waste should be disposed of per current EPA regulations. Local regulations and the Department of Transportation also track disposal of hazardous chemical waste. Many kits used in testing contain sodium azide, which can be disposed of by flushing down the drain with plenty of water to avoid buildup in plumbing.

## RADIOACTIVE HAZARDS

### General Precautions

Radioactivity is encountered in the clinical laboratory when procedures using radioisotopes, such as radioimmunoassay, are performed. The amount of radioactivity present in most medical situations is very small and represents little danger.

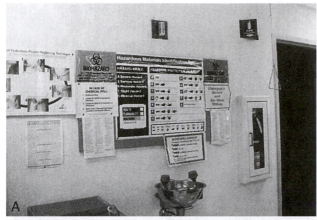

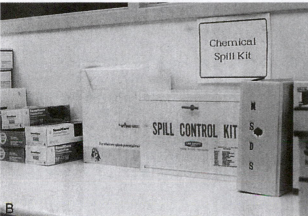

FIGURE 7–5. Examples of chemical safety equipment and information. *(From Strasinger, SK, and DiLorenzo, MA. Urinalysis and Body Fluids, ed. 4. FA Davis, Philadelphia, 2001, with permission.)*

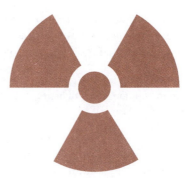

FIGURE 7–6. Radioactive symbol.

However, the effects of radiation are related to the length of exposure and are cumulative. Exposure to radiation is dependent on the combination of time, distance, and shielding. Persons working in a radioactive environment are required to wear measuring devices to determine the amount of radiation they are accumulating.

Laboratorians should be familiar with the radioactive symbol shown in **Figure 7–6.** This symbol must be displayed on the doors of all areas where radioactive material is present. Exposure to radiation during pregnancy presents a danger to the fetus, and personnel who are or who think they may be pregnant should avoid areas with this symbol.

## Radioactive Waste Disposal

Disposal of radioactive waste is regulated by the Nuclear Regulatory Commission (NRC). Such waste must be separated from other waste materials in the laboratory and may be disposed of by storing in a locked, labeled room until the background count is reduced by a specified number of half-lives. Typically, $^{125}$I is the most frequently encountered radiolabel, and this can be disposed of in this manner.

## SEROLOGICAL TESTING

### Specimen Preparation and Processing

The most frequently encountered specimen in immunological testing is serum. Blood is collected aseptically by venipuncture into a clean, dry, sterile tube. Care must be taken to avoid hemolysis, since this may produce a false-positive test. The blood specimen is allowed to clot at room temperature or at 4°C and then centrifuged. Serum should be promptly separated into another tube without transferring any cellular elements. Fresh, nonheat inactivated serum is usually recommended for testing. However, if testing cannot be performed immediately, serum may be stored between 2°C and 8°C for up to 72 hours. If there is any additional delay in testing, the serum should be frozen at –20°C or below.

### Simple Dilutions

For many tests, a measured amount of a serum sample is used directly for detection of antibodies. However, in order for a visible end point to occur in a serological reaction, the relative proportions of antigen and antibody present are important. Sometimes in a serological test, too much antibody may be present, and an end point may not be reached. In this case, serum that contains antibody must be diluted. Therefore, knowledge of **serial dilutions** is essential to understanding all serological testing in the clinical laboratory.

A dilution involves two entities: the **solute,** which is the material being diluted, and the **diluent,** which is the medium making up the rest of the solution. The relationship between these two is expressed as a fraction. For example, a 1:20 dilution implies 1 part of solute and 19 parts of diluent. The number on the bottom of the fraction is the total volume, reached by adding the volumes of the solute and diluent together.

$$1/\text{Dilution} = \text{Amount of Solute/Total Volume}$$

To create a certain volume of a specified dilution, it is helpful to know how to manipulate this relationship. An algebraic equation can be set up to find the total volume, the amount of solute, or the amount of diluent needed to make a dilution. Consider the following example:

> 2 mL of a 1:20 dilution is needed to run a specific serological test. How much serum and how much diluent are needed to make this dilution?

The equation is set up using the fraction for the dilution, indicating the relationship between the total volume and the solute, or the amount of serum needed:

$$1/20 = x/2 \text{ mL}$$

Note that the 20 represents the total number of parts in the solution and that 2 mL is the total volume desired.

Solving this equation for $x$ gives 0.1 mL for the amount of serum needed to make this dilution. The amount of diluent is obtained by subtracting 0.1 mL from 2.0 mL to give 1.9 mL of diluent. To check the answer, simply set up a proportion between the amount of solute over the total volume. This should equal the dilution desired. Thus, the correct answer has been obtained.

If, on the other hand, one knows the amount of serum to be used, a problem can be set up in the following manner:

> A 1:5 dilution of patient serum is necessary to run a serological test. There is 0.1 mL of serum that can be used. What amount of diluent is necessary to make this dilution using all of the serum?

A slightly different formula can be used to solve this problem:

$$1/\text{Dilution} - 1 = \text{Amount of Solute/Amount of Diluent}$$

$$\tfrac{1}{4} = 0.1 \text{ mL}/x$$
$$x = 0.4 \text{ mL of diluent}$$

Note that the final volume is obtained by adding 0.1 mL of solute to the 0.4 mL of diluent. Dividing the volume of the solute by the total volume of 0.5 mL yields the desired 1:5 ratio.

Depending on the unknown being solved for, either of these formulas can be used. To calculate the total volume, the total dilution factor must be used. If, however, the amount of diluent is to be calculated, the formula using dilution 21 can be used. Further problems are given at the end of the chapter to allow practice with dilution calculations.

## Compound Dilutions

The previous examples represent simple dilutions. Occasionally in the laboratory it is necessary to make a very large dilution, and it is more accurate and less costly to do this in several steps rather than all at once. Such a process is known as a *compound dilution*. The same approach is used, but the dilution occurs in several stages. For example, if a 1:500 dilution is necessary, it would take 49.9 mL of diluent to accomplish this in one step with 0.1 mL of serum. If only a small amount of solution is needed to run the test, this is wasteful; furthermore, inaccuracy may occur if the solution is not properly mixed. Therefore, it is helpful to make several smaller dilutions.

To calculate a compound dilution problem, the first step is to plan the number and sizes of simple dilutions necessary to reach the desired end point. To use the preceding example, a 1:500 dilution can be achieved by making a 1:5 dilution of the original serum, a 1:10 dilution from the first dilution, and another 1:10 dilution. This can be shown as follows:

| Serum: | | |
|---|---|---|
| 1:5 dilution | 1:10 dilution | 1:10 dilution |
| 0.1 mL serum | 0.1 mL of 1:5 dilution | 0.1 mL of 1:10 dilution |
| 0.4 mL diluent | 0.9 mL diluent | 0.9 mL diluent |

Multiplying $5 \times 10 \times 10$ equals 500, or the total dilution. Each of the simple dilutions is calculated individually by doing mental arithmetic or by using the formula given for simple dilutions. In this example, the 1:500 dilution was made using very little diluent in a series of test tubes, rather than having to use a larger volume in a flask. The volumes were kept small enough so that mixing could take place easily, and the final volume of 1.0 mL is all that is necessary to perform a test.

If, in each step of the dilution, the dilution factor is exactly the same, this is known as a *serial dilution*. Serial dilutions are often used to obtain a **titer,** or indicator of an antibody's strength. A series of test tubes is set up with exactly the same amount of diluent in each **(Fig. 7–7).** The most common serial dilution is a doubling dilution, in which the amount of serum is cut in half with each dilution. For example, six test tubes can be set up with 0.2 mL of diluent in each. If 0.2 mL of serum is added to the first tube, this becomes a 1:2 dilution.

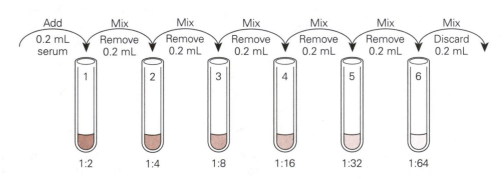

FIGURE 7–7. Serial dilution. Each tube contains 0.2 mL of diluent. Patient serum (0.2 mL) is added to tube one. This is carefully mixed, and then 0.2 mL is withdrawn and added to tube two. The process is continued until the last tube is reached. The sample is mixed, and 0.2 mL is discarded. Note that in this dilution, the amount of antibody is cut in half in each successive tube.

0.2 mL serum/0.2 mL serum + 0.2 mL
diluent = 0.2 mL/0.4 mL = 1/2

Then when 0.2 mL of the 1:2 dilution is added to 0.2 mL of diluent, a 1:4 dilution is obtained. The final dilution is obtained by counting the number of tubes and setting up a multiplication series in which the original dilution factor is raised to a power equal to the number of tubes. In this example, if the first tube contains a 1:2 dilution, the dilution in tube number six is

$$\frac{1}{2} \times \frac{1}{2} \times \frac{1}{2} \times \frac{1}{2} \times \frac{1}{2} \times \frac{1}{2} = 1/64$$

If, in this instance, an end point was reached at tube number five, the actual titer would be 1:32. To avoid confusion, this is customarily written as the reciprocal of the dilution—that is, 32. Serial dilutions do not always have to be doubling dilutions. Consider the following set of test tube dilutions:

$$1:5 \rightarrow 1:25 \rightarrow 1:125 \rightarrow 1:625 \rightarrow 1:3125$$

For each successive tube, the dilution is increased by a factor of 5, so this would indeed be considered a serial dilution. Having the ability to work with simple and compound dilutions and interpret serial dilutions is a necessary skill for laboratory work. The laboratory exercise at the end of this chapter illustrates the principle of serial dilutions.

## SUMMARY

Laboratory personnel are most frequently exposed to biological, sharp, chemical, and radiation hazards. Transmission of biological hazards that are encountered when testing patient specimens requires a chain of infection, which consists of a source, a method of transmission, and a host. Handwashing and wearing PPE are essential to prevent transmission of infectious organisms. Standard precautions should be followed at all times. Specimens, except urine, and contaminated supplies must be disposed of in a biohazard container. Sodium hypochlorite is the recommended disinfectant for blood and body fluid contamination of countertops and nondisposables. All sharps, including needles and adaptors, must be disposed of in puncture-proof containers. Recapping of needles is prohibited. Accidental exposure to blood and body fluids must be reported immediately to a supervisor. When transporting biological specimens, specific packaging requirements must be followed.

Follow specific directions when mixing chemicals, and always add acid to water, rather than water to acid. When chemical contact with skin or eyes occurs, immediately flush the area with water. An MSDS and a Chemical Hygiene Plan must be available to employees. Dispose of chemicals per EPA guidelines. Laboratorians who are pregnant should avoid areas with a radioactive symbol. Dispose of radioactive material following NRC guidelines.

Serum is typically the specimen used in serological testing to look for the presence or absence of antibody. In order for a visible end point to occur in antigen–antibody reactions, often a dilution needs to be made. Patient serum, the solute, is made weaker by adding diluent so that the antibody present is not as concentrated. The relationship between the serum and the total volume is expressed as a fraction—for example, 1:20. When several dilutions are made in which the dilution factor is the same in each case, this is called a *serial dilution*. Serial dilutions are used to determine the titer, or strength, of an antibody. The last tube in which a visible reaction is seen is considered the end point.

# CASE STUDY

The serology supervisor who has been working for the last 20 years in a small rural hospital is training a new employee. A dilution of a patient's serum must be made to run a particular test. The supervisor was having difficulty using a serological pipette, so she removed one glove. In uncapping the serum tube, a small amount of serum splashed onto the workbench. She cleaned this up with a paper towel, which she discarded in the regular paper trash. She also spilled a small amount onto her disposable lab coat. She told the new employee that since it was such a small amount, she wasn't going to worry about it, and she continued on to pipette the specimen. She then replaced the glove onto her ungloved hand and said that since it was almost break time, she would wait to wash her hands until then. Please identify all the safety violations involved.

## EXERCISE

# SERIAL DILUTIONS

## Principle

Serial dilutions are a set of dilutions in which the dilution factor is exactly the same at each step. These are used to make high dilutions with a small number of test tubes and a minimal amount of diluent. This is commonly done to determine the strength or titer of a particular antibody in patient serum as a part of the diagnosis of a disease state. Traditionally, serological pipettes have been used in this process, but now it is more common to employ micropipettes for this purpose. In this experiment, a series of doubling dilutions will be made with both serological pipettes and micropipettes, and the results will be compared.

## Sample Preparation

None

## Reagents, Materials, and Equipment

Anti-A antiserum

Serological pipettes, 1 mL

Micropipettes

Disposable plastic microtiter plates

Disposable glass test tubes, 12 × 75 mm

Saline solution (0.85 percent)

Type A red blood cells (3 to 4 percent solution)

Centrifuge

## Procedure

### Macrotiter

1. Make a 1:10 dilution of reagent anti-A antiserum by adding 1 mL of anti-A to 9 mL of saline for every 10 mL of reagent desired. Allow approximately 1.5 mL of antiserum per student. This will be enough to run the dilutions with a little extra for repeat testing.

2. If type A red blood cells are not purchased, a 4 percent solution of red blood cells can be made using type A blood collected in ethylenediaminetetraacetic acid (EDTA). Spin the collection tube in a centrifuge for approximately 10 minutes at 1500 revolutions per minute (rpm). Remove the serum and add saline to the remaining red blood cells. Transfer the solution to a disposable conical centrifuge tube that has graduations marked on it. Spin again for 10 minutes and note the color of the saline wash on top. Remove saline wash and resuspend in additional saline. Make sure all cells are uniformly resuspended. Repeat this procedure for three washes or until the saline supernatant is clear.

Note the final volume of the packed red blood cells. Make a 4 percent solution by suspending 4 mL of packed red cells in 96 mL of saline. Each student needs approximately 4 mL of the final solution.

3. Label eight 12 × 75 mm test tubes as follows: 10, 20, 40, 80, 160, 320, 640, 1280.

4. Using a 1 mL serological pipette, add 0.2 mL of saline to tubes two through eight.

5. Add 0.2 mL of anti-A antiserum to tubes one and two, using a clean serological pipette.

6. With a new serological pipette, mix tube two by drawing fluid up and down five to ten times.

7. Transfer 0.2 mL from tube two to tube three and mix.

8. Repeat the transfer and mixing process with tubes three and four, and so on through tube eight. After tube eight is mixed, discard the last 0.2 mL of the dilution.

9. Using a 1 mL serological pipette, add 0.2 mL of 4 percent type A red blood cells to each tube.

10. Centrifuge for 30 to 45 seconds.

11. Observe for agglutination by gently shaking the red blood cell button loose from the side of each test tube. A positive reaction is indicated by cells that remain clumped together after shaking. Note that the size of the clumps decreases with further dilution, but any visible clumping is considered positive.

12. Record the titer. This is the last tube in which visible agglutination can be discerned. The titer is written as the reciprocal of the dilution—that is, if the 1:160 tube is the last positive one, the titer is written as 160.

### Microtiter

1. Label one row of a microtiter plate as follows: 10, 20, 40, 80, 160, 320, 640, 1280.

2. Using a micropipette, add 20 μL of saline to wells two through eight on the microtiter plate.

3. With a new pipette tip, add 20 μL of anti-A antiserum to wells one and two.

4. Using the micropipette set to 20 μL and a new pipette tip, mix well number two by drawing up and down in the pipette several times. Wipe the outside of the pipette tip, and transfer 20 μL to well number three.

5. Repeat this process with successive wells through well number eight.

6. Add 20 μL of 4 percent type A red blood cells to all wells.

7. Rotate plate on the lab bench for 1 minute, making a concentric circular pattern. Let the plate sit for 30 minutes at room temperature.

8. Observe for agglutination with a microtiter plate reader, or carefully hold up to the light. A smooth button on the bottom of a well indicates that the red blood cells have settled out with no agglutination. If agglutination has occurred, an irregular or crenulated pattern is seen at the bottom of the well **(Fig. 7–8)**.

9. Report the titer as the last well in which agglutination can be seen. Compare the results with those from the macrotiter. The titers obtained should be within one dilution of each other (plus or minus).

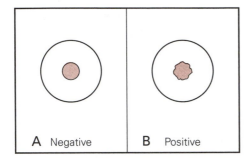

**FIGURE 7–8.** Microtiter agglutination patterns. *(A)* A negative result is indicated by a smooth button. *(B)* Agglutination is a positive result and is indicated by a ragged edge as the cells settle out.

## Interpretation of Results

This experiment introduces the student to the concept and techniques involved in making serial dilutions. This is a procedure often used to determine the titer of an antibody. The titer is defined as the reciprocal of the last tube in which a positive reaction is seen. The titer indicates the concentration of an antibody, and this is important in diagnostic testing. In some diseases, the mere presence of the antibody is enough to confirm the diagnosis. For other diseases, however, it is necessary to find a titer that is significantly elevated beyond what might be found in the normal population in order to link the antibody to an active disease state. Whenever a titer is reported, the accuracy is assumed to be plus or minus one tube.

### ACKNOWLEDGMENT

This experiment was originally designed by Dan Southern of the Clinical Laboratory Sciences Program, Western Carolina University, Cullowhee, N.C.

# LABORATORY SAFETY EXERCISE

Explore the student laboratory or the area designated by the instructor and perform the following:

1. Locate the fire extinguishers
2. State the instructions for operating the fire extinguisher
3. Locate the eyewash station
4. Locate the emergency shower
5. Locate the first-aid kit
6. Locate the master electrical panel
7. Locate the fire alarm
8. Identify the emergency exit route
9. Locate the MSDS pertaining to serology
10. Locate the emergency spill kit
11. Locate the Bloodborne Pathogen Exposure Control Plan
12. Identify the type of disinfectant available for cleaning work areas

# REVIEW QUESTIONS

1. A technologist who observes a red rash on her hands after removing her gloves

   a. should apply antimicrobial lotion to the hands.
   b. may be washing the hands too frequently.
   c. may have developed a latex allergy.
   d. should not create friction when washing the hands.

2. In the chain of infection, a contaminated work area would serve as which of the following?

   a. Source
   b. Method of transmission
   c. Host
   d. All of the above

3. The only biological waste that does not have to be discarded in a container with a biohazard symbol is

   a. urine.
   b. serum.
   c. feces.
   d. none of the above

4. Patient specimens transported by the Department of Transportation must be labeled as

   a. diagnostic specimen.
   b. clinical specimen.
   c. biological specimen, category b.
   d. All of the above

5. A technician places tightly capped serum tubes in a rack and places the rack and the specimen data in a labeled metal courier box. Is there anything wrong with this scenario?

   a. Yes, DOT requirements are not met.
   b. No, the tubes are placed in a rack.
   c. Yes, absorbent material is missing.
   d. No, the box contains the specimen data.

6. The Occupational Exposure to Bloodborne Pathogens Standard developed by OSHA requires employers to provide all of the following *except*

   a. hepatitis B immunization.
   b. safety training.
   c. hepatitis C immunization.
   d. laundry facilities for nondisposable lab coats.

7. An employee who receives an accidental needlestick should immediately

   a. apply sodium hypochlorite to the area.
   b. notify a supervisor.
   c. receive HIV prophylaxis.
   d. receive a hepatitis B booster shot.

8. The first thing to do when acid is spilled on the skin is to

   a. notify a supervisor.
   b. neutralize the area with a base.
   c. apply burn ointment.
   d. flush the area with water.

9. When combining acid and water,

   a. acid is added to water.
   b. water is added to acid.
   c. water is slowly added to acid.
   d. both solutions are added simultaneously.

10. To determine the chemical characteristics of sodium azide, an employee would consult the

    a. chemical hygiene plan.
    b. Merck manual.
    c. MSDS.
    d. NRC guidelines.

11. A technician who is pregnant should avoid working with

    a. organic chemicals.
    b. radioisotopes.
    c. HIV-positive serum.
    d. needles and lancets.

12. A 1:750 dilution of serum is needed to perform a serological test. Which of the following series of dilutions would be correct to use in this situation?

    a. 1:5, 1:15, 1:10
    b. 1:5, 1:10, 1:5
    c. 1:15, 1:10, 1:3
    d. 1:15, 1:3, 1:5

13. How much diluent needs to be added to 0.2 ml of serum to make a 1:20 dilution?

    a. 19.8 mL
    b. 4.0 mL
    c. 3.8 mL
    d. 10.0 mL

# References

1. Centers for Disease Control and Prevention. Guideline for handwashing hygiene in health-care settings. MMWR 2002:51(rr16); 1–48. http://www.cdc.gov/mmwr/PDF/rr/rr5116.pdf. Accessed September 8, 2008.
2. NIOSH Alert. Preventing allergic reactions to natural rubber latex in the workplace. DHHS (NIOSH) Publication 97–135. National Institute for Occupational Safety and Health, Cincinnati, OH, 1997.
3. Preventing transmission of infectious agents in healthcare settings 2007. http://www.cdc.gov/ncidod/dhqp/pdf/guidelines/Isolation2007.pdf. Accessed September 8, 2008.
4. Clinical Laboratory Standards Institute, formerly NACCLSs. Protection of laboratory workers from instrument biohazards and infectious disease transmitted by blood, body fluids, and tissue: Approved guideline M29-A, NCCLS, Wayne, PA, 1997.
5. Hazardous materials: Infectious Substances; harmonizing with the United Nations recommendations. Federal Register, 70 (May 19), 2005.
6. Baer, DM. Standards for transporting specimens. MLO, 37(11):38, Nokomis, FL, 2005.
7. U.S. Department of Transportation. Transporting infectious substances safely. https://hazmatonline.phmsa.dot.gov/services/publication_documents/Transporting%20Infectious%20Substances%20Safely.pdf. Accessed September 8, 2008.
8. International Air Transport Association. 2005 Diagnostic Specimen Transport Regulations. http://www.qicstat.com/Media/IATA changes_2005.pdf.
9. Occupational Exposure to Bloodborne Pathogens, Final Rule. Federal Register, 29 (Dec 6), 1991.
10. OSHA. Enforcement Procedures for the Occupational Exposure to Bloodborne Pathogens Standard. Directive 2–2.44D. Washington, DC, 1999. http://www.asha.slc.gov/oshdoc/Directive data/cpl_2–2_69.html.
11. OSHA. Needlestick requirements take effect April 18. OSHA, Washington, DC, 2001. http://www.osha.sle.gov/medic/oshnews/apr01/national-20010412.html.
12. OSHA. OSHA clarifies position on the removal of contaminated needles. OSHA, Washington, DC, 2002. http://www.osha.gov/media/oshnews/june02/trade-20020612A.html.
13. CDC, Updated U.S. Public Health Service guidelines for the management of occupational exposures to HBV, HCV, and HIV and recommendations for post-exposure prophylaxis. MMWR 2001:50(RR11), 1–42.
14. Occupational Exposure to Hazardous Chemical in Laboratories, Final Rule. Federal Register 55 (January 31), 1990.

# Precipitation Reactions

## LEARNING OBJECTIVES

*After finishing this chapter, the reader will be able to:*

1. Describe how the law of mass action relates to antigen–antibody binding.
2. Distinguish precipitation and agglutination.
3. Discuss affinity and avidity and their influence on antigen–antibody reactions.
4. Explain how the zone of equivalence is related to the lattice hypothesis.
5. Differentiate between turbidity and nephelometry and discuss the role of each in measurement of precipitation reactions.
6. Explain the difference between single diffusion and double diffusion.
7. Give the principle of the end-point method of radial immunodiffusion.
8. Determine the relationship between two antigens by looking at the pattern of precipitation resulting from Ouchterlony immunodiffusion.
9. Describe how rocket immunoelectrophoresis differs from radial immunodiffusion.
10. Compare immunoelectrophoresis and immunofixation electrophoresis regarding placement of reagents, time to obtain results, and limitations of each method.

## KEY TERMS

____ Affinity
____ Agglutination
____ Avidity
____ Cross-reactivity
____ Electrophoresis
____ Immunoelectrophoresis
____ Immunofixation electrophoresis
____ Law of mass action
____ Nephelometry
____ Ouchterlony double diffusion
____ Passive immunodiffusion
____ Postzone phenomenon
____ Precipitation
____ Prozone phenomenon
____ Radial immunodiffusion
____ Rocket immunoelectrophoresis
____ Turbidimetry
____ Zone of equivalence

# CHAPTER OUTLINE

The combination of antigen with specific antibody plays an important role in the laboratory in diagnosing many different diseases. Immunoassays have been developed to detect either antigen or antibody, and they vary from easily performed manual tests to highly complex automated assays. Many such assays are based on the principles of precipitation or agglutination. Precipitation involves combining soluble antigen with soluble antibody to produce insoluble complexes that are visible. Agglutination is the process by which particulate antigens such as cells aggregate to form larger complexes when a specific antibody is present. This chapter focuses on precipitation, and the following chapter discusses agglutination.

Precipitation was first noted in 1897 by Kraus, who found that culture filtrates of enteric bacteria would precipitate when they were mixed with specific antibody. For such reactions to occur, both antigen and antibody must have multiple binding sites for one another, and the relative concentration of each must be equal. Binding characteristics of antibodies, called *affinity* and *avidity*, also play a major role. These are discussed, along with theoretical considerations of binding, including the law of mass action and the principle of lattice formation. Such characteristics relate to the sensitivity and specificity of testing in the clinical laboratory.

## ANTIGEN–ANTIBODY BINDING

### Affinity

The primary union of binding sites on antibody with specific epitopes on an antigen depends on two characteristics of antibody known as *affinity* and *avidity*. Affinity is the initial force of attraction that exists between a single Fab site on an antibody molecule and a single epitope or determinant site on the corresponding antigen.[1] As epitope and binding site come into close proximity to each other, several types

of noncovalent bonds hold them together. These include ionic bonds, hydrogen bonds, hydrophobic bonds, and van der Waals forces.[1,2] Ionic bonds occur between oppositely charged particles. Hydrogen bonds involve an attraction between polar molecules that have a slight charge separation and in which the positive charge resides on a hydrogen atom. Hydrophobic bonds occur between nonpolar molecules that associate with one another and exclude molecules of water as they do so. Van der Waals forces occur because of the interaction between the electron clouds of oscillating dipoles. All of these are rather weak bonds that can occur only over a short distance of approximately $1 \times 10^{-7}$ mm, so there must be a very close fit between antigen and antibody.[1]

The strength of attraction depends on the specificity of antibody for a particular antigen. One antibody molecule may initially attract numerous different antigens, but it is the epitope's shape and the way it fits together with the binding sites on an antibody molecule that determines whether the bonding will be stable. Antibodies are capable of reacting with antigens that are structurally similar to the original antigen that induced antibody production. This is known as cross-reactivity. The more the cross-reacting antigen resembles the original antigen, the stronger the bond will be between the antigen and the binding site. However, if the epitope and the binding site have a perfect lock-and-key relationship, as is the case with the original antigen, the affinity will be maximal, because there is a very close fit (Fig. 8–1).

### Avidity

Avidity represents the sum of all the attractive forces between an antigen and an antibody. This involves the strength with which a multivalent antibody binds a multivalent antigen, and it is a measure of the overall stability of an antigen–antibody complex.[1,3] In other words, once

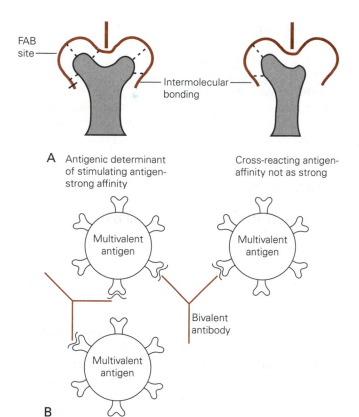

FAB site

Intermolecular bonding

**A** Antigenic determinant of stimulating antigen- strong affinity

Cross-reacting antigen- affinity not as strong

Multivalent antigen

Multivalent antigen

Bivalent antibody

Multivalent antigen

**B**

FIGURE 8–1. *Affinity and avidity. (A)* Affinity is the fit of one anti- genic determinant with one antibody binding site. The original stimulating antigen is a better fit than cross-reacting antigen. *(B)* Avidity is the sum of the forces binding multivalent antigens to multivalent antibodies.

binding has occurred, it is the force that keeps the mole- cules together. A high avidity can actually compensate for a low affinity. Stability of the antigen–antibody complex is essential to detecting the presence of an unknown, whether it is antigen or antibody.

## Law of Mass Action

All antigen–antibody binding is reversible and is governed by the **law of mass action.** This law states that free reac- tants are in equilibrium with bound reactants.[2] The equilibrium constant represents the difference in the rates of the forward and reverse reactions according to the following equation:

$$Ag + Ab \xrightleftharpoons[K_2]{K_1} AgAb$$

Where
Ag = antigen
Ab = antibody
$K_1$ = rate constant for the forward reaction
$K_2$ = rate constant for the reverse reaction

The equilibrium constant is thus

$$K = K_1/K_2 = [AgAb]/[Ab][Ag],$$

where [AgAb] = concentration of the antigen–antibody complex (mol/L)

[Ab] = concentration of antibody (mol/L)
[Ag] = concentration of antigen (mol/L)

This constant can be seen as a measure of the goodness of fit.[3] Its value depends on the strength of binding between antibody and antigen. As the strength of binding, or avidity, increases, the tendency of the antigen–antibody com- plexes to dissociate decreases, and the value of $K_2$ decreases. This increases the value of $K_1$. The higher the value of K, the larger the amount of antigen–antibody complex and the more visible or easily detectable the reaction is. The ideal conditions in the clinical laboratory would be to have an anti- body with a high affinity, or initial force of attraction, and a high avidity, or strength of binding. The higher the values are for both of these and the more antigen–antibody com- plexes that are formed, the more sensitive the test will be.

## PRECIPITATION CURVE

### Zone of Equivalence

In addition to the affinity and avidity of the antibody involved, precipitation depends on the relative proportions of antigen and antibody present. Optimum precipitation occurs in the **zone of equivalence,** in which the number of multivalent sites of antigen and antibody are approximately equal. In this zone, precipitation is the result of random, reversible reactions whereby each antibody binds to more than one antigen and vice versa, forming a stable network or lattice.[4] The lattice hypothesis, as formulated by Marrack, is based on the assumptions that each antibody molecule must have at least two binding sites, and antigen must be multivalent. As they combine, this results in a multimolec- ular lattice that increases in size until it precipitates out of solution. Heidelberger and Kendall performed the classic quantitative precipitation reactions that established proof for this theory.

As illustrated by the precipitin curve shown in **Figure 8–2,** when increasing amounts of soluble antigen are added to fixed amounts of specific antibody, the amount of precipita- tion increases up to the zone of equivalence. Then when the amount of antigen overwhelms the number of antibody- combining sites present, precipitation begins to decline.

### Prozone and Postzone

As can be seen on the precipitation curve, precipitation declines on either side of the equivalence zone due to an excess of either antigen or antibody. In the case of antibody excess, the **prozone** phenomenon occurs, in which antigen combines with only one or two antibody molecules,

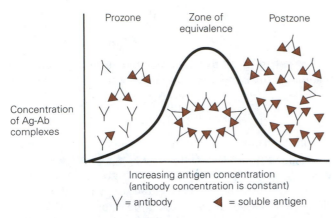

FIGURE 8–2. Precipitin curve. The precipitin curve shows how the amount of precipitation varies with varying antigen concentration when the antibody concentration is kept constant. Excess antibody is called the *prozone*, and excess antigen concentration is called the *postzone*.

and no cross-linkages are formed. This is because usually only one site on an antibody molecule is used, and many free antibody molecules remain in solution.

At the other side of the zone, where there is antigen excess, the **postzone** phenomenon occurs, in which small aggregates are surrounded by excess antigen, and again no lattice network is formed.[1] In this case, every available antibody site is bound to a single antigen, and no cross-links are formed.[4] Thus, for precipitation reactions to be detectable, they must be run in the zone of equivalence.

The prozone and postzone phenomena must be considered in the clinical setting, because negative reactions occur in both. A false-negative reaction may take place in the prozone due to high antibody concentration. If it is suspected that the reaction is a false negative, diluting out antibody and performing the test again may produce a positive result. In the postzone, excess antigen may obscure the presence of a small amount of antibody. Typically, such a test is repeated with an additional patient specimen taken about a week later. This would give time for the further production of antibody. If the test is negative on this occasion, it is unlikely that the patient has that particular antibody.

## MEASUREMENT OF PRECIPITATION BY LIGHT SCATTERING

### Turbidimetry

Precipitation is one of the simplest methods of detecting antigen–antibody reactions, because most antigens are multivalent and thus capable of forming aggregates in the presence of the corresponding antibody. When antigen and antibody solutions are mixed, the initial turbidity is followed by precipitation. Precipitates in fluids can be measured by means of turbidimetry or nephelometry. Turbidimetry is a measure of the turbidity or cloudiness of a solution. A detection device is placed in direct line with the incident

light, collecting light after it has passed through the solution. It thus measures the reduction in light intensity due to reflection, absorption, or scatter.[5] Scattering of light occurs in proportion to the size, shape, and concentration of molecules present in solution. It is recorded in absorbance units, a measure of the ratio of incident light to that of transmitted light. Measurements are made using a spectrophotometer or an automated clinical chemistry analyzer.

### Nephelometry

**Nephelometry** measures the light that is scattered at a particular angle from the incident beam as it passes through a suspension[5] **(Fig. 8–3)**. The amount of light scattered is an index of the solution's concentration. Beginning with a constant amount of antibody, increasing amounts of antigen result in an increase in antigen–antibody complexes. Thus, the relationship between antigen concentrations, as indicated by antigen–antibody complex formation, and light scattering approaches linearity.[5] Light scatter may be recorded in arbitrary units of "relative light scatter," or it may be directly extrapolated by a computer to give actual concentrations in milligrams per deciliter (mg/dL) or international units per milliliter (IU/mL), based on established values of standards. Nephelometers measure light scatter at angles ranging from 10 degrees to about 90 degrees. If a laser beam is used, light deflected only a few degrees from

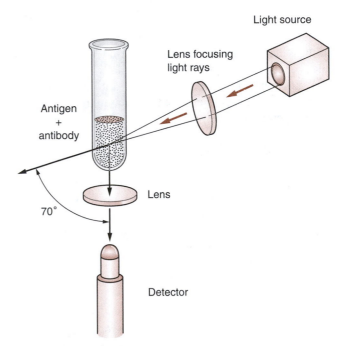

FIGURE 8–3. Principles of nephelometry. The light detection device is at an angle to the incident light, in contrast to turbidity, which measures light rays passing directly through the solution. *(From Stites, DP, et al. Clinical laboratory methods for detection of antigens and antibodies. In Stites, DP, Terr, AI, and Parslow, TG (eds): Medical Immunology, ed. 9. Appleton & Lange, Stamford, CT, 1997, p. 230, with permission.)*

the original path can be measured. Although the sensitivity of turbidity has increased, nephelometry is more sensitive, with a lower limit of detection of 1 to 10 mg/L.[2]

Nephelometry can be used to detect either antigen or antibody, but it is usually run with antibody as the reagent and the patient antigen as the unknown. In *end point nephelometry*, the reaction is allowed to run essentially to completion, but large particles tend to fall out of solution and decrease the amount of scatter. Thus, another method called *kinetic* or *rate nephelometry* was devised, in which the rate of scattering increase is measured immediately after the reagent is added. This rate change is directly related to antigen concentration if the concentration of antibody is kept constant.[6] Many automated instruments utilize this principle for the measurement of serum proteins. Quantification of immunoglobulins such as IgG, IgA, IgM, and IgE, and kappa and lambda light chains is done almost exclusively by nephelometry, because other methods are more labor-intensive.[6] Other serum proteins quantified include complement components, C-reactive protein, and several clotting factors. Nephelometry provides accurate and precise quantitation of serum proteins, and due to automation, the cost per test is typically lower than other methods.[6,7]

## PASSIVE IMMUNODIFFUSION TECHNIQUES

The precipitation of antigen–antibody complexes can also be determined in a support medium such as a gel. Agar, a high-molecular-weight complex polysaccharide derived from seaweed, and agarose, a purified agar, are used for this purpose. Agar and agarose help stabilize the diffusion process and allow visualization of the precipitin bands.[2]

Reactants are added to the gel, and antigen–antibody combination occurs by means of diffusion. When no electrical current is used to speed up this process, it is known as **passive immunodiffusion.** The rate of diffusion is affected by the size of the particles, the temperature, the gel viscosity, and the amount of hydration. An agar concentration ranging from 0.3 percent to 1.5 percent allows for diffusion of most reactants. Agarose is preferred to agar, because agar has a strong negative charge, while agarose has almost none, so interactions between the gel and the reagents are minimized. Immunodiffusion reactions can be classified according to the number of reactants diffusing and the direction of diffusion.

### Radial Immunodiffusion

James Oudin was the first to use gels for precipitation reactions, and he pioneered the technique known as *single diffusion.*[4] In single diffusion, antibody was incorporated into agarose in a test tube. The antigen was layered on top, and as the antigen moved down into the gel, precipitation occurred and moved down the tube in proportion to the amount of antigen present.[4] A modification of the single-diffusion technique, **radial immunodiffusion (RID)**, has been commonly used in the clinical laboratory. In this technique, antibody is uniformly distributed in the support gel, and antigen is applied to a well cut into the gel. As the antigen diffuses out from the well, antigen–antibody combination occurs in changing proportions until the zone of equivalence is reached and a stable lattice network is formed in the gel. The area of the ring obtained is a measure of antigen concentration, and this can be compared to a standard curve obtained by using antigens of known concentration.[1,6] **Figure 8–4** depicts some typical results.

There are two techniques for the measurement of radial immunodiffusion. The first was developed by Mancini and is known as the *end-point method*. In this technique, antigen is allowed to diffuse to completion, and when equivalence is reached, there is no further change in the ring diameter.[8] This occurs between 24 and 72 hours. The square of the diameter is then directly proportional to the concentration of the antigen. A graph is obtained by plotting concentrations of standards on the x-axis versus the diameter squared on the y-axis, and a smooth curve is fit to the points. The major drawback to this method is the time it takes to obtain results.

The Fahey and McKelvey method, also called the *kinetic method*, uses measurements taken before the point of equivalence is reached. In this case, the diameter is proportional to the log of the concentration.[9] A graph is drawn on semilog paper by plotting the antigen concentration on the log axis and the diameter on the arithmetic axis. Readings are taken at about 18 hours.

For either the end-point method or the kinetic method, it is essential that monospecific antiserum with a fairly high

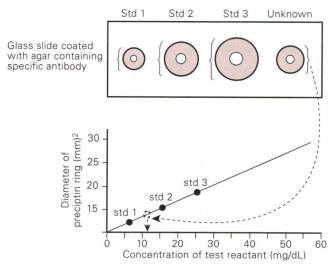

**FIGURE 8–4.** Radial immunodiffusion. The amount of precipitate formed is in proportion to the antigen present in the sample. In the Mancini end-point method, concentration is in proportion to the diameter squared. *(From Nakamura, RM, Tucker, ES III, and Carlson, IH. Immunoassays in the clinical laboratory. In Henry, JB: Clinical Diagnosis and Management by Laboratory Methods, ed. 18. WB Saunders, Philadelphia, 1991, p. 858, with permission.)*

affinity be used. This increases the clarity of the precipitation reaction. In addition, the precision of the assay is directly related to accurate measurement of samples and standards. Sources of error include overfilling or underfilling the wells, nicking the side of the wells when filling, spilling sample outside the wells, improper incubation time and temperature, and incorrect measurement. Radial immunodiffusion has been used to measure IgG, IgM, IgA, and complement components. It is simple to perform and requires no instrumentation, but it is fairly expensive to run.[6] Thus, immunodiffusion has largely been replaced by more sensitive and automated methods such as nephelometry and enzyme-linked immunosorbent assays except for low-volume analytes such as IgD or IgG subclasses.[6]

## Ouchterlony Double Diffusion

One of the older, classic immunochemical techniques is **Ouchterlony double diffusion.** In this technique, both antigen and antibody diffuse independently through a semi-solid medium in two dimensions, horizontally and vertically. Wells are cut in a gel, and reactants are added to the wells. After an incubation period of between 12 and 48 hours in a moist chamber, precipitin lines form where the moving front of antigen meets that of antibody. The density of the lines reflects the amount of immune complex formed.

Most Ouchterlony plates are set up with a central well surrounded by four to six equidistant outer wells. Antibody that is multispecific is placed in the central well, and different antigens are placed in the surrounding wells to determine if the antigens share identical epitopes.[4] The position of the precipitin bands between wells allows for the antigens to be compared with one another. Several patterns are possible: (1) Fusion of the lines at their junction to form an arc represents serological identity or the presence of a common epitope, (2) a pattern of crossed lines demonstrates two separate reactions and indicates that the compared antigens share no common epitopes, and (3) fusion of two lines with a spur indicates partial identity. In this last case, the two antigens share a common epitope, but some antibody molecules are not captured by antigen and travel through the initial precipitin line to combine with additional epitopes found in the more complex antigen. Therefore, the spur always points to the simpler antigen[1] **(Fig. 8–5).** While of more limited use because it is labor-intensive and requires experience to read, Ouchterlony double diffusion is still used to identify fungal antigens such as *Aspergillus, Blastomyces, Coccidioides,* and *Candida.*[10] In addition, this has been a classic technique to detect antibodies to extractable nuclear antigens that occur in several autoimmune diseases.[11,12] (Refer to Chapter 14 for a discussion of autoimmune diseases.)

It is important to perform this technique with care, because several problems may arise. Irregular patterns of precipitation may occur from overfilling the wells, irregular hole punching, or nonlevel incubation. Other factors affecting the accuracy of results include drying out of the

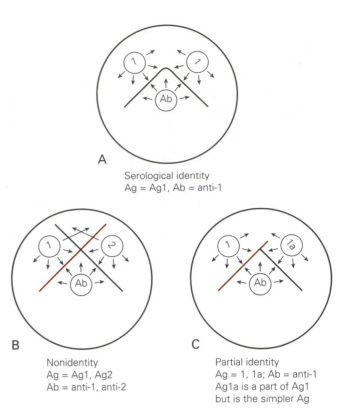

A

Serological identity
Ag = Ag1, Ab = anti-1

B

Nonidentity
Ag = Ag1, Ag2
Ab = anti-1, anti-2

C

Partial identity
Ag = 1, 1a; Ab = anti-1
Ag1a is a part of Ag1
but is the simpler Ag

**FIGURE 8–5.** Ouchterlony diffusion patterns. Antibody that is a mixture of anti-1 and anti-2 is placed in the central well. Unknown antigens are placed in the outside wells. *(A)* Serological identity. The arc indicates that the two antigens are identical. *(B)* Nonidentity. Two crossed lines represent two different precipitation reactions. The antigens share no identical determinants. *(C)* Partial identity. Antigen 1a shares a determinant that is part of antigen 1, but it is not as complex. The spur formed always points to the simpler antigen.

gels; inadequate time for diffusion, resulting in weakness of band intensity; and fungal or bacterial contamination of the gel.

## ELECTROPHORETIC TECHNIQUES

Diffusion can be combined with electrophoresis to speed up or sharpen the results. **Electrophoresis** separates molecules according to differences in their electric charge when they are placed in an electric field. A direct current is forced through the gel, causing antigen, antibody, or both to migrate. As diffusion takes place, distinct precipitin bands are formed. This technique can be applied to both single and double diffusion.

## Rocket Immunoelectrophoresis

*One-dimension electroimmunodiffusion,* an adaptation of radial immunodiffusion, was developed by Laurell in the early 1960s.[13] Antibody is distributed in the gel, and antigen is placed in wells cut in the gel, just as in RID. However, instead of allowing diffusion to take place at its own rate, electrophoresis is used to facilitate migration of the antigen into the agar. When the antigen diffuses out of the well, precipitation begins. As the concentration of antigen changes, there is dissolution and reformation of the precipitate at ever-increasing distances from the well. The end result is a precipitin line that is conical in shape, resembling a rocket, hence the name **rocket immunoelectrophoresis.** The height of the rocket, measured from the well to the apex, is directly in proportion to the amount of antigen in the sample. If standards are run, a curve can be constructed to determine concentrations of unknown specimens[2] **(Fig. 8–6).**

Rocket immunoelectrophoresis is much more rapid than RID, with results available in just a few hours.[6] It is essential, however, to determine the net charge of the molecules at the pH used for the test, because this determines the direction of migration within the gel. Typically, a pH is selected so that antibodies in the gel do not move, but the antigens become negatively charged. Antigens then migrate toward the positive anode.[4] This technique has been used to quantitate immunoglobulins, using a buffer of pH 8.6.

## Immunoelectrophoresis

**Immunoelectrophoresis** is a double-diffusion technique that incorporates electrophoresis current to enhance results. Introduced by Grabar and Williams in 1953, this is performed as a two-step process and can be used for semiquantitation of a wide range of antigens.[2,14] Typically, the source of the antigens is serum, which is electrophoresed to separate out the main protein fractions; then a trough is cut in the gel parallel to the line of separation. Antiserum is placed in the trough, and the gel is incubated for 18 to 24 hours. Double diffusion occurs at right angles to the electrophoretic separation, and precipitin lines develop where specific antigen–antibody combination takes place. These lines or arcs can be compared in shape, intensity, and location to that of a normal serum control to detect abnormalities.[5] Changes include bowing or thickening of bands, or changed mobility.[14] Interpretation may take considerable experience.

This procedure has been used as a screening tool for the differentiation of many serum proteins, including the major classes of immunoglobulins. It is both a qualitative and a semiquantitative technique and has been used in clinical

laboratories for the detection of myelomas, Waldenström's macroglobulinemia, malignant lymphomas, and other lymphoproliferative disorders.[14] (See Chapter 15 for more details on lymphoproliferative diseases.) In addition, immunodeficiencies can be detected in this manner, if no precipitin band is formed for a particular immunoglobulin. Deficiencies of complement components can also be identified. **Figure 8–7** shows examples of a normal pattern and an IgM monoclonal gammopathy, an immunoproliferative disorder. However, this technique is relatively insensitive, with a detection limit of approximately 3 to 20 uL concentration.[4] Interpretation can also be difficult and may take considerable experience. Therefore, it has largely been replaced by immunofixation electrophoresis, which gives quicker results and is easier to interpret.[2,14]

## Immunofixation Electrophoresis

**Immunofixation electrophoresis,** as first described by Alper and Johnson,[15] is similar to immunoelectrophoresis except that after electrophoresis takes place, antiserum is applied directly to the gel's surface rather than placed in a trough. Agarose or cellulose acetate can be used for this purpose. Immunodiffusion takes place in a shorter time and results in a higher resolution than when antibody diffuses from a trough. Because diffusion is only across the thickness of the gel, approximately 1 mm, the reaction usually takes place in less than 1 hour.

Most often, an antibody of known specificity is used to determine whether patient antigen is present. The unknown antigen is placed on the gel, electrophoretic separation takes place, and then the reagent antibody is applied. Immunoprecipitates form only where specific antigen–antibody combination has taken place, and the

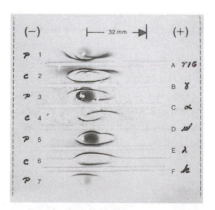

**FIGURE 8–7.** Immunoelectrophoresis film showing normal controls (odd-numbered wells) and patient serum (even-numbered wells). Trough A contains antitotal immunoglobulin, and troughs B through F contain the following monospecific antisera: B, anti-γ; C, anti-α; D, anti-μ; E, anti-λ; and F, anti-κ. The restricted electrophoretic mobility seen in well 1 with antitotal immunoglobulin and in well 5 with anti-μ and anti-λ immunoglobulins indicate that the patient has an IgM monoclonal gammopathy with λ light chains. *(From Harr, R. Clinical Laboratory Science Review, ed. 2. FA Davis, Philadelphia, 2000, Color Plate 4, with permission.)* See Color Plate 8.

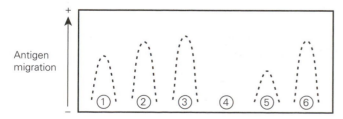

**FIGURE 8–6.** Rocket immunoelectrophoresis. Standards are in wells 1 to 3. Patient samples are in wells 4 to 6. Note that well 4 contains no antigen, because no ring is formed. Well 5 has a low concentration of antigen, and well 6 has a high concentration of antigen.

complexes have become trapped in the gel. The gel is washed to remove any nonprecipitating proteins and can then be stained for easier visibility. Typically, patient serum is applied to six lanes of the gel, and after electrophoresis, five lanes are overlaid with one each of the following antibodies: antibody to gamma, alpha, or mu heavy chains and to kappa or lambda light chains.[16] The sixth lane is overlaid with antibody to all serum proteins and serves as the reference lane. Reactions in each of the five lanes are compared to the reference lane. Hypogammaglobulinemias will exhibit faintly staining bands, while polyclonal hypergammaglobulinemias show darkly staining bands in the gamma region. Monoclonal bands, such as found in Waldenström's macroglobulinemia or multiple myeloma, have dark and narrow bands in specific lanes[16] **(Fig. 8–8).**

This method is especially useful in demonstrating those antigens present in serum, urine, or spinal fluid in low concentrations. Cerebrospinal fluid is the specimen of choice for diagnosing multiple sclerosis, and urine is used to detect the presence of Bence-Jones proteins that are found in multiple myeloma.[16,17] Although immunofixation is more sensitive than immunoelectrophoresis, dilutions may be necessary to avoid the zones of antigen excess, which may occur if concentrations of monoclonal antibody are very high.[14] Perhaps one of the best-known adaptations of this technique is the Western blot, used as a confirmatory test to detect antibodies to human immunodeficiency virus 1 (HIV-1). A mixture of HIV antigens is placed on a gel and electrophoresed to separate the individual components. The components are then transferred to nitrocellulose paper by means of blotting or laying the nitrocellulose over the gel so that the electrophoresis pattern is preserved. Patient serum is applied to the nitrocellulose and allowed to react. The strip is then washed and stained to detect precipitin bands. It is simpler to visualize the reaction on the nitrocellulose, and in this manner, antibodies to several antigens can be detected. Refer to Figure 23-1 for a specific example of a Western blot used to determine the presence of antibody to HIV-1. This technique is characteristically used to determine the presence of antibodies to organisms of complex antigenic composition. If antibodies to more than one disease-associated antigen are identified in patient serum, this usually confirms presence of the suspected disease.

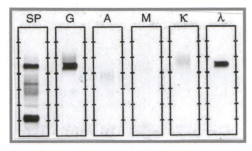

**FIGURE 8–8.** Immunofixation electrophoresis. A complex antigen mixture such as serum proteins is separated by electrophoresis. An antiserum template is aligned over the gel. Then protein fixative and monospecific antisera, IgG, IgA, IgM, κ, and λ are applied to the gel. After incubating for 30 minutes, the gel is stained and examined for the presence of paraproteins. Precipitates form where specific antigen–antibody combination has taken place. In this case, the patient has an IgG monoclonal antibody with λ chains. *(Courtesy of Helena Laboratories, Beaumont, TX ).* See Color Plate 9.

## Sources of Error in Electrophoresis

Many of the sources of error are similar for all the electrophoretic techniques, so they are discussed together here. One problem that can arise is applying the current in the wrong direction. If this occurs, samples may either run off the gel or not be separated. Incorrect pH of the buffer and incorrect electrophoresis time also hinder proper separation. Concentrations of antigen and antibody must be carefully chosen so that lattice formation and precipitation is possible. If either is too concentrated, no visible reaction will result. The amount of current applied also influences the efficiency of the separation. If the current is not strong enough, separation may be incomplete. On the other hand, if the current is too strong, heat will be generated and may denature proteins. As in diffusion techniques, wells must be carefully filled.

## COMPARISON OF PRECIPITATION TECHNIQUES

Each type of precipitation technique has its own distinct advantages and disadvantages. Some techniques are technically more demanding, and others are more automated. Each type of precipitation testing has particular applications for which it is best suited. **Table 8–1** presents a comparison of the techniques discussed in this chapter.

| Table 8–1. | Comparison of Precipitation Techniques | | |
|---|---|---|---|
| **TECHNIQUE** | **APPLICATION** | **SENSITIVITY (μg ab/mL)** | **COMMENT** |
| Nephelometry | Immunoglobulins, complement, C-reactive protein, other serum proteins | 1–10 | Automated, sensitive, expensive equipment needed |
| Radial immunodiffusion | Immunoglobulins, complement | 10–50 | Quantitative, slow, not as sensitive as nephelometry |

*Continued*

| Table 8-1. | Comparison of Precipitation Techniques—Cont'd | | |
|---|---|---|---|
| **TECHNIQUE** | **APPLICATION** | **SENSITIVITY ($\mu$g ab/mL)** | **COMMENT** |
| Ouchterlony double diffusion | Complex antigens such as fungal antigens | 20–200 | Semiquantitative, slow, may be difficult to interpret |
| Rocket electrophoresis | Immunoglobulins, complement, alpha-fetoprotein | 2 | Fast, quantitative, technically demanding |
| Immunoelectrophoresis | Differentiation of serum proteins | 20–200 | Slow, semiquantitative, difficult to interpret |
| Immunofixation electrophoresis | HIV, Lyme disease, syphilis | Variable | Fairly rapid, semiquantitative, sensitive |

HIV = Human immunodeficiency virus; Ab = antibody
Adapted from Kindt, TJ, Goldsby, RA, and Osborne, BA. Kuby Immunology, ed. 6. WH Freeman and Co., New York, 2007, p. 152.

## SUMMARY

Immunoassays in which antigen–antibody combination occurs have been developed to detect either antigen or antibody, and they play an important role in diagnosing diseases. Many such assays are based on the principle of precipitation, which involves combination of soluble antigen with soluble antibody to produce insoluble complexes that are visible.

Union of antigen and antibody depends on affinity, or the force of attraction that exists between one antibody-binding site and a single epitope on an antigen. Avidity is the sum of all attractive forces occurring between multiple binding sites on antigen and antibody. For testing purposes, it is important to have an antibody with high affinity and high avidity for the antigen in question.

Maximum binding of antigen and antibody occurs when the aggregate number of multivalent sites of antigen and antibody are approximately equal. The concentrations of antigen and antibody that yield maximum binding represent the zone of equivalence. When antibody is in excess (the prozone) or antigen is in excess (the postzone), manifestations of antigen–antibody combination such as precipitation and agglutination are present to a much lesser degree. All testing should take place in the zone of equivalence, where a reaction is most visible.

Precipitation can be detected in the laboratory by several different means. Light scatter produced by immune complexes in solution can be measured as a reduction in light intensity (turbidimetry) or as the amount of light scattered at a particular angle (nephelometry). Several automated instruments are based on these principles.

Other precipitation techniques utilize a support medium such as a gel, and antigen–antibody combination takes place by means of passive diffusion. In single diffusion, only one of the reactants travels, while the other is incorporated in the gel. An example is radial immunodiffusion, in which antibody is incorporated in a gel in a plate or a petri dish. The amount of precipitate formed is directly related to the amount of antigen present.

Ouchterlony diffusion is a double-diffusion technique in which both antigen and antibody diffuse from wells and travel toward each other. Precipitin lines may indicate identity, nonidentity, or partial identity, depending on the pattern formed.

Electrophoresis can be combined with diffusion to speed up the process and enhance the reaction patterns. Rocket immunoelectrophoresis applies an electric charge to single diffusion, with resultant precipitation patterns that look like rockets that project upward from the sample wells. In immunoelectrophoresis, the antigen is first electrophoresed by itself to separate out different components, and then antibody is placed in a trough to allow diffusion to take place. Specific reaction patterns indicate presence or absence of certain antigens. A related technique, immunofixation electrophoresis, differs in that antibody is applied directly to the gel after electrophoresis has taken place. Compared to immunoelectrophoresis, precipitation occurs in a shorter time, and bands with higher resolution are obtained.

Precipitation is adaptable to both automated technologies and individually processed testing. Thus, it is a versatile and practical method for use in the clinical laboratory.

# CASE STUDY

A 4-year-old female was hospitalized for pneumonia. She has had a history of upper-respiratory-tract infections and several bouts of diarrhea since infancy. Due to her recurring infections, the physician decided to measure her immunoglobulin levels. The following results were obtained by nephelometry:

| IMMUNOGLOBULIN | NORMAL LEVEL (3–5 yrs) (mg/dL) | PATIENT LEVEL (mg/dL) |
|---|---|---|
| IgG | 550–1700 | 800 |
| IgA | 50–280 | 20 |
| IgM | 25–120 | 75 |

## Questions

a. What do these results indicate?

b. How do they explain the symptoms?

c. How do nephelometry measurements compare with the use of RID?

# EXERCISE

## IMMUNOFIXATION ELECTROPHORESIS

### Principle

Immunofixation electrophoresis (IFE) is a two-stage procedure using agarose gel high-resolution electrophoresis in the first stage and immunoprecipitation in the second. Proteins are first separated by electrophoresis. Then, in the second stage, soluble antigen in the gel reacts with specific antibody, and the resultant antigen–antibody complexes become insoluble (as long as the antibody is in slight excess or near equivalency) and precipitate. The precipitation rate depends on the proportions of the reactants, temperature, salt concentration, and the solution's pH. The unreacted proteins are removed by a washing step, and the antigen–antibody complex is visualized by staining. The bands in the individual lanes are compared with the precipitin bands obtained with a normal control serum.

### Sample Preparation

Fresh serum or urine is the specimen of choice. Evaporation of uncovered specimens may cause inaccurate results, so specimens must be handled carefully. Plasma should not be used, because the fibrinogen may adhere to the gel matrix, resulting in a band in all patterns across the gel. If storage is necessary, samples may be kept covered at 2°C to 8°C for up to 72 hours.

### Reagents, Materials, and Equipment

Gel chamber to electrophorese, stain, destain, and then dry the gels

IFE gels

IFE protein fixative

Acid violet stain

Vials of anti-IgG, IgA, IgM kappa, and lambda antisera

Tris-buffered saline

Citric acid destain

IFE templates (20)

Blotters and blotter combs

> NOTE: The above are provided in kits available from Helena, Sebia, or the Binding Site.

Antisera template

REP prep 3100

Gel block remover

10 percent acetic acid

0.85 percent saline

Power supply capable of providing at least 350 volts

### Precautions

The gel contains barbital, which, in sufficient quantity, can be toxic. In addition, sodium azide is used as a preservative in certain reagents. To prevent the formation of toxic vapors, do not mix with acidic solutions. When discarding, always flush sink with copious amounts of water. This will prevent the formation of metallic azides, which, when highly concentrated in metal plumbing, are potentially explosive. In addition to purging pipes with water, plumbing should occasionally be decontaminated with 10 percent sodium hydroxide. The gels must be stored in the protective packaging in which they are shipped. Do not refrigerate or freeze.

### Procedure

1. Prepare all reagents, including the tris buffer, acid violet, and citric acid destain according to directions in the kit.
2. Plug the electrophoresis chamber into a power supply, and snap the electrophoresis lid into place on the chamber.
3. Dilute patient serum samples from 1:3 to 1:10, following instructions for the individual manufacturers.
4. Remove the gel from the gel pouch. Carefully detach from the plastic mold and discard the mold.
5. Dispense approximately 1 mL of REP prep onto the left side of the electrophoresis chamber.
6. Place the gel carefully into the electrophoresis chamber, making sure that any notches are aligned with pins on the chamber floor. Use a lint-free tissue to wipe around the edges of the gel backing to remove any excess REP prep. Make sure that no bubbles remain under the gel.
7. Using a blotter, gently blot the entire gel using slight fingertip pressure on the blotter. Remove the blotter.
8. Remove IFE templates from the package. Hold the template so that the small hole in the corner is toward the front right side of the chamber.
9. Carefully place the template on the gel, aligning the template slits with the marks on each side of the gel backing. The center hole in the template should align with the indention in the center of the gel.
10. Apply slight fingertip pressure to the template, making sure there are no bubbles under it.
11. Apply the appropriate serum dilution to six template slits. Wait 2 minutes after the last sample application to allow proper absorption.

12. Gently blot the excess sample from the template. Then carefully remove the template.

13. Close the lid of the chamber. Set the power to 350 volts and start the power supply. Electrophorese the gel for 7 to 8 minutes, following instructions from the kit's manufacturer.

14. Turn off the power supply and remove the lid to the electrophoresis chamber.

15. Using the gel block remover, carefully remove the two gel blocks (one on each end of the gel). Use a lint-free tissue to wipe around the edges of the gel backing to remove any excess moisture.

16. Replace the electrophoresis lid with the drying lid.

17. Holding the antisera template in the up position, place the template into the appropriate slots in the chamber.

18. Gently lower the antisera template onto the surface of the gel. No further pressure is needed.

19. Quickly pipette the fixative and antisera into the slots at the right end (anode) of each antisera channel in the template.

20. After 2 minutes (1 to 3 minutes is acceptable) incubation time, place one blotter comb into the same slots where the antisera has been applied. After 2 minutes, remove the blotter comb and the antisera template.

21. Gently blot the gel with a blotter and remove it. Place a different blotter on the surface of the gel. Place the antisera template on top of the blotter. After 5 minutes, remove the antisera template and blotter. Close the lid.

22. Dry the gel for 8 minutes by turning on only the chamber. After 8 minutes, turn the chamber off and remove the gel.

23. Fill a container with prepared stain. Fill another container with destain solution. Fill a third container with tris-buffered saline (TBS).

24. Place the gel in TBS and shake gently on a rotator for 10 minutes. Remove the gel from the TBS and allow it to drain on a blotter.

25. Place the gel into the staining dish containing the prepared stain. Leave it for 4 minutes. Remove the gel from the stain and allow it to drain on a blotter.

26. Destain the gel in two consecutive washes of destain solution. Use a gentle, alternately rocking and swirling technique. Allow the gel to remain in each wash for 1 minute. The gel background should be completely clear. Tap the gel to remove the excess destain solution.

27. Ensure that the chamber floor is clean. Replace the gel onto the chamber floor. Set a timer for 8 minutes, close the drying lid, and turn the chamber on.

28. Remove the gel from the chamber, and place it into the destain again for 1 minute. Tap the gel to remove excess destain solution.

29. Place the gel back into the chamber and dry for 5 minutes.

30. Turn off the chamber and remove the gel.

## Results

The different lanes of patient serum are compared to the normal control. One lane will have all the serum protein bands stained, and the remaining five lanes will show individual reactions with antisera to heavy chains (anti-IgG, anti-IgA, or anti-IgM) and to light chains (anti-kappa and anti-lambda). The presence of abnormal bands is indicated by an increase in size and staining activity in a particular area. Polyclonal hypergammaglobulinemia is indicated by broad, dark bands in the gamma region. A monoclonal protein band produces a pattern that is narrow and dark. Conversely, a faint band in the gamma region indicates a hypogammaglobulinemia.

## Interpretation of Results

In the clinical laboratory, immunofixation electrophoresis is primarily used for the detection of monoclonal gammopathies. A monoclonal gammopathy is a primary disease state in which a single clone of plasma cells produces elevated levels of an immunoglobulin of a single class and type. Such immunoglobulins are referred to as *monoclonal proteins*, *M-proteins*, or *paraproteins*. In some cases they are indicative of a malignancy such as multiple myeloma or Waldenström's macroglobulinemia. A monoclonal gammopathy will typically show a narrow dark band in one heavy-chain region and in one light-chain region.

Differentiation must be made between polyclonal and monoclonal gammopathies, because polyclonal gammopathies are only a secondary disease state due to clinical disorders such as chronic liver diseases, collagen disorders, rheumatoid arthritis, and chronic infections. Polyclonal gammopathies are indicated by wide bands in one or more heavy- and light-chain regions.

If there is a very high level of immunoglobulin in the patient sample, antigen excess may occur. This will result in staining of the margins, leaving the central area with little demonstrable protein stain. In this case it will be necessary to adjust the protein content of the sample by dilution.

# REVIEW QUESTIONS

1. In a precipitation reaction, how can the ideal antibody be characterized?

   a. Low affinity and low avidity
   b. High affinity and low avidity
   c. High affinity and high avidity
   d. Low affinity and high avidity

2. Precipitation differs from agglutination in which way?

   a. Precipitation can only be measured by an automated instrument.
   b. Precipitation occurs with univalent antigen, while agglutination requires multivalent antigen.
   c. Precipitation does not readily occur, because few antibodies can form aggregates with antigen.
   d. Precipitation involves a soluble antigen, while agglutination involves a particulate antigen.

3. When soluble antigens diffuse in a gel that contains antibody, in which zone does optimum precipitation occur?

   a. Prozone
   b. Zone of equivalence
   c. Postzone
   d. Prezone

4. Which of the following statements apply to rate nephelometry?

   a. Readings are taken before equivalence is reached.
   b. It is more sensitive than turbidity.
   c. Measurements are time dependent.
   d. All of the above

5. Which of the following is characteristic of the end-point method of RID?

   a. Readings are taken before equivalence.
   b. Concentration is directly in proportion to the square of the diameter.
   c. The diameter is plotted against the log of the concentration.
   d. It is primarily a qualitative rather than a quantitative method.

6. Which statement is true of measurements of turbidity?

   a. It indicates the ratio of incident light to transmitted light.
   b. Light that is scattered at an angle is detected.
   c. It is recorded in units of relative light scatter.
   d. It is not affected by large particles falling out of solution.

7. Which of the following refers to the force of attraction between an antibody and a single antigenic determinant?

   a. Affinity
   b. Avidity
   c. Van der Waals attraction
   d. Covalence

8. Which technique is typified by radial immunodiffusion combined with electrophoresis?

   a. Countercurrent electrophoresis
   b. Rocket electrophoresis
   c. Immunoelectrophoresis
   d. Southern blotting

9. Immunofixation electrophoresis differs from immunoelectrophoresis in which way?

   a. Electrophoresis takes place after diffusion has occurred.
   b. Better separation of proteins with the same electrophoretic mobilities is obtained.
   c. Antibody is directly applied to the gel instead of being placed in a trough.
   d. It is mainly used for antigen detection.

10. In which zone might an antibody-screening test be false negative?

    a. Prozone
    b. Zone of equivalence
    c. Postzone
    d. None of the above

11. If crossed lines result in an Ouchterlony immunodiffusion reaction with antigens 1 and 2, what does this indicate?

    a. Antigens 1 and 2 are identical.
    b. Antigen 2 is simpler than antigen 1.
    c. Antigen 2 is more complex than antigen 1.
    d. The two antigens are unrelated.

12. Which might affect the outcome of immunodiffusion procedures?

    a. Improper dilution of antigen in the wells
    b. Overfilling the wells
    c. Nonlevel incubation of plates
    d. All of the above

**13.** Which technique represents a single-diffusion reaction?

   a. Radial immunodiffusion

   b. Ouchterlony diffusion

   c. Immunoelectrophoresis

   d. All of the above

**14.** Which best describes the law of mass action?

   a. Once antigen–antibody binding takes place, it is irreversible.

   b. The equilibrium constant depends only on the forward reaction.

   c. The equilibrium constant is related to strength of antigen–antibody binding.

   d. If an antibody has a high avidity, it will dissociate from antigen easily.

## References

1. Kindt, TJ, Goldsby, RA, and Osborne, BA. Kuby Immunology, ed. 6. WH Freeman and Co., New York, 2007, pp. 145–167.

2. Kricka, LJ. Principles of immunochemical techniques. In Burtis, CA, Ashwood, ER, and Bruns, DE (eds): Tietz Fundamentals of Clinical Chemistry, ed. 6. Saunders Elsevier, St. Louis, 2008, pp. 155–170.

3. Ashihara, Y, Kasahara, Y, and Nakamura, RM. Immunoassays and immunochemistry. In McPherson, RA, and Pincus, MR (eds): Henry's Clinical Diagnosis and Management by Laboratory Methods, ed. 21. Saunders Elsevier, Philadelphia, 2007, pp. 793–818.

4. Mak, T, and Saunders, ME. The Immune Response: Basic and Clinical Principles. Elsevier Academic Press, Burlington, MA, 2006, pp. 147–177.

5. Kricka, LJ, and Park, JY. Optical techniques. In Burtis, CA, Ashwood, ER, and Bruns, DE (eds): Tietz Fundamentals of Clinical Chemistry, ed. 6. Saunders Elsevier, St. Louis, 2008, pp. 63–83.

6. Warren, JS. Immunoglobulin quantitation. In Detrick, B, Hamilton, RG, and Folds, JD (eds): Manual of Molecular and Clinical Laboratory Immunology, ed. 7. American Society for Microbiology Press, Washington, D.C., 2006, pp. 69–74.

7. Kang, S, Suh, J, Lee, H, Yoon, H, et al. Clinical usefulness of free light chain concentration as a tumor marker in multiple myeloma. Ann Hematol 84:588–593, 2005.

8. Mancini, G, Carbonara, AO, and Heremans, JF. Immunochemical quantitation of antigens by single radial immunodiffusion. Immunochem 2:235, 1965.

9. Fahey, JL, and McKelvey, EM. Quantitative determination of serum immunoglobulins in antibody-agar plates. J Immunol 94:84, 1965.

10. Lindsley, MD, Warnock, DW, and Morrison, CJ. Serological and molecular diagnosis of fungal infections. In Detrick, B, Hamilton, RG, and Folds, JD (eds): Manual of Molecular and Clinical Laboratory Immunology, ed. 7. American Society for Microbiology Press, Washington, D.C., 2006, pp. 569–605.

11. Reeves, WH, Satoh, M, Lyons, R, Nichols, C, et al. Detection of autoantibodies against proteins and ribonucleoproteins by double immunodiffusion and immunoprecipitation. In Detrick, B, Hamilton, RG, and Folds, JD (eds): Manual of Molecular and Clinical Laboratory Immunology, ed. 7. American Society for Microbiology Press, Washington, D.C., 2006, pp. 1007–1018.

12. Orton, SM, Peace-Brewer, A, Schmitz, JL, Freeman, K, et al. Practical evaluation of methods for detection and specificity of autoantibodies to extractable nuclear antigens. Clin Vaccine Immunol 11:297–301, 2004.

13. Laurell, CB. Antigen-antibody crossed electrophoresis. Anal Biochem 10:358–61, 1965.

14. McPherson, RA, and Massey, HD. Laboratory evaluation of immunoglobulin function and humoral immunity. In McPherson, RA and Pincus, MR (eds): Henry's Clinical Diagnosis and Management by Laboratory Methods, ed. 21. Saunders Elsevier, Philadelphia, 2007, pp. 835–848.

15. Alper, CA, and Johnson, AM. Immunofixation electrophoresis: A technique for the study of protein polymorphism. Vox Sanguinis 17:445, 1969.

16. Katzman, JA, and Kyle, RA. Immunochemical characterization of immunoglobulins in serum, urine, and cerebrospinal fluid. In Detrick, B, Hamilton, RG, and Folds, JD (eds): Manual of Molecular and Clinical Laboratory Immunology, ed. 7. American Society for Microbiology Press, Washington, D.C., 2006, pp. 88–100.

17. Keren, DF, and Humphrey, RL. Clinical indications and applications of serum and urine protein electrophoresis. In Detrick, B, Hamilton, RG, and Folds, JD (eds): Manual of Molecular and Clinical Laboratory Immunology, ed. 7. American Society for Microbiology Press, Washington, D.C., 2006, pp. 75–87.

# Agglutination

## LEARNING OBJECTIVES

*After finishing this chapter, the reader will be able to:*

1. Differentiate between agglutination and precipitation.
2. Discuss how IgM and IgG differ in ability to participate in agglutination reactions.
3. Describe physiological conditions that can be altered to enhance agglutination.
4. Describe and give an example of each of the following:
   a. Direct agglutination
   b. Passive agglutination
   c. Reverse passive agglutination
   d. Agglutination inhibition
   e. Hemagglutination inhibition
   f. Coagglutination
5. Explain and give an application for the direct Coombs' test.
6. Discuss reasons for the use of the indirect Coombs' test.
7. Describe the principle of measurement used in particle-counting immunoassay (PACIA).
8. Discuss conditions that must be met for optimal results in agglutination testing.

## KEY TERMS

____ Agglutination inhibition

____ Agglutinin

____ Coagglutination

____ Direct agglutination

____ Direct antiglobulin test

____ Hemagglutination

____ Hemagglutination inhibition

____ Indirect antiglobulin test

____ Lattice formation

____ Low ionic strength saline

____ Particle-counting immunoassay (PACIA)

____ Passive agglutination

____ Reverse passive agglutination

____ Sensitization

# CHAPTER OUTLINE

Whereas precipitation reactions involve soluble antigens, agglutination is the visible aggregation of particles caused by combination with specific antibody. Antibodies that produce such reactions are often called agglutinins. Because this reaction takes place on the surface of the particle, antigen must be exposed and able to bind with antibody. Agglutination is actually a two-step process, involving sensitization or initial binding followed by lattice formation, or formation of large aggregates. Types of particles participating in such reactions include erythrocytes, bacterial cells, and inert carriers such as latex particles. Each particle must have multiple antigenic or determinant sites, which are cross-linked to sites on other particles through the formation of antibody bridges.[1]

In 1896, Gruber and Durham published the first report about the ability of antibody to clump cells, based on observations of agglutination of bacterial cells by serum.[2] This finding gave rise to the use of serology as a tool in the diagnosis of disease, and it also led to the discovery of the ABO blood groups. Widal and Sicard developed one of the earliest diagnostic tests in 1896 for the detection of antibodies occurring in typhoid fever, brucellosis, and tularemia.[2] Agglutination reactions now have a wide variety of applications in the detection of both antigens and antibodies. Such testing is simple to perform, and the end points can easily be read visually.

Agglutination reactions can be classified into several distinct categories: direct, passive, reverse passive, agglutination inhibition, and coagglutination. Principles of each of these types of reactions are discussed, including their current use in today's clinical laboratory.

## STEPS IN AGGLUTINATION

### Sensitization

Agglutination, like precipitation, is a two-step process that results in the formation of a stable lattice network. The first reaction involves antigen–antibody combination through single antigenic determinants on the particle surface and is often called the **sensitization** step.[3] This initial reaction follows the law of mass action (see Chapter 8) and is rapid and reversible.[4] The second step is the formation of cross-links that form the visible aggregates. This represents the stabilization of antigen–antibody complexes with the binding together of multiple antigenic determinants.[4] Each stage of the process is affected by different factors, and it is important to understand these in order to manipulate and enhance end points for such reactions.

Sensitization is affected by the nature of the antibody molecules themselves. The affinity and avidity (discussed in Chapter 8) of an individual antibody determine how much antibody remains attached. The class of immunoglobulin is also important; IgM with a potential valence of 10 is over 700 times more efficient in agglutination than is IgG with a valence of 2.[5]

The nature of the antigen-bearing surface is also a key factor in the initial sensitization process. If epitopes are sparse or if they are obscured by other surface molecules, they are less likely to interact with antibody.

### Lattice Formation

The second stage, representing the sum of interactions between antibody and multiple antigenic determinants on a particle, is dependent on environmental conditions and the relative concentrations of antigen and antibody.[3] Bordet hypothesized that **lattice formation** is governed by physicochemical factors such as the milieu's ionic strength, pH, and temperature.[2] Antibody must be able to bridge the gap between cells in such a way that one molecule can bind to a site on each of two different cells. The preceding factors can be manipulated to facilitate such attachment. **Figure 9–1** depicts the two-stage process.

Erythrocytes and bacterial cells have a slight negative surface charge, and because like charges tend to repel one another, it is difficult to bring such cells together into lattice formation. Additionally, in an ionic solution, red cells surround themselves with cations to form an ionic cloud, which keeps them about 25 nm apart.[3] The ability to link cells together depends in part on the nature of the antibody.

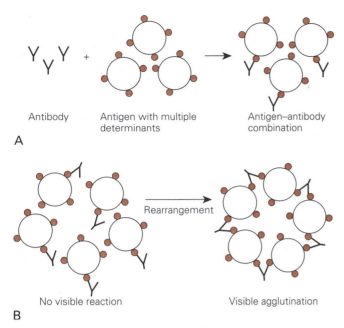

A

B

**FIGURE 9–1.** Phases of agglutination. *(A)* Sensitization. Antigen and antibody unite through antigenic determinant sites. *(B)* Lattice formation. Rearrangement of antigen and antibody bonds to form stable lattice.

Antibodies of the IgG class often cannot bridge the distance between particles, because their small size and restricted flexibility at the hinge region may prohibit multivalent binding.[1,3] IgM antibodies, on the other hand, have a diameter of about 35nm, so they are strong agglutinins.[3] Visible reactions with IgG often require the use of enhancement techniques, which vary physicochemical conditions.

## Enhancement of Lattice Formation

The surface charge must be controlled for lattice formation, or a visible agglutination reaction, to take place. One means of accomplishing this is by decreasing the buffer's ionic strength through the use of **low ionic strength saline**.[3,4] The addition of albumin in concentrations of 5 to 30 percent also helps to neutralize the surface charge and allows red cells to approach each other more closely.[4]

Other techniques that enhance agglutination, especially that of red blood cells, include increasing the viscosity, using enzymes, agitating centrifuging, and altering the temperature or the pH. Viscosity can be increased by adding agents such as dextran or polyethylene glycol (PEG). These agents reduce the water of hydration around cells and allow them to come into closer proximity for antibody to join together.[3] Bromelin, papain, trypsin, and ficin are the enzymes most often used to enhance agglutination, and these are thought to work by reducing the surface charge on red blood cells through cleaving of chemical groups and decreasing hydration.[4] Ficin cleaves sialoglycoproteins from the red blood cell surface; in addition to reducing the charge, this may change the external configuration of the membrane to reveal more antigenic determinant sites.[3] Agitation and centrifugation

provide a physical means to increase cell–cell contact and thus heighten agglutination.[4] All of these techniques plus the use of antiglobulin reagents (discussed in the section on antiglobulin testing) are used in the blood bank to better detect antigen–antibody reactions, especially in selecting blood for transfusion.

The temperature at which the antigen–antibody reaction takes place must also be considered, because it has an influence on the secondary, or aggregation, phase. Antibodies belonging to the IgG class agglutinate best at 30°C to 37°C, while IgM antibodies react best at temperatures between 4°C and 27°C. Because naturally occurring antibodies against the ABO blood groups belong to the IgM class, these reactions are best run at room temperature. Antibodies to other human blood groups usually belong to the IgG class, and reactions involving these must be run at 37°C. These latter reactions are the most important to consider in selecting compatible blood for a transfusion, because these are the ones that will actually occur in the body.

An additional physicochemical factor that can be manipulated when performing agglutination reactions is pH. Most reactions produce optimal antigen–antibody combination when the pH is between 6.5 and 7.5, but there are some exceptions, such as human anti-M and antiP1, which react best at a lower pH.[4]

## TYPES OF AGGLUTINATION REACTIONS

Agglutination reactions are easy to carry out, require no complicated equipment, and can be performed as needed in the laboratory without having to batch specimens. Batching specimens is done if a test is expensive or complicated; then a large number are run at one time, which may result in a time delay. Many kits are available for standard testing, so reagent preparation is minimal, and agglutination reactions are a frequently employed serological test. They can be used to identify either antigen or antibody. Typically, most agglutination tests are qualitative, simply indicating absence or presence of antigen or antibody, but dilutions can be made to obtain semiquantitative results. Many variations exist, and these can be categorized according to the type of particle used in the reaction and whether antigen or antibody is attached to it.

## Direct Agglutination

**Direct agglutination** occurs when antigens are found naturally on a particle. One of the best examples of direct agglutination testing involves known bacterial antigens used to test for the presence of unknown antibodies in the patient. Typically, patient serum is diluted into a series of tubes or wells on a slide and reacted with bacterial antigens specific for the suspected disease. Detection of antibodies is primarily used in diagnosis of diseases for which the bacterial agents are extremely difficult to cultivate. One such example is the Widal test, a rapid screening test to help determine the possibility of typhoid fever. The antigens used in this procedure include Salmonella O (somatic) and H (flagellar) antigens. A significant finding is a fourfold increase in antibody titer over time when paired dilutions of serum samples are tested with any of these antigens. While more specific tests are now available, this test is still considered useful in diagnosing typhoid fever in developing countries, and it remains in use in many areas throughout the world.[6,7]

If an agglutination reaction involves red blood cells, then it is called **hemagglutination.** The best example of this occurs in ABO blood group typing of human red blood cells, one of the world's most frequently used immunoassays.[1] Antisera of the IgM type can be used to determine the presence or absence of the A and B antigens, and this reaction is usually performed at room temperature without the need for any enhancement techniques. This type of agglutination reaction is simple to perform, is relatively sensitive, and is easy to read. A titer that yields semiquantitative results can be performed in test tubes or microtiter plates by making serial dilutions of the antibody. The reciprocal of the last dilution still exhibiting a visible reaction is the titer, indicating the antibody's strength.

Interpretation of the test is done on the basis of the cell sedimentation pattern. If there is a dark red, smooth button at the bottom of the microtiter well, the result is negative. A positive result will have cells that are spread across the well's bottom, usually in a jagged pattern with an irregular edge. Test tubes also can be centrifuged and then shaken to see if the cell button can be evenly resuspended. If it is resuspended with no visible clumping, then the result is negative. Positive reactions can be graded to indicate the strength of the reaction **(Fig. 9–2).** Hemagglutination kits are now available for detection of antibodies to hepatitis A virus (HAV), hepatitis B virus (HBV), hepatitis C virus (HCV), and human immunodeficiency virus (HIV) I and II, to cite just a few examples.[8–10]

## Passive Agglutination

**Passive,** or indirect, **agglutination** employs particles that are coated with antigens not normally found on their surfaces. A variety of particles, including erythrocytes, latex, gelatin, and silicates, are used for this purpose.[8] The use of synthetic beads or particles provides the advantage of consistency, uniformity, and stability.[1] Reactions are easy to read visually and give quick results. Particle sizes vary from 7 μm for red blood cells down to 0.8 μm or less for fine latex particles.[11]

Many antigens, especially polysaccharides, adsorb to red blood cells spontaneously, so they are relatively easy to manipulate. Problems encountered with the use of erythrocytes as carrier particles include the possibility of cross-reactivity, especially with heterophile antibody (see Chapter 3) if the cells used are nonhuman.

In 1955, Singer and Plotz found by happenstance that IgG was naturally adsorbed to the surface of polystyrene latex particles. While other substances such as polysaccharides and highly charged proteins are not naturally adsorbed by these particles, manipulation with certain chemicals is usually successful in coating latex particles with these substances. Latex particles are inexpensive, are relatively stable, and are not subject to cross-reactivity with other antibodies. A large number of antibody molecules can be bound to the surface of latex particles, so the number of antigen-binding sites is large.[1] Additionally, the large particle size facilitates reading of the test.[5]

Passive agglutination tests have been used to detect rheumatoid factor; antinuclear antibody occurring in the disease lupus erythematosus; antibodies to group A streptococcus antigens; antibodies to *Trichinella spiralis;* antibodies to *Treponema pallidum;* and antibodies to viruses such as cytomegalovirus, rubella, varicella-zoster, and HIV-1/HIV-2.[12–17] Because many of these kits are designed to detect

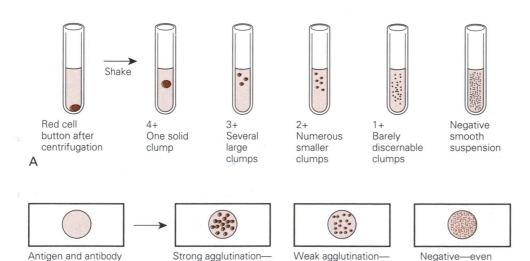

A

Red cell button after centrifugation

4+ One solid clump

3+ Several large clumps

2+ Numerous smaller clumps

1+ Barely discernable clumps

Negative smooth suspension

Shake

B

Antigen and antibody are mixed and rotated

Strong agglutination— large clumps and clear background

Weak agglutination— small clumps and cloudy background

Negative—even suspension and cloudy background

FIGURE 9–2. Grading of agglutination reactions. *(A)* Tube method. If tubes are centrifuged and shaken to resuspend the button, reactions can be graded from negative to 4+, depending on the size of clumps observed. *(B)* Slide method. Reactions can be graded from negative to strongly reactive, depending on the size of the clumps in the suspension.

IgM antibody, and there is always the risk of nonspecific agglutination caused by the presence of other IgM antibodies, reactions must be carefully controlled and interpreted. Commercial tests are usually performed on disposable plastic or cardboard cards or glass slides. Kits contain positive and negative controls, and if the controls do not give the expected results, the test is not valid. Such tests are typically used as screening tools to be followed by more extensive testing if the results are positive.

## Reverse Passive Agglutination

In **reverse passive agglutination,** antibody rather than antigen is attached to a carrier particle. The antibody must still be reactive and is joined in such a manner that the active sites are facing outward. Adsorption may be spontaneous, or it may require some of the same manipulation as is used for antigen attachment. This type of testing is often used to detect microbial antigens. **Figure 9–3** shows the differences between passive and reverse passive agglutination.

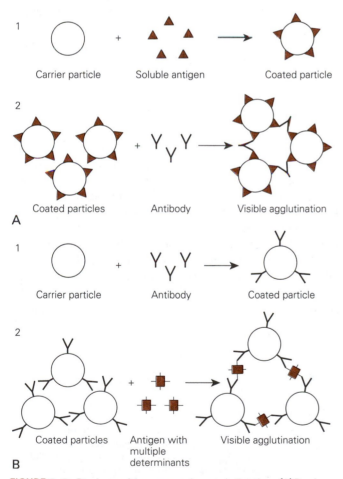

**FIGURE 9–3.** Passive and reverse passive agglutination. *(A)* Passive agglutination. Antigen is attached to the carrier particle, and agglutination occurs if patient antibody is present. *(B)* Reverse passive agglutination. Antibody is attached to the carrier particle, and agglutination occurs if patient antigen is present.

Numerous kits are available today for the rapid identification of antigens from such infectious agents as group B streptococcus, *Staphylococcus aureus*, *Neisseria meningitidis*, streptococcal groups A and B, *Haemophilus influenzae*, rotavirus, *Cryptococcus neoformans*, *Vibrio cholera* 01, and *Leptospira*.[7,18–24] Rapid agglutination tests have found the widest application in detecting soluble antigens in urine, spinal fluid, and serum.[8] The principle is the same for all these tests: Latex particles coated with antibody are reacted with a patient sample containing the suspected antigen. In some cases, an extraction step is necessary to isolate antigen before the reagent latex particles are added. Organisms can be identified in a few minutes with fairly high sensitivity and specificity, although this varies for different organisms. For example, the sensitivity of latex agglutination kits for the detection of cryptococcal antigen has been reported to be as high as 99 percent, while the specificity of testing for *Candida albicans* is much lower.[24] Use of monoclonal antibodies has greatly cut down on cross-reactivity, but there is still the possibility of interference or nonspecific agglutination. Such tests are most often used for organisms that are difficult to grow in the laboratory or for instances when rapid identification will allow treatment to be initiated more promptly. Direct testing of specimens for the presence of viral antigens has still not reached the sensitivity of enzyme immunoassays, but for infections in which a large amount of viral antigen is present, such as rotavirus and enteric adenovirus in infants, latex agglutination tests are extremely useful.[22,25] Reverse passive agglutination testing has also been used to measure levels of certain therapeutic drugs, hormones, and plasma proteins such as haptoglobin and C-reactive protein. In all of these reactions, rheumatoid factor will cause a false positive as it reacts with any IgG antibody, so this must be taken into account.

## Agglutination Inhibition

**Agglutination inhibition** reactions are based on competition between particulate and soluble antigens for limited antibody-combining sites, and a lack of agglutination is an indicator of a positive reaction. Typically, this type of reaction involves haptens that are complexed to proteins; the hapten–protein conjugate is then attached to a carrier particle. The patient sample is first reacted with a limited amount of reagent antibody that is specific for the hapten being tested. Indicator particles that contain the same hapten one wishes to measure in the patient are then added. If the patient sample has no free hapten, the reagent antibody is able to combine with the carrier particles and produce a visible agglutination. In this case, however, agglutination is a negative reaction, indicating that the patient did not have sufficient hapten to inhibit the secondary reaction **(Fig. 9–4).** Either antigen or antibody can be attached to the particles. The sensitivity of the reaction is governed by the avidity of the antibody itself. It can be a highly sensitive assay capable of detecting small quantities of antigen.[1] Detection of illicit drugs such as cocaine or heroin

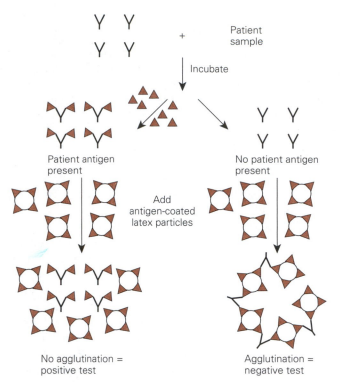

FIGURE 9–4. Agglutination inhibition. Reagent antibody is added to the patient sample. If patient antigen is present, antigen–antibody combination results. When antigen-coated latex particles are added, no agglutination occurs, which is a positive test. If no patient antigen is there, the reagent antibody combines with latex particles, and agglutination results, which is a negative test.

are examples of very sensitive agglutination inhibition tests.

**Hemagglutination inhibition** reactions use the same principle, except red blood cells are the indicator particles. This type of testing has been used to detect antibodies to certain viruses, such as rubella, mumps, measles, influenza, parainfluenza, HBV, herpesvirus, respiratory syncytial virus, and adenovirus.[1,8,10] Red blood cells have naturally occurring viral receptors. When virus is present, spontaneous agglutination occurs, because the virus particles link the red blood cells together. Presence of patient antibody inhibits the agglutination reaction.

To perform a hemagglutination inhibition test, patient serum is first incubated with a viral preparation. Then red blood cells that the virus is known to agglutinate are added to the mixture. If antibody is present, this will combine with viral particles and prevent agglutination, so a lack of or reduction in agglutination indicates presence of patient antibody. Controls are necessary, because there may be a factor in the serum that causes agglutination, or the virus may have lost its ability to agglutinate.

## Coagglutination

**Coagglutination** is the name given to systems using bacteria as the inert particles to which antibody is attached. *Staphylococcus aureus* is most frequently used, because it has a protein on its outer surface, called *protein A*, which naturally adsorbs the fragment crystallizable (Fc) portion of antibody molecules. The active sites face outward and are capable of reacting with specific antigen **(Fig. 9–5)**. These particles exhibit greater stability than latex particles and are more refractory to changes in ionic strength. However, because bacteria are not colored, reactions are often difficult to read. Such testing is highly specific, but it may not be as sensitive for detecting small quantities of antigen, as is latex agglutination.[11] Coagglutination reagents have been used in identification of streptococci, *Neisseria meningitidis*, *Neisseria gonorrhoeae*, *Vibrio cholera* 0139, and *Haemophilus influenzae*.[7,11]

## ANTIGLOBULIN-MEDIATED AGGLUTINATION

The antihuman globulin test, also known as the *Coombs' test*, is a technique that detects nonagglutinating antibody by means of coupling with a second antibody. It remains one of the most widely used procedures in blood banking. The key component of the test is antibody to human globulin that is made in animals or by means of hybridoma techniques.[3] Such antibody will react with the Fc portion of the human antibody attached to red blood cells. Agglutination takes place because the antihuman globulin is able to bridge the distance between cells that IgG alone cannot do. The strength of the reaction is proportional to the amount of

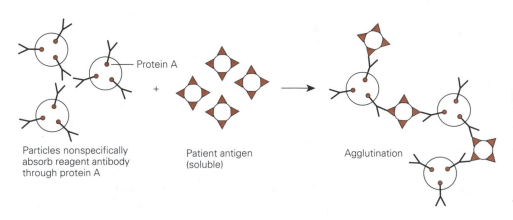

FIGURE 9–5. Coagglutination with *Staphylococcus aureus*. *Staphylococcus aureus* particles nonspecifically bind the Fc portion of immunoglobulin molecules. When reagent antibody is used, combination with patient antigen produces a visible agglutination reaction.

antibody coating the red blood cells. The Coombs' test can be divided into two different types, direct and indirect, each of which has a different purpose.

## Direct Antiglobulin Test

The **direct antiglobulin test** is used to demonstrate in vivo attachment of antibody or complement to an individual's red blood cells. This test serves as an indicator of autoimmune hemolytic anemia, hemolytic disease of the newborn, sensitization of red blood cells caused by the presence of drugs, or a transfusion reaction.[4] The test is called *direct*, because red blood cells are tested directly as they come from the body. A blood sample is obtained from the patient, the red blood cells are washed to remove any antibody that is not specifically attached, and then cells are tested directly with antibody to IgG or complement components. If IgG or complement is present on the red blood cells, the antihuman globulin (Coombs' reagent) is able to bridge the gap between red blood cells and cause a visible agglutination (Fig. 9–6A).

Polyspecific antiserum will react with IgG and with complement component C3d. Antibodies to C3b, C4b, or C4d may also be present.[3] If such a reaction is positive, then monospecific antibody, which will react with only one component, is used. This will differentiate between IgG and individual complement components on the patient's red blood cells. A positive test indicates that an immune reaction is taking place in that individual.

## Indirect Antiglobulin Test

The **indirect antiglobulin test,** or indirect Coombs' test, is used to determine the presence of a particular antibody in a patient, or it can be used to type patient red blood cells for specific blood group antigens. This is a two-step process, in which washed red blood cells and antibody are allowed to combine at 37°C, and the cells are then carefully washed again to remove any unbound antibody. When antihuman globulin is added, a visible reaction occurs where antibody has been specifically bound.

This test is most often used to check for the presence of clinically significant alloantibody in patient serum when performing compatibility testing for a blood transfusion.[4] In this case, patient serum is used to combine with reagent red blood cells of known antigenicity. All reactions are run at 37°C to detect clinically significant antibodies. Cells are then washed, and antihuman globulin is added. Tubes are centrifuged and read for agglutination (see Fig. 9–6B).

Possible sources of error in performing the Coombs' test include failure to wash cells, improper centrifugation, failure to add test serum or antihuman globulin, and use of expired reagents or those that have not been properly stored.[3] In addition, an improper concentration of red cells may alter the results. Too heavy a red cell concentration may mask agglutination, while too light a concentration will

A

B

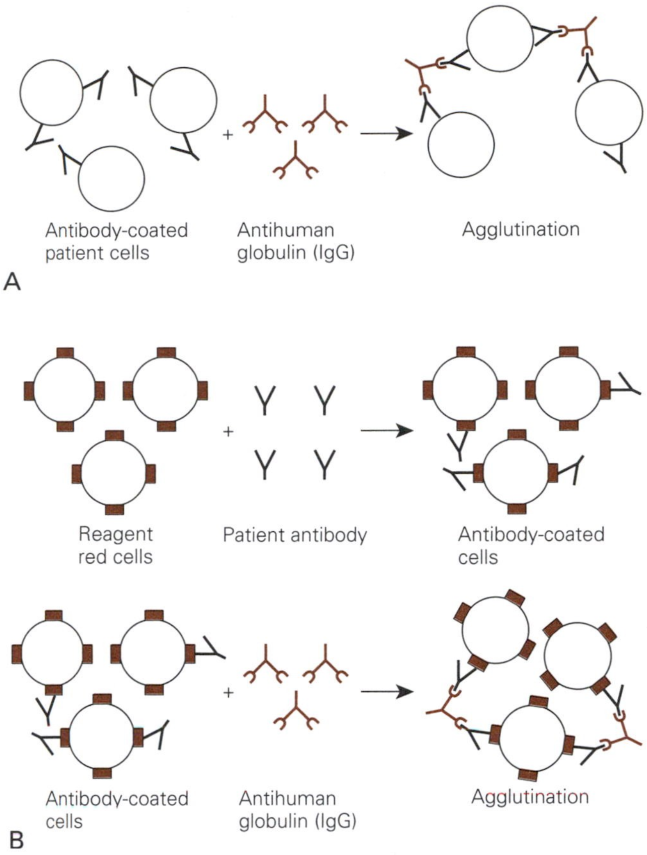

**FIGURE 9–6.** Direct and indirect antiglobulin tests. *(A)* Direct antiglobulin test (DAT). Antihuman globulin is combined with patient cells that have become coated with antibody in vivo. *(B)* Indirect antiglobulin test (IAT). Reagent cells are reacted with patient antibody. These are washed, and then antihuman globulin is added to enhance agglutination.

make the reaction hard to read.[3] Thus, it is important to use quality controls and to interpret results carefully.

## INSTRUMENTATION

While agglutination reactions require no complicated instrumentation to read, several systems have been developed using automation to increase sensitivity. Many of these use turbidimetry, which is based on the principle that as particles combine, light scatter increases, and the absorbance of the solution increases proportionally. (Refer to Chapter 8 for further discussion of the principles of turbidimetry.) Nephelometry has also been applied to the reading of agglutination reactions, and the term *particle-enhanced immunoassay* is used to describe such reactions. Nephelometry without the use of particles is capable of detecting soluble antigen–antibody complexes at a sensitivity of between 1 and 10 µg/mL.[9] If particles are used, the sensitivity can be increased to nanograms/mL.[8,9] For this type of reaction, small latex particles with a diameter of less than 1 µm are used. One such type of instrumentation system is called a PACIA.

**Particle-counting immunoassay (PACIA)** involves measuring the number of residual nonagglutinating particles in a specimen. These are counted by means of a laser beam in an optical particle counter similar to one that is designed to count blood cells. Nephelometric methods are used to measure forward light scatter. Very large and very small particles are excluded by setting certain thresholds on the instrument.

Latex particles are coated with whole antibody molecules or with $F(ab)_2$ fragments. Use of the latter reduces interference and nonspecific agglutination. If antigen is present, complexes will form and will be screened out by the counter because of their large size. An inverse relationship exists between the number of unagglutinated particles counted and the amount of unknown in the patient specimen. Measurements are made by looking at the rate at which the number of unagglutinated particles decrease, called a *rate assay*, or the total number of unagglutinated particles left at the end, known as an *end-point assay*.[9] PACIAs have been used to measure several serum proteins, therapeutic drugs, tumor markers, and viral antigens, such as those associated with measles, herpes simplex, and hepatitis B surface antigen.[8] Particle immunoassays are approximately three orders of magnitude more sensitive than standard manual agglutination methods.[8] One disadvantage, however, is the need to invest in expensive equipment.

## QUALITY CONTROL AND QUALITY ASSURANCE

Although agglutination reactions are simple to perform, interpretation must be carefully done. Techniques must be standardized as to concentration of antigen, incubation time, temperature, diluent, and the method of reading. The possibility of cross-reactivity and interfering antibody should always be considered. Cross-reactivity is caused by the presence of antigenic determinants that resemble one another so closely that antibody formed against one will react with the other. Most cross-reactivity can be avoided through the use of monoclonal antibody directed against an antigenic determinant that is unique to a particular antigen.

Heterophile antibody and rheumatoid factor are two interfering antibodies that may produce a false-positive result. Heterophile antibodies (see Chapter 3) are most often a consideration when red blood cells are used as the carrier particle. Patients may have an antibody that is capable of reacting with an antigen on the red blood cell other than the antigen that is being tested for. Such cross-reactions can be controlled by preadsorption of test serum on red blood cells without the test antigen or by treating red blood cells to remove possible interfering antigens. Rheumatoid factor, as mentioned previously, will react with any IgG present and is especially a problem in reverse passive agglutination tests. If this is suspected, samples can be treated with pronase or the reducing agent 2-mercaptoethanol to reduce false-positive results due to the IgM rheumatoid factor.[8] The use of positive and negative control sera is essential in agglutination testing, but it cannot rule out all false-positive reactions.

Other considerations include proper storage of reagents and close attention to expiration dates. Reagents should never be used beyond the expiration date. Each new lot should be evaluated before use, and the manufacturer's instructions for each kit should always be followed. The sensitivity and specificity of different kits may vary and thus must be taken into account.

Advantages of agglutination reactions include rapidity; relative sensitivity; and the fact that if the sample contains a microorganism, it does not need to be viable. In addition, most tests are simple to perform and require no expensive equipment. Test are conducted on cards, tubes, and microtiter plates, all of which are extremely portable. A wide variety of antigens and antibodies can be tested for in this manner. It must be kept in mind, however, that agglutination tests are screening tools only and that a negative result does not rule out presence of the disease or the antigen. The quantity of antigen or antibody may be below the sensitivity of the test system. Refer to **Table 9–1** for a list of false-positive and false-negative reactions. While the number of agglutination tests have decreased in recent years, they continue to play an important role in the identification of rare pathogens such as *Francisella* and *Brucella* and more common organisms such as rotavirus and *Cryptococcus*, for which other testing is complex or unavailable.[8]

## Table 9-1.   Causes of False-Positive and False-Negative Reactions in Agglutination Testing

| CAUSE | CORRECTION |
|---|---|
| **False-Positive Reactions** | |
| Overcentrifugation: Button is packed too tight and is difficult to resuspend. | Regulate centrifuge to proper speed and time. |
| Contaminated glassware, slides, or reagents: Contaminants (dust, dirt, or fingerprints) may cause cells to clump. | Keep supplies covered in storage and handle with care. |
| Autoagglutination: Test cells clump without specific antibody present; mainly a problem with red cells. | Use a control with saline and no antibody present. If the control is positive, test is invalidated. |
| Saline stored in glass bottles: Colloidal silica may leach out and cause agglutination. | Store saline in plastic containers. |
| Presence of cross-reactivity. | Use purified antigen preparations and specific monoclonal antibody whenever possible. |
| Presence of rheumatoid factor. | Test specifically for rheumatoid factor to rule out its presence. If rheumatoid factor is present, agglutination results must be interpreted carefully. |
| Presence of heterophile antibody: This occurs mainly when red blood cells are used as the carrier particle. | Preabsorb serum with red blood cells without specific antigen, or pretreat red blood cells to remove other antigens. |
| Delay in reading a slide test: Dried out antigen may look like agglutination. | Follow directions and read reactions immediately after incubation. |
| **False-Negative Reactions** | |
| Under centrifugation: If sample is undercentrifuged, cells may not be close enough to interact. | Regulate centrifuge to proper speed and time. |
| Inadequate washing of cells, especially in antiglobulin testing: Unbound immunoglobulins may neutralize the antihuman globulin. | Wash cells thoroughly, according to the procedure being followed. Use control cells on negative reactions. |
| Reagents not active: This may be caused by improper storage. | Refrigerate antisera, but do not freeze because loss of activity may occur. |
| Delays in testing procedures: This especially pertains to antiglobulin testing. Antibody may be eluted from red blood cells. | Once a procedure is begun, follow through to the end without delay. |
| Incorrect incubation temperature: Too low a temperature may result in the lack of association of antigen and antibody. | Check temperature at which test is carried out. |
| Insufficient incubation time: Antigen and antibody may not have time for association. | Follow instructions carefully. |
| Prozone phenomenon: Too much patient antibody for amount of test. | If this is suspected, dilute antibody and repeat the test. |
| Failure to add antiglobulin reagent: This occurs mainly in direct and indirect antiglobulin testing. | Add check cells that are antibody-coated to see if agglutination occurs after a negative test. If there is still no agglutination, disregard the results and repeat. |

## SUMMARY

Agglutination, first observed in 1896 when antibody was found to react with bacterial cells, is a versatile technique that is simple to perform. The process of agglutination can be divided into two steps: (1) sensitization or initial binding, which depends on the nature of the antibody and the antigen-bearing surface, and (2) lattice formation, which is governed by such factors as pH, ionic strength, and temperature. Decreasing the ionic strength of the milieu, running the reaction at a pH between 6.7 and 7.2, and choosing the correct temperature for the particular immunoglobulin type can all enhance lattice formation. Many of these manipulations are necessary to overcome the fact that many particles in solution are charged, and like charges tend to repel one another. Due to its larger size, IgM is usually able to effect lattice formation without additional enhancement, while for IgG, such measures are necessary to see a visible reaction.

Agglutination reactions can be divided into several distinct categories: (1) direct, (2) passive, (3) reverse passive, (4) agglutination inhibition, and (5) coagglutination. In direct agglutination, antigens are found naturally on the indicator particle, but in passive agglutination, antigens are artificially attached to such a particle. Reverse passive agglutination is so called because antibody is attached to the indicator particle. Agglutination inhibition is based on competition between antigen-coated particles and soluble patient antigen for a limited number of antibody sites. This is the only instance in which agglutination represents a negative test. Coagglutination uses bacteria as the carrier particle to which antibody is attached.

Coombs' tests involve the use of antihuman globulin to enhance agglutination. Two distinct techniques, direct and indirect testing, are frequently used in the blood bank, and each has a specific purpose. The direct Coombs' test is used to detect in vivo coating of patient cells with antigen. The indirect Coombs' test amplifies in vitro antigen–antibody combination. Typically, it is employed to detect unexpected patient antibody to red blood cells intended for a transfusion.

Several automated agglutination techniques have been employed in the clinical laboratory to increase the sensitivity of agglutination reactions. PACIA looks at residual nonagglutinating particles by means of nephelometry. As agglutination occurs, clumps of antigens increase in size, and these large clumps are not counted. The amount of unknown in a patient specimen is therefore indirectly proportional to the number of unagglutinated particles, because an increase in unknown results in a decrease in particles that do not agglutinate.

Quality control is an important aspect of the performance of agglutination reactions. Concentration of antigen, incubation time, temperature, diluent used, and the method of reading should be standardized for each particular test done. This helps to cut down on the occurrence of false-positive and false-negative results. Agglutination reactions are typically used as screening tests; they are fast and sensitive and can yield valuable information when interpreted correctly.

# CASE STUDY

A 25-year-old female who was 2 months pregnant went to her physician for a prenatal workup. She had been vaccinated against rubella, but her titer was never established. She was concerned because a friend of hers who had never been vaccinated for rubella thought she might have the disease. The patient had previously been on an all-day shopping trip with her friend. The physician ordered a rubella test as a part of the prenatal workup. The results on an undiluted serum specimen were positive.

Questions

a. What does the positive rubella test indicate?

b. How should this be interpreted in the light of the patient's condition?

c. Is a semiquantitative test indicated?

# EXERCISE

## LATEX AGGLUTINATION SLIDE TEST FOR RUBELLA

### Principle

Rubella virus is the etiologic agent of German measles. It generally causes a mild viral infection with a slight rash. However, it is recommended that all women of childbearing age be tested for the presence of rubella antibodies to determine their immune status, because viral infection during the first trimester of pregnancy can result in birth defects or stillbirth. Manual card tests used to determine the presence of antibodies to rubella are based on the principle of passive agglutination. Latex particles that are coated with solubilized rubella virus allow a visible observation of the antigen–antibody reaction. When patient serum is mixed with the latex reagent, a visible agglutination reaction will result if specific antibody is present.

### Specimen Collection

Collect blood aseptically by venipuncture into a clean, dry, sterile tube and allow it to clot. Separate the serum without transferring any cellular elements. Do not use grossly hemolyzed, excessively lipemic, or bacterially contaminated specimens. Fresh non–heat inactivated serum is recommended for the test. However, if the test cannot be performed immediately, serum may be stored between 2°C and 8°C for up to 48 hours. If there is any additional delay, freeze the serum at –20°C.

For diagnosis of current or recent rubella infection, paired sera (acute and convalescent) should be obtained. The acute sera should be collected as soon after rash onset as possible or at the time of exposure. Convalescent sera should be obtained 7 to 21 days after the onset of the rash or at least 30 days after exposure if no clinical symptoms appear. Test acute and convalescent sera simultaneously using the semiquantitative procedure.

### Reagents, Materials, and Equipment

Kit containing the following:

Latex antigen

Dilution buffer

High reactive control

Low reactive control

Negative control

Plastic stirrers

Disposable slides

   Materials required but not provided:

A pipette or pipettes capable of providing 10, 20, 35, and
   50 μL volumes.

Timer

### Precautions

Latex reagent controls and buffer contain 0.1 percent sodium azide as a preservative. Sodium azide may react with lead and copper plumbing to form highly explosive metal azides. On disposal, flush with a large volume of water to prevent azide buildup.

The virus strain used in the preparation of the latex reagent has been previously inactivated. However, it is recommended that users follow the same safety precautions in effect for the handling of other types of potentially infectious material.

Each donor unit used in the preparation of control material was tested by an FDA-approved method for the presence of antibodies to HIV, HBV surface antigen, and HCV and was found to be negative. However, the controls should be handled as recommended for any potentially infectious human serum or blood specimen.

### Procedure*

#### Qualitative Slide Test

1. Allow reagents, controls, and specimens to reach room temperature.
2. Label test slide for each sample and control to be tested. Avoid touching surface inside the circles.
3. Pipette 10 to 25 μL of sample or control (depending upon the particular kit) into the appropriate circle.
4. Using a new plastic stirrer for each circle, spread the serum to fill the entire circle.
5. Resuspend the latex reagent by gently mixing the vial until the suspension is homogeneous. Using the dropper provided, hold the dropper perpendicular to the slide, and place one drop of latex reagent onto each circle containing the serum or control.
6. Rotate the slide back and forth in a figure-eight pattern, slowly and evenly, for 2 minutes. Alternately, place the card on a rotator under a moistened humidifying cover for the time specified in the kit.
7. Immediately following rotation, place the slide on a flat surface and observe for agglutination using a direct light source.

---

\* This is a generalized procedure that is used in kits such as the RUBAscan, Sure-Vue Rubella, Remel Color Slide Rubella, and others.

## Semiquantitative Slide Test

If a positive reaction is obtained, the specimen may be serially diluted with diluent to obtain a semiquantitative estimate of the rubella antibody level.

1. Label the test slide using twofold serial dilutions (e.g., 1:2, 1:4, 1:8) for the high positive control and for each positive serum sample to be tested. The low positive control and negative control are not subject to serial twofold dilutions.

2. Prepare dilutions according to instructions for the particular kit.

3. Using a separate plastic stirrer for each set of samples or controls, mix each specimen or control until the entire area of each oval is filled. Start at the highest dilution of each sample or control, and proceed to the next lower dilution with the same stirrer until all circles are spread.

4. Resuspend the latex reagent by gently mixing the vial until the suspension is homogeneous. Using the dropper provided, hold it perpendicular to the slide and place one drop of latex reagent onto each circle.

5. Rotate the slide back and forth in a figure-eight pattern, slowly and evenly, for 2 minutes. Alternately, place the card on a rotator under a moistened humidifying cover for the time specified in the kit.

6. Immediately following rotation, place the slide on a flat surface and observe for agglutination using a direct light source.

## Results

The presence of any visible agglutination significantly different from the negative control indicates the presence of antibodies against rubella virus in the serum sample. Both the low and high positive controls should show agglutination different from the uniform appearance of the negative control. The negative control should show no agglutination. In the semiquantitative test, the rubella titer will correspond to the highest serum dilution that produces visible agglutination. The high positive control should give a titer within one doubling dilution of that indicated on the label.

## Interpretation of Results

Undiluted serum will give a positive reaction if at least $10 \pm 1$ IU/mL of antibody is present. This indicates that the individual has immunity to rubella. When a semiquantitative test is performed with acute and convalescent sera from the same patient, a fourfold increase in titer is considered to be significant. This typically indicates infection. Some individuals previously exposed to rubella may demonstrate a rise in antibody titer. Seroconversion can also be seen after a vaccination procedure. All test results must be evaluated by a physician in light of the clinical symptoms shown by the patient.

# REVIEW QUESTIONS

1. Which of the following best describes agglutination?
   a. A combination of soluble antigen with soluble antibody
   b. A combination of particulate antigen with soluble antibody
   c. A reaction that produces no visible end point
   d. A reaction that requires instrumentation to read

2. All of the following could be used to enhance an agglutination reaction *except*
   a. increasing the viscosity of the medium.
   b. using albumin.
   c. increasing the ionic strength of the medium.
   d. centrifugation.

3. Agglutination of dyed bacterial cells represents which type of reaction?
   a. Direct agglutination
   b. Passive agglutination
   c. Reverse passive agglutination
   d. Agglutination inhibition

4. In which of the following circumstances would the indirect Coombs' test be employed?
   a. Identification of the ABO blood groups
   b. Identification of cold-reacting antibody
   c. Identification of an unexpected IgG antibody
   d. Identification of hemolytic disease of the newborn

5. In an agglutination reaction, if cells are not centrifuged long enough, which of the following might occur?
   a. False-negative result
   b. False-positive result
   c. No effect
   d. Slight effect but can be ignored

6. Agglutination inhibition could best be used for which of the following types of antigens?
   a. Large cellular antigens such as erythrocytes
   b. Soluble haptens
   c. Bacterial cells
   d. Antigen attached to latex particles

7. Which of the following correctly describes reverse passive agglutination?
   a. It is a negative test.
   b. It can be used to detect autoantibodies.
   c. It is used for identification of bacterial antigens.
   d. It is used to detect sensitization of red blood cells.

8. In which of the following tests is patient antigen determined by measuring the number of nonagglutinating particles left after the reaction has taken place?
   a. Direct agglutination
   b. Coagglutination
   c. PACIA
   d. Coombs' testing

9. Reactions involving IgG may need to be enhanced for which reason?
   a. It is only active at 25°C.
   b. It may be too small to produce lattice formation.
   c. It has only one antigen-binding site.
   d. It is not able to produce visible in vitro agglutination.

10. For which of the following tests is a lack of agglutination a positive reaction?
    a. Hemagglutination
    b. Passive agglutination
    c. Reverse passive agglutination
    d. Agglutination inhibition

11. All of the following would be considered good quality-control procedures *except*
    a. storing reagents properly.
    b. standardizing temperature of reactions.
    c. allowing the reaction to go as long as possible.
    d. using monoclonal antibody to avoid cross-reactivity.

12. A positive direct Coombs' test could occur under which circumstances?
    a. Hemolytic disease of the newborn
    b. Autoimmune hemolytic anemia
    c. Antibodies to drugs that bind to red cells
    d. Any of the above

# References

1. Kindt, TJ, Goldsby, RA, and Osborne, BA. Kuby Immunology, ed. 6. WH Freeman, New York, 2007, pp. 145–167.

2. Tinghitella, TJ, and Edberg, SC. Agglutination tests and limulus assay for the diagnosis of infectious diseases. In Balows, A, Hausler, WJ, and Hermann, KL, et al. (eds): Manual of Clinical Microbiology, ed. 5. American Society for Microbiology, Washington, D.C., 1991, pp. 61–72.

3. Brecher, ME (ed). The 50th Anniversary AABB Edition 1953–2003 Technical Manual, ed. 14. American Association of Blood Banks, Bethesda, 2002, pp. 253–269.

4. Beadling, WV, and Cooling, L. Immunohematology. In McPherson, RA, and Pincus, MR (eds): Henry's Clinical Diagnosis and Management by Laboratory Methods, ed. 21. Saunders Elsevier, Philadelphia, 2007, pp. 618–669.

5. Mak, TW, and Saunders, ME. The Immune Response: Basic and Clinical Principles. Elsevier, Burlington, MA, 2006, pp. 147–178.

6. Taiwo, SS, Fadiora, SO, Oparinde, DP, and Olowe, OA. Widal agglutination titres in the diagnosis of typhoid fever. West Afr J Med 26:97–101, 2007.

7. Pasetti, MF, Nataro, JP, and Levine, MM. Immunologic methods for diagnosis of infections caused by diarrheagenic *Enterobacteriaceae* and *Vibrionaceae*. In Detrick, B, Hamilton, RG, and Folds, JD (eds): Manual of Molecular and Clinical Laboratory Immunology, ed. 7. ASM Press, Washington, DC, 2006, pp. 448–461.

8. Carpenter, AB. Immunoassays for the diagnosis of infectious diseases. In Murray, PR, Baron, EJ, Jorgensen, JH, Landry, ML, et al. (eds): Manual of Clinical Microbiology, ed. 9. ASM Press, Washington, D.C., 2007, pp. 257–270.

9. Ashihara, Y, Kasahara, Y, and Nakamura, RM. Immunoassay and immunochemistry. In McPherson, RA, and Pincus, MR (eds): Henry's Clinical Diagnosis and Management by Laboratory Methods, ed. 21. Saunders Elsevier, Philadelphia, 2007, pp. 793–818.

10. Forbes, BA, Sahm, DF, and Weissfeld, AS. Bailey and Scott's Diagnostic Microbiology, ed. 12. Mosby Elsevier, St. Louis, 2007, pp. 159–171.

11. Forbes, BA, Sahm, DF, and Weissfeld, AS. Bailey and Scott's Diagnostic Microbiology, ed. 12. Mosby Elsevier, St. Louis, 2007, pp. 147–158.

12. Shet, A, and Kaplan, E. Diagnostic methods for group A streptococcal infection. In Detrick, B, Hamilton, RG, and Folds, JD (eds): Manual of Molecular and Clinical Laboratory Immunology, ed. 7. ASM Press, Washington, DC, 2006, pp. 428–433.

13. Jenson, HB. Epstein-Barr virus. In Detrick, B, Hamilton, RG, and Folds, JD (eds): Manual of Molecular and Clinical Laboratory Immunology, ed. 7. ASM Press, Washington, DC, 2006, pp. 637–647.

14. Linde, A, and Falk, KI. Epstein-Barr virus. In Murray, PR, Baron, EJ, Jorgensen, JH, Landry, ML, et al. (eds): Manual of Clinical Microbiology, ed. 9. ASM Press, Washington, D.C., 2007, pp. 1564–1573.

15. Bellini, WJ, and Icenogle, JP. Measles and rubella viruses. In Murray, PR, Baron, EJ, Jorgensen, JH, Landry, ML, et al. (eds): Manual of Clinical Microbiology, ed. 9. ASM Press, Washington, D.C., 2007, pp. 1378–1391.

16. Li, H, Ketema, F, Sill, AM, Kreisel, KM, et al. A simple and inexpensive particle agglutination test to distinguish recent from established HIV-1 infection. Int J Infect Dis 11:459–465, 2007.

17. Creegan, L, Bauer, HM, Samuel, MC, Klausner, J, et al. An evaluation of the relative sensitivities of the venereal disease research laboratory test and the *Treponema pallidum* particle agglutination test among patients diagnosed with primary syphilis. Sex Transm Dis 34:1016–1018, 2007.

18. Senthilkumar, TMA, Subathra, M, Phil, M, Ramadass, P, et al. Rapid serodiagnosis of Leptospirosis by latex agglutination test and flow-through assay. Indian J Med Microbiol 26:45–49, 2008.

19. Bannerman, TL, and Peacock, SJ. Staphylococcus, Micrococcus, and other catalase-positive cocci. In Murray, PR, Baron, EJ, Jorgensen, JH, Landry, ML, et al. (eds): Manual of Clinical Microbiology, ed. 9. ASM Press, Washington, D.C., 2007, pp. 390–411.

20. Spellerberg, B, and Bryant, C. *Streptococcus*. In Murray, PR, Baron, EJ, Jorgensen, JH, Landry, ML, et al. (eds): Manual of Clinical Microbiology, ed. 9. ASM Press, Washington, D.C., 2007, pp. 412–429.

21. Park, CH et al. Detection of group B streptococcal colonization in pregnant women using direct latex agglutination testing of selective broth. J Clin Micro 39:408–409, 2001.

22. de Goes, AC, de Moraes, MT, deCastro Silveira, W, Araujo, It, et al. Development of a rapid and sensitive latex agglutination-based method for detection of group A rotavirus. J Virol Methods 148:211–217, 2008.

23. Janda, WM, and Gaydos, CA. Neisseria. In Murray, PR, Baron, EJ, Jorgensen, JH, Landry, ML, et al. (eds): Manual of Clinical Microbiology, ed. 9. ASM Press, Washington, D.C., 2007, pp. 601–620.

24. Lindsley, MD, Warnock, DW, and Morrison, CJ. Serological and molecular diagnosis of fungal infections. In Detrick, B, Hamilton, RG, and Folds, JD (eds): Manual of Molecular and Clinical Laboratory Immunology, ed. 7. ASM Press, Washington, DC, 2006, pp. 569–605.

25. Landry, ML. Rapid viral diagnosis. In Detrick, B, Hamilton, RG, and Folds, JD (eds): Manual of Molecular and Clinical Laboratory Immunology, ed. 7. ASM Press, Washington, DC, 2006, pp. 610–616.

# 10 Labeled Immunoassays

# CHAPTER OUTLINE

The need to develop rapid, specific, and sensitive assays to determine the presence of important biologically active molecules ushered in a new era of testing in the clinical laboratory. Labeled immunoassays are designed for antigens and antibodies that may be small in size or present in very low concentrations. The presence of such antigens or antibodies is determined indirectly by using a labeled reactant to detect whether or not specific binding has taken place.

The substance to be measured is known as the **analyte.** Examples include bacterial antigens, hormones, drugs, tumor markers, specific immunoglobulins, and many other substances. Analytes are bound by molecules that react specifically with them. Typically, this is antibody. One reactant, either the antigen or the antibody, is labeled with a marker so that the amount of binding can be monitored. Labeled immunoassays have made possible rapid quantitative measurement of many important entities such as viral antigens in patients infected with HIV. This ability to detect very small quantities of antigen or antibody has revolutionized the diagnosis and monitoring of numerous diseases and has led to more prompt treatment for many such conditions.

## CHARACTERISTICS OF LABELED ASSAYS

### Competitive versus Noncompetitive Assays

Current techniques include the use of fluorescent, radioactive, chemiluminescent, and enzyme labels. The underlying principles of all these techniques are essentially the same. There are two major formats for all labeled assays: competitive and noncompetitive. In a **competitive immunoassay,** all the reactants are mixed together simultaneously, and labeled antigen competes with unlabeled patient antigen for a limited number of antibody-binding sites. The amount of bound label is inversely proportional to the concentration of the labeled antigen. This means that the more label detected, the less there is of patient antigen.

In a typical **noncompetitive immunoassay,** antibody, often called *capture antibody,* is first passively absorbed to a solid phase. Unknown patient antigen is then allowed to react with and be captured by the antibody. After washing to remove unbound antigen, a second antibody with a label is added to the reaction. In this case, the amount of label measured is directly proportional to the amount of patient antigen.

In both types of assays, the label must not alter the reactivity of the molecule, and it should remain stable for the shelf life of the reagent. Radioactivity, enzymes, fluorescent compounds, and chemiluminescent substances have all been used as labels. Each of these is discussed in a later section.

### Antibodies

In any assay, it is essential for the antibody used to have a high affinity for the antigen in question. As discussed in Chapter 8, affinity is the strength of the primary interaction between a single antibody-combining site and an antigenic determinant or epitope. In competitive binding assays, there is random interaction between individual antigen and antibody molecules. Therefore, the higher the affinity of antibody for antigen, the larger the amount of antigen bound to antibody and the more accurately specific binding can be measured. The ultimate sensitivity of the immunoassay, in fact, depends largely on the magnitude of affinity.[1,2]

The antibody used should also be very specific for the antigen involved in the reaction. The discovery of monoclonal antibodies has made available a constant source of highly specific antibody that has increased the ability to detect small amounts of analyte with great accuracy.[3]

## Standards or Calibrators

Standards, also known as *calibrators*, are unlabeled analytes that are made up in known concentrations of the substance to be measured. They are used to establish a relationship between the labeled analyte measured and any unlabeled analyte that might be present in patient specimens.[4] Differing amounts of standards are added to antibody–antigen mixtures to ascertain their effect on binding of the labeled reagent. Most instruments then extrapolate this information and do a best-fit curve (one that is not absolutely linear) to determine the concentration of the unknown analyte.

## Separation Methods

In most assays, once the reaction between antigen and antibody has taken place, there must be a partitioning step, or a way of separating reacted from unreacted analyte. Currently, most immunoassays use a *solid-phase* vehicle for separation. Numerous materials, such as polystyrene test tubes, microtiter plates, glass or polystyrene beads, magnetic beads, and cellulose membranes, have been used for this purpose. Antigen or antibody is attached by physical adsorption, and when specific binding takes place, complexes remain attached to the solid phase. This provides a simple way to separate bound and free reactants.

If a separation step is employed in an assay, the efficiency of the separation is critical to the accuracy of the results. The bound and unbound fractions are usually separated by physical means, including decanting, centrifugation, or filtration. This is followed by a washing step to remove any remaining unbound analyte. Great care must be taken to perform this correctly, because incomplete washing leads to incomplete removal of the labeled analyte and inaccurate results.[4]

## Detection of the Label

The last step common to all immunoassays is detection of the labeled analyte. For radioimmunoassays, this involves a system for counting radioactivity, while for other labels such as enzymes, fluorescence, or chemiluminescence, typically a change in absorbance in a substrate is measured by spectrophotometry. All systems must use stringent quality controls.

## Quality Control

When measuring analytes that are present in very limited quantities, it is essential to establish quality-control procedures. Because the goal of testing is to determine whether patient levels are increased or decreased over normal values, test performance must be monitored to limit random errors. One means of doing this is to run a blank tube, usually phosphate-buffered saline, with every test. This is not expected to have any detectable label but serves as a check for nonspecific adsorption and for inadequate washing between steps. Any readings indicative of label in the blank are known as *background*. If the background is too high, wash steps need to be made more efficient.[4]

A negative control and a high and a low positive control should be run in addition. This serves as a check on the quality of the reagents to make sure the label is readily detectable under current testing conditions. All controls and the patient sample are usually run in duplicate. If any controls are out of range, test values should not be reported. Automated procedures have cut down on many performance variables. Individual testing procedures are now considered in the following sections.

## RADIOIMMUNOASSAY

### Competitive Binding Assays

The first type of immunoassay developed was **radioimmunoassay (RIA)**, pioneered by Yalow and Berson in the late 1950s. It was used to determine the level of insulin–anti-insulin complexes in diabetic patients.[5,6] A radioactive substance is used as a label. Radioactive elements have nuclei that decay spontaneously, emitting matter and energy. Several radioactive labels, including $^{131}I$; $^{125}I$; and tritiated hydrogen, or $^{3}H$, have been used, but $^{125}I$ is the most popular.[5] It has a half-life of 60 days, and because it has a higher counting rate than that of $^{3}H$, the total counting time is less. It is easily incorporated into protein molecules, and it emits gamma radiation, which is detected by a gamma counter. Very low quantities of radioactivity can be easily measured.[2]

RIA was originally based on the principle of competitive binding. Thus, the analyte being detected competes with a radiolabeled analyte for a limited number of binding sites on a high-affinity antibody.[1,5] The concentration of the radioactive analyte is in excess, so all binding sites on antibody will be occupied. If patient antigen is present, some of the binding sites will be filled with unlabeled analyte, thus decreasing the amount of bound radioactive label **(Fig. 10–1)**. When bound and free radiolabeled antigens are separated and a washing step has occurred, the amount of label in the bound phase is indirectly proportional to the amount of patient antigen present. This can be illustrated by the following equation:

$$6Ag^* + 2Ag + 4Ab \rightarrow 3Ag^*Ab + 1AgAb + 3Ag^* + 1Ag$$

In this example, labeled and unlabeled antigens occur in a 3:1 ratio. Binding to a limited number of antibody sites will take place in the same ratio. Thus, on the right side of the equation, three of the four binding sites are occupied by labeled antigen, while one site is filled by unlabeled

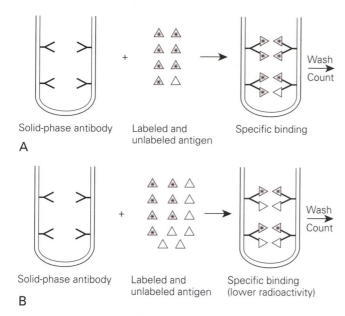

Solid-phase antibody    Labeled and    Specific binding
                        unlabeled antigen

**A**

Solid-phase antibody    Labeled and    Specific binding
                        unlabeled antigen    (lower radioactivity)

**B**

**FIGURE 10–1.** Principle of RIA. Labeled antigen competes with patient antigen for a limited number of binding sites on solid-phase antibody. *(A)* Very little patient antigen is present, making radioactivity of the solid phase high. *(B)* More patient antigen is present, and the radioactivity of the solid phase is reduced in proportion to the amount of patient antigen bound.

antigen. As the amount of patient antigen increases, fewer binding sites will be occupied by labeled antigen, as demonstrated by the next equation:

$$6Ag^* + 18Ag + 4Ab \rightarrow 1Ag^*Ab + 3AgAb + 5Ag^* + 15Ag$$

In this case, the ratio of labeled to unlabeled antigen is 1:3. Binding to antibody sites takes place in the same ratio, and the amount of bound label is greatly decreased in comparison to the first equation. In this type of RIA, use of a constant amount of radiolabeled antigen with standards of known concentration will result in a standard curve that can be used to extrapolate the concentration of the unknown patient antigen.[5] The detection limits of competitive assays are largely determined by the affinity of the antibody.[2] These limits have been calculated to be as low as 10 fmol/L, or 600,000 molecules in a sample volume of 100 μL.[1]

## Advantages and Disadvantages of Radioimmunoassay

Examples of substances that are measured by RIA include thyroid-stimulating hormone and total serum IgE.[2,7] RIA is an extremely sensitive and precise technique for determining trace amounts of analytes that are small in size.

However, chief among the disadvantages of all RIA techniques is the health hazard involved in working with radioactive substances. Laboratories have found it more and more difficult and expensive to maintain a license and to comply with federal regulations. In addition, disposal problems, short shelf life, and the need for expensive equipment has caused laboratorians to explore other techniques

for identifying analytes in low concentration.[2] Enzyme immunoassays have largely replaced RIA because of their comparable sensitivity and the availability of automated instrumentation that allows for processing of a large number of samples in less time.[3]

## ENZYME IMMUNOASSAY

Enzymes are naturally occurring molecules that catalyze certain biochemical reactions. They react with suitable substrates to produce breakdown products that may be chromogenic, fluorogenic, or luminescent. Some type of spectroscopy can then be used to measure the changes involved. As labels for immunoassay, they are cheap and readily available, have a long shelf life, are easily adapted to automation, and cause changes that can be measured using inexpensive equipment.[2] Sensitivity can be achieved without disposal problems or the health hazards of radiation. Because one molecule of enzyme can generate many molecules of product, little reagent is necessary to produce high sensitivity.[1,3] Enzyme labels can either be used qualitatively to determine the presence of an antigen or antibody or quantitatively to determine the actual concentration of an analyte in an unknown specimen. Assays based on the use of enzymes can be found in such diverse settings as clinical laboratories, doctors' offices, and at-home testing.

Enzymes used as labels for immunoassay are typically chosen according to the number of substrate molecules converted per molecule of enzyme, ease and speed of detection, and stability.[2] In addition, availability and cost of enzyme and substrate play a role in the choice of a particular enzyme as reagent. Typical enzymes that have been used as labels in colorimetric reactions include horseradish peroxidase, glucose-6-phosphate dehydrogenase, alkaline phosphatase, and β-D-galactosidase.[1,4] Alkaline phosphatase and horseradish peroxidase have the highest turnover (conversion of substrate) rates, high sensitivity, and are easy to detect, so they are most often used in such assays.[2]

Enzyme assays are classified as either heterogeneous or homogeneous on the basis of whether a separation step is necessary. **Heterogeneous enzyme immunoassays** require a step to physically separate free from bound analyte. In **homogeneous immunoassays,** on the other hand, no separation step is necessary, because enzyme activity diminishes when binding of antibody and antigen occurs. The principles underlying each of these types of assays are discussed next.

### Heterogeneous Enzyme Immunoassay

#### Competitive·EIA

The first enzyme immunoassays (EIAs) were competitive assays based on the principles of RIA. Enzyme-labeled antigen competes with unlabeled patient antigen for a limited number of binding sites on antibody molecules that are attached to a solid phase. After carefully washing to remove any nonspecifically bound antigen, enzyme activity is determined. Enzyme activity is inversely proportional to the concentration of the test substance, meaning that the more patient antigen is bound, the less enzyme-labeled antigen can attach. In this manner, a sensitivity of nanograms ($10^{-9}$ g)/mL can be achieved.[3] This method is typically used for measuring small antigens that are relatively pure, such as insulin and estrogen.[3]

## Noncompetitive EIA

Although competitive tests have a high specificity, the tendency in the laboratory today is toward the use of noncompetitive assays, because they have a higher sensitivity.[1] Many such assays are capable of detecting concentrations of less than 1 pg/mL, achieving a sensitivity actually higher than most RIAs.[3] Noncompetitive assays are often referred to as indirect **enzyme-linked immunosorbent assays (ELISA),** because the enzyme-labeled reagent does not participate in the initial antigen–antibody binding reaction. This type of assay is one of the most frequently used immunoassays in the clinical laboratory due to its sensitivity, specificity, simplicity, and low cost.[1,3,8] Either antigen or antibody may be bound to solid phase. A variety of solid-phase supports are used, including microtiter plates, nitrocellulose membranes, and magnetic latex beads. When antigen is bound to solid phase, patient serum with unknown antibody is added and given time to react. After a wash step, an enzyme-labeled antiglobulin is added. This second antibody reacts with any patient antibody that is bound to solid phase. If no patient antibody is bound to the solid phase, the second labeled antibody will not be bound. After a second wash step, the enzyme substrate is added. The amount of enzyme label detected is directly proportional to the amount of antibody in the specimen **(Fig. 10–2).**

This type of assay has been used to measure antibody production to infectious agents that are difficult to isolate in the laboratory and has been used for autoantibody testing.[2] Viral infections especially are more easily diagnosed by this method than by other types of testing.[1] This technique remains the preferred screening method for detecting antibody to HIV, hepatitis A, and hepatitis C.[9-12] ELISA-based tests are also

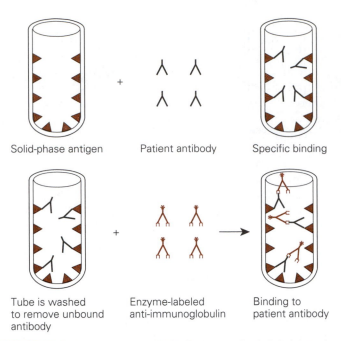

**FIGURE 10–2.** Noncompetitive ELISA. Patient antibody is incubated with solid-phase antigen. After a wash step, enzyme-labeled anti-immunoglobulin is added. This will bind to the patient antibody on solid phase. A second wash step is performed to remove any unbound anti-immunoglobulin, and substrate for the enzyme is added. Color development is directly proportional to the amount of patient antibody present.

used to identify Epstein-Barr–specific antibodies produced in infectious mononucleosis.[13]

## Capture Assays

If antibody is bound to the solid phase, these assays are often called **sandwich immunoassays,** or **capture assays.** Antigens captured in these assays must have multiple epitopes. Excess antibody attached to solid phase is allowed to combine with the test sample to capture any antigen present. After an appropriate incubation period, enzyme-labeled antibody is added. This second antibody recognizes a different epitope than the solid-phase antibody and completes the "sandwich." Enzymatic activity is directly proportional to the amount of antigen in the test sample **(Fig. 10–3).**

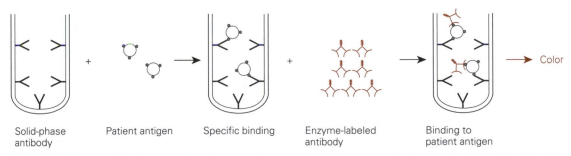

**FIGURE 10–3.** Noncompetitive ELISA: sandwich technique with solid-phase antibody. Patient antigen is incubated with solid-phase antibody. After washing, enzyme-labeled immunoglobulin is added, which combines with additional determinant sites on the bound patient antigen. After a second wash step, substrate for the enzyme is added. Color development is directly proportional to the amount of patient antigen present.

Capture assays are best suited to antigens that have multiple determinants, such as antibodies, polypeptide hormones, proteins, tumor markers, and microorganisms, especially viruses.[2] When used with microorganisms, the epitope must be unique to the organism being tested, and it must be present in all strains of that organism. Use of monoclonal antibodies has made this a very sensitive test system. Rotavirus in stool and respiratory syncytial virus in respiratory tract secretions are two examples of capture assays.[14–16] In addition, recently developed ELISAs have made it much easier to detect parasites such as *Giardia lamblia* and *Cryptosporidium* in the stool.[17–19] Antigen-detection tests have also proved useful for identifying fungi such as *Aspergillus*, *Candida*, and *Cryptococcus*.[17,20–22]

Another major use of capture assays is in the measurement of immunoglobulins, especially those of certain classes. For instance, the presence of IgM can be specifically determined, thus indicating an acute infection. Measurement of IgE, including allergen-specific IgE, which appears in minute quantities in serum, can also be accomplished with this system.[23] (Chapter 13 provides a more detailed discussion on detection of IgE.) When capture assays are used to measure immunoglobulins, the specific immunoglobulin class being detected is actually acting as antigen, and the antibody is antihuman immunoglobulin.

Indirect ELISA tests are more sensitive than their direct counterparts, because all patient antigen has a chance to participate in the reaction. However, there is more manipulation than in direct tests, because there are two incubations and two wash steps.

Heterogeneous enzyme assays, in general, achieve a sensitivity similar to that of RIA.[1] In sandwich assays, capture antibody on solid phase must have both a high affinity and a high specificity for this test system to be effective. However, there may be problems with nonspecific protein binding or the presence of antibodies to various components of the testing system.[3] If this is suspected, serum can be pretreated to avoid this problem. Sandwich assays are also subject to the hook effect, an unexpected fall in the amount of measured analyte when an extremely high concentration is present.[24] This typically occurs in antigen excess, where the majority of binding sites are filled, and the remainder of patient antigen has no place to bind. If this condition is suspected, serum dilutions must be made and then retested.

## Rapid Immunoassays

### Membrane-Based Cassette Assays

Membrane-based cassette assays are a relatively new type of enzyme immunoassay. They are rapid, easy to perform, and give reproducible results.[2] Although designed primarily for point-of-care or home testing, many of these have been modified for increased sensitivity and can be made semiquantitative for use in a clinical laboratory. Typically these are designed as single-use, disposable

assays in a plastic cartridge. The membrane is usually nitrocellulose, which is able to easily immobilize proteins and nucleic acids.[3] The rapid flow through the membrane and its large surface area enhance the speed and sensitivity of ELISA reactions.[1] Either antigen or antibody can be coupled to the membrane, and the reaction is read by looking for the presence of a colored reaction product. Some test devices require the separate addition of patient sample, wash reagent, labeled antigen or antibody, and the substrate.

Another type of rapid assay, called *immunochromatography*, combines all the previously mentioned steps into one. The analyte is applied at one end of the strip and migrates toward the distal end, where there is an absorbent pad to maintain a constant capillary flow rate.[2] The labeling and detection zones are set between the two ends. As the sample is loaded, it reconstitutes the labeled antigen or antibody, and the two form a complex that migrates toward the detection zone. An antigen or antibody immobilized in the detection zone captures the immune complex and forms a colored line for a positive test **(Fig. 10–4)**. This may be in the form of a plus sign. Excess labeled immunoreactant migrates to the absorbent pad. This type of test device has been used to identify microorganisms such as *Streptococcus pyogenes* and *Streptococcus agalactiae* and has been used to test for pregnancy, for troponin in a heart attack, and for hepatitis B surface antigen, to name just a few examples. Test results are most often qualitative rather than quantitative.

## Homogeneous Enzyme Immunoassay

A homogeneous enzyme immunoassay is any antigen–antibody system in which no separation step is necessary. Homogeneous assays are generally less sensitive than heterogeneous assays, but they are rapid, simple to perform, and adapt easily to automation.[1,2] No washing steps are necessary. Their chief use has been in the determination of low-molecular-weight analytes such as hormones, therapeutic drugs, and drugs of abuse in both serum and urine.[1,24] An

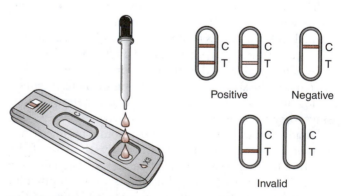

**FIGURE 10–4.** Example of a membrane cassette assay. © Inverness Medical. Used by permission. One line represents the positive control, and the second line indicates a positive test.

example of a homogeneous immunoassay is the enzyme-multiplied immunoassay technique (EMIT) developed by the Syva Corporation.

Homogeneous assays are based on the principle of change in enzyme activity as specific antigen–antibody combination occurs. Reagent antigen is labeled with an enzyme tag. When antibody binds to specific determinant sites on the antigen, the active site on the enzyme is blocked, resulting in a measurable loss of activity. Free analyte (antigen) competes with enzyme-labeled analyte for a limited number of antibody-binding sites, so this is a competitive assay. Enzyme activity is directly in proportion to the concentration of patient antigen or hapten present in the test solution. A physical separation of bound and free analyte is thus not necessary.

The sensitivity of homogeneous assays is determined by the following: (1) detectability of enzymatic activity; (2) change in that activity when antibody binds to antigen; (3) strength of the antibody's binding; and (4) susceptibility of the assay to interference from endogenous enzyme activity, cross-reacting antigens, or enzyme inhibitors. Typically, a sensitivity of micrograms per milliliter is reached, far less than that achievable by heterogeneous enzyme assays, because the amplification properties of enzymes are not utilized.[24] This technique is usually applied only to detection of small molecules that could not be easily measured by other means.

Other considerations include the fact that only certain enzymes are inhibited in this manner. Enzymatic activity may be altered by steric exclusion of the substrate, or there may also be changes in the conformation structure of the enzyme, especially in the region of the active site. Two enzymes that are frequently used in this type of assay are malate dehydrogenase and glucose-6-phosphate dehydrogenase.[2]

## Advantages and Disadvantages of Enzyme Immunoassay

Enzyme immunoassays have achieved a sensitivity similar to that of RIA without creating a health hazard or causing disposal problems. The use of nonisotopic enzyme labels with high specific activity in noncompetitive assays increases sensitivity and does so using shorter incubation times than the original RIAs.[2] There is no need for expensive instrumentation, because most assays can be read by spectrophotometry or by simply noting the presence or absence of color. Reagents are inexpensive and have a long shelf life. Although homogeneous assays are not as sensitive as heterogeneous assays, they are simple and require no separation step.

Disadvantages include the fact that some specimens may contain natural inhibitors. Additionally, the size of the enzyme label may be a limiting factor in the design of some assays. Nonspecific protein binding is another difficulty encountered with the use of enzyme labels.[3] However, this technique has been successfully applied to a wide range of assays, and its use will continue to increase.

## FLUORESCENT IMMUNOASSAY

In 1941, Albert Coons demonstrated that antibodies could be labeled with molecules that fluoresce.[5,25] These fluorescent compounds are called *fluorophores* or *fluorochromes*. They can absorb energy from an incident light source and convert that energy into light of a longer wavelength and lower energy as the excited electrons return to the ground state. Fluorophores are typically organic molecules with a ring structure, and each has a characteristic optimum absorption range. The time interval between absorption of energy and emission of fluorescence is very short and can be measured in nanoseconds.

Ideally, a fluorescent probe should exhibit high intensity, which can be distinguished easily from background fluorescence.[2] It should also be stable. The two compounds most often used are fluorescein and rhodamine, usually in the form of isothiocyanates, because these can be readily coupled with antigen or antibody. Fluorescein absorbs maximally at 490 to 495 nm and emits a green color at 517 to 520 nm. It has a high intensity, good photostability, and a high quantum yield. Tetramethylrhodamine absorbs at 550 nm and emits red light at 580 to 585 nm. Because their absorbance and emission patterns differ, fluorescein and rhodamine can be used together. Other compounds used are phycoerythrin, europium (β-naphthyl trifluoroacetone), and lucifer yellow VS.[1,5]

Fluorescent tags or labels were first used for histochemical localization of antigen in tissues. This technique is called **immunofluorescent assay (IFA),** a term restricted to qualitative observations involving the use of a fluorescence microscope. In this manner, many types of antigens can be detected either in fixed tissue sections or in live cell suspensions with a high degree of sensitivity and specificity.

The presence of a specific antigen is determined by the appearance of localized color against a dark background. This method is used for rapid identification of microorganisms in cell culture or infected tissue, tumor-specific antigens on neoplastic tissue, transplantation antigens, and CD antigens on T and B cells through the use of cell flow cytometry.[26] (See Chapter 12 for a more complete discussion of the principles of cell flow cytometry.)

### Direct Immunofluorescent Assays

Fluorescent staining can be categorized as direct or indirect, depending on whether the original antibody has a fluorescent tag attached. In a **direct immunofluorescent assay,** antibody that is conjugated with a fluorescent tag is added directly to unknown antigen that is fixed to a microscope slide. After incubation and a wash step, the slide is read using a fluorescence microscope. Antigens are typically visualized as bright apple green or orange-yellow objects against a dark background. Direct immunofluorescent assay is best suited to antigen detection in tissue or body fluids, while indirect assays can be used for both antigen and antibody identification.[3,25] Examples of antigens detected by this method include *Legionella pneumophila*, *Pneumocystis carinii*, *Chlamydia trachomatis*, and respiratory syncytial virus (RSV)[26,27] **(Fig. 10–5).**

## Indirect Immunofluorescent Assays

**Indirect immunofluorescent assays** involve two steps, the first of which is incubation of patient serum with a known antigen attached to a solid phase. The slide is washed, and then an antihuman immunoglobulin containing a fluorescent tag is added. This combines with the first antibody to form a sandwich, which localizes the fluorescence. In this manner, one antibody conjugate can be used for many different types of reactions, eliminating the need for numerous purified, labeled reagent antibodies. Indirect assays result in increased staining, because multiple molecules can bind to each primary molecule, thus making this a more sensitive technique.[5] Such assays are especially useful in antibody

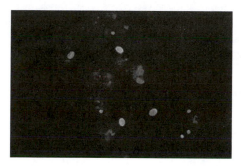

FIGURE 10–5. Direct fluorescent antibody test for *Giardia* and *Cryptosporidium* in stool. Larger oval bodies are *Giardia lamblia* cysts, and the smaller round bodies are *Cryptosporidium sp.* cysts. *(Courtesy of Meridian Bioscience, Cincinnati, OH.) See Color Plate 10.*

identification and have been used to detect treponema, antinuclear, chlamydial, and toxoplasma antibodies, as well as antibodies to such viruses such as herpes simplex, Epstein-Barr, and cytomegalovirus.[3,25,28,29] **Figure 10–6** depicts the difference between the two techniques.

Both techniques allow for a visual assessment of the adequacy of the specimen. This is especially helpful in testing for chlamydia and RSV antigens.[26] Immunofluorescent assays in general, however, face the issue of subjectivity in the reading of slides. Only experienced clinical laboratorians should be responsible for reporting out slide results.

## Other Fluorescent Immunoassays

Quantitative fluorescent immunoassays (FIAs) can be classified as heterogeneous or homogeneous, corresponding to similar types of enzyme immunoassays. In this case, the label is fluorescent, and such a label can be applied to either antigen or antibody. Solid-phase heterogeneous fluorescent assays have been developed for the identification of antibodies to nuclear antigen, toxoplasma antigen, rubella virus, and numerous other virus antigens.[2] In addition, fluorescent assays are used to detect such important biological compounds as cortisol, progesterone, and serum thyroxine (T4).[2]

However, many of the newer developments in fluorescent immunoassay have been related to homogeneous immunoassays. Homogeneous FIA, just like the corresponding EIAs, requires no separation procedure, so it is rapid and simple to perform. There is only one incubation step and no wash step, and usually competitive binding is involved. The basis for this technique is the change that occurs in the fluorescent label on antigen when it binds to specific antibody. Such changes may be related to wavelength

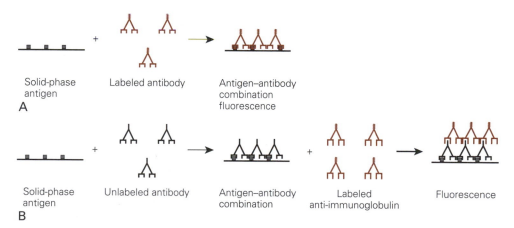

FIGURE 10–6. Direct versus indirect immunofluorescent assays. *(A)* Direct fluorescent assay. Solid-phase antigen fixed to a microscope slide is incubated directly with a fluorescent-labeled antibody. The slide is washed to remove unbound antibody. If specific antigen is present in the patient sample, fluorescence will be observed. *(B)* Indirect fluorescence. Patient antibody is reacted with specific antigen fixed to a microscope slide. A wash step is performed, and a labeled antihuman immunoglobulin is added. After a second wash step to remove any uncombined anti-immunoglobulin, fluorescence of the sample is determined. The amount of fluorescence is directly in proportion to the amount of patient antibody present.

emission, rotation freedom, polarity, or dielectric strength. There is a direct relationship between the amount of fluorescence measured and the amount of antigen in the patient sample. As binding of patient antigen increases, binding of the fluorescent analyte decreases, and hence more fluorescence is observed.

One of the most popular techniques developed is **fluorescence polarization immunoassay (FPIA),** which is based on the change in polarization of fluorescent light emitted from a labeled molecule when it is bound by antibody.[24] Incident light directed at the specimen is polarized with a lens or prism so the waves are aligned in one plane. If a molecule is small and rotates quickly enough, the emitted light is unpolarized after it is excited by polarized light.[1,3] If, however, the labeled molecule is bound to antibody, the molecule is unable to tumble as rapidly, and it emits an increased amount of polarized light. Thus, the degree of polarized light reflects the amount of labeled analyte that is bound.

In FPIA, labeled antigens compete with unlabeled antigen in the patient sample for a limited number of antibody binding sites. The more antigen that is present in the patient sample, the less the fluorescence-labeled antigen is bound and the less the polarization that will be detected. Hence, the degree of fluorescence polarization is inversely proportional to concentration of the analyte **(Fig. 10–7).**

This technique is limited to small molecules that tumble freely in solution, usually those analytes with a molecular weight under 2000 d.[2,3] An additional consideration is nonspecific binding of the labeled conjugate to

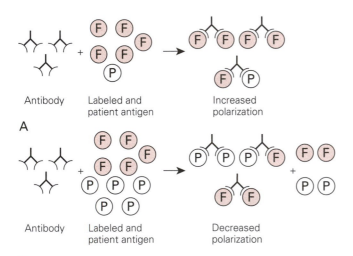

**A**

**B**

**FIGURE 10–7.** Fluorescence polarization immunoassay. Reagent antibody is combined with patient antigen and fluorescent-labeled antigen. *(A)* If little or no patient antigen is present, antibody will bind to the labeled antigen. Binding causes these molecules to rotate more slowly in solution, increasing the amount of polarized light that they return. *(B)* When patient antigen is present, more labeled antigen will be unbound. These molecules will rotate more quickly in solution, giving off light in many directions, and polarization will be decreased.

other proteins in serum. Binding to these molecules would increase polarization, thus falsely decreasing values. FPIA has been used mainly to determine concentrations of therapeutic drugs and hormones. It requires sophisticated instrumentation and is the basis for several automated analyzers on the market today.

## Advantages and Disadvantages of Fluorescent Immunoassay

In principle, the use of fluorescence has the potential for high sensitivity and versatility.[24] The methodology is fairly simple, and there is no need to deal with and dispose of hazardous substances. The main problem, however, has been separation of the signal on the label from autofluorescence produced by different organic substances normally present in serum. Another difficulty encountered is the fact that nonspecific binding to substances in serum can cause quenching or diminishing of the signal and change the amount of fluorescence generated. Fluorescence polarization has been developed to overcome some of these problems, and this technique has seen more widespread use.[3] It does, however, require expensive dedicated instrumentation, which may limit its use in smaller laboratories.

## CHEMILUMINESCENT IMMUNOASSAYS

### Principle of Chemiluminescence

**Chemiluminescence** is another technique employed to follow antigen–antibody combination. It is the emission of light caused by a chemical reaction, typically an oxidation reaction, producing an excited molecule that decays back to its original ground state.[3] A large number of molecules are capable of chemiluminescence, but some of the most common substances used are luminol, acridinium esters, ruthenium derivatives, and nitrophenyl oxalates.[1–3] When these substances are oxidized, typically using hydrogen peroxide and an enzyme for a catalyst, intermediates are produced that are of a higher energy state. These intermediates spontaneously return to their original state, giving off energy in the form of light.[30] Light emissions range from a rapid flash of light to a more continuous glow that can last for hours. Acridinium esters, for example, emit a quick burst or flash of light, while the light remains for a longer time with luminol and dioxetane.[30] Different types of instrumentation are necessary for each kind of emission.

This type of labeling can be used for heterogeneous and homogeneous assays, because labels can be attached to either antigen or antibody. In heterogeneous assays, competitive and sandwich formats are the ones most often used. Smaller analytes such as therapeutic drugs and steroid hormones are measured using competitive assays, while the sandwich format is used for larger analytes such as protein hormones.

## Advantages and Disadvantages of Chemiluminescent Assays

Chemiluminescent assays have an excellent sensitivity, comparable to EIA and RIA, and the reagents are stable and relatively nontoxic.[2,30] The sensitivity of some assays has been reported to be in the range of attamoles ($10^{-18}$ mol) to zeptomoles ($10^{-21}$ mol).[1,3] Because very little reagent is used, they are also quite inexpensive to perform. The relatively high speed of detection also means a faster turnaround time. Detection systems basically consist of photomultiplier tubes, which are simple and relatively inexpensive.

However, false results may be obtained if there is lack of precision in injection of the hydrogen peroxide or if some biological materials such as urine or plasma cause quenching of the light emission. This method has begun to be more widely applied to immunologic testing and has great potential for the future.

## SUMMARY

Labeled immunoassays were developed to measure antigens and antibodies that may be small in size or present in very low concentrations. The substance that is being measured is the analyte. Labeling techniques include the use of radioactivity, enzymes, fluorescence, and chemiluminescence. There are two major types of immunoassays: competitive and noncompetitive. In competitive assays, all the reactants are added at the same time, and labeled antigen competes with patient antigen for a limited number of antibody-binding sites. Noncompetitive assays, on the other hand, allow any antigen present to combine with an excess of antibody attached to a solid phase. Then a second antibody bearing a label is added and binds wherever there is patient antigen.

Antibodies used in immunoassays must be very specific and have a high affinity for the antigen in question. Specificity helps to cut down on cross-reactivity, and the affinity determines how stable the binding is between antigen and antibody. These two factors help to determine the sensitivity of such assays. Bound and unbound label are separated by using a sold-phase surface, such as glass beads, cellulose membranes, polystyrene test tubes, or microtiter plates, to attach either antigen or antibody.

Radioimmunoassay was the first type of immunoassay to be applied to quantitative measurements of analytes in the clinical laboratory. The original technique was based on competition between labeled and unlabeled antigen for a limited number of antibody-binding sites. The more analyte that is present in the patient sample, the lower the amount of radioactivity that is detected.

Enzymes can be used as labels in much the same manner as radioactivity. Competitive assays involve the use of labeled analyte and a limited number of antibody-binding sites. Once separation of bound and unbound analyte has been achieved, substrate for the enzyme is added to the reaction mix, and the presence of the enzyme is detected by a color change in the substrate.

Most enzyme assays used in the laboratory today are noncompetitive. Often, it is antigen that is bound to solid phase and patient antibody that is being detected. After allowing sufficient time for binding to occur, a second enzyme-labeled antibody is added. The sensitivity of noncompetitive assays is greater than that of competitive assays.

Simple one-step formats have been developed for heterogeneous enzyme assays. Rapid flow-through test devices are able to capture antigen or antibody in a certain spot on a membrane. The results are easy to interpret.

Homogeneous enzyme assays require no separation step. They are based on the principle that enzyme activity changes as specific antigen–antibody binding occurs. When antibody binds to enzyme-labeled antigen, steric hindrance results in a loss in enzyme activity.

Fluorochromes are fluorescent compounds that are used as markers in immunologic reactions. Direct immunofluorescent assays involve antigen detection through a specific antibody that is labeled with a fluorescent tag. In indirect immunofluorescent assays, the original antibody is unlabeled. Incubation with antigen is followed by addition of a second labeled anti-immunoglobulin that detects antigen–antibody complexes.

Heterogeneous fluorescent immunoassays are similar to those described for other labels. Recent research has been directed toward improvement of homogeneous fluorescent immunoassays to reduce the background fluorescence normally found in serum. FPIA takes advantage of the fact that when an antigen is bound to antibody, polarization of light increases.

Chemiluminescence is the production of light energy by certain compounds when they are oxidized. Substances that do this can be used as markers in reactions that are similar to RIA and EIA.

Each type of system has advantages and disadvantages related to the particular nature of the label. Some are better for large multivalent antigens, while others are capable of detecting only small haptens. These limitations must be kept in mind when choosing the technique that is most sensitive and best suited for a particular analyte.

# CASE STUDY

A 2-year-old male child has symptoms that include fatigue, nausea, vomiting, and diarrhea. These symptoms have persisted for several days. Stool cultures for bacteria pathogens such as *Salmonella* and *Shigella* were negative. The stool was also checked for ova and parasites, and the results were negative. The day-care center that the child attends has had a previous problem with contaminated water, and the physician is suspicious that this infection might be caused by *Cryptosporidium*, a waterborne pathogen. However, because no parasites were found, he is not certain how to proceed.

## Questions

a. Does a negative finding rule out the presence of a parasite?

b. What other type of testing could be done?

c. How does the sensitivity of testing such as enzyme immunoassay compare with visual inspection of stained slides?

d. What are other advantages of enzyme immunoassay tests?

# EXERCISE

## ENZYME IMMUNOASSAY DETERMINATION OF HUMAN CHORIONIC GONADOTROPIN

### Principle

Membrane cassette tests for pregnancy determination are one-step solid-phase enzyme immunoassays designed to detect the presence of hCG in urine or serum. hCG is a hormone secreted by the trophoblast of the developing embryo; it rapidly increases in the urine or serum during the early stages of pregnancy. In a normal pregnancy, hCG can be detected in serum as early as 7 days following conception, and the concentration doubles every 1.3 to 2 days. It is subsequently excreted into the urine. Levels of hCG reach a peak of approximately 200,000 mIU/mL at the end of the first trimester.

Because the test cassette contains all necessary reagents, this is called *immunochromatography*. The test band region is precoated with anti-alpha hCG antibody to trap hCG as it moves through the membrane caused by capillary action. When the patient specimen is added, it reconstitutes an anti-beta hCG antibody, which is complexed to colloidal gold particles. This complex is trapped by the anti-alpha hCG and forms a colored complex in the test region. This may be in the form of a straight line or a plus sign. A positive test results if a minimum concentration of approximately 25 mIU/mL is present. The control region contains a second antibody directed against the anti-beta hCG antibody. This second antibody reacts with the excess anti-beta hCG antibody gold particles to indicate that the test is working correctly.

### Sample Preparation

Serum, plasma, or urine may be used for testing. Any urine specimen may be used, but the first morning specimen is preferable, because it is the most highly concentrated. Plasma collected with ethylenediaminetetra-acetic acid, heparin, or citrate may be used. Specimens may be stored for up to 72 hours at 2°C to 8°C. If specimens need to be held longer, freezing at 220°C is recommended. Freezing and thawing is not recommended.

### Reagents, Materials, and Equipment

Test kit containing test cassettes

Marked pipettes or sample dispensers

Urine control

Serum control

Timer

NOTE: There are numerous kits on the market. Examples are SureStep, QuickView, Concise, and Clearview.

### Procedure

1. Remove the test device from its protective pouch.
2. Allow the test device to equilibrate to room temperature.
3. Draw sample up to the mark on the pipette.
4. Dispense a certain number of drops or the entire contents of the pipette, depending on kit instructions.
5. Wait for the sample to completely run through the membrane.
6. Colored bands will usually appear in 1 to 3 minutes.
7. A colored band should also appear in the control region. If it does not, the test is invalidated.

### Results

A sample is positive if a line forms in the test region. A negative specimen will produce a line in the control region only. If no color develops in the control region, either the reagents are not active or the test procedure was incorrect.

### Interpretation of Results

The hCG hormone consists of two subunits, called *alpha* and *beta*. The beta subunit is unique to hCG, while the alpha subunit can be found in other hormones. In this test system, as soon as a patient sample containing hCG is added, it binds to monoclonal anti-beta hCG antibody, which is complexed to an indicator such as colloid gold particles. The monoclonal antibody to the alpha portion of hCG on the cassette membrane binds the hCG complex as the patient sample travels along the membrane. A second antibody directed against the anti-beta hCG antibody is bound in the control region.

False negatives caused by cross-reactivity with other hormones such as luteinizing hormone and follicle-stimulating hormone are avoided through the use of monoclonal antibody that is directed against the β chain of hCG. Note that the actual procedure and reagents present will vary slightly with individual kits. This type of testing is a visual qualitative test only.

NOTE: There are other kits on the market that can be used to demonstrate EIA reactions readily. Some of these are available for infectious agents such as *Streptococcus pyogenes* and *Streptococcus agalactiae*. Another alternative is an EIA kit that simulates HIV testing, available from Edvotek, Inc. (See Chapter 23 for the procedure.)

# REVIEW QUESTIONS

1. Which of the following statements accurately describes competitive binding assays?

   a. Excess binding sites for the analyte are provided.
   b. Labeled and unlabeled analyte are present in equal amounts.
   c. The concentration of patient analyte is inversely proportional to bound radioactive label.
   d. All the patient analyte is bound in the reaction.

2. How do heterogeneous assays differ from homogeneous assays?

   a. Heterogeneous assays require a separation step.
   b. Heterogeneous assays are easier to perform than homogeneous assays.
   c. The concentration of patient analyte is directly proportional to bound label in homogeneous assays.
   d. Homogeneous assays are more sensitive than heterogeneous ones.

3. In the following equation, what is the ratio of bound radioactive antigen (Ag*) to bound patient antigen (Ag)?

   $$12Ag^* + 4Ag + 4Ab \rightarrow :\underline{\quad}Ag^*Ab + \underline{\quad}AgAb + Ag^* + \underline{\quad}Ag$$

   a. 1:4
   b. 1:3
   c. 3:1
   d. 8:4

4. Which of the following characterizes a capture or sandwich enzyme assay?

   a. Less sensitive than competitive enzyme assays
   b. Requires two wash steps
   c. Best for small antigens with a single determinant
   d. A limited number of antibody sites on solid phase

5. Advantages of EIA over RIA include all *except* which one of the following?

   a. Decrease in hazardous waste
   b. Shorter shelf life of kit
   c. No need for expensive equipment
   d. Ease of adaptation to automated techniques

6. Which of the following is characteristic of direct fluorescent assays?

   a. The anti-immunoglobulin has the fluorescent tag.
   b. Antibody is attached to a solid phase.
   c. Microbial antigens can be rapidly identified by this method.
   d. The amount of color is in inverse proportion to the amount of antigen present.

7. Which of the following is true of fluorescence polarization immunoassay?

   a. Both antigen and antibody are labeled.
   b. Large molecules polarize more light than smaller molecules.
   c. When binding occurs, there is quenching of the fluorescent tag.
   d. The amount of fluorescence is directly proportional to concentration of the analyte.

8. All of the following are desirable characteristics of antibodies used in immunoassays *except*

   a. high affinity.
   b. high specificity.
   c. high cross-reactivity.
   d. not found in the patient sample.

9. In a noncompetitive enzyme immunoassay, if a negative control shows the presence of color, which of the following might be a possible explanation?

   a. No reagent was added.
   b. Washing steps were incomplete.
   c. The enzyme was inactivated.
   d. No substrate was present.

10. Which of the following best characterizes chemiluminescent assays?

    a. Only the antigen can be labeled.
    b. Tests can be read manually.
    c. These are only homogeneous assays.
    d. A chemical is oxidized to produce light.

11. Immunofluorescent assays may be difficult to interpret for which reason?

    a. Autofluorescence of substances in serum
    b. Nonspecific binding to serum proteins
    c. Subjectivity in reading results
    d. Any of the above

12. Which statement best describes flow-through immunoassays?

    a. Results are quantitative.
    b. Reagents must be added separately.
    c. They are difficult to interpret.
    d. They are designed for point-of-care testing.

# References

1. Kricka, LJ. Principles of immunochemical techniques. In Burtis, CA, Ashwood, ER, and Bruns, DE (eds): Tietz Fundamentals of Clinical Chemistry, ed. 6. Saunders Elsevier, St. Louis, 2008, pp. 155–170.

2. Ashihara, Y, Kasahara, Y, and Nakamura, RM. Immunoassays and immunochemistry. In McPherson, RA, and Pincus, MR (eds): Henry's Clinical Diagnosis and Management by Laboratory Methods, ed. 21. Saunders Elsevier, Philadelphia, 2007, pp. 793–818.

3. Carpenter, AB. Immunoassays for the diagnosis of infectious diseases. In Murray, PR, et al. (eds): Manual of Clinical Microbiology, ed. 9. ASM Press, Washington, DC, 2007, pp. 257–269.

4. Mak, TW, and Saunders, ME. The Immune Response: Basic and Clinical Principles. Elsevier, Burlington, MA, 2006, pp. 147–176.

5. Kindt, TJ, Goldsby, RA, and Osborne, BA. Kuby Immunology, ed. 6. WH Freeman and Co., New York, 2007, pp. 145–167.

6. Yalow, RS, and Berson, SA. Immunoassay of endogenous plasma insulin in man. J Clin Invest 39:1157, 1960.

7. Fleischer, DM, and Wood, RA. Tests for immunological reactions to foods. In Detrick, B, Hamilton, RG, and Folds, JD (eds): Manual of Molecular and Clinical Laboratory Immunology, ed. 7. ASM Press, Washington, DC, 2006, pp. 975–973.

8. Meriggioli, MN. Use of immunoassays in neurological diagnosis and research. Neurological Res 27:734, 2005.

9. Dewar, R et al. Principles and procedures of human immunodeficiency virus serodiagnosis. In Detrick, B, Hamilton, RG, and Folds, JD (eds): Manual of Molecular and Clinical Laboratory Immunology, ed. 7. ASM Press, Washington, DC, 2006, pp. 834–846.

10. Bendinelli, M et al. Viral hepatitis. In Detrick, B, Hamilton, RG, and Folds, JD (eds): Manual of Molecular and Clinical Laboratory Immunology, ed. 7. ASM Press, Washington, DC, 2006, pp. 724–745.

11. Pearlman, BL. Hepatitis C: A clinical review. South Med J 97:364, 2004.

12. Wong, T, and Lee, SS. Hepatitis C: A review for primary care physicians. CMAJ 174:649, 2006.

13. Jenson, HB. Epstein-Barr virus. In Detrick, B, Hamilton, RG, and Folds, JD (eds): Manual of Molecular and Clinical Laboratory Immunology, ed. 7. ASM Press, Washington, DC, 2006, pp. 637–647.

14. Feng, N, and Matsui, SM. Rotaviruses and noroviruses. In Detrick, B, Hamilton, RG, and Folds, JD (eds): Manual of Molecular and Clinical Laboratory Immunology, ed. 7. ASM Press, Washington, DC, 2006, pp. 746–755.

15. Piedra, PA, and Boivin, G. Respiratory syncytial virus, human metapneumovirus, and the parainfluenza viruses. In Detrick, B, Hamilton, RG, and Folds, JD (eds): Manual of Molecular and Clinical Laboratory Immunology, ed. 7. ASM Press, Washington, DC, 2006, pp. 700–706.

16. Murata, Y, and Falsey, AR. Respiratory syncytial virus infection in adults. Antivir Ther 12:659, 2007.

17. Nutman, TB. Mycotic and parasitic diseases: Introduction. In Detrick, B, Hamilton, RG, and Folds, JD (eds): Manual of Molecular and Clinical Laboratory Immunology, ed. 7. ASM Press, Washington, DC, 2006, pp. 555–556.

18. Leber, Al, and Novak-Weekley, S. Intestinal and urogenital amebae, flagellates, and ciliates. In Murray, PR, et al. (eds): Manual of Clinical Microbiology, ed. 9. ASM Press, Washington, DC, 2007, pp. 2092–2112.

19. Xiao, L, and Cama, V. Cryptosporidium. In Murray, PR, et al. (eds): Manual of Clinical Microbiology, ed. 9. ASM Press, Washington, DC, 2007, pp. 1745–1761.

20. Lindsley, MD, Warnock, DW, and Morrison, CJ. Serological and molecular diagnosis of fungal infections. In Detrick, B, Hamilton, RG, and Folds, JD (eds): Manual of Molecular and Clinical Laboratory Immunology, ed. 7. ASM Press, Washington, DC, 2006, pp. 569–605.

21. Shea, YR. Algorithms for detection and identification of fungi. In Murray, PR et al. (eds): Manual of Clinical Microbiology, ed. 9. ASM Press, Washington, DC, 2007, pp. 257–269.

22. Sable, C. Advances in antifungal therapy. Ann Rev Med 59:361, 2008.

23. Homburger, HA. Allergic diseases. In McPherson, RA, and Pincus, MR (eds): Henry's Clinical Diagnosis and Management by Laboratory Methods, ed. 21. Saunders Elsevier, Philadelphia, 2007, pp. 962–971.

24. Remaley, AT, and Hortin, GL. Protein analysis for diagnostic applications. In Detrick, B, Hamilton, RG, and Folds, JD (eds): Manual of Molecular and Clinical Laboratory Immunology, ed. 7. ASM Press, Washington, DC, 2006, pp. 7–21.

25. Collins, AB, Colvin, RB, Nousari, CH, and Anhalt, GJ. Immunofluorescence methods in the diagnosis of renal and skin diseases. In Detrick, B, Hamilton, RG, and Folds, JD (eds): Manual of Molecular and Clinical Laboratory Immunology, ed. 7. ASM Press, Washington, DC, 2006, pp. 414–423.

26. Forbes, BA, Sahm, DF, and Weissfeld, AS. Bailey and Scott's Diagnostic Microbiology, ed. 12. Mosby Elsevier, St. Louis, 2007, pp. 147–158.

27. Forbes, BA, Sahm, DF, and Weissfeld, AS. Bailey and Scott's Diagnostic Microbiology, ed. 12. Mosby Elsevier, St. Louis, 2007, pp. 510–524.

28. Von Muhlen, CA, and Nakamura, RM. Clinical and laboratory evaluation of rheumatic diseases. In McPherson, RA, and Pincus, MR (eds): Henry's Clinical Diagnosis and Management by Laboratory Methods, ed. 21. Saunders Elsevier, Philadelphia, 2007, pp. 916–932.

29. Forbes, BA, Sahm, DF, and Weissfeld, AS. Bailey and Scott's Diagnostic Microbiology, ed. 12. Mosby Elsevier, St Louis, 2007, pp. 533–541.

30. Jandreski, MA. Chemiluminescence technology in immunoassays. Lab Med 29:555–560, 1998.

# 11 Molecular Diagnostic Techniques

*Susan M Orton, PhD, MT(ASCP), D (ABMLI)*

## LEARNING OBJECTIVES

*After finishing this chapter, the reader will be able to:*

1. Describe the structure and function of deoxyribonucleic acid (DNA) and ribonucleic acid (RNA) within a cell.
2. Explain what a nucleic acid probe is and how it is used.
3. Define *hybridization* and discuss the conditions that influence its specificity.
4. Differentiate dot-blot from a Southern blot.
5. Describe the role of restriction endonucleases in DNA analysis.
6. Explain the basis of DNA chip technology.
7. Discuss the principles and major steps of the polymerase chain reaction (PCR).
8. Discuss the advantages of real-time PCR.
9. Describe the major difference between end-point and real-time PCR.
10. Differentiate target amplification from probe amplification and give examples of each.
11. Compare the relative advantages and disadvantages of amplification systems in general.
12. Correlate individual nucleic acid techniques with actual use in clinical settings.
13. Determine when nucleic acid technology is appropriate for clinical testing.

## KEY TERMS

____ Branched DNA (bDNA) signal amplification
____ Deoxyribonucleic acid (DNA)
____ DNA sequencing
____ Dot-blot
____ Gel electrophoresis
____ Hybridization
____ In situ hybridization
____ Ligase chain reaction (LCR)
____ Northern blot
____ Nucleic acid probe
____ Nucleic acid sequence
____ based amplification
____ (NASBA)
____ Polymerase chain
____ reaction (PCR)
____ Primers
____ Purine
____ Pyrimidine
____ Real-time PCR
____ Restriction endonuclease
____ Restriction fragment length
____ polymorphisms (RFLPs)
____ Reverse transcriptase
____ Ribonucleic acid (RNA)
____ Sandwich hybridization
____ Southern blot
____ Strand displacement
____ amplification (SDA)
____ Stringency
____ Transcription
____ Transcription-mediated
____ amplification (TMA)
____ Translation

# CHAPTER OUTLINE

## CHARACTERISTICS OF NUCLEIC ACIDS

Molecular diagnostic assays are powerful new tools used to gain information to aid in diagnosis and monitoring of disease. These techniques are based on the detection of specific nucleic acid sequences in microorganisms or particular cells. Molecular techniques used in the clinical lab to identify unique nucleic acid sequences include enzymatic cleavage of nucleic acids, gel electrophoresis, enzymatic amplification of target sequences, and hybridization with nucleic acid probes. All of these techniques are discussed in this chapter in addition to an overview of the structure and functions of deoxyribonucleic acid (DNA) and ribonucleic acid (RNA). Advantages and disadvantages of each type of detection method will be presented along with examples of use in actual clinical settings.

### Composition of DNA and RNA

The two main types of nucleic acids are **deoxyribonucleic acid (DNA)** and **ribonucleic acid (RNA).** DNA carries the primary genetic information within chromosomes found in each cell. Genes are sequences of DNA that encode information for the translation of nucleic acid sequence into amino acid sequence, resulting in protein production. The entire sequence of the human genome is more than 3 billion DNA bases long.[1] However, the actual number of encoded genes, approximately 30,000, is much lower than originally predicted. DNA is packaged into genes, which are all packaged within duplicate pairs of chromosomes. Humans have 23 pairs of chromosomes and 1 pair of sex chromosomes, giving us a total of 46 chromosomes.

RNA, on the other hand, is an intermediate nucleic acid structure that helps convert the genetic information encoded within DNA into proteins that are the primary cellular component. DNA acts as the template for synthesis of RNA.

Both nucleic acid structures are polymers made up of repeating nucleotides, or bases, that are linked together to form long molecules. Each nucleotide consists of a cyclic, 5-carbon sugar, with a phosphate group at the 5′ C and one of four nitrogenous bases at the 1′ C. The sugar deoxyribose is present in DNA, while ribose is the primary sugar found in RNA.

DNA and RNA have the same two **purine** bases, adenine and guanine, but the **pyrimidine** bases differ. DNA uses cytosine and thymine, while in RNA, uracil replaces thymine. DNA exists primarily as a double-stranded molecule with very specific base pair linkages: Adenine pairs with thymine, and cytosine pairs with guanine. Any other combinations of base pairs are either too large or too small and do not fit together. The nitrogenous bases are found on the inside of the molecule, and the sugars are linked together via alternating phosphate groups to form the outside backbone. Nucleotides are joined together by phosphodiester bonds that link the 5′ phosphate group of one sugar to the 3′ hydroxyl group of an adjacent sugar.[2] The two strands are twisted into an alpha helix **(Fig. 11–1).** Hydrogen bonding between adjacent bases holds the two chains together.

### Replication of DNA

DNA is a very stable molecule, which makes it ideal for a clinical specimen. It loses its conformational structure only under extremes of heat, pH, or the presence of destabilizing agents.[2] Replication of the DNA molecule is very straightforward. It is characterized as a *semi-conservative* process, because one strand of the molecule acts as a template for creation of a complementary strand. Two daughter molecules result, each of which is an exact copy of the original molecule. This process can be replicated in the laboratory, because the hydrogen bonds that hold the two

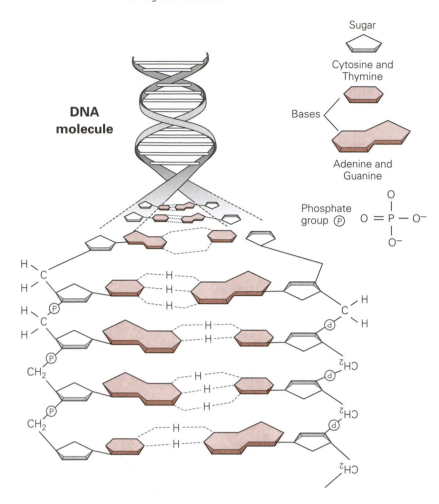

Sugar

Bases — Cytosine and Thymine

Adenine and Guanine

Phosphate group ℗

$$O = P - O^-$$

**DNA molecule**

**FIGURE 11–1.** DNA molecule. The double helix of DNA is shown along with details of how the bases, sugars, and phosphates connect to form the structure of the molecule. DNA is a double-stranded molecule twisted into a helix (think of a spiral staircase). Each spiraling strand, composed of a sugar-phosphate backbone and attached bases, is connected to a complementary strand by noncovalent hydrogen bonding between paired bases. The bases are adenine (A), thymine (T), cytosine (C), and guanine (G). A and T are connected by two hydrogen bonds. G and C are connected by three hydrogen bonds.

strands together are relatively weak.[3] The double helix can easily be separated or *denatured* using heat or an alkaline solution. When heat is used to separate the strands, the process is known as *melting*. When DNA strands cool to normal physiological conditions, complementary strands spontaneously rejoin or *anneal*. It is these characteristics that are exploited in molecular testing. Going from a genetic sequence encoded within DNA into a functional protein involves two major processes: transcription and translation. **Transcription** is the generation of a strand of messenger RNA (mRNA) that codes for the gene that is to be expressed as a protein. In turn, **translation** occurs when the mRNA travels from the nucleus into the cytoplasm of the cell to ribosomes, where the mRNA sequence is "translated" into an amino acid sequence that makes the protein encoded for by DNA in the nucleus.

### Types of RNA

One strand of DNA, the coding strand, serves as the template for the production of mRNA. All forms of RNA are single-stranded polymers with an irregular three-dimensional structure and are of much shorter lengths than DNA. Messenger RNA is used to translate the DNA code into making functional proteins. The two other types of RNA

are transfer RNA (tRNA), which transports different amino acids to make proteins, and ribosomal RNA (rRNA), which acts as the site for protein synthesis directed by the mRNA. RNA is less stable than DNA because it is single stranded; this makes it more susceptible to alkaline hydrolysis. RNA is also rapidly degraded by RNase enzymes, which appear in abundance everywhere in the environment.[2] However, RNA can easily be replicated and is also used in molecular diagnostic techniques.

### HYBRIDIZATION TECHNIQUES

Spontaneous pairing of complementary DNA strands forms the basis for techniques that are used to detect and characterize genes. Probe technology is typically the basis for identification of individual genes or DNA sequences. A **nucleic acid probe** is a short strand of DNA or RNA of a known sequence that is used to identify the presence of its complementary DNA/RNA in a patient specimen. Binding of two such complementary strands is known as **hybridization** and is very specific. The two strands should share at least 16 to 20 consecutive bases of perfect complementarity to form a stable hybrid.[1] The probability of such a match occurring by chance is less than 1 in 1 billion, so there is an extraordinary degree of specificity to this process.[1] Probes are labeled with a marker such as a radioisotope, a fluorochrome, an enzyme, or a chemiluminescent substrate to make detection of hybridization possible. Hybridization can take place either in a solid support medium or in solution.

## Solid Support Hybridization

Dot-blot and sandwich hybridization assays are the simplest types of solid support hybridization assays.[1] In the **dot-blot** assay, clinical samples are applied directly to a membrane surface. The membrane is heated to denature or separate DNA strands, and then labeled probes are added. After careful washing to remove any unhybridized probe, presence of remaining probe is detected by autoradiography or enzyme assays **(Fig. 11–2)**. A positive result indicates presence of a specific sequence of interest. This permits qualitative testing of a clinical specimen, because it only indicates presence or absence of a particular genetic sequence. It is much easier to handle multiple samples in this manner.[4] However, there may be difficulty with the interpretation of weak positive reactions, because there can be background interference.[5]

**Sandwich hybridization** is a modification of the dot-blot procedure. It was designed to overcome some of the background problems associated with the use of unpurified samples.[2] The technique uses two probes, one of which is bound to the membrane and serves to capture target sample DNA. The second probe anneals to a different site on the target DNA, and it has a label for detection. The sample nucleic acid is thus sandwiched in between the capture probe on the membrane and the signal-generating probe.[2] Because two hybridization events must take place, specificity is increased. Sandwich hybridization assays have been developed using microtiter plates instead of membranes, which has made the procedure more adaptable to automation.[2]

To characterize DNA present in a patient sample in a more detailed fashion, enzymes called **restriction endonucleases** are often used. These enzymes cleave both strands of a double-stranded DNA at specific recognition sites that are approximately 4 to 6 base pairs long.[1] Human DNA may yield millions of unique fragments.[1] The resulting fragments are separated from each other on the basis of size and charge by a procedure known as **gel electrophoresis.** Digested cellular DNA from a patient blood or tissue sample is placed in wells in an agarose gel and covered with buffer. The

molecules migrate through the gel under the influence of an electrical field, and they are separated on the basis of molecular weight. Smaller fragments migrate faster, while the larger fragments remain closer to the origin. The gel can either be stained with ethidium bromide and viewed under ultraviolet (UV) light to see the entire pattern of fragments, or specific nucleic acid sequences can be identified through the use of DNA probes **(Fig. 11–3)**.

Differences in restriction patterns are referred to as **restriction fragment length polymorphisms (RFLPs).**

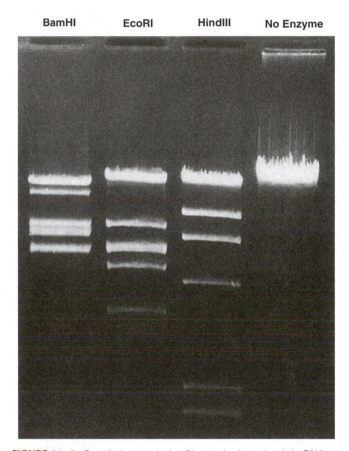

**FIGURE 11–3.** Restriction analysis of bacteriophage lambda DNA. Three enzymes—BamHI, EcoRI, and HindIII—are used to cleave DNA at specific sites. Each produces a different pattern when the DNA is electrophoresed. Ethidium bromide is used to help visualize the DNA under UV light. (*From Restriction Enzyme and DNA Kit, Carolina Biological Supply Company, Burlington, NC, with permission.*)

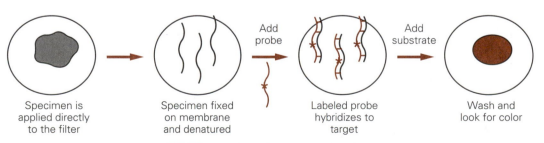

**FIGURE 11–2.** Dot-blot hybridization assay.

This is caused by variations in nucleotides within genes that change where the restriction enzymes cleave the DNA. When such a mutation occurs, different-sized pieces of DNA are obtained. Such RFLP patterns can be used to identify specific microorganisms, to establish strain relatedness, to detect polymorphisms in major histocompatibility complex (MHC) genes, or to obtain a DNA fingerprint of a particular individual.[6]

Analysis of DNA fragments using probes is typically carried out using a technique known as a *Southern hybridization assay,* or **Southern blot,** named after its discoverer, E. M. Southern. After DNA fragments are separated out by gel electrophoresis, the fragments are denatured using alkali and then transferred, or "blotted," onto a nitrocellulose or nylon membrane for the hybridization reaction to take place. The transfer is accomplished by placing the membrane on top of the gel and allowing the buffer plus DNA to wick onto the membrane. Traditionally, this procedure takes overnight, but newer methods using vacuum and pressure systems have significantly increased the speed of the transfer.[2]

Once the DNA is on the nitrocellulose membrane, heating or UV light is used to cross-link the strands onto the membrane, thus immobilizing them. A labeled probe, whose sequence is complimentary to the sequence of interest, is then added to the membrane for hybridization to take place. The membrane is then washed, and the amount of bound probe remaining is determined by detection of the label **(Fig. 11–4)**. Several nonradiolabeled probes, including enzyme, chemiluminescent, and acridinium labels, have been developed for use, and these appear to be as sensitive as the original radiolabeled probes. The use of these probes avoids

the hazards associated with use of radioactivity.[7] The absence of any visible bands indicates an absence of the sequence of interest.

Southern blots are useful to analyze alterations of large spans of DNA, where amplification by the polymerase chain reaction (PCR) may not be practical. Southern blot analysis can reveal polymorphisms in DNA sequence based upon the RFLP profile made visible by the probes. Southern blots have been used to determine the clonal composition of lymphocyte populations. Only when a large number of cloned cells are present do rearranged genes specific for T-cell receptors or immunoglobulins appear in sufficient quantity to produce a detectable band that is different from the normal or germ-line DNA. This is typically an indicator of a lymphoid malignancy such as B-cell lymphoma, chronic myelogenous leukemia, or hairy cell leukemia.[1,4] Detection of a malignant clone can help distinguish between reactive lymphocytes seen in an inflammatory process and true malignancies. DNA testing is especially helpful in both diagnosis and classification of T-cell malignancies.[4] It has had a tremendous impact on diagnosis of non-Hodgkin's lymphomas.[8] Molecular testing can also be used to monitor therapy and remission of lymphomas. If tissue from separate lymphomatous lesions are from the same original source or clone, they usually show identical DNA rearrangements and produce identical bands on a Southern blot.[1] In general, however, Southern blots are complex, time-consuming to perform, and require a relatively large sample, which can limit its clinical usefulness.[5]

**Northern blots** are performed in a similar manner, but in this technique, RNA is extracted and separated. This tool

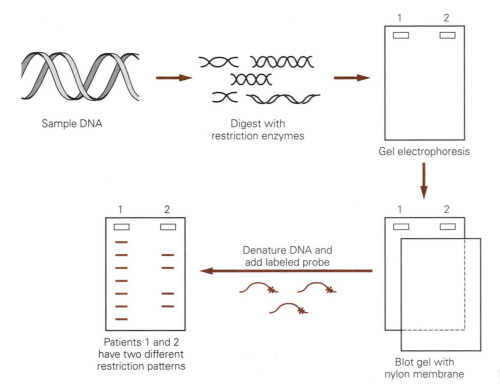

Sample DNA

Digest with restriction enzymes

Gel electrophoresis

Denature DNA and add labeled probe

Patients 1 and 2 have two different restriction patterns

Blot gel with nylon membrane

**FIGURE 11–4.** Southern blot.

is used most often to determine the level of expression of a particular messenger RNA species to see if a gene is actually being expressed.[2] Because RNA is a short, single-stranded molecule, it does not have to be digested before electrophoresis, but it has to be denatured to ensure that it is in an unfolded, linear form. Probes are then used to identify the presence of specific bands.

## Solution Hybridization

Hybridization assays can also be performed in a solution phase. In this type of setting, both the target nucleic acid and the probe are free to interact in a reaction mixture, resulting in increased sensitivity compared to that of solid support hybridization.[5] It also requires a smaller amount of sample, although the sensitivity is improved when target DNA is extracted and purified.[5]

For solution hybridizations, the probe must be single-stranded and incapable of self-annealing.[4] Several unique detection methods exist. In one of these, an S1 nuclease is added to the reaction mix. This will digest only unannealed or single-stranded DNA, leaving the hybrids intact. Double-stranded DNA can then be recovered by precipitation with trichloroacetic acid or by binding it to hydroxyapatite columns.[1,9]

A second and less technically difficult means of solution hybridization is the hybridization protection assay (HPA). For this assay, a chemiluminescent acridinium ester is attached to a probe. After the hybridization reaction takes place, the solution is subjected to alkaline hydrolysis, which hydrolyzes the chemiluminescent ester if the probe is not attached to the target molecule. If the probe is attached to the target DNA, the ester is protected from hydrolysis. Probes that remain bound to a specific target sequence give off light when exposed to a chemical trigger such as hydrogen peroxide at the end of the assay.

An additional type of solution phase hybridization assay uses an antibody specific for DNA/RNA hybrids to "capture" and detect the hybrids that are formed during the solution hybridization. Digene's Hybrid Capture 2 (Digene Corp., Gaithersburg, MD) assay, used to detect human papillomavirus (HPV), is an example of this type of assay. HPV DNA in the sample is hybridized with an unlabeled RNA probe, and the viral DNA-RNA hybrids are then captured by the antibody.

Solution phase hybridization assays are fairly adaptable to automation, especially those using chemiluminescent labels. Assays can be performed in a few hours.[4] However, low positive reactions are difficult to interpret because of the possibility of cross-reacting target molecules.[9]

## In Situ Hybridization

**In situ hybridization** represents a third type of hybridization reaction in which the target nucleic acid is found in intact cells. It provides information about the presence of specific DNA targets in relation to its distribution within the tissues. This technique is the same as immunohistochemistry except that nucleic acids instead of antibodies are used as probes. For probes to reach the nucleic acid, they must be small enough, usually limited to 500 bases or less, to penetrate the cells in question.[4] Formalin-fixed and paraffin-embedded tissue sections are typically used for this procedure. Because preparation of tissue specimens can vary greatly in each lab, it is recommended that an endogenous control probe be used.[5] This probe will react positively with all cells and is used to indicate that penetration of the sample has occurred.

Probes have typically been labeled with radioactive substances, but the trend today is toward using fluorescent or enzyme labels. If a fluorescent tag is used, the procedure is called *fluorescent in situ hybridization*, or *FISH*. After completion of the procedure, evaluation should be performed by an experienced histopathologist.[5] This technique is used to detect a number of malignancies linked to chromosomal abnormalities, such as chronic myelogenous leukemia, in which there is a translocation from chromosome 9 to chromosome 22, and inherited disorders that occur as a result of chromosomal abnormalities. When FISH is used on metaphase chromosome spreads or interphase nuclei, it can detect numerical alterations or translocation of chromosomal material.

## DNA Chip Technology

Previously, genetic studies examined individual gene expression by northern blotting or examined polymorphisms by gel-based restriction digests and sequence analysis, but with advances in microchips and bead-based array technologies, high-throughput analysis of genetic variation is now possible. Biochips, also called *microarrays*, are very small devices used to examine DNA, RNA, and other substances. These chips allow thousands of biological reactions to be performed at once.[10] Typically, a biochip consists of a small rectangular solid surface that is made of glass or silicon with short DNA or RNA probes anchored to the surface.[11] The number of probes on a biochip surface can vary from 10 to 20 up to hundreds of thousands.[10,11] Usually, the nucleic acid in the sample is amplified before it is analyzed. After amplification, the sample, labeled with a fluorescent tag, is loaded onto the chip. Hybridization occurs on the chip's surface, allowing thousands of hybridization reactions to occur at one time. Unbound strands of the target sample are then washed away. The fluorescent-tagged hybridized samples are detected using a fluorescent detector[10] **(Fig. 11–5)**. The intensity of the fluorescent signal at a particular location is proportional to the sequence homology at a particular locus. Complete sequence matches results in bright fluorescence, while single-base mismatches result in a dimmer signal, indicative of a point mutation. Since most single nucleotide polymorphisms (SNPs) are silent and have no apparent functional consequence, the challenge is to

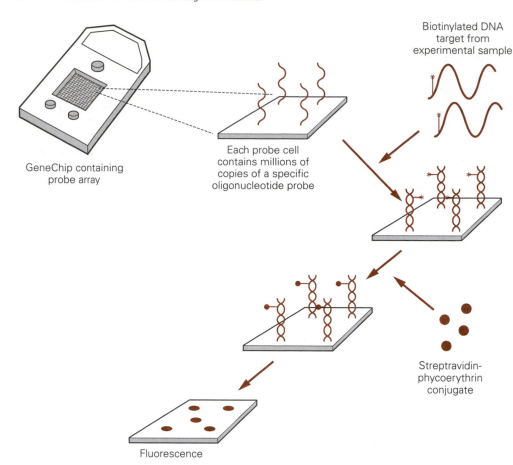

FIGURE 11–5. Analysis of HIV-I. Labeled patient DNA is placed on the biochip or microarray. In this case, the label is biotin. Hybridization takes place, followed by a washing step. Strepavidin conjugated to a fluorescent dye is added. This will complex with any patient DNA present. The resulting fluorescent pattern can pick up mutations associated with drug resistance.

identify the set of SNPs that are directly related to or that cause disease. Detection of point mutations can be used for classifying leukemias, molecular staging of tumors, and characterizing microbial agents.[12] One prime example is the determination of genes associated with drug resistance in HIV testing. Identification of such genes guides the physician in selecting a proper drug regimen for a particular patient.

## Drawbacks of Hybridization Techniques

In any of the previously mentioned hybridization techniques, conditions of the reaction itself may determine how sensitive and specific the technique is. Under the conditions in which most assays are conducted, two nucleic acid strands must share at least 16 to 20 consecutive bases of perfect complementarity to form a stable hybrid.[12] **Stringency,** or correct pairing, is most affected by the salt concentration, the temperature, and the concentration of destabilizing agents such as formamide or urea. Decreasing the salt concentration, increasing the temperature, and increasing the concentration of formamide or urea all help to ensure that only the most perfectly matched strands will remain paired in a stable hybrid. If the conditions are not carefully controlled, however, mismatches can occur, and the results may not be valid.

In addition, even under carefully controlled conditions, often the amount of nucleic acid in a patient specimen may present in very low quantity, which may be below the threshold for probe detection. The sensitivity of these assays can be increased by amplifying the sequence of interest. There are other amplification techniques as well, and they fall into three general categories: target amplification, probe amplification, and signal amplification. Each of these will be discussed and relevant clinical examples given.

## DNA SEQUENCING

**DNA sequencing** is considered the "gold standard" for many molecular applications, from mutation detection to genotyping, but it requires proper methodology and interpretation to prevent misidentification. The sequence should be analyzed on both DNA strands to provide even greater accuracy. Patient sequences are compared to known reference sequences to detect mutations. Most sequencing strategies include PCR amplification as the first step to amplify the region of interest to be sequenced. The sequencing reaction itself is based upon the dideoxy chain termination reaction developed by Sanger and colleagues in 1977.[13] If any one of the four dideoxynucleotides are incorporated into a growing DNA chain, synthesis is halted. This results in fragments of varying lengths depending upon where incorporation of the dideoxynucleotide bases has occurred. These nucleotides lack the 3′ and 2′ hydroxyl (OH) group on the pentose ring, and because DNA chain elongation requires the addition of deoxynucleotides to the 3′OH group, incorporation of the dideoxynucleotide terminates chain length.

The most commonly used form of this sequencing method in the clinical lab uses "cycle sequencing," which is similar to a PCR reaction in that the steps involved include denaturing, annealing of a primer, chain extending, and terminating by varying the temperature of the reaction. The newly generated fragments are tagged with a fluorescent dye and separated, based upon size, by denaturing gel or capillary electrophoresis and are spotted by fluorescence detectors as the fragments pass through the detector **(Fig. 11–6)**. Using this automated method with capillary electrophoresis, about 600 base pairs can be sequenced in 2.5 hours.[6] DNA sequencing is most commonly used to detect mutations. For example, in infectious disease testing such as sequencing of HIV for drug resistance, information about the particular strain is used to establish appropriate therapy and make treatment decisions.

## TARGET AMPLIFICATION

Target amplification systems are in vitro methods for the enzymatic replication of a target molecule to levels at which it can be readily detected.[5] This allows the target sequence to be identified and further characterized. There are numerous different types of target amplification. Examples include polymerase chain reaction (PCR), transcription mediated amplification (TMA), strand displacement amplification (SDA), and nucleic acid sequence-based amplification (NASBA). Of these, PCR is by far the best-known and most widely used technique in clinical laboratories.[6] However, the other non-PCR methods have become more popular in recent years.

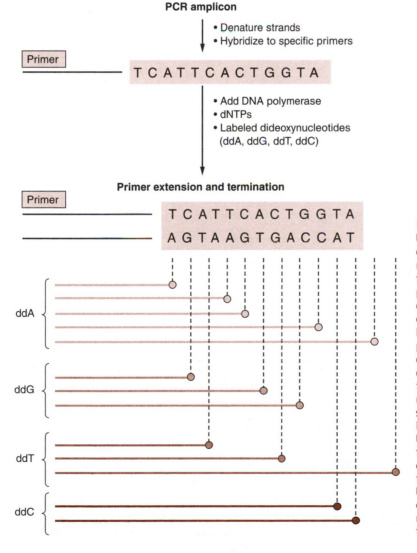

FIGURE 11–6. DNA sequencing based upon the Sanger dideoxy chain termination reaction. The region of interest is first amplified using PCR. Sequence-specific primers then hybridize with the denatured amplicons followed by extension of the new strand by DNA polymerase. At various points in the DNA extension, a dideoxy base (ddA, ddG, ddT, or ddC) is incorporated, which stops further extension of DNA. This results in a mixture of newly synthesized products of various lengths. Each dideoxy terminator base is labeled with a specific fluorescent tag that can be detected by a fluorescent detector. The fragments are separated based on their size, and fluorescence is read on each strand, resulting in the sequence of the DNA.

## Polymerase Chain Reaction

The **polymerase chain reaction (PCR)** is capable of amplifying tiny quantities of nucleic acid up to levels that can be later detected with various strategies, usually involving a hybridization reaction using nucleic acid probes. Kary Mullis was awarded the Nobel Prize in 1993 for developing this technique. Cellular DNA is isolated from the clinical sample (either the patient's own DNA or DNA from an infectious organism). PCR requires several components for the reaction to occur: (1) a thermostable DNA polymerase (originally isolated from the bacterium *Thermus aquaticus*, thus "Taq" polymerase), (2) deoxynucleotides of each base (referred to as *dNTPs*), (3) the DNA of interest containing the target sequence, and (4) oligonucleotide **primers,** short segments of DNA that are between 20 and 30 nucleotides long, that are complimentary to opposite strands that flank the sequence of interest to be amplified and detected.

Each PCR cycle consists of three steps: denaturing, annealing, and extending at different temperatures. During denaturation, the double-stranded DNA is heated to 95°C to separate or denature the DNA into single strands. The mixture is then cooled slightly to 52°C, at which time the primers bind to or anneal to the complimentary sequences on the separate DNA strands. During the third step, elongation, which is typically at 72°C, the heat-stable DNA polymerase binds to the 3′ end of each primer and synthesizes a new strand of DNA using the original sample DNA as a template.[12,14] The usual span between primers is between 50 and 1500 nucleotide bases.[5] Amplification of PCR products is an exponential process in which, under optimal conditions, each cycle results in a doubling of product **(Fig. 11–7).** With newer technology, one cycle takes approximately 60 to 90 seconds, resulting in a rapid process. The resulting DNA fragments, referred to as *amplicons*, are detected using various methods. Initially, amplicons were detected by visualization on agarose gels. For most clinical applications, amplicons are detected using labeled nucleic acid probes. In this manner, a target sequence present at fewer than 100 copies can be detected.[15,16]

RNA can also be amplified with the addition of a step prior to the PCR reaction itself. The enzyme **reverse transcriptase** is used to generate copy DNA (cDNA) using the RNA as a template. This reverse transcription step must be performed, since the DNA polymerase used in the PCR reaction recognizes only DNA sequences and not RNA.

The need for quicker turnaround times and ways to reduce contamination led to the development of automated

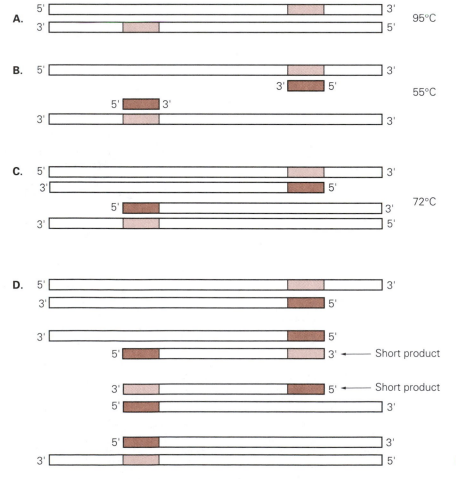

FIGURE 11–7. Principles of PCR.

methods that use "closed-tube" technology to prevent contamination of unamplified samples with amplified amplicons from other samples. The most recent development in PCR technology is the ability to measure the generation of amplicons in "real time," which reduces the amount of time it takes to run a PCR reaction. **Real-time PCR** is facilitated by using fluorescent dyes or probes and thermal cyclers that can take fluorescence readings during each cycle instead of waiting until all the cycles have been completed before analyzing all the amplicons (end-point PCR).

PCR is an extremely sensitive technique that is used to amplify a target sequence present in low amounts. It is often used for organisms such as viruses that are hard to grow in the laboratory, and it is so sensitive that it can actually detect nonreplicating viral genomes. One of the major uses for PCR is in testing for the presence of HIV. Because HIV is an RNA virus, an initial enzyme, reverse transcriptase, must be added to convert the original RNA into DNA. This is known as *reverse transcriptase PCR (RT-PCR)*. A blood sample of less than 1 mL is sufficient to perform this test, making it ideal for testing neonates.[17] It is also useful in detecting infected individuals during the period before antibody appears, in predicting prognosis, and in monitoring treatment.[17,18] Currently, there are several FDA-approved assays for quantitation of HIV-1 in human plasma **(Table 11–1)**.

RT-PCR is also considered the gold standard for detecting hepatitis C virus and monitoring therapy in those infected.[19] Additional uses for PCR include identifying *Mycobacterium tuberculosis* and diagnosing early initial infection with cytomegalovirus (CMV).[19]

Another important use of PCR in immunology is the identification of human leukocyte antigens (HLAs) for tissue transplantation, especially bone marrow transplantation in which the nature of the match determines the success or failure of the transplant. PCR is used to amplify HLA gene sequences so that donors and recipients can be matched at the allele level.[19,20] This is especially helpful in identifying polymorphisms at the HLA DP locus, which is specifically related to graft versus host reactivity in bone marrow transplants. HLA typing for class I antigens had traditionally

been done using serological methods, but this was not helpful in identification of HLA class II antigens. It has been reported that at least 25 percent of serologically identified class II antigens were incorrectly identified.[4] Matching of class II antigens at the allelic level has proved to increase the success rate of bone marrow transplants.[20]

HLA antigens can be identified by PCR using several different methods. *Sequence specific oligonucleotide probe hybridization (SSOPH)* creates millions of copies of HLA genes in a test tube using a generic primer for the whole region.[4,21] The amplified DNA is then tested with a series of probes. The level of resolution is controlled by the choice and number of probes used in testing.[21] Numerous probes are required for clear resolution of HLA antigens to the allele level. This is currently the most commonly used method for DNA-based typing.[21] It is utilized for high-resolution typing by the National Marrow Donor Program registry.

A second method, called *sequence specific primer typing*, uses only PCR to identify specific HLA alleles. There are unique primer pairs for each gene locus, so when electrophoresis is done, presence of a band indicates that a particular gene is there.[4] The PCR product can also be subjected to direct sequence base typing to detect exact alleles present. The latter is more complex and more expensive.

The activity of cytokines (see Chapter 5) can also be measured using PCR. Because cytokines tend to have a short half-life, identification of messenger RNA is a more sensitive method of determining cytokine production. RT-PCR is a highly sensitive method that requires only a few hours to perform and needs only a nanogram of total RNA. Measurement of cytokines is a very new field and has great potential for monitoring and treating numerous hematologic diseases.

However, the extreme sensitivity of PCR can be detrimental, because carryover of previously amplified DNA into unamplified samples may cause false-positive results. A single copy can cause sample contamination if amplicon is aerosolized.[9] Automation has reduced the potential for contamination by decreasing the number of manual steps and developing "closed" systems in which amplified products

| Table 11–1. | FDA Approved Quantitive HIV-1 (Viral Load) Assays* | | |
|---|---|---|---|
| **MANUFACTURER** | **TEST NAME** | **METHOD** | **LINEAR RANGE (copies/mL)** |
| Roche Molecular Diagnostics | Amplicor HIV-1 Monitor | RT-PCR[1] | 400–750,000 standard<br>50–100,000 ultrasensitive |
| BioMerieux, Inc. | Nuclisens | NASBA[2] | $176–3.47 \times 10^6$ |
| Siemens Health Care Diagnostics | VERSANT HIV-1 RNA 3.0 | bDNA[3] | 75–500,000 |
| Abbott Molecular, Inc. | Abbott Real-Time HIV-1 | Real-time PCR | $40–10 \times 10^6$ |

[1]RT-PCR: reverse transcriptase PCR
[2]NASBA: Nucleic Acid Sequence-Based Amplification
[3]bDNA: Branched DNA
*The Association for Molecular Pathology maintains an up-to-date listing of "FDA Cleared/Approved Molecular Diagnostic Tests." To access this list, please visit http://amp.org/, under "Resources."

are detected in the same tube as the PCR reaction. Automation has also significantly reduced turnaround time and costs per test. With the availability of reagents in kit form and the lower cost of oligonucleotide probes, many more labs are starting to perform molecular assays.[5] Although it may not be suitable for routine screening, when used as an adjunct to standard testing, PCR can be extremely helpful. It will play a more significant role in diagnosis as further developments and refinements are made.

False-positives can be decreased by physically separating areas of sample preparation from amplification areas. UV light can be used to inactivate DNA within a hood and on pipettes, test tubes, and reaction mixes.[9] Additionally, 10 percent bleach (7 mM sodium hypochlorite) is also effective and widely used to decontaminate nonporous work surfaces, including bench tops, hoods, or other areas that might come into contact with nucleic acid–contaminated material.

There is also a widely used chemical method to prevent contamination of unamplified samples with previously amplified PCR products. This method is the dUTP-UNG system in which dTTP is substituted with dUTP in the PCR reaction master mix. This results in dUTP being incorporated into the newly synthesized amplicon. At the beginning of each PCR, the enzyme uracil-N-glycosylase (UNG) is added to the reaction mixture. This enzyme degrades any nucleic acid containing uracil, such as with a sample contaminated with previously amplified products. UNG is added initially and allowed to react for 2 to 10 minutes at 50°C prior to the PCR reaction. Upon the initial denaturation step, the UNG is degraded so that it will not affect subsequently synthesized products that incorporate the dUTP in the master mix.[22,23] The use of appropriate positive and negative controls is also essential.

## Transcription–Based Amplification

In 1989, Kwoh and colleagues developed the first non-PCR nucleic acid amplification method, which was a transcription-based amplification system (TAS) that amplified an RNA target.[24] The reaction was a two-step process that involved generation of cDNA from the target RNA followed by reverse transcription of the cDNA template into multiple copies of RNA. Multiple cycles result in amplification of the target. From this system, two other non-PCR target amplification methods have been developed that are currently used in clinical assays: nucleic acid sequence based amplification (NASBA) and transcription mediated amplification (TMA). The advantage of these two methods is that they are both isothermal reactions that do not require the use of a thermal cycler.

**Nucleic acid sequence based amplification (NASBA)** uses the enzymes reverse transcriptase, RNase H, and bacteriophage T7 DNA-dependent RNA polymerase to isothermally amplify an RNA target. Initially, cDNA is formed from target RNA using sequence-specific primers, one of which contains a T7 RNA polymerase binding site at its 5′ end. RNase H in the reaction degrades the initial strands of target RNA in the RNA/DNA hybrids. A second primer binds to and extends the newly synthesized cDNA, resulting in the formation of double-stranded cDNAs with one strand containing the template for the T7 RNA polymerase to bind and generate multiple RNA transcripts that can then serve as target RNA to which the primers bind and synthesize more cDNA **(Fig. 11–8)**. Organon Teknika (now BioMerieux, Durham, NC) developed an electrochemiluminescence-based solid-phase sandwich hybridization system to automate the detection of amplified products generated by NASBA. This system can be adapted to detect various targets; the NucliSENS system is FDA-approved for quantitation of HIV-1.

**Transcription-mediated amplification (TMA)** is another transcription-based amplification method that, like NASBA, is also isothermal.[15] However, TMA uses only two enzymes to drive the reaction: an RNA polymerase and a reverse transcriptase, unlike NASBA, which uses three enzymes.[25] In addition, two primers are used to target a particular nucleic acid sequence. One of the primers contains a promotor sequence for RNA polymerase.

The first step is to produce a DNA template for RNA transcription by hybridizing the promotor primer to the target rRNA at a particular site. Reverse transcriptase creates a DNA copy, called *cDNA*, of the target rRNA. The original RNA strand is destroyed by the RNase activity of the reverse transcriptase. A new strand of DNA is synthesized from the DNA copy, thus making a double-stranded DNA molecule. RNA polymerase recognizes the promotor sequence in the DNA template and begins transcription of multiple copies.[15]

Again, each newly synthesized RNA molecule serves as a template for a new round of replication. This initiates an autocatalytic cycle in which up to 10 billion RNA molecules can be transcribed from the DNA template in less than 1 hour.[4,25,26] Gen-Probe (San Diego, CA) has developed and patented this technique for detection of *Chlamydia trachomatis*, *Neisseria gonorrhoeae*, *Mycobacterium tuberculosis*, *Mycobacterium avium*, HIV-1, HBV, and HCV from various types of samples.[15,16,27,28]

## Strand Displacement Amplification (SDA)

**Strand displacement amplification (SDA)** was originally developed and patented by Becton Dickinson, Inc. (Franklin Lakes, NJ) in 1991.[29,30,31] One set of primers incorporates a specific restriction enzyme site that is later attacked by an endonuclease. The resulting "nick" created in only one strand by the restriction enzyme allows for displacement of the amplified strands that then, in turn, serve as targets for further amplification and nick digestion. A modified deoxynucleotide (dATPαS; one of the oxygen molecules in the triphosphate moiety has been replaced with sulfur) is used to synthesize a double-stranded, hemiphosphorothioated DNA recognition site for the restriction enzyme cleavage that allows only single-strand

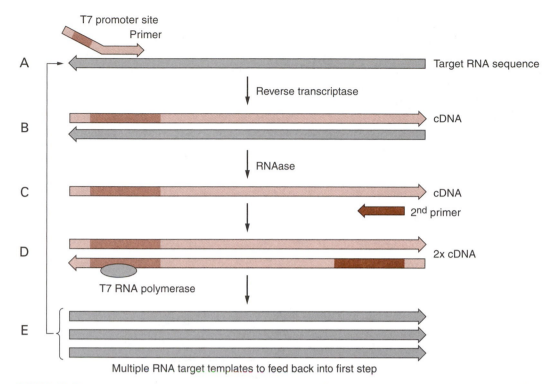

**FIGURE 11–8.** Transcription-based amplification systems. Non-PCR method of amplifying RNA targets. NASBA and TMA are based upon this methodology; NASBA uses three enzymes (reverse transcriptase, RNase H, and T7 DNA-dependent RNA polymerase) while TMA uses only RNA polymerase and a reverse transcriptase with inherent RNase H activity. Initial steps in the procedure involve generation of cDNAs from the target RNA using primers (which incorporate a T7 RNA polymerase binding site; A and B). RNase H then destroys the initial strands of target RNA from the RNA cDNA hybrids (C). The cDNA then serves as template for the generation of double-stranded cDNA, with one strand (containing the T7 binding site) serving as the template for reverse transcription and synthesis of multiple copies of RNA using the T7 RNA polymerase (D). The RNAs then serve as templates for more cDNA templates to be made, and the cycles continue (E).

nicking of the unmodified strand instead of cutting through both strands. Becton Dickinson currently markets this methodology under the label BD ProbeTec and is FDA-approved for the detection of *Legionella pneumophila* and a combination kit for *Chlamydia trachomatis* and *Neisseria gonorrhoeae*.[32]

## PROBE AMPLIFICATION

Rather than directly amplifying the target, there are several techniques that amplify the detection molecule or probe itself. The ligase chain reaction is one example of this technique.

DNA ligase amplification, or the **ligase chain reaction (LCR),** patented by Abbott Laboratories, represents one main type of probe amplification technique.[33] DNA ligase enzyme is a repairing enzyme that links preexisting DNA strands together by joining the 5′ end of one strand to the 3′ end of another strand.[1] In this case, the enzyme is used to join two pairs of oligonucleotide probes only after they have bound to the complementary target sequence, which will hold them in precise end-to-end alignment.[1] Each pair of probes must hybridize to opposite ends (3′ and 5′) of the target DNA molecule. Once the probes are in place, the ligase joins the two together. After this has occurred, each linked pair of probes can be made single-stranded and then act as

a template for ligation of additional probes **(Fig. 11–9)**. The thermostable ligase enzyme from *T aquaticus* remains active throughout the thermal cycling process. This technique has been used for detection of *Borrelia burgdorferi*, *Mycobacteria* species, and *Neisseria gonorrhoeae*.[15]

Ligation reactions are very specific, because a single base pair mismatch at the junction of the oligonucleotide probe keeps ligation from occurring.[2] Disadvantages, however, include the possibility of blunt-end ligation of probes without the target being present. Thus, the exact sequence of the region to be amplified must be known to help prevent false-positive results from occurring.

## SIGNAL AMPLIFICATION

The last category of amplification is based upon amplification of the signal generated by the probe hybridizing to a specific target RNA or DNA. This technique uses a reporter group (the labeled tag) being attached in greater numbers to the probe molecule or increasing the signal intensity generated by each labeled tag.[15] Because the patient nucleic acid itself is not replicated or amplified, this type of technique is less prone to contamination problems. However, the sensitivity may be lower than for enzyme amplification methods, so it may have a more limited use in cases of low numbers of target copies.[15]

Perhaps the best known of the signal amplification systems is the **branched DNA (bDNA) signal amplification** system originally developed by Chiron Corporation and now sold through Siemens Healthcare Diagnostics (Tarrytown, NJ). This technique employs multiple probes and several simultaneous hybridization steps. It has been compared to decorating a Christmas tree and involves several sandwich hybridizations. In the first step, target-specific oligonucleotide probes capture the target sequence to a solid support. Then a second set

of target-specific probes called *extenders* hybridize to adjoining sequences and act as binding sites for a large piece called the *branched amplification multimer.* Each branch of the amplification multimer has multiple side branches capable of binding numerous (up to 10,000) enzyme labeled oligonucleotides onto each target molecule.[4,15] The most recent bDNA system has high specificity and can provide quantitative detection over a range of several orders of magnitude ($10^2$ to $10^5$ copies/mL; **Fig. 11–10).**

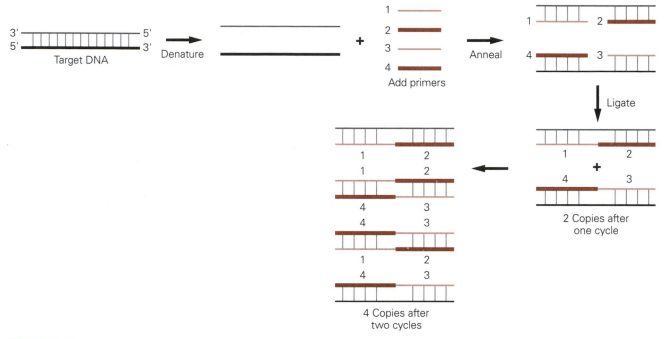

FIGURE 11–9. LCR. Two pairs of probes are used to hybridize to the target DNA molecule. They are joined together by a ligase enzyme. Once bound, the ligated probes can act as a template for additional DNA replication.

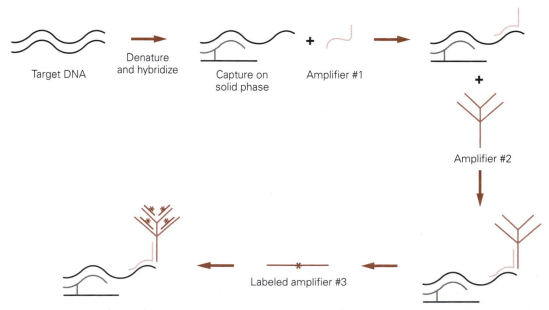

FIGURE 11–10. Branched chain amplification. Several different probes are used to amplify the signal rather than the target DNA itself. The first probe captures the target. Amplifier 1 binds in a different place and forms the base for amplifier 2, the branched chain. Amplifier 3 contains the signal.

Branched DNA systems are well suited to detecting nucleic acid target with sequence heterogeneity, such as hepatitis C and HIV, because if one or two of the capture or extender probes fail to hybridize, the signal-generating capacity is not lost as a result of the presence of several remaining probe complexes. Additionally, the need for several independent probe-target hybridization events provides a great deal of specificity. The danger of false-positive results caused by carryover of target material is decreased, as the target itself is not amplified. However, nonspecific localization of reagents can result in background amplification.[2] Assays for hepatitis B and C, HIV-1, and CMV have been developed using this method.[15] This system is also used to quantitate HIV-1 with a lower limit of detection at 75 copies/mL **(Table 11–1)**.[32] It has been validated for the quantitation of viral load testing of all the subtypes. Therefore, this technique can be used for quantitation and to help monitor the therapeutic response.

## DRAWBACKS OF AMPLIFICATION SYSTEMS

Amplification systems in general are subject to several potential problems. The greatest of these is the potential for false-positive results caused by contaminating nucleic acids. In the case of PCR, LCR, and SDA, DNA products are the main source of contamination. For NASBA and TMA, RNA products are the possible contaminants. Therefore, it is necessary to use some form of product inactivation as part of a quality-control program.[15] Separating sample preparation areas from amplification areas and using inactivation systems, such as UV light and dUTP-UNG chemical system in PCR, help to alleviate contamination. Recent advances in automated amplification systems employ closed systems where amplification and detection occur in the same tube, resulting in much less potential for contamination and reducing turnaround times and labor costs.

The exquisite sensitivity of these techniques can present a problem in that very small numbers of pathogens present may not be significant. Amplification procedures can determine if RNA or DNA from a particular organism are present but reveals nothing about the viability of the organism. There is also the possibility that inhibiting substances in clinical specimens may affect enzymatic amplification methods and cause false-negative reactions.

## FUTURE OF MOLECULAR DIAGNOSTIC TECHNIQUES

When molecular testing first became available for clinical laboratory testing in the late 1980s, it was restricted to a relatively few high-volume laboratories in the areas of infectious disease testing, human genetics, and histocompatibility. Those early assays were specialty tests and did not replace conventional laboratory assays. They tended to be cost-prohibitive and very complex. However, at the beginning of the 21st century, more and more laboratories began performing molecular diagnostic testing; in some cases, it is now considered mainstream. This virtual explosion of molecular testing in clinical labs is due to several factors, including more readily available reagents, both FDA-approved and analyte-specific reagents (ASRs), the trend toward real-time amplification technologies, more choices in automated specimen processing (nucleic acid extraction), and now the fact that molecular procedures are the "gold standard" for diagnosis of many diseases and infections.[4] For example, in many labs testing for *Chlamydia trachomatis* and *Neisseria gonorrhoeae*, nucleic acid–based testing is performed instead of conventional assays. Molecular-based assays for these agents are competitively priced, provide superior sensitivity, and are relatively easy to perform. Molecular testing can be cost-effective in other ways as well. For example, rapid identification of mycobacteria can reduce patient/hospital costs by eliminating the need for unnecessary respiratory isolation for patients suspected of having tuberculosis.[15] Detection of multidrug-resistant strains of *Mycobacterium tuberculosis* may lead to more timely public health control measures. Identification of genes for antimicrobial resistance in other organisms will help in more effective treatment for severe infections.[16] HCV genotyping and pretreatment viral load testing in newly diagnosed infections provides the physician with valuable information to determine therapy regimens.[33] HIV viral load testing can play a role in diagnosis of HIV in neonates born to HIV-infected mothers and in the diagnosis of acute HIV infections, which are defined as the period after exposure to the virus but before seroconversion.[34]

In addition to direct detection of infectious microorganisms, there are numerous applications in immunology and hematology. Molecular HLA typing has revolutionized histocompatibility testing.[4] The impact on class II typing has resulted in a significant decrease in morbidity and mortality in bone marrow transplants. Hematologic diseases can also be followed more easily now, and molecular technology likely will influence treatment choices in acute leukemia cases.[4]

The problem of contamination is beginning to be addressed in numerous ways. Multiple closed systems have been developed so that both amplification and detection take place in the same test tube. These newer techniques are also more suitable to automation, which has brought down labor costs and should continue to do so in the future. As diagnostic kits and reagents become more widely available, use of these techniques will rise.

The increased specificity and sensitivity of molecular testing will become the standard of practice in immunology and microbiology. Rapid turnaround time plus increasing automation will bring down the cost and will allow such techniques to be used in smaller hospitals and in larger medical centers. Molecular techniques will not replace culture for those organisms that are easily grown and identified in the laboratory, nor will it replace hematologic procedures that are standardized and efficient. However, for esoteric organisms and diseases, molecular techniques will most likely replace serological techniques that are subject to cross-reactivity and the unpredictability of the antibody response in individual patients.

## SUMMARY

The unique characteristics of DNA and RNA make them ideal tools to use as diagnostic indicators of disease. Both are made up of nucleotides that occur in very specific sequences in different cells and microorganisms. They can be used to determine the presence of microorganisms, particular genes that would indicate cancerous or precancerous states, and much more. DNA exists as a double-stranded molecule with very specific base pair linkages: Adenine pairs with thymine, and guanine pairs with cytosine. When the DNA molecule is replicated, the strands are separated, and a new strand is created that is complementary to the parent strand. This exact base pairing forms the basis for identification of unknown sequences through the use of known short nucleic acid sequences called probes. Hybridization is the pairing of a probe with a complementary DNA strand. The probe is labeled with a marker for detection. Dot-blots and sandwich hybridization techniques are used to directly identify specific sequences in patient samples.

Detailed characterization of DNA can be accomplished through the use of enzymes called restriction endonucleases that cleave DNA at specific recognition sites. Then when the DNA is electrophoresed, the resulting fragments can be separated on the basis of size. Individuals or specific microorganisms can be identified on the basis of unique patterns obtained, called RFLPs. If the resulting electrophoretic pattern is transferred to a membrane for use in hybridization, this is known as a Southern blot. Northern blots involve separation of RNA in a similar manner. Individual fragments can also be isolated and sequenced to identify single nucleotide polymorphisms (SNPs), also important for identification purposes.

Hybridization of probes with target nucleic acids can also take place in solution or in intact cells. The hybridization protection assay is an example of the former. The label on the probe is only protected from degradation if it is attached to the target nucleic acid. If intact cells or tissue is used, this is called in situ hybridization.

DNA/RNA chips represent a microenvironment in which thousands of hybridization reactions are possible. Chips are used to identify particular strains of viruses such as HIV and help determine resistance to particular therapeutic drugs. Chip technology is also being used more extensively to identify alterations of genes in various cancers.

If there is not enough nucleic acid in a specimen for detection, analysis amplification methods can be used to increase either the target or the detection system. Polymerase chain reaction (PCR) is the most widely used method of target amplification. Specific primers coupled with a thermostable DNA polymerase are used to make copies of the original DNA strands. Each cycle results in a doubling of a specific target sequence, and approximately 30 cycles produce millions of copies of the original molecules. This technique is used clinically to identify viruses such as hepatitis B, hepatitis C, and HIV, and to perform HLA typing and measure cytokine activity.

TMA, NASBA, and SDA are target amplification methods based on the use of a DNA template to make numerous RNA copies of the target sequence. *Chlamydia trachomatis*, *Mycobacterium tuberculosis*, *Mycobacterium avium*, and HIV are some examples of microorganisms identified by this method.

Probes rather than target nucleic acid can be amplified by the ligase chain reaction (LCR). LCR actually splices two DNA probes together to make a single-strand copy of the target nucleic acid sequences.

Signal amplification is another means of detecting small amounts of target nucleic acid. The branched DNA method uses a series of hybridization steps, including a capture probe, an extender probe, and a multimer probe to enhance the signal to a detectable level.

All amplification techniques are subject to false-positive reactions resulting from either contamination with previously amplified products or background reactivity. In addition, quality-control procedures and laboratory standardization need to be developed. However, molecular techniques are exceedingly specific and rapid and will eventually replace serological techniques for identification of organisms that are difficult to culture and antigens such as HLA, in which small differences must be distinguished.

# CASE STUDY

A 23-year-old male presented himself to an urgent care center with urethral discharge and a red rash on his feet and forearms. He stated that he had had unprotected sex with a prostitute within the past 2 weeks. He was treated empirically for chlamydia, gonorrhea (GC), and Rocky Mountain spotted fever (RMSF). The following laboratory tests were ordered: Chlamydia/GC PCR; RPR; serology testing for RMSF; hepatitis B, C; and HIV. All test results were negative except for Chlamydia PCR.

Fourteen days later, the patient presents to an infectious disease clinic with a headache, a fever of 38.1°C, nausea and vomiting, myalgia, 2 weeks of fatigue and mouth ulcers, and a 10 lb weight loss within the past 3 weeks. Laboratory tests at this time reveal the patient is lymphocytopenic, and his liver function enzymes are slightly elevated.

## Questions

a. What is the most likely diagnosis of this patient: Chlamydia, HIV, HSV, syphilis, hepatitis B, or hepatitis C?

b. What laboratory test would you like repeated on the second visit, and why?

c. What molecular test could have been ordered on the patient's first visit that may have likely been able to provide a diagnosis for him?

# EXERCISE

## GEL ELECTROPHORESIS OF DNA

### Principle

This experiment will demonstrate the use of restriction enzymes to cleave DNA from the bacteriophage lambda (48,502 base pairs in length). The resulting fragments will be separated out using gel electrophoresis. The three restriction endonucleases used are BamHI, EcoRI, and HindIII. BamHI and HindIII are from *Haemophilus influenzae*, and EcoRI is from *Escherichia coli*. Three sample tubes of lambda DNA are prepared and incubated at 37°C with one of the enzymes in each tube. A fourth tube, the negative control, is incubated without an endonuclease.

The DNA samples are then loaded into wells of an agarose gel and are electrophoresed. An electrical field applied across the gel causes the DNA fragments in the samples to migrate through the gel toward the positive electrode. The smaller DNA fragments migrate faster than the larger ones. Each enzyme will produce a different set of bands, representing different-sized fragments. Only one band should be produced from the control tube, in which no enzymatic digestion took place. The resulting pattern for each is called a *DNA fingerprint*. After electrophoresis, a compound that binds to DNA is used to make the bands visible. A Polaroid camera can be used to make a permanent record of the results.

### Sample Preparation

Dehydrated DNA is reconstituted by adding distilled or deionized water. The dehydrated DNA and enzymes used in the kit can be stored at room temperature for up to 2 years. DNA and the enzymes are not of human origin, but they should be handled using standard safety precautions.

### Reagents, Materials, and Equipment

Kit from Carolina Biological Supply Company, which contains the following:

Vials of lambda DNA

6 vials BamHI

6 vials EcoRI

6 vials HindIII

6 vials loading dye

6 control reaction tubes

Tris-borate-ethylenediaminetetraacetic acid (TBE) buffer concentrate

6 staining trays

15 1.5 mL tubes

Agarose (3.2 grams for 400 mL)

Floating tube rack

Additional equipment needed:

Micropipettors (0–10 μL or 0–20 μL)

Micropipette tips

Gel electrophoresis chambers and power supplies

Boiling water bath or microwave oven

Water bath at 60°C

Water bath at 37°C

White light box/UV light box with mid or long wavelength for viewing stained gels

0.25 N HCl and 0.25 N NaOH for decontaminating ethidium bromide staining solution

Optional equipment:

Polaroid gun camera or other camera for recording results

> **CAUTION:** Ethidium bromide is a mutagen and a suspected carcinogen. If it is used for staining, gloves should be worn at all times, and staining should be confined to a small area of the laboratory. After staining, a funnel can be used to decant as much ethidium bromide as possible from the staining tray back into the storage container. The stain may be reused to stain 15 or more gels. Used staining solutions and gels need to be disabled first before discarding. The steps for doing so are listed in the procedure.

### Procedure*

A. Restriction Digest

1. To reconstitute the DNA, add 280 μL of distilled or deionized water to each of two tubes of DNA provided. Allow to sit for 5 minutes.

2. Hold each closed tube firmly at the top, and flick the side of the tube repeatedly to mix the contents. Do this for 1 full minute.

3. Allow tubes to stand for an additional 5 minutes. The DNA solution should look slightly opaque. It is very important that the DNA be totally dissolved.

4. Aliquot 90 μL of DNA into each of six 1.5 mL tubes to be used by each laboratory group.

5. Select four 0.2 mL tubes, each of which contains a different enzyme. The blue tube contains BamHI, the pink tube contains EcoRI, the green tube contains HindIII, and the yellow tube has no enzyme at all.

---

*Procedure is taken from the Teacher's Manual included with the kit called Restriction Enzyme and DNA Kit from Carolina Biological Supply Company, Burlington, NC.

6. Add 20 μL of DNA into each of the colored tubes. Mix the DNA and enzymes by pipetting up and down several times. There should be no concentration of the blue color in the bottom of the tube if DNA and enzymes are mixed sufficiently. Use a fresh pipette tip when adding DNA into each reaction tube to prevent cross-contamination.

7. Incubate all reaction tubes for a minimum of 20 minutes at 37°C.

B. Preparation of Cast Agarose Gel

1. Prepare the TBE buffer solution by pouring the contents of the 20X TBE concentrate into a 3 L flask or carboy. Add 2850 mL of distilled or deionized water for a final volume of 3 L. Stir for 1 to 2 minutes.

2. Prepare 0.8 percent agarose solution by adding 3.2 grams of agarose to 400 mL of TBE buffer in a clean 1 L flask. Cover with aluminum foil and heat in a boiling water bath for 10 to 20 minutes. Swirl to ensure that no undissolved agarose remains. Alternatively, prepare four individual flasks of agarose by weighing out 0.8 grams of agarose for each flask and adding it to 100 mL of buffer in a 250 mL flask. Cover flasks with parafilm, and heat one individually in a microwave until the solution becomes clear.

3. Place flasks in a 60°C water bath to cool the agarose to 60°C before pouring.

4. Seal ends of gel-casting tray with tape, or use a self-sealing tray. Insert the well-forming comb.

5. Carefully pour enough agarose solution into the casting tray to fill it to a depth of about 5 mm. The gel should cover only about one-third the height of comb teeth. While the agarose is still liquid, a pipette tip or toothpick can be used to move large bubbles or solid debris to the sides or end of tray.

6. Let gel solidify without disturbing for about 20 minutes. Gel will become cloudy as it solidifies.

7. Unseal ends of casting tray, and place the gel in the gel box for electrophoresis with the comb at the negative (black) end.

8. Fill gel box with 1X TBE buffer to a level that just covers the entire surface of the gel.

9. Gently remove comb by pulling straight up, being careful not to rip the wells.

10. Make sure that the wells are completely covered with buffer. If there are any dimples, slowly add buffer until the dimples disappear.

C. Electrophoresis

1. Add 2 μL of loading dye to each reaction tube, and mix dye with digested DNA by tapping the tube on the lab bench, or pulse with a microcentrifuge.

2. Use a micropipette to load contents of each reaction tube into a separate well in the gel. Load wells by steadying pipette with two hands. Expel any air in the micropipette tip end before loading gel. Place pipette tip through surface of buffer, and position the tip over a well. Slowly expel the mixture. The loading dye should cause the sample to sink to the bottom of the well.

3. Close the top of the electrophoresis chamber, and connect electrical leads to a power supply, anode to anode and cathode to cathode.

4. Turn on power supply, and set voltage for approximately 125 volts. Note that this voltage will allow for adequate separation on mini-gels in approximately 1 hour.

5. Allow the DNA to migrate until the bromphenol blue band from the loading dye is near the end of the gel.

6. Turn off power supply, disconnect leads from the inputs, and remove the top of the electrophoresis chamber.

7. Carefully remove casting tray, and slide gel into staining tray.

8. Flood gel with ethidium bromide solution, and allow to stain for 10 to 15 minutes. Decant stain back into the container, using a funnel.

9. Rinse gel and tray under running water to remove excess ethidium bromide solution.

10. Place on UV light box for viewing and photography.

> **NOTE:** Another version of this kit comes with Carolina BLU dye, which avoids the hazards of working with ethidium bromide and which can be viewed with a regular light box instead of one with a UV light source.

## Disabling the Gels and Used Staining Solution

1. Add one volume of 0.05 M $KMnO_4$, and mix carefully.

2. Add one volume of 0.25 N HCl, and mix carefully. Let stand at room temperature for several hours.

3. Add one volume of 0.25 N NaOH, and mix carefully.

4. Discard disabled solution down sink. Discard gels in the regular trash.

## Interpretation of Results

Digestion with BamHI should produce five fragments, EcoRI should produce five fragments, and HindIII should produce six fragments. Because each enzyme recognizes a distinctive base pair sequence, a different pattern will be obtained with each enzyme, and no separation will take place in the control tube. This same technique is used with human DNA to obtain a DNA fingerprint or to look for particular mutations that result in differences in numbers of bands.

# REVIEW QUESTIONS

1. Which technique is based on probe amplification rather than amplification of the target in question?

    a. PCR
    b. TMA
    c. Dot-blot
    d. Branched chain amplification

2. How are DNA and RNA different?

    a. Only RNA contains uracil.
    b. Only DNA contains cytosine.
    c. DNA is less stable than RNA.
    d. RNA is usually double-stranded.

3. All of the following are true of a nucleic acid probe *except*

    a. it is a short nucleic acid chain.
    b. it can be made up of either DNA or RNA.
    c. it is labeled with a marker for detection.
    d. it attaches to double-stranded DNA.

4. Which of the following techniques uses restriction enzymes, electrophoresis, and then transfer of DNA fragments onto a solid matrix, followed by probing with labeled probes?

    a. Dot-blot
    b. Southern blot
    c. Hybridization protection assay
    d. LCR

5. All of the following would be advantages of nucleic acid amplification techniques *except*

    a. detection of nonviable organisms.
    b. extreme sensitivity.
    c. early detection of disease.
    d. low cost.

6. Which best describes the principle of DNA chip technology?

    a. Chips contain multiple probes on their surface.
    b. Chips contain multiple copies of one unique probe.
    c. The sample is labeled with a fluorescent tag.
    d. Hybridization is detected by the presence of radioactivity.

7. A hybridization reaction involves which of the following?

    a. Binding of two complementary DNA strands
    b. Cleaving of DNA into smaller segments
    c. Separating DNA strands by heating
    d. Increasing the number of DNA copies

8. Which best describes the PCR?

    a. Two probes are joined by a ligating enzyme.
    b. RNA copies of the original DNA are made.
    c. Extender probes are used to detect a positive reaction.
    d. Primers are used to make multiple DNA copies.

9. During PCR, what happens in the annealing step?

    a. The primers bind to the target DNA.
    b. Strands are separated by heating.
    c. An RNA copy is made.
    d. Protein is made from the DNA strands.

10. What is the function of restriction endonucleases?

    a. They splice short DNA pieces together.
    b. They cleave DNA at specific sites.
    c. They make RNA copies of DNA.
    d. They make DNA copies from RNA.

11. To what does *in situ hybridization* refer?

    a. Nucleic acid probes react with intact cells within tissues.
    b. Probes are protected from degradation if hybridized.
    c. RNA polymerase copies messenger RNA.
    d. Hybridization takes place in solution.

12. What is PCR used for in clinical settings?

    a. Detection of early HIV infection
    b. Determination of specific HLA antigens
    c. Measurement of cytokines
    d. All of the above

# References

1. Parslow, TG. Molecular genetic techniques for clinical analysis of the immune system. In Stites, DP, Terr, AI, and Parslow, TG (eds): Medical Immunology, ed. 9. Appleton & Lange, Stamford, CT, 1997, pp. 309–318.

2. Lo, DYM, and Chiu, RWK. Principles of molecular biology. In Burtis, CA, Ashwood, ER, and Bruns, DE (eds): Tietz Textbook of Clinical Chemistry and Molecular Diagnostics, ed. 4. Elsevier Saunders, St. Louis, 2006, pp. 1393–1406.

3. Wisecarver, J. The ABCs of DNA. Lab Med 28:48, 1997.

4. Podzorski, RP. Molecular methods. In Detrick, B, Hamilton, RG, and Folds, JD, et al. (eds): Manual of Molecular and Clinical Laboratory Immunology, ed. 7. American Society for Microbiology, Washington, DC, 2006, pp. 26–52.

5. Tenover, FC, and Unger, ER. Nucleic acid probes for detection and identification of infectious agents. In Persing, DH, Smith, TF, and Tenover, FC, et al. (eds): Diagnostic Molecular Microbiology: Principles and Applications. American Society for Microbiology, Washington, D.C., 1993, pp. 3–25.

6. Forbes, BA, Sahm, DF, and Weissfeld, AS. Bailey and Scott's Diagnostic Microbiology, ed. 10. Mosby, St. Louis, 1998, pp. 188–207.

7. Whetsell, AJ, Drew, JB, and Milman, G, et al. Comparison of three nonradioisotopic polymerase chain reaction-based methods for detection of human immunodeficiency virus type 1. J Clin Microbiol 30:845, 1992.

8. Hansen, CA. Clinical applications of molecular biology in diagnostic hematology. Lab Med 24:562, 1993.

9. Unger, ER, and Piper, MA. Molecular diagnostics: Basic principles and techniques. In Henry, JB (ed): Clinical Diagnosis and Management by Laboratory Methods, ed. 20. WB Saunders, Philadelphia, 2001, pp. 1275–1295.

10. Friedrich, MJ. New chip on the block. Lab Med 30:180, 1999.

11. Check, W. Clinical microbiology eyes nucleic acid-based technologies. ASM News 64:84, 1998.

12. Schrenzel, J, Hibbs, JR, and Persing, DH. Hybridization array technologies. In Henry, JB (ed): Clinical Diagnosis and Management by Laboratory Methods, ed. 20. WB Saunders, Philadelphia, 2001, pp. 1296–1302.

13. Sanger, F, Nicklen, S, and Coulson, AR. DNA sequencing with chain terminating inhibitors. Proc Natl Acad Sci USA 74:5463, 1977.

14. Wittwer, CT, and Kusukawa, N. Nucleic acid techniques. In Bruns, DE, Ashwood, ER, and Buris, CA (eds): Fundamentals of Molecular Diagnostics. Saunders Elsevier, St. Louis, 2007, pp. 46–79.

15. Persing, DH. In vitro nucleic acid amplification techniques. In Persing, DH, Smith, TF, and Tenover, FC, et al. (eds): Diagnostic Molecular Microbiology: Principles and Applications. American Society for Microbiology, Washington, DC, 1993, pp. 51–87.

16. Mitchell, PS, and Persing, DH. Current trends in molecular microbiology. Lab Med 30:263, 1999.

17. Constantine, N, and Zhao, R. Molecular based laboratory testing and monitoring for human immunodeficiency virus infections. Clin Lab Sci 18(4):263–270, 2005.

18. Weikersheimer, PB. Viral load testing for HIV: Beyond the CD4 count. Lab Med 30:102, 1999.

19. Eisenbrey, AB. Choosing appropriate methodologies on the clinical environment: Immunological techniques versus molecular methods. In Rose, NR, De MacArio, EC, and Folds, JD, et al. (eds): Manual of Clinical Laboratory Immunology, ed. 5. American Society for Microbiology, Washington, DC, 1997, pp. 108–115.

20. Perkins, HA. HLA typing for transplantation of stem cells form unrelated donors. Lab Med 28:451, 1997.

21. Schmitz, JL. HLA typing using molecular methods. In Coleman, WB, and Tsongalis, GJ (eds): Molecular Diagnostics for the Clinical Laboratorian, ed. 2. Humana Press, Totowa, NJ, 2006, pp. 485–493.

22. Pang, J, Modlin, J, and Yolken, R. Use of modified nucleotides and uracil-DNA glycosylase (UNG) for the control of contamination in the PCR-based amplification of RNA. Mol Cell Probes 6(3):251–256, 1992.

23. Pruvost, M, Grange, T, and Geigl, EM. Minimizing DNA contamination by using UNG-coupled quantitative real-time PCR on degraded DNA samples: Application to ancient DNA studies. Biotechniques 38(4):569–575, 2005.

24. Kwoh, DY, Davis, GR, Whitfield, KM, Chapelle, LJ, DiMichele, LJ, and Giangeas, TR. Transcription-based amplification system and detection of amplified human immunodeficiency virus type 1 with a bead-based sandwich hybridization format. Proc Natl Acad Sci USA 86:1173–1177, 1989.

25. Hill, CS. Molecular diagnostics for infectious diseases. J Clin Lig Assay 19:43,1996.

26. New directions in molecular diagnostic testing. Gen-Probe Inc., San Diego, pp. 1–12.

27. http://www.gen-probe.com/prod_serv/clinical.asp, accessed November 1, 2007.

28. Nelson, NC. Molecular tools for building nucleic acid IVDs. IVD Technology, March/April 1997.

29. Little, MC, Andrews, J, Moore, R, Bustos, S, Jones, L, Embres, C, Durmowicz, G, et al. Strand displacement amplification and homogenous real-time detection incorporated in a second-generation DNA probe system. BDProbe TecET Clin Chem, 45:777–784, 1999.

30. Walker, GT, Fraiser, ML, Schram, JL, Little, MC, Nadequ, JG, and Malinowski, DP. Strand displacement amplification—an isothermal in vitro DNA amplification technique. Nucl Acid Res 20:1691–1696, 1992.

31. Walker, GT, Little, MC, Nadeau, JG, and Shank, DD. Isothermal in vitro amplification of DNA by a restricion enzyme/DNA polymerase system. Proc Natl Acad Sci USA, 89:392–396, 1992.

32. http://www.amp.com/resources, accessed November 30, 2007.

33. Zein, NN. Clinical significance of hepatitis C virus genotypes. Clin Micro Rev 13:223–235, 2000.

34. Ferreira-Gonzalez, A, Versalovic, J, Habecbu, S, and Caliendo, AM. Molecular methods in diagnosis and monitoring of infectious diseases. In Bruns, DE, Ashwood, ER, and Burtis, CA (eds): Fundamentals of Molecular Diagnostics. Saunders Elsevier, St. Louis, 2007, 171–196.

# Flow Cytometry and Laboratory Automation

*Susan M. Orton, PhD, MT (ASCP), D (ABMLI)*

## LEARNING OBJECTIVES

*After finishing this chapter, the reader will be able to:*

1. List and describe the function of each of the major components of a flow cytometer.
2. Discuss the difference between intrinsic and extrinsic parameters in flow cytometry.
3. List the advantages and disadvantages of automated testing in a clinical immunology lab.
4. Discuss the principle of hydrodynamic focusing within the flow cytometer.
5. Define the concept of fluorescence in flow cytometry.
6. Explain the difference between forward-angle light scatter (FSC) and side scatter (SSC).
7. Discuss the difference between analyzing flow cytometry data using single-parameter histograms and dual-parameter dot plots.
8. List several clinical applications for flow cytometry.
9. Apply knowledge of various T- and B-cell surface antigens to identify various cell populations.
10. Discuss advantages and disadvantages of automated immunoassay analyzers.
11. Describe the difference between a random access and a batch analyzer.
12. Define *accuracy, precision, reportable range, analytic sensitivity, analytic specificity, reportable range, reference interval.*

## KEY TERMS

___ Accuracy
___ Analytic sensitivity
___ Analytic specificity
___ Automatic sampling
___ Batch analyzer
___ Dual-parameter dot plot
___ Extrinsic parameter
___ Flow cytometer
___ Forward-angle light scatter
___ Gate
___ Immunophenotyping
___ Intrinsic parameter
___ Laser light source
___ Monoclonal antibodies
___ Precision
___ Random access analyzer
___ Reference interval
___ Reportable range
___ Right-angle light scatter
___ Single-parameter histogram

# CELL FLOW CYTOMETRY

## Principle

The first true **flow cytometers** were developed in the 1960s, primarily for research purposes. However, in the early 1980s, physicians started seeing patients with a new mysterious disease characterized by a drop in circulating helper T cells, and flow cytometry was brought into the clinical laboratory. Since that time, flow cytometry has been routinely used to identify infection with HIV, and **immunophenotyping** cells—identifying their surface antigen expression—has become a major component of the workload in most clinical immunology laboratories.

Cell flow cytometry is an automated system in which single cells in a fluid suspension are analyzed in terms of their intrinsic light-scattering characteristics and are simultaneously evaluated for extrinsic properties (i.e., the presence of specific surface proteins) using fluorescent labeled antibodies or probes. By using several different fluorochromes, cytometers can simultaneously measure multiple cellular properties. Another significant advantage of flow cytometry is that because the flow rate of cells within the cytometer is so rapid, thousands of cells can be analyzed in seconds, allowing for the accurate detection of very rare cells. The major components of a flow cytometer include the fluidics, the **laser light source,** the optics and photodetectors, and a computer for data analysis and management.[1]

## Instrumentation

### Fluidics

For cellular parameters to be accurately measured in the flow cytometer, it is crucial that cells pass through the laser one at a time in single file. Cells are processed into a suspension, and the cytometer draws up the cell suspension and injects the sample inside a carrier stream of isotonic saline (sheath fluid) to form a laminar flow. The sample stream is constrained by the carrier stream and is thus hydronamically focused so that the cells pass single file through the intersection of the laser light source (**Fig. 12–1**).

### Laser Light Source

Each cell is interrogated by a light source that typically consists of one or more small air-cooled lasers. The wavelength of monochromatic light emitted by the laser in turn dictates which fluorochromes can be used. A fluorochrome, or fluorescent molecule, is one that absorbs light across a spectrum of wavelengths and emits light of lower energy across a spectrum of longer wavelengths. Each fluorochrome has a distinctive spectral pattern of absorption (excitation) and emission. Not all fluorochromes can be used with all lasers, because each fluorochrome has distinct spectral characteristics. Therefore, the choice of fluorochromes to be used in an assay depends on the light source used for excitation (**Table 12–1**). Most clinical flow cytometers have at least one laser, typically argon, that emits at 488 nm. Newer cytometers also have a second laser, helium-neon (He-Ne), that emits at 633 nm. This allows more fluorochromes to be analyzed in a single tube at one time. As a result of a cell passing through the laser, light is scattered in many directions. The amount and type of light scatter (LS) can provide valuable information about a cell's physical properties. Light at two specific angles is measured by the flow cytometer: **forward-angle light scatter (FSC),** and orthogonal **right-angle light scatter,** or 90-degree-angle light scatter (SSC).

| Table 12–1. | Fluorochromes Commonly Used in Clinical Flow Cytometry | |
| --- | --- | --- |
| **EXCITATION WAVELENGTH** | **FLUOROCHROME OR DYE** | **EMISSION WAVELENGTH** |
| 488 nm (argon laser) | Fluorescein isothiocyanate (FITC) | 530 |
| | Phycoerythrin (PE) | 580 |
| | Propidium iodide (PI) | 620 |
| | Peridinin chlorophyll (PerCP) | 670 |
| 633 nm (He-Ne laser) | Allophycocyanin (APC) | 670 |
| | Cy-5 | 670 |

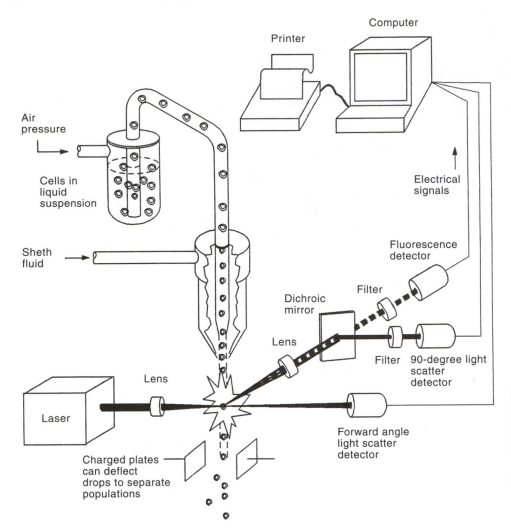

**FIGURE 12–1.** Flow cytometry. Components of a laser-based flow cytometer include the fluidics system for cell transportation, a laser for cell illumination, photodetectors for signal detection, and a computer-based management system. Both forward and 90-degree LS are measured, indicating cell size and type.

FSC, or light scattered at less then 90 degrees, is considered an indicator of size, while the SSC signal is indicative of granularity or intracellular complexity of the cell. Thus, these two values, which are considered **intrinsic parameters,** can be used to characterize different cell types. If one looks at a sample of whole blood on a flow cytometer, where all the red blood cells have been lysed, the three major populations of white blood cells (lymphocytes, monocytes, and granulocytes) can be roughly differentiated from each other based solely on their intrinsic parameters (FSC and SSC; **Fig. 12–2**).

Unlike FSC and SSC, which represent light-scattering properties that are intrinsic to the cell, **extrinsic parameters** require the addition of a fluorescent probe for their detection. Fluorescent labeled antibodies bound to the cell are interrogated by the laser. By using fluorescent molecules with various emission wavelengths, the laboratorian can simultaneously evaluate an individual cell for several extrinsic properties. The clinical utility of such multicolor analysis is enhanced when the fluorescent data are analyzed in conjunction with FSC and SSC.[2]

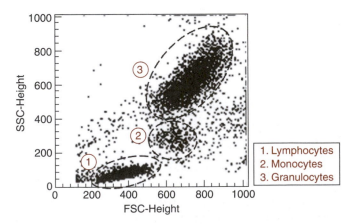

**FIGURE 12–2.** Peripheral blood leukocyte analysis by simultaneous evaluation of forward-angle light scatter (FCS) and 90-degree LS (SSC). Based on the intrinsic characteristics of size (FSC) and granularity (SSC) only, the three main populations of white cells (lymphocytes, monocytes, and granulocytes) can be discriminated into individual populations.

## Optics

The various signals (light scatter and fluorescence) generated by the cells' interaction with the laser are detected by photomultiplier tubes and detectors. The number of fluorochromes capable of being measured simultaneously is limited by the number of photodetectors in the flow cytometer. The specificity of each photodetector for a given band length of wavelengths is achieved by the arrangement of a series of optical filters that are designed to maximize collection of light derived from a specific fluorochrome while minimizing collection of light from other fluorochromes used to stain the cells. The newer flow cytometers actually use fiber-optic cables to direct light to the detectors. Most clinical flow cytometers in use today are capable of three- to six-color detection using one to two lasers.

When fluorescent light reaches the photomultiplier tubes, it creates an electrical current that is converted into a voltage pulse. The voltage pulse is then converted (using various methods depending on the manufacturer) into a digital signal. The digital signals are proportional to the intensity of light detected. The intensity of these converted signals is measured on a relative scale that is generally set into 1 to 256 channels, from lowest energy level or pulse to the highest level.

## Data Acquisition and Analysis

Once the intrinsic and extrinsic cellular properties of many cells (typically 10,000 to 20,000 "events" are collected for each sample) have been collected and the data digitalized, it is ready for analysis by the operator. Each parameter can be analyzed independently or in any combination. Graphics of the data can be represented in multiple ways. The first level of representation is the **single-parameter histogram,** which plots a chosen parameter (generally fluorescence) on the x-axis versus the number of events on the y-axis, so only a single parameter is analyzed using this type of graph **(Fig. 12–3)**. The operator can then set a marker to differentiate between cells that have low levels of fluorescence (negative) from cells that have high levels of fluorescence (positive) for a particular fluorochrome labeled antibody. The computer will then calculate the percentage of "negative" and "positive" events from the total number of events collected.

The next level of representation is the bivariant histogram, or **dual-parameter dot plot,** where each dot represents an individual cell or event. Two parameters, one on each axis, are plotted against each other. Each parameter to be analyzed is determined by the operator. Using dual-parameter dot plots, the operator can then draw a "gate" around a population of interest and analyze various parameters (extrinsic and intrinsic) of the cells contained within the gated region **(Fig. 12–4)**. This allows the operator to screen out debris and isolate subpopulations of cells of interest.

When analyzing a population of cells using a dual-parameter dot plot, the operator chooses which parameters

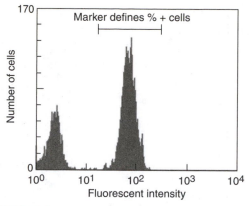

**FIGURE 12–3.** Example of a single parameter flow histogram. The y-axis consists of the number of events. The x-axis is the parameter to be analyzed, which is chosen by the operator, usually an extrinsic parameter, such as a fluorescent labeled antibody. The operator can then set a marker to isolate the positive events. The computer will then calculate the percent positive events within the designated markers.

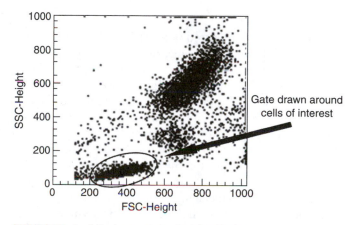

**FIGURE 12–4.** A dual-parameter dot plot. Both parameters on the x- and y-axes are chosen by the operator. In this case, lysed whole blood is analyzed on FSC (x-axis) and SSC (y-axis). The operator then draws a "gate" or isolates the population of interest (e.g., lymphocytes) for further analysis.

to analyze on both the x- and y-axes. He or she then divides the dot plot into four quadrants, separating the positives from the negatives in each axis **(Fig. 12–5)**. Quadrant 1 consists of cells that are positive for fluorescence on the y-axis and negative for fluorescence on the x-axis. Quadrant 2 consists of cells that are positive for fluorescence on both the x- and y-axes. Quadrant 3 consists of cells that are negative for fluorescence on both the x- and y-axes. And quadrant 4 consists of cells that are positive for fluorescence on the x-axis and negative for fluorescence on the y-axis. The computer will then calculate the percentage of cells in each quadrant based on the total number of events counted (typically 10,000 to 20,000 events per sample). For example, a gate can be drawn around a population of cells based on their FSC versus SSC characteristics, and the extrinsic

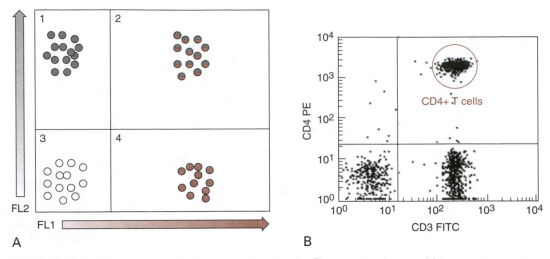

**FIGURE 12–5.** Quadrant analysis of a dual-parameter dot plot. The operator chooses which parameters to analyze on each axis. *(A)* On each axis there are positive (fluorescence positive) and negative (fluorescence negative) cells. *(B)* Example of a dual-parameter dot plot to identify CD4+ T cells: CD3 on the x-axis and CD4 on the y-axis. The cells in quadrant 2 that are both positive for CD3 and CD4 are true CD4+ T cells.

characteristics of the gated population can be analyzed—that is, lymphocytes can be gated, and then the subpopulations of T cells (CD3+ and CD4+ or CD2+) and B cells (CD2−, CD19+) can be analyzed **(Fig. 12–6)**. The absolute count of a particular cell type—for instance, CD4+ T lymphocytes—is obtained by multiplying the absolute cell count of the population of interest (e.g., lymphocytes) derived from a hematology analyzer by the percentage of the population of interest in the sample (CD3+ and CD4+ lymphocytes).[1,2]

Detailed phenotypic analysis can determine the lineage and clonality, as well as the degree of differentiation and activation of a cell population. This is useful for differential diagnosis or clarification of closely related lymphoproliferative disorders.

## Sample Preparation

Samples commonly used for analysis include whole blood, bone marrow, and fluid aspirates. Whole blood should be collected into ethylenediaminetetraacetic acid (EDTA), the anticoagulant of choice for samples processed within 30 hours of collection. Heparin can also be used for whole blood and bone marrow and can provide improved stability in samples over 24 hours old. Blood should be stored at room temperature (20°C to 25°C) prior to processing and should be well mixed before being pipetted into staining tubes.[2,3] Hemolyzed or clotted specimens should be rejected. Peripheral blood, bone marrow, and other samples with large numbers of red cells require erythrocyte removal to allow for efficient analysis of white cells.

Historically, density gradient centrifugation with Ficoll-Hypaque (Sigma, St. Louis, MO) was used to generate a cell suspension enriched for lymphocytes or blasts. However, this method results in selective loss of some cell populations.[4] Alternatively, there are numerous erythrocyte lysis techniques available, both commercial and noncommercial.[4]

Tissue specimens are best collected and transported in tissue culture medium (RPMI 1640) at either room temperature or 4°C, if analysis will be delayed. The specimen is then disaggregated to form a single cell suspension, either by mechanical dissociation or by enzymatic digestion. Mechanical disaggregation, or "teasing," is preferred and is accomplished by the use of either a scalpel and forceps, a needle and syringe, or wire mesh screen.[5] Antibodies are then added to the resulting cellular preparation and processed for analysis. The antibodies used are typically monoclonal, each with a different fluorescent tag.

## Clinical Applications

Routine applications of flow cytometry in the clinical laboratory include immunophenotyping of peripheral blood lymphocytes, enumeration of CD34+ stem cells in peripheral blood and bone marrow for use in stem cell transplantation, and immunophenotypic characterization of acute leukemias, non-Hodgkin's lymphomas, and other lymphoproliferative disorders.

Immunophenotyping by flow cytometry has become an important component of initial evaluation and subsequent post-therapeutic monitoring in leukemia and lymphoma management. Flow cytometric findings have been incorporated into current leukemia and lymphoma classifications, beginning with the Revised European-American Lymphoma classification in 1994 and, more recently, in the proposed World Health Organization (WHO) classifications.[6,7] One of the most important components of flow cytometric analysis is the stratification of hematopoietic malignancies by

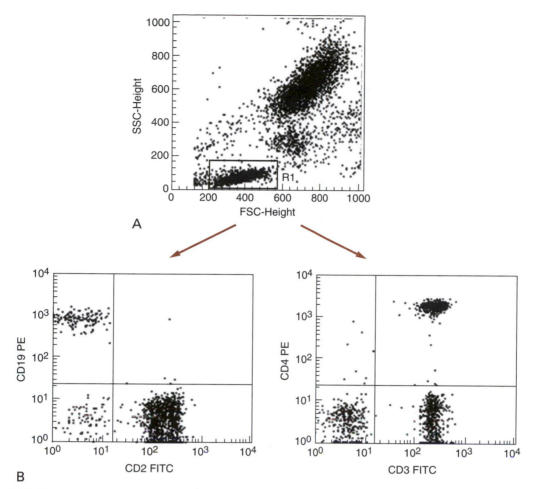

**FIGURE 12–6.** Gating strategy to analyze lymphocyte subsets in a sample of whole blood. Whole blood is incubated with fluorescent-labeled antibodies specific for CD2, CD3, CD4, and CD19. The sample is washed, RBCs are lysed, and the sample is analyzed on the flow cytometer. To analyze using gating strategies, the sample is first plotted on FSC versus SSC. (A) A gate, or region, is drawn around the lymphocyte population. (B) On the subsequent plots of fluorescent markers, only the lymphocyte population is analyzed. The dot plot is divided into four quadrants to isolate positive from negative populations. The computer calculates the percent positive cells in each quadrant. Example of a flow pattern analyzing two different cell surface markers. CD3 identifies the T-cell population. CD4 identifies the percentage of the T-cell population that are T helper cells (CD4+). Three distinct populations are identified: CD3+ CD4+ in the upper right quadrant; CD3+ CD4− in the lower right quadrant; and CD3− CD4− in the lower left quadrant.

their lineage (i.e., B cell, T cell, or myeloid) and the degree of differentiation. Some of the more common cell-differentiation antigens are listed in **Table 12–2** and include CD2, CD3, CD4, CD7, CD8 found on T cells, CD19, CD20, CD22 found on B cells, CD11b, CD13, CD15, CD16 on myeloid cells, and CD11b, CD14, HLA-DR (MHC class II) on monocytoid cells.[8,9]

CD45 is a pan-leukocyte marker present on all white cells but with varying levels of expression; this results in varying levels of fluorescence. This variance in expression is based on the cell's maturity. Blasts express lower levels of CD45 (low fluorescence) but show an increase of CD45 expression as the cell matures, so mature white cells have much brighter fluorescence compared to their earlier progenitor stages. This varying level of CD45 expression is useful in differentiating various populations of white cells.

Immunophenotyping of white blood cell populations is essential when an immunodeficiency is suspected. Enumeration of peripheral blood CD4+ T cells in HIV-infected patients remains the highest volume test performed in the flow cytometry laboratory, because it is used in classifying stages of HIV disease and determining treatment options.[10,11] HIV type 1 infections cause a rapid, profound decrease in CD4+ T cell numbers and an expansion of CD8+ T-cell levels during the early course (12 to 18 months) of the illness.[12,13] Some individuals continue to rapidly lose CD4+ T cells and progress to AIDS, while others maintain relatively stable CD4+ T-cell counts and remain AIDS-free for years. During this chronic phase of HIV-1 disease, the decline in CD4+ T cells can be slow over many years due to maintenance of homeostatic mechanisms. However, as these homeostatic mechanisms start to fail,

## Table 12–2.    Surface Markers on T and B Cells

| ANTIGEN | CELL TYPE | FUNCTION |
|---|---|---|
| CD2 | Thymocytes, T cells, NK cells | Involved in T-cell activation |
| CD3 | Thymocytes, T cells | Associated with T-cell antigen receptor; role in TCR signal transduction |
| CD4 | Helper T cells, monocytes, macrophages | Coreceptor for MHC class II; receptor for HIV |
| CD5 | Mature T cells, thymocytes, subset of B cells (B1) | Positive or negative modulation of T- and B-cell receptor signaling |
| CD8 | Thymocyte subsets, cytotoxic T cells | Coreceptor for MHC class I |
| CD10 | B- and T-cell precursors, bone marrow stromal cells | Protease; marker for pre-B CALLA |
| CD11b | Myeloid an NK cells | $\alpha$ M subunit of integrin CR3, binds complement component iC3b, |
| CD13 | Myelomonocytic cells | Zinc metalloprotease |
| CD14 | Monocytic cells | Lipopolysaccharide receptor |
| CD15 | Neutrophils, eosinophils, monocytes | Terminal trisaccharide expressed on glycolipids |
| CD16 | Macrophages, NK cells, neutrophils | Low affinity Fc receptor, mediates phagocytosis and ADCC |
| CD19 | B cells, follicular dendritic cells | Part of B-cell coreceptor, signal transduction molecule that regulates B-cell development and activation |
| CD21 | B cells, follicular dendritic cells, subset of immature thymocytes | Receptor for complement component C3d; part of B-cell coreceptor with CD 19 |
| CD23 | B cells, monocytes, follicular dendritic cells | Regulation of IgE synthesis; triggers release of Il-1, Il-6, and GM-CSF from monocytes |
| CD25 | Activated T cells, B cells, monocytes | Receptor for IL-2 |
| CD44 | Most leukocytes | Adhesion molecule mediating homing to peripheral lymphoid organs |
| CD45 | All hematopoietic cells | Tyrosine phosphatase, augments signaling |
| CD45R | Different forms on all hematopoietic cells | Essential in T- and B-cell antigen-stimulated activation |
| CD 56 | NK cells, subsets of T cells | Not known |
| CD 94 | NK cells, subsets of T cells | Subunit of NKG2-A complex involved in inhibition of NK cell cytotoxicity |

NK = Natural killer; TCR = CD3-$\alpha\beta$ receptor complex; MHC = major histocompatibility class; HIV = human immunodeficiency virus; CALLA = common acute lymphoblastic leukemia antigen; Fc = Fragment crystallizable; ADCC = antibody-dependent cell cytotoxicity; IgE = immunoglobulin E; GM-CSF = granulocyte-macrophage colony-stimulating factor.

there is a further decline in CD4+ T and CD8+ T cells, which eventually leads to the development of AIDS.[14] CD4+ T-cell levels are used to stage HIV disease progression, are prognostic for the development of AIDS, and are used to monitor response to antiretroviral therapy. The Centers for Disease Control and Prevention (CDC) guidelines stage HIV-1 disease by CD4+ T-cell level into three groups: >500 CD4 cells/mm3, or >28 percent CD4 cells within lymphocytes; 200 to 500 CD4 cells/mm3, or 14 to 28 percent CD4 cells; and <200 CD4 cells/mm3, or <14 percent CD4 cells.[11]

Additional examples of flow cytometry use include the determination of DNA content, or ploidy status of tumor cells. This can provide the physician with important prognostic information.[15] Monitoring patients who have been treated for leukemia or lymphoma for "minimal residual disease" has also become another important function of the flow cytometer, since statistically significant rare cell events can be easily detected. In the case of a fetal–maternal hemorrhage, using flow cytometry to detect hemoglobin F positive cells is much more sensitive than the traditional Kleihauer-Betke method.[16,17] Flow cytometry is also being used in human leukocyte antigen typing and cross-matching for solid organ transplantation.[1,15]

Immunophenotyping by flow cytometry, in whatever capacity that it is used, is not possible without the use of fluorescent-labeled monoclonal and polyclonal antibodies. **Monoclonal antibodies** specific for various surface antigens are preferable to using polyclonal antibodies. The ability to produce monoclonal antibodies through hybridoma and recombinant DNA techniques has contributed greatly to the accuracy of flow cytometry and has widened its use. (See Chapter 4 for a discussion of monoclonal antibody production.)

# IMMUNOASSAY AUTOMATION

In addition to the use of flow cytometry, advances in automated technology are becoming more evident in clinical immunology labs with the advent of immunoassay analyzers. Reliable immunoassay instrumentation, excluding radioimmunoassay, was first available in the early 1990s. Using a solid support for separating free and bound analytes, these instruments have made it possible to automate heterogeneous immunoassays even for low-level peptides, such as peptide hormones.[18] Currently there are over two dozen different types of automated immunoassay analyzers that are capable of performing almost all common diagnostic immunoassays,[19] and they have largely replaced manual testing, especially in larger laboratories. The driving motivation for the development of immunoassay analyzers has been the need to create an automated system capable of reducing or eliminating the many manual tasks required to perform analytical procedures. Eliminating manual steps decreases the likelihood of error, since the potential error due to fatigue or erroneous sampling is reduced.[20] Laboratory professionals are also trying to streamline test performance to reduce turnaround time and the cost per test. Automation, in some cases, is much more accurate and precise compared to manual methods and, depending on the assay platform, may be more sensitive as well. Other potential benefits of immunoassay automation include the ability to provide more service with less staff; saving on controls, duplicates, dilutions, and repeats; longer shelf life of reagents and less disposal due to outdating; and the potential for automation of sample delivery with bar codes for better sample identification.[21]

Due to the wide variety of automated immunoassay analyzers available, it can be difficult to determine the best instrument for any given laboratory. There are many factors to consider other than the analytic quality of assays that are available. **Table 12–3** offers a partial list of factors to consider in determining what type of analyzer will fulfill a laboratory's needs. It is important for all those involved in the instrument's selection to prioritize the properties of any analyzer to meet the demands of the laboratory.

There are currently two main types of immunoassay analyzers on the market: batch analyzers and random access analyzers **(Table 12–4)**. **Batch analyzers** can examine multiple samples and provide access to the test samples for the formation of subsequent reaction mixtures. However, such batch analyzers permit only one type of analysis at a time. In some cases, this may be considered a drawback; stat samples cannot be loaded randomly, and there cannot be multiple analyses on any one sample. Partially for those reasons, the next generation of analyzers was designed in a modular system that could be configured to measure multiple analytes from multiple samples. These types of analyzers are called **random access analyzers,** in which multiple test samples can be analyzed, and multiple testing can be performed on any test sample.[22]

| **Table 12–3.** | **Factors for Consideration in Selecting an Automated Immunoassay Instrument** |
|---|---|
| **CATEGORY** | **FACTOR** |
| Analytical | Sensitivity |
| | Precision |
| | Accuracy/test standardization |
| | Linearity |
| | Interferences |
| | Carryover effects |
| Economic | Purchase cost |
| | Lease options |
| | Maintenance costs |
| | Reagent costs |
| | Operator time and costs |
| | Disposable costs |
| Instrument | Maintenance requirements |
| | Automation compatibility |
| | Space requirements |
| | Utility requirements |
| | Reliability |
| | Clot error detection |
| Manufacturer | Future product plans |
| | Reputation |
| | Technical support |
| | Menu expansion plans |
| Operational | Test menu |
| | Throughput |
| | Reagent capacity |
| | Reagent stability |
| | STAT capability |
| | Reflex testing ability |
| | Reagent kit size |
| | Training requirements |
| | Operating complexity |
| | Waste requirements |
| | Reagent storage requirements |
| | Downtime plans |

Reprinted from Remaley, AT, and Hortin, GL. Protein analysis for diagnostic applications. In Detrick, B, Hamilton, RG, and Folds, JD, et al. (eds): Manual of Molecular and Clinical Laboratory Immunology, ed. 7. American Society for Microbiology, Washington, DC, 2006, p. 15.

## Table 12–4.   Automated Immunoassay Analyzers

| MANUFACTURER | INSTRUMENT | OPERATIONAL TYPE | ASSAY PRINCIPLE |
| --- | --- | --- | --- |
| Abbott Diagnostics | AxSym | Continuous Random Access | FPIA, MEIA |
| | Architect | Batch, random access, cont. random access | Enhanced chemiluminescence |
| Beckman Coulter | Access | Cont. random access | Chemiluminescence |
| BioMérieux | VIDAS | Batch, random access | Fluorescence/EIA coated SPR |
| The Binding Site, Inc. | DSX automated system | Batch | EIA |
| Bio-Rad Labs, Clin. Diag. Group | BioPlex | Cont. random access | Bead flow cytometric (multiplex) |
| | PhD System | Batch | EIA |
| Diamedix Corp. | Mago Plus Automated EIA Processor | Batch, random access | EIA |
| Diasorin, Inc. | ETI-Max | Batch, random access | EIA |
| Hycor Biomedical, Inc. | HY-TEC | Random batches | EIA |
| Inverness Medical Professional Diagnostics | AIMS | Batch | EIA, multiplexing/bead |
| Ortho-Clinical Diag., a J&J Co. | VITROS | Cont. random access | Chemiluminescence (enhanced) |
| Phadia | ImmunoCAP | Cont. random access | FEIA |
| Siemens Medical Solutions Diag. | ADVIA Centaur | Cont. random access | Chemiluminescence |
| | IMMULITE | Cont. random access | Chemiluminescence |
| TOSOH Bioscience, Inc. | AIA | Cont. random access | Fluorescence, EIA |

Source: CAP Today, June 2007.

EIA = enzyme immunoassay; FEIA = fluoroenzyme immunoassay; FPIA = fluorescent polarization immunoassay; MEIA = microparticle enzyme immunoassay; SPR = solid phase receptacle

Automation can and does occur in all three stages of laboratory testing: the preanalytical, analytical, and postanalytical stages. For the purposes of this chapter, discussion is limited to automation within the analytical stage of testing.

The tasks to be considered during the analytical stage include introducing sample, adding reagent, mixing reagent and sample, incubating, detecting, calculating, and reporting readout or results. All or some of these tasks may be automated on various immunoassay analyzers. **Automatic sampling** can be accomplished by several different methods: peristaltic pumps (older technology) and positive-liquid displacement pipettes (newer technology) are two examples. In most systems, samples are pipetted using thin, stainless-steel probes. Issues to consider with probe technology are the inclusion of clot detectors that will automatically reject a sample if a clot is detected and the ability of the sample probe to detect the amount of the sample liquid, using a liquid level sensor. This latter sensor must be able to detect the lack of sample in a tube, usually because of a short draw, and reject such samples. Another issue associated with reusable pipette probes is carryover or contamination of one sample with material from the previous samples. Various methods have been developed to reduce carryover, including the use of disposable pipette tips to initially transfer samples.

Reagent use in automated immunoassay analyzers requires consideration of the following factors: handling, preparing and storing, and dispensing. Some reagents come ready for use, but if not, the analyzer must be able to properly dilute reagents before they can be used. Most reagents come with bar codes that are read by the analyzer to reduce operator error, so if the wrong reagent is loaded into the analyzer by mistake, the analyzer will detect the error and generate an error message.

After reagents have been added to the samples, the next concern is proper mixing to obtain reliable results. Analyzers use different methods for mixing, including magnetic stirring, rotation paddles, forceful dispensing, and vigorous lateral shaking. Whichever method used, it is imperative that there be no splashing between sample wells to prevent erroneous results.

Timed incubation is then carried out at ambient temperatures, or analyzers need to have built-in incubators for temperature-controlled incubation. Heated metal blocks are widely used to incubate reagent wells or cuvets.

Detection of the final analyte depends on the chemistry involved in the immunoassay. In the past, colorimetric absorption spectroscopy has been the principle means of measurement, due to the ability to measure a wide variety of compounds. Other methods of detection include fluorescence and chemiluminescence, both of which require fluorescence detectors.

## Validation

Regardless of the instrumentation considered, proper validation of new instrumentation or methodology must always be performed. The laboratory needs to determine how it will meet Clinical Laboratory Improvement Amendment (CLIA) regulations for verifying the manufacturer's performance specifications. The regulations apply to each nonwaived test or test system brought into the laboratory for the first time. Validation of the new instrument or method must be completed before patient results using that instrument can be reported. There are multiple resources available on the topic of method validation. The Centers for Medicare and Medicaid Services has an overview of the CLIA (available at http://www.cms.hhs.gov/CLIA). The specific requirements for method validation for nonwaived and modified tests (Subpart K) can be found at http://www.cms.hhs.gov/CLIA/downloads/apcsubk1.pdf. **Table 12–5** lists other governmental websites with information regarding method/instrument validation.[23]

As designated by CLIA, the required verifications to be determined for a new method are accuracy, precision, analytic sensitivity, analytic specificity to include interfering substances, reportable range, and reference intervals. **Accuracy** refers to the test's ability to actually measure what it claims to measure. For example, the assay may be tested using previously known positives or negatives as provided by proficiency testing or interlaboratory exchange. Also, parallel testing with an alternative method or technology is a form of accuracy testing. **Precision** refers to the ability to consistently reproduce the same result on repeated testing of the same sample. CLIA '88 specifies that the standard deviation and coefficient of variation should be calculated from 10 to 20 day-to-day quality-control results.[24] At least one normal and one abnormal control should be included in the analysis. **Analytic sensitivity** is defined as the lowest measureable amount of an analyte, while **analytic specificity** is the assay's ability to generate a negative result when the analyte is not present. The **reportable range** is defined as the range of values that will generate a positive result for the specimens assayed by the test procedure. Note that this may not include the entire dynamic range of the analytic instrument used to produce the result. Finally, the **reference interval** is the range of values found in healthy individuals who do not have the condition that is detected by the assay. This is used to define the expected value of a negative test.

Choosing an automated immunoassay analyzer is complicated and depends greatly on the main tasks to be performed in a particular laboratory. Batch analyzers may work best if only one type of testing is performed on a large scale. Random access analyzers allow for more flexibility, include rapid processing of stat samples. In either case, any new instrument requires extensive validation before patient results can be reported with confidence. Instrumentation can increase turnaround time for testing, remove the possibility of manual errors, and allow for greater sensitivity in determining the presence of low-level analytes.

## SUMMARY

Flow cytometry is a powerful tool to identify and enumerate various cell populations. It was first used in clinical laboratories to perform CD4+ T-cell counts in HIV-infected individuals. A flow cytometer measures multiple properties of cells suspended in a moving fluid medium. As each cell or particle passes single file through a laser light source, it produces a characteristic light pattern that is measured by multiple detectors for scattered light (forward and 90 degrees) and fluorescent emissions (if the cell is stained with a fluorochrome). Forward scatter is a measure of cell size, while side scatter determines a cell's internal complexity, or granularity.

Determining an individual's lymphocyte population is essential in diagnosing such conditions as lymphomas, immunodeficiency diseases, unexplained infections, or acquired immune diseases such as AIDS. Lymphocytes are identified using monoclonal antibodies directed against specific surface antigens. Reactions can be identified manually by employing a fluorescence microscope or by immunoenzyme staining methods. However, flow cytometry is the most commonly used method for immunophenotyping of lymphocyte populations.

Other instrumentation in the clinical immunology laboratory includes a variety of automated immunoassay analyzers that are currently available. They have replaced manual immunoassay procedures in many laboratories. These automated systems can generate more accurate, precise, and sensitive analysis of many analytes compared to manual immunoassays. There are many factors to consider in determining which analyzer will fill the needs of a particular

| Table 12–5. | CLIA-Related Governmental Websites | |
|---|---|
| **AGENCY** | **WEBSITE** |
| Centers for Disease Control and Prevention | www.phppo.cdc.gov/clia/default.aspx |
| Food and Drug Administration | www.fda.gov/cdrh/CLIA/index/html |
| The College of American Pathologists Laboratory Accreditation Program Inspection Checklist for Chemistry | www.cap.org/apps/docs/ laboratory_accreditation/checklists/ chemistry_and_toxicology_ april2006.pdf |
| Clinical Laboratory Standards Institute Evaluation Protocol | www.clsi.org |

laboratory, including deciding whether a batch or a random access analyzer can best serve testing needs.

Automation is incorporated in all stages of laboratory testing: preanalytical, analytical, and postanalytical. Once an analyzer has been purchased, a thorough validation of all assays to be performed must be done to ensure quality. The validation should include at least a determination of accuracy, precision, reportable range, reference range, analytic sensitivity, and analytic specificity. Automated analyzers are costly but can reduce turnaround time and hands-on time by the technical staff and can provide sensitive and precise results.

# CASE STUDIES

1. A laboratory has just purchased a new immunoassay analyzer, and validation is being done before patient results can be reported out. Twenty random patient samples are run by both the old and new methodology. According to the newer instrumentation, three samples that were negative by the old method are positive by the new instrument.

## Questions

a. What sort of possible error—that is, sensitivity, specificity, accuracy, or precision—does this represent?

b. What steps should be taken to resolve this discrepancy?

2. A 3-year-old female is sent for immunologic testing because of recurring respiratory infections, including several bouts of pneumonia. The results show decreased immunoglobulin levels, especially of IgG. Although her white blood cell count was within the normal range, the lymphocyte count was low. Flow cytometry was performed to determine if a particular subset of lymphocytes was low or missing. **Figure 12–7** shows the flow cytometry results obtained.

## Questions

a. What do the flow cytometry patterns indicate about the population of lymphocytes affected?

b. How can this account for the child's recurring infections?

c. What further type of testing might be indicated?

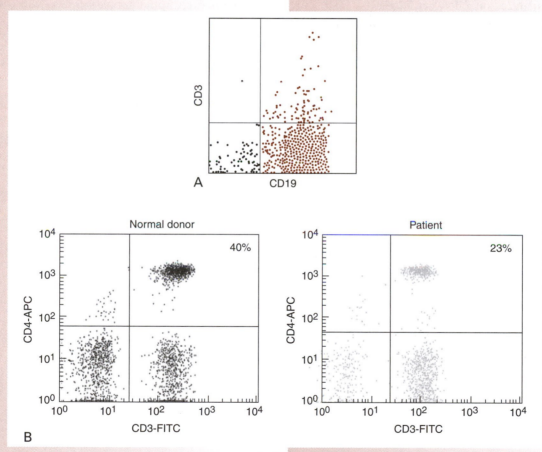

**FIGURE 12–7.** Flow cytometry patterns for case study. *(A)* Plot of CD3 versus CD19. *(B)* Plot of CD3 versus CD4.

# REVIEW QUESTIONS

1. Flow cytometry separates cells on the basis of which of the following?
   a. Forward and 90-degree side scatter of an interrupted beam of light
   b. Front-angle scatter only of an interrupted light beam
   c. Absorbance of light by different types of cells
   d. Transmittance of light by cells in solution

2. Forward-angle light scatter is an indicator of cell
   a. granularity.
   b. density.
   c. size.
   d. number.

3. What is the single most important requirement for samples to be analyzed on a flow cytometer?
   a. Whole blood is collected into a serum-separator tube.
   b. Cells must be in a single-cell suspension.
   c. Samples must be fixed in formaldehyde prior to processing.
   d. Blood must be kept refrigerated while processing.

4. Which represents the best explanation for a flow cytometer's ability to detect several cell surface markers at the same time?
   a. The forward scatter can separate out cells on the basis of complexity.
   b. One detector can be used to detect many different wavelengths.
   c. For each marker, a specific fluorochrome–antibody combination is used.
   d. Intrinsic parameters are separated out on the basis of amount of side scatter.

5. Which of the following cell surface markers would be present on a population of T helper cells?
   a. CD3 and CD4
   b. CD3 and CD8
   c. CD3 only
   d. CD4 only

6. Which cell surface marker is termed the *common acute lymphoblastic leukemia marker*?
   a. CD19
   b. CD10
   c. CD23
   d. CD21

7. All of the following are clinical applications for flow cytometry *except*
   a. fetal hemoglobin.
   b. immunophenotyping of lymphocyte subpopulations.
   c. HIV viral load analysis.
   d. enumeration of stem cells in a peripheral blood mononuclear cell product.

8. Which type of analyzer allows one to measure multiple analytes from multiple samples, loaded at any time?
   a. Batch analyzer
   b. Random access analyzers
   c. Front-end loaded analyzers
   d. Sequential access analyzers

9. All of the following are benefits of automation *except*
   a. greater accuracy.
   b. increased turnaround time.
   c. savings on controls.
   d. less disposal of outdated reagents.

10. If an analyzer gets different results each time the same sample is tested, what type of problem does this represent?
    a. Sensitivity
    b. Specificity
    c. Accuracy
    d. Precision

# References

1. Marti, GE, Steler-Stevenson, M, Bleesing, JJH, and Fleisher, TA. Introduction to flow cytometry. Seminars in Hem 38(2):93, 2001.
2. National Committee for Clinical Laboratory Standards. Clinical applications of flow cytometry quality assurance and immunophenotyping of peripheral blood lymphocytes. H42-A. National Committee for Clinical Laboratory Standards, Wayne, PA, 1998.
3. Renzi, P, and Ginns, LC. Analysis of T cell subsets in normal adults. Comparison of whole blood lysis technique to Ficoll-Hypaque separation by flow cytometry. Immunol Methods 98:53–56, 1987.
4. Carter, PH, Resto-Ruiz, S, Washington, GC, Ethridge, S, Palini, A, Vogt, R, Waxdal, M, Fleisher, T, Noguchi, PD, and Marti, GE. Flow cytometric analysis of whole blood lysis, three anticoagulants, and five cell preparations. Cytometry 13:68–74, 1992.
5. Braylon, RC, and Benson, NA. Flow cytometric analysis of lymphomas. Arch Pathol Lab Med 113:627–633, 1989.
6. Harris, HL, Jaffe, ES, Stein, H, Banks, PM, Chan, JKC, Cleary, ML, DEelsol, G, et al. A revised European-American classification of lymphoid neoplasms: A proposal from the International Lymphoma Study Group. Blood 84:1361–1392, 1994.
7. Harris, NLE, Jaffe, ES, Diebold, J, Flandrin, G, Muller-Hermelink, HK, Vardiman, J, Lister, TA, and Bloomfield, CD. The World Health Organization classification of neoplastic diseases of the hematopoietic and lymphoid tissues. Report of the clinical Advisory Committee meeting, Airlie House, Virginia. Ann Oncol 10:1419–1432, 1999.
8. Wood, BL. Immunophenotyping of leukemia and lymphoma by flow cytometry. In Detrick, B, Hamilton, RG, and Folds, JD, et al. (eds): Manual of Molecular and Clinical Laboratory Immunology, ed. 7. American Society for Microbiology, Washington, DC, 2006, pp. 171–186.
9. Bleesing, JJH, and Fleisher, TA. Immunophenotyping. Seminars in Hem 38(2):100, 2001.
10. Centers for Disease Control and Prevention. 1997 revised guidelines for performing CD4+T cell determinations in persons infected with human immunodeficiency virus (HIV). Morb Mortal Wkly Rep 46:1–29, 1997.
11. Centers for Disease Control. 1993 revised classification system for HIV infections and expanded case definition for AIDS among adolescents and adults. Morb Mort Wkly Rep 41:1–19, 1992.
12. Giorgi, JVA, Kesson, M, and Chou, CC. Immunodeficiency and infectious diseases. In Rose, NL, deMacario, CE, Fahey, JL, Friedman, H, and Penn, GM (eds): Manual of Clinical Laboratory Immunology, ed. 4. American Society for Microbiology, Washington, D.C., 1992, pp. 174–181.
13. Zaunders, J, Carr, A, McNally, L, Penny, R, and Cooper, DA. Effects of primary HIV-1 infections on subsets of CD4+ and CD8+ T lymphocytes. AIDS 9:561–566, 1995.
14. Margolick, JB, Munoz, A, Donnenberg, A, Park, LP, Galai, N, Giorgi, JV, O'Gorman, MRG, and Ferbas, J. Failure of T-cell homeostasis preceding AIDS in HIV infection. Nat Med 1:674–680, 1995.
15. Diguiseppe, JA. Flow cytometry. In Coleman, WB, and Tsongalis, GJ (eds): Molecular Diagnostics: For the Clinical Laboratorian, ed. 2. Humana Press, Inc., Totowa, NJ, 2006, pp. 163–172.
16. Chen, JC, Davis, BH, Wood, B, and Warzynski, MJ. Multicenter clinical experience with flow cytometric method for fetomaternal hemorrhage detection. Ctyometry 50:285–290, 2002.
17. Fernandes, BJ, vonDadelszen, P, Fazal, I, Bansil, N, and Ryan, G: Flow cytometric assessment of feto-maternal hemorrhage; a comparison with Betke-Kleihauer. Prenat Diagn 27(7):641–643, 2007.
18. Remaley, AT, and Hortin, GL. Protein analysis for diagnostic applications. In Detrick, B, Hamilton, RG, and Folds, JD, et al. (eds). Manual of Molecular and Clinical Laboratory Immunology, ed. 7. American Society for Microbiology, Washington, DC, 2006, pp. 7–21.
19. Wheeler, MJ. Automated immunoassay analysers. Ann Clin Biochem 38:217, 2001.
20. Sunheimer, RL, and Threatte, G. Analysis: Clinical laboratory automation. In McPherson, RA, and Pincus, MR (eds): Henry's Clinical Diagnosis and Management by Laboratory Methods, ed. 21. Saunders Elsevier, Philadelphia, 2007, pp. 56–63.
21. Turgeon, ML. Automated procedures. In Immunology and Serology in Laboratory Medicine, ed. 3. Mosby, St. Louis, 2003, pp.157–164.
22. http://www.patentstorm.us/patents/5358691-description.html, last accessed March 2, 2008.
23. Moon, TC, and Legrys, VA. Teaching method validation in the clinical laboratory science curriculum. Clin Lab Sci21(1):19–24, 2008.
24. Association for Molecular Pathology. Association for Molecular Pathology Statement: Recommendations for in-house development and operation of molecular diagnostic tests. Am J Clin Path 111:449–463, 1999.

# Immune Disorders

# 13 Hypersensitivity

## LEARNING OBJECTIVES

*After finishing this chapter, the reader will be able to:*

1. Define *hypersensitivity*, *atopy*, and *allergen*.
2. Discuss the key immunologic reactant involved in immediate hypersensitivity.
3. Describe the changes that take place in IgE-coated mast cells and basophils when binding with a specific antigen occurs.
4. Relate clinical manifestations of immediate hypersensitivity to specific mediators released from mast cells and basophils.
5. Describe anaphylaxis.
6. Discuss the advantages and disadvantages of skin testing for immediate hypersensitivity.
7. Compare total IgE and allergen-specific IgE testing as to sensitivity and the significance of the diagnostic findings.
8. Discuss how cellular damage occurs in type II hypersensitivity.
9. Give examples of type II hypersensitivity reactions.
10. Explain the significance of a positive direct antiglobulin test.
11. Distinguish between type II and type III hypersensitivity reactions on the basis of the nature of the antigen involved and the mechanisms of cellular injury.
12. Discuss the Arthus reaction and serum sickness as examples of type III hypersensitivity reactions.
13. Relate how type IV sensitivity differs from the other three types of hypersensitivity reactions.
14. Explain the nature of the immunologic reaction in contact dermatitis and hypersensitivity pneumonitis.

## KEY TERMS

___ Anaphylaxis
___ Arthus reaction
___ Atopy
___ Cold autoagglutinins
___ Contact dermatitis
___ Delayed hypersensitivity
___ Eosinophil chemotactic factor of anaphylaxis (ECF-A)
___ Hemolytic disease of the newborn (HDN)
___ Histamine
___ Hypersensitivity
___ Hyposensitization
___ Immediate hypersensitivity
___ Isohemagglutinin
___ Neutrophil chemotactic factor
___ Passive cutaneous anaphylaxis
___ Radioallergosorbent test (RAST)
___ Radioimmunosorbent test (RIST)
___ Serum sickness
___ Warm autoimmune hemolytic anemia

# CHAPTER OUTLINE

In previous chapters, the immune response has been described as a defense mechanism by which the body rids itself of potentially harmful antigens. In some cases, however, this process can end up causing damage to the host. When this type of reaction occurs, it is termed **hypersensitivity,** which can be defined as a heightened state of immune responsiveness. Typically, it is an exaggerated response to a harmless antigen that results in injury to the tissue, disease, or even death. British immunologists P. G. H. Gell and R. R. A. Coombs devised a classification system for such reactions based on four different categories.

In type I reactions, cell-bound antibody reacts with antigen to release physiologically active substances. Type II reactions are those in which free antibody reacts with antigen associated with cell surfaces. In type III hypersensitivity, antibody reacts with soluble antigen to form complexes that precipitate in the tissues. In these latter two types, complement plays a major role in producing tissue damage. Type IV hypersensitivity differs from the other three, because sensitized T cells rather than antibody are responsible for the symptoms that develop. **Figure 13–1** gives an illustrative comparison of the four main types of hypersensitivity.

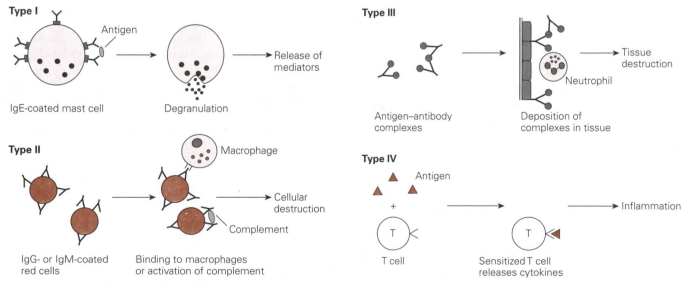

**FIGURE 13–1.** Comparison of hypersensitivity reactions for types I to IV. *(Type I)* Antigen-specific IgE is bound to mast cells. Antigen bridges adjacent antibody molecules, causing disruption of the cell membrane with release of mediators. *(Type II)* Antibody is directed against cellular antigens. Complement is activated, and target cells are destroyed. *(Type III)* Soluble antigens combine with antibody to form immune complexes. These are deposited in tissues. Complement activation and exocytosis cause tissue damage. *(Type IV)* T cells become sensitized to antigen and release lymphokines on second exposure to that antigen. A localized inflammatory reaction occurs.

Although some disease manifestations may overlap among these categories, knowledge of the general characteristics of each will help in understanding the immune processes that trigger such tissue damage. Types I through III have previously been referred to as immediate hypersensitivity, because symptoms develop within a few minutes to a few hours. Type IV hypersensitivity has been called delayed hypersensitivity, because its manifestations are not seen until 24 to 48 hours after contact with antigen. For each of the four main reaction types, the nature of the immune reactants is discussed, examples are given, and relevant testing is reviewed. Refer to **Table 13–1** for a summary of the main characteristics that distinguish each class.

## TYPE I HYPERSENSITIVITY

The distinguishing feature of type I hypersensitivity is the short time lag, usually seconds to minutes, between exposure to antigen and the onset of clinical symptoms. The key reactant present in type I, or immediate sensitivity reactions, is IgE. Antigens that trigger formation of IgE are called *atopic antigens,* or *allergens.* **Atopy** refers to an inherited tendency to respond to naturally occurring inhaled and ingested allergens with continued production of IgE.[1] The prevalence of allergic diseases has increased greatly in developed countries in the last 20 to 30 years, and it is estimated that as much as 30 percent of the U.S. population have some type of allergic symptoms.[2,3] Typically, patients who exhibit allergic or immediate hypersensitivity reactions produce a large amount of IgE in response to a small concentration of antigen. IgE levels appear to depend on the interaction of both genetic and environmental factors.

Carl Wilhelm Prausnitz and Heinz Küstner were the first researchers to show that a serum factor was responsible for type I reactions. Serum from Küstner, who was allergic to fish, was injected into Prausnitz. A later exposure to fish antigen at the same site resulted in an allergic skin reaction.[1]

This type of reaction is known as **passive cutaneous anaphylaxis.** It occurs when serum is transferred from an allergic individual to a nonallergic individual, and then the second individual is challenged with specific antigen. Although this experiment was conducted in 1921, it was not until 1967 that the serum factor responsible, namely IgE, was identified. Characteristics of IgE are described in Chapter 4.

## Triggering of Type I Reactions by IgE

IgE is primarily synthesized in the lymphoid tissue of the respiratory and gastrointestinal tracts. Normal levels are in the range of approximately 150 ng/mL.[1,4] The regulation of IgE production appears to be a function of a subset of T cells called *type 2 helper cells (Th2).*[1,5] The normal immune response to microorganisms and possible allergens is a function of type 1 helper cells (Th1), which produce interferon-gamma (IFN-γ). IFN-γ, along with interleukin-12 and interleukin-18, which are produced by macrophages, may actually suppress production of IgE type antibodies.[4] However, in people with allergies, Th2 cells respond instead and produce interleukin-3 (IL-3), interleukin-4 (IL-4), interleukin-5 (IL-5), interleukin-9 (IL-9), and interleukin-13 (IL-13).[4] See Chapter 5 for a discussion of cytokines. IL-4 and IL-13 are responsible for the final differentiation that occurs in B cells, initiating the transcription of the gene that codes for the epsilon-heavy chain of immunoglobulin molecules belonging to the IgE class.[1,4,5] IL-5 and IL-9 are involved in the development of eosinophils, while IL-4 and IL-9 promote development of mast cells. IL-4, IL-9, and IL-13 all act to stimulate overproduction of mucus, a characteristic of most allergic reactions.

This propensity to secrete cytokines that promote production of IgE is linked to a gene locus on chromosome 5 that encodes cytokines IL-3, IL-4, IL-5, IL-9, IL-13, and granulocyte-monocyte colony stimulating factor (GM-CSF).[6] All of these cytokines are key to a switch to a Th2 response. Il-4 and IL-13 activate transcription of the epsilon gene in B cells when they bind to specific receptors.[4,7]

| Table 13–1. | Comparison of Hypersensitivity Reactions | | | |
|---|---|---|---|---|
| | **TYPE I** | **TYPE II** | **TYPE III** | **TYPE IV** |
| **Immune Mediator** | IgE | IgG | IgG or IgM | T cells |
| **Antigen** | Heterologous | Autologous or heterologous | Autologous or heterologous | Autologous or heterologous |
| **Complement Involvement** | No | Yes | Yes | No |
| **Immune Mechanism** | Release of mediators from mast cells and basophils | Cytolysis due to antibody and complement | Deposits of antigen–antibody complexes | Release of cytokines |
| **Examples** | Anaphylaxis, hay fever, food allergies, asthma | Transfusion reactions, autoimmune hemolytic anemia, HDN | Serum sickness, Arthus reaction, lupus erythematosus | Contact dermatitis, tuberculin test, pneumonitis |

HDN = hemolytic disease of the newborn

Although actual antibody synthesis is regulated by the action of cytokines, the tendency to respond to specific allergens appears to be linked to inheritance of certain major histocompatibility complex (MHC) genes. Various human leukocyte antigen (HLA) class II molecules, especially HLA-DR2, DR4, and DR7, seem to be associated with a high response to individual allergens.[7] HLA-D molecules are known to play a role in antigen presentation (see Chapter 3), and thus individuals who possess particular HLA molecules are more likely to respond to certain allergens.[6]

In addition, individuals who are prone to allergies exhibit certain variations in the gene found on chromosome 11q that codes for receptors for IgE found on several types of cells.[5-7] It is thought that polymorphisms in the beta chain of these receptors are linked to atopy. These high-affinity receptors, named FCε-RI receptors, bind the fragment crystallizable (FC) region of the epsilon-heavy chain and are found on basophils and mast cells. A single cell may have as many as 200,000 such receptors.[4,6] Other cells, such as monocytes, eosinophils, Langerhans cells, and dendritic cells, also have receptors for IgE, but their concentration is low. However, Langerhans and dendritic cells internalize and process allergens from the environment and transport the allergen-MHC class II complex to local lymphoid tissue, where synthesis of IgE occurs.[4] Binding of IgE to cell membranes increases the half-life of IgE from 2 or 3 days up to at least 10 days. Once bound, IgE serves as an antigen receptor on mast cells and basophils. Cross-linking of at least two antibody molecules by antigen triggers release of mediators from these cells. When cross-linking occurs, intracellular signaling events due to multiple phosphorylation reactions cause an increase in calcium. The influx of calcium promotes synthesis of arachidonic acid from membrane lipids. It also promotes cytokine synthesis and release of preformed mediators due to degranulation.[1] **Figure 13–2** depicts this reaction.

## Role of Mast Cells and Basophils

Mast cells are the principle effector cells of immediate hypersensitivity, and they are derived from precursors in the bone marrow that migrate to specific tissue sites to mature. Although they are found throughout the body, they are most prominent in connective tissue, the skin, the upper and lower respiratory tract, and the gastrointestinal tract.[1] In most organs, mast cells tend to be concentrated around the small blood vessels, the lymphatics, the nerves, and the glandular tissue.[7] These cells contain numerous cytoplasmic granules that are enclosed by a bilayered membrane. Histamine, which comprises approximately 10 percent of the total weight of granular constituents, is found in 10 times greater supply per cell than in basophils.[6]

Mast cell populations in different sites differ in the amounts of allergic mediators that they contain and in their sensitivity to activating stimuli and cytokines. All types of cells are triggered in the same manner, however. They release a variety of cytokines and other mediators that enhance the allergic response.[1]

Basophils represent approximately 1 percent of the white blood cells in peripheral blood. They have a half-life of about 3 days. They contain histamine-rich granules and high-affinity receptors for IgE, just as in mast cells. They respond to chemotactic stimulation and tend to accumulate in the tissues during an inflammatory reaction. In the presence of IgE, the number of receptors has been found to increase, indicating a possible mechanism of upregulation during an allergic reaction.[4,6]

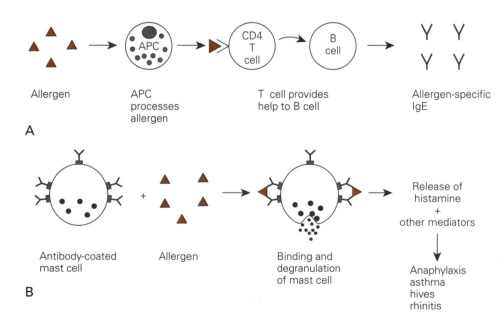

A

B

FIGURE 13–2. Type I hypersensitivity. *(A)* Sensitization. Formation of antigen-specific IgE that attaches to mast cells. *(B)* Activation. Reexposure to specific antigen with subsequent degranulation of mast cells and release of mediators. (APC = antigen-processing cell.)

## Mediators Released from Granules

### Preformed Mediators

Cross-linking of surface-bound IgE on basophils and mast cells by a specific allergen causes changes in the cell membrane that result in the release of mediators from the cytoplasmic granules. These preformed or primary mediators include histamine, heparin, eosinophil chemotactic factor of anaphylaxis (ECF-A), **neutrophil chemotactic factor,** and proteases.[4] Release of these substances is responsible for the early phase symptoms seen in allergic reactions, which occur within 30 to 60 minutes after exposure to the allergen. The effect of each of these mediators is discussed and a summary is presented in **Table 13–2.**

**Histamine,** a major component of mast cell granules, is a low-molecular-weight vasoactive amine. Its effects, which appear within 30 to 60 seconds after release, are dependent on activation of four different types of receptors found on cells in various types of tissue.[8] Activation of $H_1$ receptors results in contraction of smooth muscle in bronchioles, blood vessels, and the intestines, and generally induces proinflammatory activity.[6,8] In addition, there is increased capillary permeability, altered cardiac contractility, and increased mucous gland secretion in the upper-respiratory tract. Binding to $H_2$ receptors increases gastric acid secretion, airway mucus production, and permeability of capillaries and venules.[6] $H_3$ receptors are found on central and peripheral neural tissue. Bone marrow cells, mast cells, and peripheral blood cells such as eosinophils, neutrophils, and basophils all have $H_4$ receptors.[6,8] $H_4$ receptors appear to be involved in immune regulation, including chemotaxis of mast cells; recruitment of eosinophils, neutrophils, and basophils; and cytokine secretion.[8]

In the skin, histamine is responsible for local erythema or redness and wheal and flare formation. Contraction of the smooth muscle in the bronchioles may result in airflow obstruction. Increased vascular permeability may cause hypotension or shock. Depending on the route by which an individual is exposed to the triggering allergen, one or more of these effects may be seen.

**Eosinophil chemotactic factor of anaphylaxis (ECF-A)** is another preformed factor released from granules. This attracts eosinophils to the area and induces expression of eosinophil receptors for C3b.[7] Eosinophils have granules that contain major basic protein, eosinophil cationic protein, eosinophil peroxidase, eosinophil derived neurotoxins, histaminases, and phospholipase D.[4] All of these products are toxic to bronchial epithelial cells and to helminth parasites. Killing of parasites is thought to be the reason that IgE production evolved.

One of the proteolytic enzymes released is *tryptase*. Tryptase cleaves kininogen to generate bradykinin, which induces prolonged smooth muscle contraction and increases vascular permeability and secretory activity.[1] Complement split products are also released when C3 is converted to C3a and C3b.

### Newly Synthesized Mediators

In addition to immediate release of preformed mediators, mast cells and basophils are triggered to synthesize certain

| Table 13–2. | Mediators of Immediate Hypersensitivity | | |
|---|---|---|---|
| | **MEDIATOR** | **STRUCTURE** | **ACTIONS** |
| Preformed | Histamine | MW 111 | Smooth muscle contraction, vasodilation, increased vascular permeability |
| | ECF-A | MW 380–2000 | Chemotactic for eosinophils |
| | Neutrophil chemotactic factor | MW 600,000 | Chemotactic for neutrophils |
| | Proteases | MW 130,000 | Convert C3 to C3b, mucus production, activation of cytokines |
| Newly Synthesized | $PGD_2$ | Arachidonic acid derivative | Vasodilation, increased vascular permeability |
| | $LTB_4$ | Arachidonic acid derivative | Chemotactic for neutrophils, eosinophils |
| | $LTC_4$, $LTD_4$, $LTE_4$ | Arachidonic acid derivatives | Increased vascular permeability, bronchoconstriction, mucous secretion |
| | Platelet activating factor | MW 300–500 | Platelet aggregation |
| | Cytokines IL-1, TNF-a, IL-3, IL-4, IL-5, IL-6, IL-9, IL-13, IL-14, IL-16, GM-CSF | Small MW proteins | Increase inflammatory cells in area, and increase IgE production |

MW = molecular weight; ECF-A = eosinophil chemotactic factor of anaphylaxis; PGD = prostaglandin; LT = leukotriene

other reactants from the breakdown of phospholipids in the cell membrane. These products are responsible for a late-phase allergic reaction seen within 6 to 8 hours after exposure to antigen. Newly formed mediators include platelet-activating factor (PAF); prostaglandin (PG) $D_2$; leukotrienes (LT) $B_4$, $C_4$, $D_4$, and $E_4$); and cytokines.[1,4,5,7] Prostaglandins and leukotrienes are derived from arachidonic acid, a membrane lipid, by two separate metabolic pathways. In one pathway, the enzyme 5-lipoxygenase cleaves arachidonic acid to generate leukotrienes. The other pathway uses cyclooxygenase, which results in prostaglandin production.

$PGD_2$ is the major product of the cyclooxygenase pathway. When released by mast cells, it mimics the effects of histamine, causing bronchial constriction and vasodilation.[1,6] It is much more potent than histamine, but it is released in smaller quantities. In skin reactions, $PGD_2$ triggers wheal and flare formation. Thus, the overall effect is to enhance and potentiate the action of histamine.

Leukotrienes, resulting from the 5-lipoxygenase pathway of arachidonic acid metabolism, are also responsible for late-phase symptoms of immediate sensitivity. Leukotrienes $C_4$, $D_4$, and $E_4$ were originally collectively named the *slow-reacting substances of anaphylaxis (SRS-A)*. $LTC_4$ and $LTD_4$ are 1000 times more potent than histamine in causing increased vascular permeability, bronchoconstriction, and increased mucous secretion in small airways.[1,6] In the intestines, leukotrienes induce smooth muscle contraction. Systemically, they may produce hypotension as a result of diminished cardiac muscle contractility and lessened blood flow.

$LTB_4$ is a potent chemotactic factor for neutrophils and eosinophils. The appearance of eosinophils is especially important as a negative feedback control mechanism. Eosinophils release histaminase, which degrades histamine, and phospholipase D, which degrades PAF. Additionally, superoxides created in both eosinophils and neutrophils cause the breakdown of leukotrienes. Eosinophil products can also have a damaging effect. Eosinophil cationic protein and eosinophil-derived neurotoxin contribute to extensive tissue destruction.[1,7]

PAF is a phospholipid released by monocytes, macrophages, neutrophils, eosinophils, mast cells, and basophils. The effects of PAF include platelet aggregation, chemotaxis of eosinophils and neutrophils, increased vascular permeability, and contraction of smooth muscle in the lungs and intestines.[5]

Cytokines released from mast cells include IL-1, IL-3, IL-4, IL-5, IL-6, IL-9, IL-13, IL-14, IL-16, GM-CSF, and TNF-$\alpha$.[1,9] These cytokines alter the local microenvironment, leading to an increase in inflammatory cells such as neutrophils, eosinophils, and macrophages. IL-3 and IL-4 increase IgE production to further amplify the Th2 response.[1,6] In addition, IL-3 is a growth factor for mast cells and basophils, and IL-4 recruits T cells, basophils, eosinophils, and monocytes.[7] IL-5 also recruits eosinophils. A high concentration of TNF-$\alpha$ may contribute to the symptoms of shock seen in systemic anaphylaxis.

The newly formed mediators are responsible for a late phase reaction in 4 to 6 hours after exposure to the allergen, during which numerous cells such as eosinophils, neutrophils, Th2 cells, mast cells, basophils, and macrophages exit the circulation and infiltrate the allergen-filled tissue. They release further mediators that prolong the hyperactivity and may lead to tissue damage.[7]

## Clinical Manifestations of Immediate Hypersensitivity

Type I hypersensitivity is a widespread health problem, as it is estimated that up to 25 percent of the population suffers from some sort of allergy.[3,7] The clinical manifestations caused by release of both preformed and newly synthesized mediators from mast cells and basophils vary from a localized skin reaction to a systemic response known as anaphylaxis. Symptoms depend on such variables as route of exposure, dosage, and frequency of exposure. If an allergen is inhaled, it is most likely to cause respiratory symptoms such as asthma or rhinitis. Ingestion of an allergen may result in gastrointestinal symptoms, and injection into the bloodstream can trigger a systemic response.

Anaphylaxis is the most severe type of allergic response, because it is an acute reaction that simultaneously involves multiple organs. It may be fatal if not treated promptly. Coined by biologists Paul-Jules Portier and Charles Robert Richet in 1902, the term literally means "without protection." Anaphylactic reactions are typically triggered by glycoproteins or large polypeptides. Smaller molecules, such as penicillin, are haptens that may become immunogenic by combining with host cells or proteins. Typical agents that induce anaphylaxis include venom from bees, wasps, and hornets; drugs such as penicillin; and foods such as shellfish, peanuts, or dairy products.[1,7,10] Additionally, latex sensitivity is now a significant cause of anaphylaxis among health-care workers and in patients who have had multiple surgery procedures, such as children with spina bifida.[11,12] It is estimated that approximately 10 percent of all health-care workers have been sensitized to latex, due to the implementation of OSHA regulations requiring gloves for laboratory procedures and for working with patients.[11,12]

Clinical signs of anaphylaxis begin within minutes after antigenic challenge and may include bronchospasm and laryngeal edema, vascular congestion, skin manifestations such as urticaria (hives) and angioedema, diarrhea or vomiting, and intractable shock because of the effect on blood vessels and smooth muscle of the circulatory system. The severity of the reaction depends on the number of previous exposures to the antigen with consequent buildup of IgE on mast cells and basophils. Massive release of reactants, especially histamine, from the granules is responsible for the ensuing symptoms. Death may result from asphyxiation due to upper-airway edema and congestion, irreversible shock, or a combination of these symptoms.

Rhinitis is the most common form of atopy, or allergy. It affects about 15 to 20 percent of children in developed countries.[2] Symptoms include paroxysmal sneezing; rhinorrhea, or runny nose; nasal congestion; and itching of the nose and eyes.[13] Although the condition itself is merely annoying, complications such as sinusitis, otitis media (ear infection), eustachian tube dysfunction, and sleep disturbances may result. Pollen, mold spores, animal dander, and particulate matter from house dust mites are examples of airborne foreign particles that act directly on the mast cells in the conjunctiva and respiratory mucous membranes to trigger rhinitis.

Particles no larger than 2 to 4 μm in diameter such as pollen, dust, or fumes, may reach the lower-respiratory tract to cause asthma.[1,14] *Asthma* is derived from the Greek word for "panting" or "breathlessness." It can be defined clinically as recurrent airflow obstruction that leads to intermittent sneezing, breathlessness, and, occasionally, a cough with sputum production. The airflow obstruction is due to bronchial smooth muscle contraction, mucosal edema, and heavy mucous secretion. All of these changes lead to an increase in airway resistance, making it difficult for inspired air to leave the lungs. This trapped air creates the sense of breathlessness.

Food allergies are another example of type I immediate hypersensitivity reactions. Some of the most common food allergies involve cow's milk, peanuts, and eggs.[2,13] Symptoms limited to the gastrointestinal tract include cramping, vomiting, and diarrhea, while spread of antigen through the bloodstream may cause hives and angioedema on the skin, as well as asthma or rhinitis. Eczema, an itchy red skin rash, may be caused by food allergens or exposure to house dust mites.[13]

## Treatment of Immediate Hypersensitivity

Avoidance of known allergens is the first line of defense. This includes environmental interventions such as encasing mattresses and pillows in allergen-proof covers and not allowing pets inside the house.[14] Drugs used to treat immediate hypersensitivity vary with the severity of the reaction. Localized allergic reactions, such as hay fever, hives, or rhinitis, can be treated easily with antihistamines and decongestants. Asthma is often treated with a combination of therapeutic reagents, including antihistamines and bronchodilators, followed by inhaled corticosteroids.[13,14] Systemic reactions require the use of epinephrine to quickly reverse symptoms.

Another approach to treatment involves immunotherapy or **hyposensitization.** Very small quantities of sensitizing antigen are injected into the patient with the idea of building up IgG antibodies. Individuals with moderate to severe symptoms are given weekly doses of antigen that gradually increases in strength.[15] The blocking antibodies formed circulate in the blood and combine with antigen before it can reach IgE-coated cells. In addition, it appears that T cell–mediated suppression occurs due to the action of T regulatory cells, thus decreasing synthesis of IgE.[1]

A new approach involves use of an anti-IgE monoclonal antibody. This antibody combines with IgE at the same site

that IgE would normally use to bind to receptors on mast cells. Blocking of this site does not allow IgE to bind to mast cells, thus helping to alleviate allergic symptoms.[16–18] Omalizumab was the first such antibody to be approved for therapeutic use in the United States.[19] In addition to blocking the release of mediators from mast cells, down-regulation of FcεRI receptors occurs, thus curtailing the response.[20] Anti-IgE therapy has been successful in treating moderate to severe asthma and shows much promise for the future.[6,16,18,20]

## Testing for Immediate Hypersensitivity

### In Vivo Skin Tests

Testing for allergies or immediate hypersensitivity can be categorized as in vivo or in vitro methods. In vivo methods involve direct skin testing, which is the least expensive and most specific type of testing.[21] Cutaneous and intradermal tests are the two skin tests most often used. In cutaneous testing, or a prick test, a small drop of material is injected into the skin at a single point. After 15 minutes, the spot is examined, and the reaction is recorded. A positive reaction is formation of a wheal that is 3 mm greater in diameter than the negative control.[21] A negative saline control and a positive control of histamine should always be included.[10,21] Cutaneous testing uses a thousandfold higher concentration than intradermal tests, but a lesser amount of antigen is used, thus decreasing the chances of an anaphylactic response.[6,21]

Intradermal tests use a greater amount of antigen and are more sensitive than cutaneous testing. However, they are usually performed only if prick tests are negative and allergy is still suspected. An extremity, such as an arm, to which a tourniquet can be applied, is used to stop an unexpected systemic reaction. A 1 mL tuberculin syringe is used to administer 0.01 to 0.05 mL of test solution between layers of the skin. The test allergen is diluted 100 to 1000 times more than the solution used for cutaneous testing. After 15 to 20 minutes, the site is inspected for erythema and wheal formation. A wheal 3 mm greater than the negative control is considered a positive test.[6]

Skin testing is relatively simple and inexpensive, and it lends itself to screening for a number of allergens. However, antihistamines must be stopped 24 to 72 hours before testing, and there is the danger that a systemic reaction can be triggered. In addition, skin testing is not recommended for children under 3 years of age.

### In Vitro Tests: Total IgE

#### Testing Principles

In vitro tests involve measurement of either total IgE or antigen-specific IgE. These are less sensitive than skin testing but usually are less traumatic to the patient. Total IgE testing has become more important as a screening test before a patient is referred to an allergy specialist, because it is a good indicator of the likelihood of allergic disease.[6] The first test developed for the measurement of total IgE was the competitive **radioimmunosorbent test (RIST).** The RIST used radiolabeled IgE to compete with patient IgE for binding sites on a solid phase coated with anti-IgE. RIST has largely been replaced by noncompetitive solid-phase immunoassays due to the expense and difficulty of working with radioactivity.[6,19]

In noncompetitive solid-phase immunoassay, antihuman IgE is bound to a solid phase such as cellulose, a paper disk, or a microtiter well. Patient serum is added and allowed to react, and then a labeled anti-IgE is added to detect the bound patient IgE. This label is an enzyme or a fluorescent tag. The second anti-IgE antibody recognizes a different epitope than that recognized by the first antibody. The resulting "sandwich" of solid-phase anti-IgE, serum IgE, and labeled anti-IgE is washed, and the label is measured. In this case, the amount of label detected is directly proportional to the IgE content of the serum **(Fig. 13–3)**. Although the second incubation doubles the time of the assay, the sensitivity of this type of testing is excellent, and the results are minimally affected by the presence of nonspecific serum factors.[19]

Total serum IgE testing is used clinically to aid in diagnosis of allergic rhinitis, asthma, or other allergic conditions that may be indicated by patient symptoms.[19] It serves as a screening test to determine if more specific allergy testing is indicated. It is also important in diagnosis of parasitic infections; bronchopulmonary aspergillosis; and hyper-IgE syndrome, a condition in which excessive amounts of IgE are produced.[19]

## Interpretation of Total IgE Results

Total IgE values are reported in kilo international units (IU) per liter. One IU is equal to a concentration of 2.4 ng of protein per milliliter. IgE concentration varies with the individual's age, sex, and smoking history and his or her family history of allergy. Levels also vary as a function of exposure to allergens. In infants, normal serum levels of IgE are less than 2 k IU/L; increases up to 10 kIU/L are indicative of allergic disease.[6,14] After the age of 14 years, IgE levels in the range of 400 kIU/L are considered to be abnormally elevated.[14] A cutoff point of 100 IU, however, is frequently used in testing to identify individuals with allergic tendencies.[6] Although two-thirds of adults who have allergic

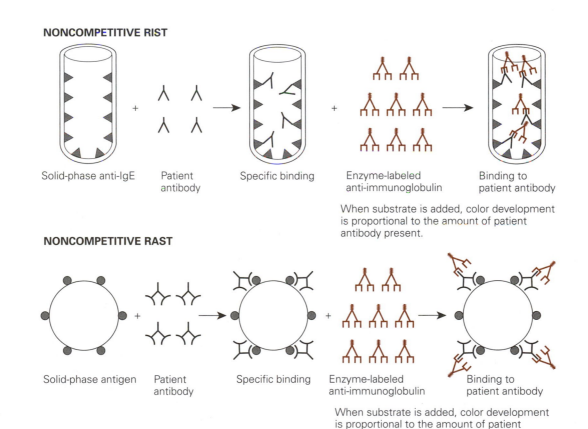

**NONCOMPETITIVE RIST**

Solid-phase anti-IgE | Patient antibody | Specific binding | Enzyme-labeled anti-immunoglobulin | Binding to patient antibody

When substrate is added, color development is proportional to the amount of patient antibody present.

**NONCOMPETITIVE RAST**

Solid-phase antigen | Patient antibody | Specific binding | Enzyme-labeled anti-immunoglobulin | Binding to patient antibody

When substrate is added, color development is proportional to the amount of patient antibody present.

**FIGURE 13–3.** Comparison of RIST and RAST. RIST measures total IgE by capturing the antibody with solid-phase anti-IgE. A second anti-IgE immunoglobulin with an enzyme label is used to produce a visible reaction. RAST measures antigen-specific IgE by using solid-phase antigen to capture patient antibody. Then a second antibody, enzyme-labeled anti-IgE immunoglobulin, is added. This combines with any bound IgE to produce a visible reaction in the presence of substrate.

symptoms would fall into this category, the other one-third might be incorrectly diagnosed. Additionally, IgE levels may be elevated due to other conditions, such as helminth infections, Wiskott-Aldrich syndrome, DiGeorge syndrome, and hyper-IgE syndrome.[19] Thus, total IgE levels must be interpreted in light of the patient's personal and family history, and they should not be regarded as an absolute predictor of allergy. Although measurement of total IgE levels can be a useful screening tool, allergen-specific IgE is more helpful in actual treatment of the individual.

### Antigen-Specific IgE Testing

#### Testing Principles

The original commercial testing method for determining specific IgE was known as the **radioallergosorbent test (RAST),** introduced in 1966. Principles of the test remain the same, but newer testing methods involve the use of enzyme or fluorescent labels rather than radioactivity. Allergen-specific IgE testing is safer to perform than skin testing and is easier on some patients, especially children or apprehensive adults, and the sensitivity now approaches that of skin testing.[15] It is especially useful in detecting allergies to common triggers such as ragweed, trees, grasses, molds, animal dander, milk, and egg albumin.

Allergen-specific IgE testing is a noncompetitive solid-phase immunoassay in which the solid phase is coated with specific allergen and reacted with patient serum. A carbohydrate solid phase, such as paper cellulose disks, agarose beads, or microcrystalline cellulose particles, seems to work best. After washing to remove unbound antibody, a labeled anti-IgE is added. Traditional RAST used a radioactive label, while newer tests use an enzyme or fluorometric label. A second incubation occurs, and then, after a washing step, the amount of label in the sample is measured. The amount of label detected is directly proportional to the amount of specific IgE in the patient's serum. Controls and standards are run in parallel with patient serum. Figure 13–3 shows a comparison of the total and allergen-specific IgE testing.

#### Interpretation of Allergen-Specific IgE Results

Newer commercially available testing systems such as Pharmacia and Upjohn's ImmunoCAP and Diagnostic Products Corporation IMMULITE have greatly increased the sensitivity of in vitro allergy testing.[22,23] IgE can now be measured quantitatively, and concentrations as low as 0.35 KIU/L can be detected.[6] It is important to run positive and negative controls to aid in the interpretation of test results. A negative test may be used to confirm the absence of a specific atopic disease, and this has a higher negative predictive value than total IgE testing.[19] However, in a positive test, the quantity of antibody measured does not necessarily correlate with the severity of disease.[19] This type of testing is very useful to determine common food allergies and sensitivity to the venom of stinging insects such as honey bees, yellow jackets, wasps, and hornets, but it is more difficult to determine inhalant allergies.[6] The cutoff for a positive test

also varies with the particular allergen.[24] Thus, results must be interpreted in conjunction with patient symptoms.

#### Microarray Testing

The newest generation of allergy testing involves the use of microarrays. This miniaturization of diagnostic testing allows for multiallergen diagnosis with a low sample volume and a high throughput capacity.[25]

Microarrays can be attached to a standard microscope slide, using only a few picograms of each allergen to be tested.[26] In this manner, at least 5000 allergens can be tested for at once, using a minimal amount of serum, approximately 20µL.[3] The principle is the same as noncompetitive immunoassays, in that patient serum with possible IgE is allowed to react with the microarray of allergens, and then an anti-IgE with a fluorescent tag is added. After careful washing, slides are read automatically. The presence of color indicates a positive test for that allergen.

Recombinant DNA technology has greatly contributed to the development of successful microarrays. It is now possible to characterize and create allergens at the molecular level, which enhances specificity. Up to this point, allergy testing involved use of extracts of allergens, which may not have been completely pure. Identification of DNA coding for specific allergens has allowed creation of purified antigens for both testing and immunotherapy purposes.[26] This same testing system can be used to look for increases in IgG to indicate the efficacy of immunotherapy treatment.[3] Use of microarrays with recombinant allergens will significantly enhance the value of specific IgE testing.

## TYPE II HYPERSENSITIVITY

The reactants responsible for type II hypersensitivity, or cytotoxic hypersensitivity, are IgG and IgM. They are triggered by antigens found on cell surfaces. These antigens may be altered self-antigens or heteroantigens. Antibody coats cellular surfaces and promotes phagocytosis by both opsonization and activation of the complement cascade. Macrophages, neutrophils, and eosinophils have Fc receptors that bind to the Fc region of antibody on target cells, thus enhancing phagocytosis. Natural killer (NK) cells also have Fc receptors, and if these link to cellular antigens, cytotoxicity results. If the complement cascade is activated, complement can trigger cellular destruction in two ways: (1) by coating cells with C3b, thus facilitating phagocytosis through interaction with specific receptors on phagocytic cells, or (2) by complement-generated lysis if the cascade goes to completion. Hence, complement plays a central role in the cellular damage that typifies type II reactions.

### Transfusion Reactions

Transfusion reactions are examples of cellular destruction that result from antibody combining with heteroantigens. There are more than 29 different blood group systems, with a total of more than 700 different red cell antigens.[27,28] Some antigens are stronger than others and are more likely to stimulate antibody production. Major groups involved in transfusion reactions include the ABO, Rh, Kell, Duffy, and Kidd systems.[27,29] Certain antibodies are produced naturally with no prior exposure to red blood cells, while other antibodies are produced only after contact with cells carrying that antigen.

The ABO blood group is of primary importance in considering transfusions. Anti-A and anti-B antibodies are naturally occurring antibodies, or **isohemagglutinins,** probably triggered by contact with identical antigenic determinants on microorganisms. Individuals do not form such antibodies to their own red blood cells. Thus, a person who has type A blood has anti-B in the serum, and a person with type B blood has anti-A antibodies. An individual with type O blood has both anti-A and anti-B in the serum, because O cells have neither of these two antigens. The antibody formed typically belongs to the IgM class, but IgG may also be made.

If a patient is given blood for which antibodies are already present, a transfusion reaction occurs. This can range from acute massive intravascular hemolysis to an undetected decrease in red blood cell survival. The extent of the reaction depends on the following factors: (1) the temperature at which the antibody is most active, (2) the plasma concentration of the antibody, (3) the particular immunoglobulin class, (4) the extent of complement activation, (5) the density of the antigen on the red blood cell, and (6) the number of red blood cells transfused.[30] It is most important to detect antibodies that react at 37°C. If a reaction occurs only below 30°C, it can be disregarded, because such antigen–antibody complexes tend to dissociate at 37°C.

Acute hemolytic transfusion reactions may occur within minutes or hours after receipt of incompatible blood. In this case, the individual has been exposed to the antigen before and has preformed antibodies to it. Reactions that begin immediately are most often associated with ABO blood group incompatibilities, and antibodies are of the IgM class.[1,30] As soon as cells bearing that antigen are introduced into the patient, intravascular hemolysis occurs because of complement activation, and it results in the release of hemoglobin and vasoactive and procoagulant substances into the plasma. This may induce disseminated intravascular coagulation (DIC), vascular collapse, and renal failure. Symptoms in the patient may include fever, chills, nausea, lower back pain, tachycardia, shock, and hemoglobin in the urine.[29,30]

Delayed hemolytic reactions occur within the first 2 weeks following a transfusion and are caused by a secondary response to the antigen to which the patient has previously been exposed. The type of antibody responsible is IgG, which was initially present in such low titer that it was not detectable with an antibody screen. Antigens most involved in delayed reactions include those in the Rh, Kell, Duffy, and Kidd blood groups.[1,31] Rh, Kell, and Duffy antigens may also be involved in immediate transfusion reactions. In a delayed reaction, antibody-coated red blood

cells are removed extravascularly in the spleen or in the liver, and the patient may experience a mild fever, low hemoglobin, mild jaundice, and anemia. Intravascular hemolysis does not take place to any great extent, because IgG is not as efficient as IgM in activating complement. (See Chapter 4 for further details.)

## Hemolytic Disease of the Newborn

**Hemolytic disease of the newborn (HDN)** appears in infants whose mothers have been exposed to blood-group antigens on the baby's cells that differ from their own. The mother makes IgG antibodies in response, and these cross the placenta to destroy fetal red cells. Severe HDN is called *erythroblastosis fetalis.* The most common antigen involved in severe reactions is the D antigen, a member of the Rh blood group. HDN due to ABO incompatibility is actually more common, but the disease is milder because the majority of antibodies formed are IgM, which cannot cross the placenta.[32] Other antibodies associated with HDN include anti-c, anti-C, anti-E, anti-e, and less commonly those associated with the Kell, Duffy, and Kidd blood groups.[33]

Exposure usually occurs during the birth process, where fetal cells leak into the mother's circulation. Typically the first child is unaffected, but the second and later children have an increased risk of the disease due to an anamnestic response. The extent of the first fetal-maternal bleed influences whether antibodies will be produced. If enough of the baby's red cells get into the mother's circulation, memory B cells develop. These become activated upon re-exposure to the same red cell antigen, and IgG is then produced. This crosses the placenta and attaches to the fetal red blood cells in a subsequent pregnancy.

Depending on the degree of antibody production in the mother, the fetus may be aborted, stillborn, or born with evidence of hemolytic disease as indicated by jaundice. As red blood cells are lysed and free hemoglobin released, this is converted to bilirubin, which builds up in the plasma. There is too much of it to be conjugated in the liver, so it accumulates in the tissues. Bilirubin levels above 20 mg/dL are associated with deposition in tissue such as the brain and result in a condition known as kernicterus. Treatment for severe HDN involves an exchange transfusion to replace antibody-coated red cells. If serum antibody titrations during the pregnancy indicate a high level of circulating antibody, intrauterine transfusions can be performed.[1,32]

To prevent the consequences of HDN, all women should be screened at the onset of pregnancy. If they are Rh-negative, they should be tested for the presence of anti-D antibodies on a monthly basis. In current practice, anti-D immune globulin, called Rhogam, is administered prophylactically at 28 weeks of gestation and within 72 hours following delivery.[32,34] It is assumed that the immune globulin inhibits production of antibody by combining with and destroying the D+ red blood cells, thus preventing them from being antigenic **(Fig. 13–4)**. This practice has

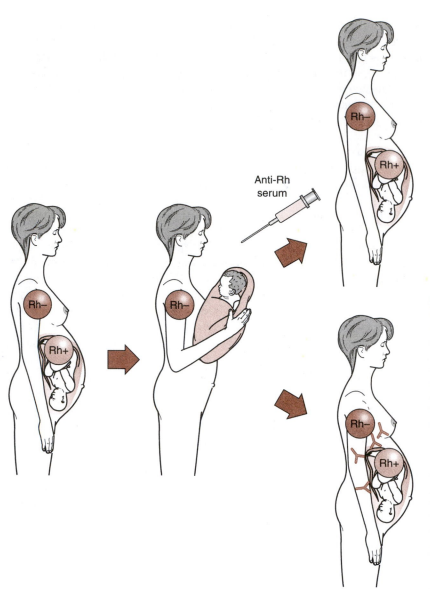

Anti-Rh
serum

**FIGURE 13-4.** Passive immunization to prevent hemolytic disease of the newborn. An Rh-negative mother is exposed to Rh antigens during pregnancy with an Rh-positive fetus. If passively immunized with anti-Rh sera at 7 months and on delivery, the maternal anti-Rh immune response is suppressed. A subsequent pregnancy (upper right) is uncomplicated by HDN. If passive immunization is not practiced, the mother may develop anti-Rh antibodies, and a second Rh-positive fetus is likely to exhibit destruction of red blood cells characteristic of HDN. *(From Barrett, JT. Textbook of Immunology, ed. 5. Mosby, St. Louis, 1988 p. 339, with permission.)*

dramatically reduced the number of women who form anti-D antibodies, now affecting a little over 1 percent.[35]

## Autoimmune Hemolytic Anemia

Autoimmune hemolytic anemia is an example of a type II hypersensitivity reaction directed against self-antigens, because individuals with this disease form antibodies to their own red blood cells. Symptoms include malaise, lightheadedness, weakness, and possibly mild jaundice. Such antibodies can be categorized into two groups: warm reactive antibodies, which react at 37°C, and cold reactive antibodies, which react only below 30°C. Autoimmune hemolytic anemia occurs in approximately 1 in 80,000 individuals.[32]

**Warm autoimmune hemolytic anemia,** accounting for more than 70 percent of autoimmune anemias, is characterized by formation of IgG antibody, which reacts most strongly at 37°C.[32] Some of these antibodies may be primary with no other disease association, or they may be secondary to another disease process. Associated diseases may include some of the following: viral or respiratory infections, such as infectious mononucleosis, cytomegalovirus, or chronic active hepatitis, or immunoproliferative diseases such as chronic lymphocytic leukemia and lymphomas.[32,36] In addition, certain drugs can be adsorbed onto red blood cells and are capable of stimulating antibody production. Examples include acetaminophen, penicillins, cephalosporins, rifampin, sulfonamides, and methyldopa.[1,37,38] Often, however, the underlying cause of antibody production is unknown, so this is referred to as *idiopathic autoimmune hemolytic anemia.*

Typically, the patient exhibits symptoms of anemia because of clearance of antibody-coated red blood cells by the liver and spleen. Hemolysis is primarily extravascular, because IgG is not as efficient as IgM in activating complement, but intravascular hemolysis can also occur if complement does become activated. Patients with warm autoimmune hemolytic anemia are usually treated with corticosteroids or splenectomy in more serious cases.[37] A newer treatment with anti-CD 20 (rituximab or alemtuzumab) is now available for cases that are refractory to corticosteroids.[37,39] This antibody attaches to B cells, causing down-regulation of antibody production and other effector cell activity.

**Cold autoagglutinins**, a less frequent cause of immune hemolytic anemias, typically are found in persons in their fifties and sixties.[32] These are thought to be triggered by antigens on microorganisms, because antibodies have been known to occur following *Mycoplasma* pneumonia and infectious mononucleosis.[37] Cold autoagglutinins have also been seen in such diseases as chronic lymphocytic leukemia, non-Hodgkin's lymphoma, myelodysplastic syndrome, or connective tissue diseases such as systemic lupus erythematosus.[32] In children, such antibodies have been associated with virus and respiratory infections.

These cold-reacting antibodies belong to the IgM class, and most are specific for the Ii blood groups on red cells.[31,37] These antibodies usually don't cause clinical symptoms. Reactions are seen only if the individual is exposed to the cold and the temperature in the peripheral circulation falls below 30°C. Peripheral necrosis may result. Although complement activation begins in the cold, it can proceed at body temperature. If the entire complement sequence is activated, intravascular hemolysis may occur.[32,37] If red blood cells become coated with C3b, this helps macrophages to bind, and these cells are rapidly cleared in the liver, further decreasing the number of circulating red blood cells. A simple treatment is to keep the patient warm, especially the hands and feet, to prevent complement activation.

## Type II Reactions Involving Tissue Antigens

All the reactions that have been discussed so far deal with individual cells that are destroyed when a specific antigen–antibody combination takes place. Some type II reactions involve destruction of tissues because of combination with antibody. Organ-specific autoimmune diseases in which antibody is directed against a particular tissue are in this category. Goodpasture's syndrome is an example of such a disease (see Chapter 14 for details). The antibody produced during the course of this disease reacts with basement membrane protein. Usually the glomeruli in the kidney and pulmonary alveolar membranes are affected.[1] Antibody binds to glomerular and alveolar capillaries, triggering the complement cascade, which provokes inflammation. An evenly bound linear deposition of IgG in glomerular basement membrane, as detected by fluorescent-labeled anti-IgG, is indicative of Goodpasture's syndrome. Treatment usually involves the use of corticosteroids or other drugs to suppress the immune response.

Other examples of reactions to tissue antigens include some of the organ-specific autoimmune diseases such as Hashimoto's disease, myasthenia gravis, and insulin-dependent diabetes mellitus. Immunologic manifestations and detection of these diseases are presented in Chapter 14.

## Testing for Type II Hypersensitivity

As discussed in Chapter 9, Coombs's discovery of the antiglobulin test in 1945 made possible the detection of antibody or complement on red blood cells. Direct antiglobulin testing (DAT) is performed to detect transfusion reactions, hemolytic disease of the newborn, and autoimmune hemolytic anemia. (Refer to the exercise at the end of the chapter for details.) Polyspecific antihuman globulin is a mixture of antibodies to IgG and complement components such as C3b and C3d, and it is used for initial testing. If the test is positive, then it should be repeated using monospecific anti-IgG, anti-C3b, and anti-C3d to determine which of these is present.[31] If an autoimmune hemolytic anemia is caused by IgM antibody, only the test for complement components would be positive.

The indirect Coombs' test is used in the crossmatching of blood to prevent a transfusion reaction. It is used either to determine the presence of a particular antibody in a patient or to type patient red blood cells for specific blood group antigens. In vitro binding of antibody to red cells, rather than in vivo binding, is detected by this method. This is a two-step process, in which red blood cells and antibody are allowed to combine at 37°C, and then the cells are carefully washed to remove any unbound antibody. Antihuman globulin is added to cause a visible reaction if antibody has been specifically bound. Any negative tests are confirmed by quality-control cells, which are coated with antibody. Refer to Chapter 9 for additional details on indirect antiglobulin testing.

## TYPE III HYPERSENSITIVITY

Type III hypersensitivity reactions are similar to type II reactions in that IgG or IgM is involved and destruction is complement mediated. However, in the case of type III diseases, the antigen is soluble. When soluble antigen combines with antibody, complexes are formed that precipitate out of the serum. Normally such complexes are cleared by phagocytic cells, but if the immune system is overwhelmed, these complexes deposit in the tissues. There they bind complement, causing damage to the particular tissue. Deposition of antigen–antibody complexes is influenced by the relative concentration of both components. If a large excess of antigen is present, sites on antibody molecules become filled before cross-links can be formed. In antibody excess, a lattice cannot be formed because of the relative scarcity of antigenic determinant sites. The small complexes that result in either of the preceding cases remain suspended or may pass directly into the urine. Precipitating complexes, on the other hand, occur in mild antigen excess, and these are the ones most likely to deposit in the tissues. Sites in which this typically occurs include the glomerular basement membrane, vascular endothelium, joint linings, and pulmonary alveolar membranes.[1]

Complement binds to these complexes in the tissues, causing the release of mediators that increase vasodilation and vasopermeability, attract macrophages and neutrophils, and enhance binding of phagocytic cells by means of C3b deposited in the tissues. If the target cells are large and cannot be engulfed for phagocytosis to take place, granule and lysosome contents are released by a process known as *exocytosis.* This results in the damage to host tissue that is typified by type III reactions. Long-term changes include loss of tissue elements that cannot regenerate and accumulation of scar tissue.

## Arthus Reaction

The classic example of a localized type III reaction is the **Arthus reaction,** demonstrated by Maurice Arthus in 1903. Using rabbits that had been immunized to produce an abundance of circulating antibodies, Arthus showed that when these rabbits were challenged with an intradermal injection of the antigen, a localized inflammatory reaction resulted. This reaction, characterized by erythema and edema, peaks within 3 to 8 hours and is followed by a hemorrhagic necrotic lesion that may ulcerate.[1] The inflammatory response is caused by antigen–antibody combination and subsequent formation of immune complexes that deposit in small dermal blood vessels. Complement is fixed, attracting neutrophils and causing aggregation of platelets. Neutrophils release toxic products such as oxygen-containing free radicals and proteolytic enzymes. Activation of complement is essential for the Arthus reaction, because the C3a and C5a generated activate mast cells to release permeability factors; consequently, immune complexes localize along the endothelial cell basement membrane. The Arthus reaction is rare in humans (**Fig. 13–5**).

## Serum Sickness

Serum sickness is a generalized type III reaction that is seen in humans, although not as frequently as it used to be. **Serum sickness** results from passive immunization with animal serum, usually horse or bovine, used to treat such infections as diphtheria, tetanus, and gangrene. Vaccines and bee stings may also trigger this type of reaction.[1] Generalized symptoms appear in 7 to 21 days after injection of the animal serum and include headache, fever, nausea, vomiting, joint pain, rashes, and lymphadenopathy. Recovery takes between 7 and 30 days.

In this disease, the sensitizing and the shocking dose of antigen are one and the same, because antibodies develop while antigen is still present. High levels of antibody form immune complexes that deposit in the tissues. Usually this is a benign and self-limiting disease, but previous exposure to animal serum can cause cardiovascular collapse on reexposure. These symptoms have occurred with monoclonal

THE ARTHUS PHENOMENOM

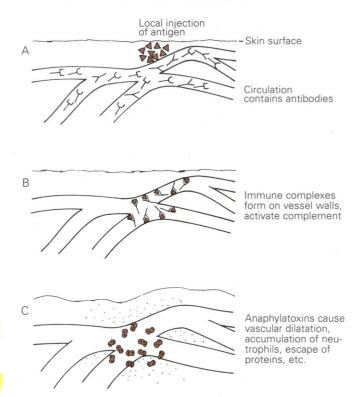

**FIGURE 13–5.** The Arthus phenomenon. *(A)* Antigen is injected into the skin of an individual who has circulating antibody of that specificity. *(B)* Immune complexes are formed and deposit on the walls of blood vessels, activating complement. *(C)* Complement fragments cause dilation and increased permeability of blood vessels, edema, and accumulation of neutrophils. *(From Widmann, FK. An Introduction to Clinical Immunology. FA Davis, Philadelphia, 1989, p. 228, with permission.)*

antibody treatment using mouse antibodies to human cells. Now, however, monoclonal antibodies are genetically engineered human antibodies, and such reactions do not occur.

## Autoimmune Diseases

Type III hypersensitivity reactions can be triggered by either autologous or heterologous antigens. Several of the autoimmune diseases fall into this category. Systemic lupus erythematosus (SLE) and rheumatoid arthritis are two such examples. In SLE, antibodies are directed against constituents such as DNA and nucleohistones, which are found in most cells of the body. Immune complex deposition involves multiple organs, but the main damage occurs to the glomerular basement membrane in the kidney.

In rheumatoid arthritis, an antibody called *rheumatoid factor* is directed against IgG. Immune complex deposition occurs in the membranes of inflamed joints. Complement enhances tissue destruction in both diseases. See Chapter 14 for a more detailed discussion of these two conditions.

## Testing for Type III Hypersensitivity

In specific diseases such as SLE and rheumatoid arthritis, the presence of antibody can be detected by agglutination reactions using antigen-coated carrier particles, including red blood cells or latex particles, or enzyme immunoassays. Fluorescent staining of tissue sections has also been used to determine deposition of immune complexes in the tissues. The staining pattern seen, and the particular tissue affected, helps to identify the disease and determine its severity.

A more general method of determining immune complex diseases is by measuring complement levels. Decreased levels of individual components or decreased functioning of the pathway may be indicative of antigen–antibody combination. The results must be interpreted with regard to other clinical findings, however. Refer to Chapter 6 for a discussion of complement testing.

## TYPE IV HYPERSENSITIVITY

Type IV, or delayed, hypersensitivity was first described in 1890 by Robert Koch, who observed that individuals infected with *Mycobacterium tuberculosis* (Mtb) developed a localized inflammatory response when injected intradermally with a filtrate from the organism.[1] Type IV hypersensitivity differs from the other three types of hypersensitivity in that sensitized T cells, usually a subpopulation of Th1 cells, play the major role in its manifestations. Antibody and complement are not directly involved. There is an initial sensitization phase of 1 to 2 weeks that takes place after the first contact with antigen. Then, upon subsequent exposure to the antigen, symptoms typically take several hours to develop and reach a peak 48 to 72 hours after exposure to antigen.[40] The reaction cannot be transferred from one animal to another by means of serum, but only through transfer of T lymphocytes. Langerhans cells in the skin and macrophages in the tissue capture and present antigen to T helper cells of the Th1 subclass. Th1 cells are activated and release cytokines, including IL-3, interferon gamma (IFN-γ., tumor necrosis factor-beta (TNF-β), and tumor necrosis factor-alpha (TNF-α), that recruit macrophages and neutrophils, produce edema, promote fibrin deposition, and generally enhance an inflammatory response.[1,40] Cytotoxic T cells are also recruited, and they bind with antigen-coated target cells to cause tissue destruction. Allergic skin reactions to bacteria, viruses, fungi, and environmental antigens such as poison ivy typify this type of hypersensitivity.

## Contact Dermatitis

**Contact dermatitis** is a form of delayed hypersensitivity that accounts for a significant number of all occupationally acquired illnesses. It is estimated that 15 to 20 percent of the Western-world population is allergic to one or more chemicals in the environment.[41,42] Reactions are usually due to low-molecular-weight compounds that touch the skin.

The most common causes include poison ivy, poison oak, and poison sumac, all of which give off urushiol in the plant sap and on the leaves. Allergic dermatitis due to contact with these three plants affects between 10 and 50 million Americans every year.[43] Other common compounds that produce allergic skin manifestations include nickel; rubber; formaldehyde; hair dyes and fabric finishes; cosmetics; and medications applied to the skin, such as topical anesthetics, antiseptics, and antibiotics.[41,44] In addition, latex allergy has been reported to affect between 3.8 and 17 percent of all health-care workers in the United States.[12] Most of these substances probably function as haptens that bind to glycoproteins on skin cells. The Langerhans cell, a skin macrophage, functions as the antigen-presenting cell at the site of antigen contact.[42] It appears that Langerhans cells may migrate to regional lymph nodes and generate sensitized Th1 cells there. This sensitization process takes several days, but once it occurs, its effects last for years.[1]

After repeat exposure to the antigen, cytokine production causes macrophages to accumulate. A skin eruption characterized by erythema, swelling, and the formation of papules appears anywhere from 6 hours to several days after the exposure. The papules may become vesicular, with blistering, peeling, and weeping. There is usually itching at the site **(Fig. 13–6)**. The dermatitis is first limited to skin sites exposed to the antigen, but then it spreads out to adjoining areas. The duration of the reaction depends upon the degree of sensitization and the concentration of antigen absorbed. Dermatitis can last for 3 to 4 weeks after the antigen has been removed.[42]

Simple redness may fade of its own accord within several days. If the area is small and localized, a topical steroid may be used for treatment. Otherwise, systemic corticosteroids may be administered. The patient also needs to avoid contact with the offending allergen.

## Hypersensitivity Pneumonitis

Recent evidence shows that hypersensitivity pneumonitis is mediated predominantly by sensitized T lymphocytes that

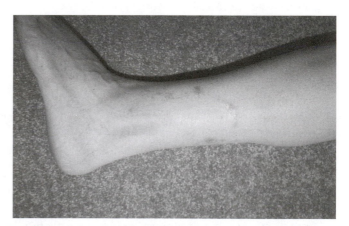

**FIGURE 13–6.** Contact hypersensitivity. Formation of papules after exposure to poison ivy.

respond to inhaled allergens. IgG and IgM antibodies are formed, but these are thought to play only a minor part. This is an allergic disease of the lung parenchyma, characterized by inflammation of the alveoli and interstitial spaces. It is caused by chronic inhalation of a wide variety of antigens, and it is most often seen in men between the ages of 30 and 50 years.[45] Depending on the occupation and the particular antigen, the disease goes by several names, including farmer's lung, pigeon breeder's disease, and humidifier lung disease. The reaction is most likely due to microorganisms, especially bacterial and fungal spores, that individuals are exposed to from working with moldy hay, pigeon droppings, compost, moldy tobacco, infested flour, and moldy cheese, to name just a few examples. Symptoms include a dry cough, shortness of breath, fever, chills, weight loss, and general malaise, which may begin within 4 to 8 hours after exposure to a high dose of the offending allergen.[7,45] Alveolar macrophages and lymphocytes trigger a chronic condition characterized by interstitial fibrosis with alveolar inflammation. Systemic corticosteroid therapy is used for treatment.

## Tuberculin–Type Hypersensitivity

Testing for exposure to tuberculosis is a classic example of a delayed hypersensitivity reaction. This is based on the principle that soluble antigens from *Mycobacterium tuberculosis* induce a reaction in people who have or have had tuberculosis. When challenged with antigen intradermally, previously sensitized individuals develop an area of erythema and induration at the injection site. This is the result of infiltration of T lymphocytes and macrophages into the area. The blood vessels become lined with mononuclear cells, and the reaction reaches a peak by 72 hours after exposure.

The tuberculin skin test uses a *Mycobacterium tuberculosis* antigen prepared by making a purified filtrate from the cell wall of the organism. This purified protein derivative (PPD) is injected under the skin, and the reaction is read at 48 to 72 hours. A positive test indicates that the individual has previously been exposed to *Mycobacterium tuberculosis* or a related organism, but it does not necessarily mean there is a presently active case.

## Testing for Delayed Hypersensitivity

The patch test is considered the gold standard in testing for contact dermatitis.[42,44] This must be done when the patient is free of symptoms or when he or she at least has a clear test site. A nonabsorbent adhesive patch containing the suspected allergen is applied on the patient's back, and the skin is checked for a reaction over the next 48 hours. Redness with papules or tiny blisters is considered a positive test. Final evaluation is conducted at 96 to 120 hours. All readings should be done by a skilled evaluator. False negatives can result from inadequate contact with the skin.

Another type of skin test for delayed hypersensitivity, the Mantoux method, is performed in much the same manner as testing for the presence of IgE. Typically, 0.1 mL of the antigen is injected intradermally, using a syringe and a fine needle.[7,46] The test site is read at 48 and 72 hours for the presence of induration. An induration of 5 mm or more is considered a positive test.[46] Antigens typically used for testing are *Candida albicans*, tetanus toxoid, tuberculin, and fungal antigens such as trichophyton and histoplasmin.[46]

## SUMMARY

Hypersensitivity reactions are exaggerated reactions to antigens that are typically not harmful. Usually there is destruction of host tissue in the process of attempting to destroy the antigen. Gell and Coombs devised a system of classification for such reactions based on immune mediators and the nature of the triggering antigen. Type I hypersensitivity, or immediate hypersensitivity, is manifested within minutes of exposure to antigen. The principle mediator is IgE, which does not remain free in the serum but binds to mast cells and basophils. When cell-bound antibody binds antigen, the resulting degranulation of the effector cells releases mediators that enhance the inflammatory response. Preformed mediators that are released include histamine, eosinophil chemotactic factor of anaphylaxis, neutrophil chemotactic factor, and proteolytic enzymes such as tryptase. Together, these factors are responsible for contraction of smooth muscle in the bronchioles, blood vessels, and intestines; increased capillary permeability; increased concentration of eosinophils and neutrophils in the area; and decreased coagulability of blood. Newly synthesized mediators, such as prostaglandins, leukotrienes, and PAF, potentiate the effects of histamine and other preformed mediators.

Clinical manifestations of immediate hypersensitivity include localized wheal and flare skin reactions; rhinitis; and systemic anaphylactic responses, which can be life-threatening. Tests to determine the potential for incurring such reactions include both in vitro and in vivo methods. The noncompetitive RIST measures total IgE by using radiolabeled anti-IgE that binds to patient's IgE on solid phase. RAST is a noncompetitive or capture method to determine antibody to specific allergens. In vivo skin tests such as the prick or intradermal tests are done by exposing the patient directly to a very small amount of allergen injected under the skin. A positive test produces a wheal and flare reaction.

The reactants responsible for type II hypersensitivity are IgG and IgM. They react with antigens located on cellular surfaces and trigger activation of the complement cascade. Target cells are damaged or destroyed by the opsonizing effect of antibody or complement components or by complement-generated lysis if the cascade goes to completion. Examples of type II reactions due to exogenous antigens include autoimmune hemolytic anemia, transfusion reactions, and HDN.

The DAT is used to screen for transfusion reactions, autoimmune hemolytic anemia, and hemolytic disease of the newborn. Washed patient red blood cells are combined with antihuman globulin and observed for agglutination, indicating the presence of IgG or complement components on the cells.

Goodpasture's syndrome is an example of a type II reaction directed against a self-antigen in tissue. This syndrome is the result of antibody that reacts with the basement membrane of the glomerulus. Complement is activated, causing tissue damage and eventual loss of renal function.

In type III hypersensitivity reactions, IgG, IgM, and complement are also involved, but the reaction is directed against soluble rather than cellular antigens. If mild antigen excess occurs, the antigen–antibody complexes precipitate out and deposit in the tissues. The sites most affected are the basement membrane in the kidneys, the linings of blood vessels, and the joint linings. When complement binds to these complexes, phagocytic cells are attracted to the area. If the target cells cannot be engulfed, a reverse-phagocytic process called exocytosis takes place. The Arthus reaction, characterized by deposition of antigen–antibody complexes in the blood vessels, is a classic example of a type III reaction. Other examples include serum sickness and autoimmune diseases such as SLE and rheumatoid arthritis. Specific tests can be performed to determine the nature of the antibody involved.

Type IV, or delayed, hypersensitivity differs from the other three categories in that antibody and complement do not play a major role. Activation of T cells with the subsequent release of cytokines is responsible for the tissue damage seen in this type of reaction. Contact dermatitis resulting from exposure to poison ivy, poison oak, or a metal such as nickel is an example of haptens triggering a reaction to self-antigens. Skin testing and lymphocyte activation are used to determine sensitivity to particular antigens.

All four types of hypersensitivity represent defense mechanisms that stimulate an inflammatory response to cope with and react to antigen that is seen as foreign. In many cases, the antigen is not harmful, but the response to it results in tissue damage. This necessitates treatment to limit the damage.

# CASE STUDIES

1. A 13-year-old male had numerous absences from school in the spring due to cold symptoms that included head congestion and cough. He had been on antibiotics twice, but he seemed to go from one cold to the next. A complete blood cell (CBC) count showed no overall increase in white blood cells, but a mild eosinophilia was present. Because he had no fever or other signs of infection, his physician suggested that a total IgE screening test be run. The total IgE value was 250 IU/mL, which was within high-normal limits.

## Questions

a. What would account for the eosinophilia noted?

b. What conclusions can be drawn from the total IgE value?

c. What other tests might be indicated?

2. A 55-year-old male went to his physician complaining of feeling tired and run down. Two months previously, he had pneumonia and was concerned that he might not have completely recovered. He indicated that his symptoms only become noticeable if he goes out in the cold. A CBC count was performed, showing that his white cell count was within normal limits, but his red cell count was just below normal. A DAT performed on red blood cells was weakly positive after incubating at room temperature for 5 minutes. When the DAT was repeated with monospecific reagents, the tube with anti-C3d was the only one positive.

## Questions

a. What does a positive DAT indicate?

b. What is the most likely class of the antibody causing the reaction?

c. Why was the DAT positive only with anti-C3d when monospecific reagents were used?

# EXERCISE

## DIRECT ANTIGLOBULIN TEST

### Principle

The direct antiglobulin test (DAT) is used to detect in vivo coating of red blood cells with antibody, usually IgG, or complement degradation products such as C3d or C3dg. Presence of complement products indicates that antigen–antibody combination triggered the complement pathway and produced split products. DAT testing helps to diagnose autoimmune hemolytic anemia, HDN, transfusion reactions, or other type II hypersensitivity reactions.

### Sample Preparation

Collect blood by venipuncture using aseptic technique and avoiding hemolysis. Use ethylenediaminetetraacetic acid (EDTA) as the anticoagulant.

### Reagents, Materials, and Equipment

Polyspecific antihuman globulin reagent (AHG)

Bovine albumin, 22 percent

12 × 75 mm disposable glass test tubes

Disposable plastic blood bank pipettes

### Procedure

1. Prepare a 2 to 5 percent suspension of patient red cells by using saline.
2. Prepare a 6 percent suspension of bovine albumin by diluting the 22 percent suspension. To make 10 ml of a 6 percent suspension, add 2.7 mL of 22 percent bovine albumin to 7.3 mL of saline.
3. Place one drop of the red cell suspension in each of two labeled test tubes.
4. Fill each tube with saline, and centrifuge in a blood bank centrifuge for approximately 1 minute.
5. Decant tube, add saline to completely resuspend the cell button, and recentrifuge. Repeat this procedure three more times for a total of four washes.
6. Completely decant the final wash, and immediately add one or two drops of polyspecific AHG (as specified by the manufacturer) to one tube. Add one or two drops of 6 percent bovine albumin to the other tube.
7. Mix and centrifuge for approximately 30 seconds.
8. Dislodge the button from the bottom of the tube by gently tilting back and forth until no cells remain at the bottom of the tube.
9. Examine the tube carefully for agglutination by tilting back and forth and looking for clumps.

10. Leave any nonreactive tests for 5 minutes at room temperature, and then centrifuge and read again.
11. Add one drop of IgG-coated red cells to any nonreactive tube.
12. Centrifuge and examine the cells for agglutination. Any previously negative tube should be positive when the control cells are added.

### Interpretation

This is a screening test for the presence of immunoglobulin, namely either IgG or IgM on red cells. It also detects breakdown products of complement activation, namely C3d, indicating that complement activation has taken place. C3d is a breakdown product of C3b, the most abundant complement component. If C3d is present, this indicates that antigen–antibody combination must have taken place to initiate the complement cascade.

In either case, a positive test indicates that red cells have been coated in vivo and that a type II hypersensitivity reaction has occurred. Typically, coating with antibody usually causes an immediate reaction, while if only complement products are present, the reaction may need to be incubated and reread in 5 minutes.

A negative result is confirmed by the use of check cells or control cells. These red cells have been coated with IgG by the manufacturer. When antibody-coated cells are added to a tube that is negative, the antihuman globulin that is still present and not bound will bind to the control cells. When centrifuged, a tube with control cells should show at least a 2+ agglutination. This ensures that the patient cells have been properly washed to get rid of any residual immunoglobulins in the serum. It also confirms that reactive AHG was added.

A positive DAT would be found in the case of autoimmune hemolytic anemia, in which the patient produces an antibody to his or her own red cells. In the case of a transfusion reaction, a positive DAT indicates that the patient had preformed antibody to the red cells that were transfused. If cord blood cells are tested and found to be positive, this is an indicator of HDN, in which the mother's antibodies have coated the baby's red cells.

Positive results with polyspecific antiglobulin can be followed up by repeating the entire procedure with monospecific reagents (i.e., one that is specific for IgG and one that reacts with C3d). A reaction with only anti-C3d indicates that the antibody triggering the reaction is likely of the IgM class.

# REVIEW QUESTIONS

1. Which of the following is a general characteristic of hypersensitivity reactions?

   a. Immune responsiveness is depressed.
   b. Antibody is involved in all reactions.
   c. Either self-antigen or heterologous antigen may be involved.
   d. The antigen triggering the reaction is a harmful one.

2. Which of the following is associated with an increase in IgE production?

   a. Transfusion reaction
   b. Activation of Th1 cells
   c. Reaction to poison ivy
   d. HDN

3. Which of the following would cause a positive DAT test?

   a. Presence of IgG on red cells
   b. Presence of C3b or C3d on red cells
   c. A transfusion reaction due to preformed antibody
   d. Any of the above

4. All of the following are associated with type I hypersensitivity *except*

   a. release of preformed mediators from mast cells.
   b. activation of complement.
   c. cell-bound antibody bridged by antigen.
   d. an inherited tendency to respond to allergens.

5. Which newly synthesized mediator has a mode of action similar to that of histamine?

   a. $LTB_4$
   b. Heparin
   c. ECF-A
   d. $PGD_2$

6. Which of the following is associated with anaphylaxis?

   a. Buildup of IgE on mast cells
   b. Activation of complement
   c. Increase in cytotoxic T cells
   d. Large amount of circulating IgG

7. To determine if a patient is allergic to rye grass, the best test to perform is

   a. total IgE testing.
   b. skin prick test.
   c. DAT.
   d. complement fixation.

8. Which condition would result in HDN?

   a. Buildup of IgE on mother's cells
   b. Sensitization of cytotoxic T cells
   c. Exposure to antigen found on both mother and baby red cells
   d. Prior exposure to foreign red cell antigen

9. What is the immune mechanism involved in type III hypersensitivity reactions?

   a. Cellular antigens are involved.
   b. Deposition of immune complexes occurs in antibody excess.
   c. Only heterologous antigens are involved.
   d. Tissue damage results from exocytosis.

10. What is the immune phenomenon associated with the Arthus reaction?

    a. Tissue destruction by cytotoxic T cells
    b. Removal of antibody-coated red blood cells
    c. Deposition of immune complexes in blood vessels
    d. Release of histamine from mast cells

11. Contact dermatitis can be characterized by all of the following *except*

    a. formation of antigen–antibody complexes.
    b. generation of sensitized T cells.
    c. Langerhans cells acting as antigen-presenting cells.
    d. complexing of a hapten to self-antigen.

12. Which of the following conclusions can be drawn about a patient whose total IgE level is determined to be 150 IU/mL?

    a. The patient definitely has allergic tendencies.
    b. The patient may be subject to anaphylactic shock.
    c. Further antigen-specific testing should be done.
    d. The patient will never have an allergic reaction.

13. Which of the following explains the difference between type II and type III hypersensitivity reactions?

    a. Type II involves cellular antigens.
    b. Type III involves IgE.
    c. IgG is involved only in type III reactions.
    d. Type II reactions involve no antibody.

14. A 37-year-old woman received two units of packed red blood cells following a surgical procedure. She had been transfused once before. Five days after surgery, she experienced a slight fever and some hemoglobin in her urine, indicating a delayed transfusion reaction. A DAT test on a blood sample was positive. Which of the following statements best describes this reaction?

    a. The patient had IgM antibody to the red cells transfused.
    b. The patient's reaction was due to an amnestic response.
    c. Only IgE was coating the transfused red blood cells.
    d. The antibody present reacted best at room temperature.

# References

1. Kindt, TJ, Goldsby, RA, and Osborne, BA. Kuby Immunology, ed. 6. WH Freeman and Company, New York, 2007, pp. 371–400.

2. Host, A, Andraes, S, Charkin, S, Diaz-Vaquez, C, et al. Allergy testing in children: Why, who, when, and how. Allergy 58: 559–569, 2003.

3. Mothes, N, Valenta, R, and Spitzauer, S. Allergy testing: The role of recombinant allergens. Clin Chem Lab Med 44: 125–132, 2006.

4. Gould, HJ, Sutton, BJ, Beavil, AJ, Beavil, RL, et al. The biology of IgE and the basis of allergic disease. Ann Rev Immunol 21:579–628, 2003.

5. Kay, AB. Allergy and allergic diseases, Part I. N Engl J Med 344:30–37, 2001.

6. Homberger, HA. Allergic diseases. In McPherson, RA, and Pincus, MR (eds): Henry's Clinical Diagnosis and Management by Laboratory Methods, ed. 21. Saunders Elsevier, Philadelphia, 2007, pp. 961–971.

7. Mak, TW, and Saunders, ME. The Immune Response: Basic and Clinical Principles. Elsevier Academic Press, Burlington, MA, 2006, pp. 923–962.

8. Jutel, M, Blaser, K, and Akdis, CA. Histamine in allergic inflammation and immune modulation. Int Arch Allergy Immunol 137:82–92, 2005.

9. Abramson, J, and Pecht, I. Regulation of the mast cell response to the type 1 Fc epsilon receptor. Immunol Rev 217:231–254, 2007.

10. Li, JT. Allergy testing. Am Fam Physician 66:621–624, 2002.

11. Taylor, JS, and Erkek, E. Latex allergy: Diagnosis and management. Dermatol Ther 17:289–301, 2004.

12. Zak, HN, Kaste, LM, Schwarzenberger, K, et al. Health-care workers and latex allergy. Arch Environ Health 55:336–347, 2000.

13. Berger, WE. Monoclonal anti-IgE antibody: A novel therapy for allergic airways disease. Ann Allergy, Asthma, Immunol 88:152–160, 2002.

14. Kay, AB. Allergy and allergic diseases, Part II. N Engl J Med 344:109–113, 2001.

15. Platts-Mills, T, Leung, DYM, and Schatz, M. The role of allergens in asthma. Am Fam Physician 76:675–680, 2007.

16. Plaut, M, and Valentine, MD. Allergic rhinitis. N Engl J Med 353:1934–44, 2005.

17. Hughes, ATD. Anti-IgE antibody may help treat some asthma patients. JAMA 284:2859–2890, 2000.

18. Milgrom, H, Fick, RB Jr., Su, JQ, et al. Treatment of allergic asthma with monoclonal anti-IgE antibody. N Engl J Med 341(26):1966–1973, 1999.

19. Hamilton, RG. Immunological methods in the diagnostic allergy clinical and research laboratory. In Detrick, B, Hamilton, RG, and Folds, JD (eds): Manual of Molecular and Clinical Laboratory Immunology, ed. 7. ASM Press, Washington, DC, 2006, pp. 955–963.

20. Milgrom, H. Is there a role for treatment of asthma with omalizumab? Arch Dis Child 88:71–74, 2003.

21. Damin, DA, and Peebles, Jr., RS. In vivo diagnostic allergy testing. In Detrick, B, Hamilton, RG, and Folds, JD (eds): Manual of Molecular and Clinical Laboratory Immunology, ed. 7. ASM Press, Washington, DC, 2006, pp. 947–954.

22. Cobbaert, CM, and Jonker, GJ. Allergy testing on the Immulite 2000 random-access immunoanalyzer—a clinical evaluation study. Clin Chem Lab Med 43:772–781, 2005.

23. Smits, WM, Letz, KL, Evans, TS, and Giese, JK. Evaluating the response of patients undergoing both allergy skin testing and in vitro allergy testing with the ImmunoCAP technology system. J Am Acad Nurse Pract 15:415–423, 2003.

24. Fleischer, DM, and Wood, RA. Tests for immunological reactions to foods. In Detrick, B, Hamilton, RG, and Folds, JD (eds): Manual of Molecular and Clinical Laboratory Immunology, ed. 7. ASM Press, Washington, DC, 2006, pp. 975–983.

25. Renault, NK, Mirotti, L, and Alcocer, MJC. Biotechnologies in new high-throughput food allergy tests: Why we need them. Biotechnol Lett 29:333–339, 2007.

26. Harwanegg, C, Laffer, S, Hiller, R, Mueller, MW, et al. Microarrayed recombinant allergens for diagnosis of allergy. Clin Exp Allergy 33:7–13, 2003.

27. Garratty, G, Dzik, W, Issitt, PD, et al. Terminology for blood group antigens and genes—historical origins and guidelines in the new millennium. Transfusion 40:477–489, 2000.

28. Storry, JR, and Olsson, ML. Genetic basis of blood group diversity. Brit J Haematol 126:759–771, 2004.

29. Dzieckowski, JS, and Anderson, KC. Transfusion biology and therapy. In Kasper, DL, Braunwald, E, Fauci, AE, Hauser, SL, et al. (eds): Harrison's Principles of Internal Medicine, ed. 16. McGraw-Hill, New York, 2005, pp. 662–667.

30. Davenport, RD, and Mintz, PD. Transfusion medicine. In McPherson, RA, and Pincus, MR (eds): Henry's Clinical Diagnosis and Management by Laboratory Methods, ed. 21. Saunders Elsevier, Philadelphia, 2007, pp. 669–684.

31. Beadling, WV, and Cooling, L. Immunohematology. In McPherson, RA, and Pincus, MR (eds): Henry's Clinical Diagnosis and Management by Laboratory Methods, ed. 21. Saunders Elsevier, Philadelphia, 2007, pp. 617–668.

32. Reddy, VVB. Extracorporal defects leading to increased erythrocyte destruction—immune causes. In Rodak, BF, Fritzma, GA, and Doig, K (eds): Hematology: Clinical Principles and Applications. Saunders Elsevier, St. Louis, 2007, pp. 325–332.

33. Garratty, G, Glynn, SA, and McEntire, R. ABO and Rh(D) phenotype frequencies of different racial/ethnic groups in the United States. Transfusion 44:703–706, 2004.

34. Mak, TW, and Saunders, ME. The Immune Response: Basic and Clinical Principles. Elsevier Academic Press, Burlington, MA, 2006, pp. 696–749.

35. Murray, NA, and Roberts, IAG. Haemolytic disease of the newborn. Arch Dis Child 92:F83–F88, 2007.

36. Elghetany, MT, and Banki, K. Erythrocytic disorders. In McPherson, RA, and Pincus, MR (eds): Henry's Clinical Diagnosis and Management by Laboratory Methods, ed. 21. Saunders Elsevier, Philadelphia, 2007, pp. 504–544.

37. Bunn, HF, and Rosse, W. Hemolytic anemias and acute blood loss. In Kasper, DL, Braunwald, E, Fauci, AE, Hauser, SL, et al. (eds): Harrison's Principles of Internal Medicine, ed. 16. McGraw-Hill, New York, 2005, pp. 607–616.

38. Garvey, B. Rituximab in the treatment of autoimmune haematological disorders. Brit J Haematol 141:149–169, 2008.

39. D'Arena, G, Taylor, RP, Cascavilla, N, and Lindorfer, MA. Monoclonal antibodies: New therapeutic agents for autoimmune hemolytic anemia? Endocr Metab Immune Disord 8:62–68, 2008.

40. Jacob, SE, and Zapolanski, T. Systemic contact dermatitis. Dermatitis 19:9–15, 2008.

41. Thyssen, JP, Johansen, JD, and Menne, T. Contact allergy epidemics and their controls. Contact Dermatitis 56:185–195, 2007.

42. Karlberg, A, Bergstrom, MA, Borje, A, Luthman, K, et al. Allergic contact dermatitis—formation, structural requirements, and reactivity of skin sensitizers. Chem Res Toxicol 21:53–69, 2008.

43. Gladman, AC. *Toxicodendron* dermatitis: Poison ivy, oak, and sumac. Wilderness and Environ Med 17:120–128, 2006.

44. Jacob, SE, and Steele, T. Allergic contact dermatitis: Early recognition and diagnosis of important allergens. Dermatol Nurs 18:433–446, 2006.

45. Merrill, W. Hypersensitivity pneumonitis: Just think about it. Chest 120:1055–1058, 2001.

46. McCormick, T, and Shearer, W. Delayed-type hypersensitivity skin testing. In Detrick, B, Hamilton, RG, and Folds, JD (eds): Manual of Molecular and Clinical Laboratory Immunology, ed. 7. ASM Press, Washington, DC, 2006, pp. 234–240.

# 14 Autoimmunity

## KEY TERMS

____ Antinuclear antibody (ANA)

____ Autoimmune disease

____ Autoimmune thyroid disease (AITD)

____ Central tolerance

____ Fluorescent antinuclear antibody (FANA) testing

____ Graves' disease

____ Hashimoto's thyroiditis

____ Molecular mimicry

____ Multiple sclerosis (MS)

____ Myasthenia gravis (MG)

____ Peripheral tolerance

____ Rheumatoid arthritis (RA)

____ Rheumatoid factor (RF)

____ Systemic lupus erythematosus (SLE)

____ Thyroid-stimulating hormone (TSH)

____ Thyroid-stimulating hormone receptor antibody (TSHRab)

____ Thyrotoxicosis

____ Type I diabetes mellitus

## LEARNING OBJECTIVES

*After finishing this chapter, the reader will be able to:*

1. Describe the factors that contribute to the development of autoimmunity.
2. Distinguish organ-specific and systemic autoimmune diseases, giving an example of each.
3. Describe the effects of systemic lupus erythematosus (SLE) on the body.
4. Discuss the immunologic mechanisms known for SLE.
5. List four types of autoantibodies found in lupus, and describe the pattern seen with each in immunofluorescence testing.
6. Differentiate screening tests from antibody-specific tests for lupus.
7. Discuss the symptoms of rheumatoid arthritis (RA).
8. Describe characteristics of the key antibodies found in RA.
9. Discuss screening tests for rheumatoid factor (RF) and anti-CCP, explaining the limitations of current testing procedures.
10. Differentiate Hashimoto's thyroiditis and Graves' disease on the basis of laboratory findings and immune mechanisms.
11. List the main antibodies tested for in Graves' and Hashimoto's diseases, and describe testing procedures.
12. Relate genetic susceptibility to the development of insulin-dependent diabetes mellitus.
13. Explain immunologic mechanisms known to cause destruction of β cells in type I diabetes mellitus.
14. Discuss the immunologic findings in multiple sclerosis (MS).
15. Describe how the finding of oligoclonal bands in cerebrospinal fluid can help in diagnosis of multiple sclerosis.
16. Explain how the symptoms that occur in myasthenia gravis (MG) are related to the presence of auotantibodies.
17. Discuss how Goodpasture's syndrome differs from glomerulonephritis due to nonspecific deposition of immune complexes.

# CHAPTER OUTLINE

**Autoimmune diseases** are conditions in which damage to organs or tissues results from the presence of autoantibody or autoreactive cells. Such diseases affect 5 to 7 percent of the population and are thought to be caused by the loss or breakdown of self-tolerance.[1] In the early 1900s, Ehrlich described this phenomenon as "horror autotoxicus," literally meaning "fear of self-poisoning." Thus, it was recognized early on that under normal circumstances, the immune response was held in check so that self-antigens were not destroyed.

Self-tolerance is believed to be brought about by several mechanisms, including clonal deletion of relevant effector cells and active regulation by T cells. As described in Chapter 2, during the maturation process of T cells, the great majority of undifferentiated lymphocytes that are processed through the thymus do not survive. It is thought that this is where potentially self-reactive T-cell clones are destroyed. The same process happens with B cells as they mature in the bone marrow. This destruction of potentially self-reactive lymphocytes is referred to as **central tolerance.** The process is not totally effective, however, as normal individuals do possess self-reactive lymphocytes.

Thus, in the secondary lymphoid organs, **peripheral tolerance** is maintained by a delicate balance between the T helper cell type 1 (Th1) and T helper cell type 2 (Th2) populations.[1] In animal models of autoimmune disease, the Th1 cells have been implicated as primary mediators of autoimmune disease, because they release proinflammatory cytokines.[1] The reaction to foreign antigens is typically a Th2 response, and the accompanying cytokines do not cause the same type of destruction as Th1 cells. Recent findings indicate that regulatory T cells (Tregs) play a central role in maintaining this balance and eliminating harmful autoimmune

responses. (See Chapter 5 for details about regulatory T cells.)

Major histocompatibility complex (MHC) products also seem to influence antigen recognition or nonrecognition by determining the type of peptides that can be presented to the T cells. There is a close fit between an antigenic peptide and the groove of an individual MHC molecule, as discussed in Chapter 3. Therefore, inheritance of a gene coding for a specific MHC molecule may make an individual more susceptible to a particular autoimmune disease. In addition, the expression of class II molecules on cells where they are not normally found may result in the presentation of self-antigens for which no tolerance has been established. In several of the diseases presented in this chapter, there are examples of host cells that exhibit class II molecules on their surfaces after an inflammatory response. The strongest link found to date between certain HLA molecules and specific diseases is between HLA-B27 and ankylosing spondylitis. Individuals who possess HLA-B27 have a 90 times greater chance of developing the disease than the normal population.[1] Other associations between inheritance of certain MHC genes and the tendency to develop particular autoimmune diseases are discussed in the chapter.

Several other mechanisms are thought to contribute to autoimmunity: release of sequestered antigens, molecular mimicry, and polyclonal B-cell activation. Antigens that are protected from encountering the circulation are not exposed to potentially reactive lymphocytes. Examples of these are myelin basic protein, normally sequestered by the blood–brain barrier, and sperm. Trauma to the tissue by means of an accident or infection may introduce such antigens to the general circulation. In the case of sperm, vasectomy can induce autoantibody formation.

**Molecular mimicry** refers to the fact that many individual viral or bacterial agents contain antigens that closely resemble self-antigens. Exposure to such foreign antigens may trigger antibody production that in turn reacts with similar self-antigens. Examples are poliovirus VP2 and acetylcholine (ACH) receptors, measles virus P3 and myelin basic protein, and papilloma virus E2 and insulin receptors.[1] Further examples are discussed with individual diseases.

The last major factor is polyclonal B-cell activation. B-cell defects include the abnormal expression or function of key signaling molecules, dysregulation of cytokines, and changes in B-cell developmental subsets.[2] One defect in particular, Fc receptor polymorphisms, the receptor for antibody that normally down-regulates antibody production, may cause continual B-cell stimulation.[2] These defects may be enhanced by organisms such as gram-negative bacteria and several viruses, including cytomegalovirus and Epstein-Barr virus (EBV), which are polyclonal activators. They induce proliferation of numerous clones of B cells that express IgM in the absence of T helper (Th) cells.[1] In this process, B cells that may be reactive to self-antigens can be activated.

Besides the factors mentioned previously, several others must be taken into account in the etiology of autoimmune diseases. Some of these are defects in the immune system, the influence of hormones, and environmental conditions. Defects in natural killer cells, in the secretion of cytokines, in apoptosis (or killing of cells), and in complement components all may contribute to the loss of self-tolerance. Hormones, especially estrogens, may also play a role, because they are known to affect cytokine production and may influence which T cells, either Th1 or Th2, are more active in a particular response.[3] This explains in part why women are more prone to autoimmune diseases. Thus, there is not one cause but many contributing factors that are responsible for the pathological conditions found in autoimmune diseases.

Autoimmune diseases can be classified as systemic or organ-specific. There is often a good bit of overlap between the two, because some diseases that start out as organ-specific later affect other organs. **Table 14–1** lists some of the more important autoimmune diseases. Many of the key diseases for which serological testing is available are discussed in this chapter.

## SYSTEMIC LUPUS ERYTHEMATOSUS

**Systemic lupus erythematosus (SLE)** represents the prototype of human autoimmune diseases. It is a chronic systemic inflammatory disease marked by alternating exacerbations and remissions, affecting between 15 and 50 individuals out of 100,000 in the United States.[4,5] Incidence of the disease has tripled over the last four decades.[4] The peak age of onset is usually between 20 and 40 years. Women are much more likely than men to be stricken, by a margin of approximately 10 to 1.[1,5] It is also more common in African Americans and Hispanics than in whites.[5] With earlier diagnosis and improved treatments, the 5-year survival rate has increased to greater than 90 percent.[6]

The immune response is directed against a broad range of target antigens, as the typical patient has an average of three circulating autoantibodies.[5] It appears that there is an interplay between genetic susceptibility and environmental factors. In whites, there is a strong association with human leukocyte antigens (HLA) DR and DQ. As discussed in

| Table 14–1. | Spectrum of Autoimmune Diseases | |
|---|---|---|
| **SPECIFICITY** | **DISEASE** | **TARGET TISSUE** |
| **Organ-Specific** | Hashimoto's thyroiditis | Thyroid |
| | Graves' disease | Thyroid |
| | Pernicious anemia cells | Gastric parietal |
| | Addison's disease | Adrenal glands |
| | Type I diabetes mellitus | Pancreas |
| | MG | Nerve-muscle synapses |
| | MS | Myelin sheath of nerves |
| | Autoimmune hemolytic anemia | Red blood cells |
| | Idiopathic thrombocytopenic purpura | Platelets |
| | Goodpasture's syndrome | Kidney, lungs |
| | RA | Joints, lungs, skin |
| | Scleroderma | Skin, gut, lungs, kidney |
| **Systemic** | SLE | Skin, joints, kidney, brain, heart, lungs |

MG = myasthenia gravis; MS = multiple sclerosis; RA = rheumatoid arthritis; SLE = systemic lupus erythematosus

Chapter 3, the HLA antigens play a role in presentation of foreign or self-antigens to T and B cells. Additionally, lupus has been associated with inherited deficiencies of complement components C1q, C2, and C4. (See Chapter 6 for a discussion of complement factors.) Abnormalities of Fc γ receptors on B cells, macrophages, dendritic cells, and neutrophils that bind IgG and prevent excess immune reactions have also been found.[7] Environmental factors include exposure to ultraviolet light, certain medications, and infectious agents.[8] Hormones are also important, because they may influence the regulation of transcription of genes that are central to the SLE expression.[8] In fact, use of estrogen-containing contraceptives or hormone replacement therapy has been found to double the risk of developing lupus.[5]

## Clinical Signs

The clinical signs are extremely diverse, and nonspecific symptoms such as fatigue, weight loss, malaise, fever, and anorexia are often the first to appear. Joint involvement seems to be the most frequently reported manifestation, because over 90 percent of patients with SLE are subject to polyarthralgias or arthritis.[9] Typically, the arthritis is symmetric and involves the small joints of the hands, wrists, and knees.

After joint involvement, the next most common signs are skin manifestations. An erythematous rash may appear on any area of the body exposed to ultraviolet light. Less common but perhaps more dramatic is the appearance of the classic butterfly rash across the nose and cheeks. This is what is responsible for the name *lupus*, derived from the Latin term meaning "wolflike." This rash appears in only about 30 to 40 percent of all patients **(Fig. 14–1)**. In discoid lupus, skin lesions have central atrophy and scarring.

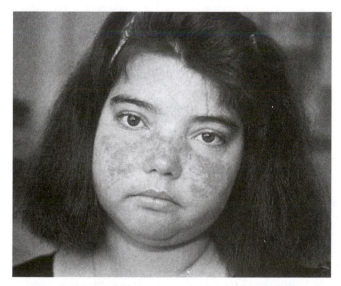

**FIGURE 14–1.** Butterfly rash in SLE. Characteristic rash over the cheekbones and forehead is diagnostic of SLE. The disease often begins in young adulthood and may eventually involve many organ systems. *(From Steinman, L. Autoimmune disease. Sci Am 269:107, 1993, with permission.)*

One-half to two-thirds of all patients exhibit evidence of renal involvement. There are several types of lesions, but the most dangerous is diffuse proliferative glomerulonephritis (DPGN), in which there is cellular proliferation in at least 50 percent of the glomeruli.[5] Twenty percent of individuals with DPGN will die or develop end-stage renal disease within 10 years of diagnosis.[9] Other conditions may include deposition of immune complexes in the subendothelial tissue and thickening of the basement membrane. All of these can lead to renal failure, the most frequent cause of death in patients with SLE.

Other systemic effects may include cardiac involvement with pericarditis, tachycardia, or ventricular enlargement; pleuritis with chest pain; neuropsychiatric manifestations such as seizures, mild cognitive dysfunction, psychoses, or depression; or hematologic abnormalities such as anemia, leukopenia, thrombocytopenia, or lymphopenia.[9,10] In order for a clinical diagnosis of lupus to be made, four of eleven specific criteria must be present: malar rash, discoid rash, photosensitivity, oral ulcers, arthritis, serositis, renal disorders, neurological disorders, hematologic disorders, immunologic disorders, and presence of antinuclear antibodies.[5] Within the category of immunologic disorders are antibodies to double-stranded DNA, to Smith antigen, and to phospholipids.

## Immunologic Findings

The first clue in the mystery of lupus was the discovery of the LE cell by Malcolm Hargraves in 1948. The LE cell is a neutrophil that has engulfed the antibody-coated nucleus of another neutrophil. This phenomenon, which mainly appears in vitro, occurs when cells are damaged and release nuclear material. Nine years after the LE cell was discovered, the first anti-DNA antibody was identified. Now it is known that SLE is associated with more than 25 autoantibodies. Some of the more common ones are listed in **Table 14–2.**

The large number of possible autoantibodies reflects a generalized dysregulation of the immune system.[11,12] There is an uncontrolled autoreactivity of T and B cells leading to the production of autoantibodies. This activity may be due to a deficiency of regulatory T cells, as discussed in Chapter 2. Regulatory T cells (Tregs) play a crucial role in the maintenance of self-tolerance in peripheral lymphoid organs, as they suppress T-cell proliferation.[13] Tregs in lupus seem to be more sensitive to apoptosis, or programmed cell death.[13] In addition, altered Fc receptors for IgG on B cells keep them from being switched off, so they continue to produce antibody.[7] Dysfunctional processing in the routine nonimmunologic clearing of cellular debris may also be a key to the pathogenesis of SLE.[12] Abnormal apoptosis of certain types of cells may occur, releasing excess amounts of cellular constituents such as DNA and ribonucleic acid (RNA). Individuals who inherit certain HLA genes are more likely to respond to such self-antigens.

## Table 14–2.   Common Antinuclear Antibodies

| AUTOANTIBODY | CHARACTERISTICS OF ANTIGEN | IMMUNOFLUORESCENT PATTERN | DISEASE ASSOCIATION |
|---|---|---|---|
| Anti–ds-DNA | ds-DNA | Homogeneous | SLE |
| Anti–ss-DNA | Related to purines and pyrimidines | Not detected on routine screen | SLE, many other diseases |
| Anti-histone | Different classes of histones | Homogeneous | Drug-induced SLE, other diseases |
| Anti-DNP | DNA-histone complex | Homogeneous | SLE, drug-induced SLE |
| Anti-Sm | Extractable nuclear antigen (RNA component) | Speckled | Diagnostic for SLE |
| Anti-RNP | Proteins complexed with nuclear RNA | Speckled | SLE, mixed connective tissue diseases |
| Anti-SS-A (Ro) | Proteins complexed to RNA | Finely speckled | SLE, Sjögren's syndrome, others |
| Anti-SS-B (La) | Phosphoprotein complexed to RNA polymerase | Finely speckled | SLE, Sjögren's syndrome, others |
| Anti-nucleolar | RNA polymerase, nucleolar protein | Homogeneous staining of nucleolus | SLE, systemic sclerosis |
| Anti-Scl-70 | DNA topoisomerase I | Atypical speckled | Systemic sclerosis, Scleroderma |
| Anti–Jo-1 | Histidyl-tRNA synthetase | Fine cytoplasmic speckling | Polymyositis |

Adapted from Bradwell, AR, Hughes, RG, and Karim, AR. Immunofluorescent antinuclear antibody tests. In Detrick, B, Hamilton, RG, and Folds, JD (eds): Manual of Molecular and Clinical Laboratory Immunology, ed. 7. ASM Press, Washington, DC, 2006, pp. 996–97.
DNA = deoxyribonucleic acid; SLE = systemic lupus erythematosus; DNP = deoxyribonucleoprotein; RNA = ribonucleic acid; RNP = ribonucleoprotein

Constant presence of antigenic material triggers polyclonal activation of B cells, one of the main immunologic characteristics in lupus. There is an accompanying alteration in the function of both Th1 and Th2 helper cells, resulting in enhanced production of certain cytokines that contribute to up-regulation of antibody production by B cells.[14] In particular, increased production of interleukin-10 (IL-10), which normally serves an immunosuppressive role, correlates with increased antibody production and with disease activity. IL-10 appears to trigger an increase in antibodies directed against DNA and stimulate production of platelet-activating factor.[15,16]

Once immune complexes are formed, they cannot be cleared as well from the circulation because of other possible deficiencies. These include defects in complement receptors on phagocytic cells; defects in receptors for the Fc portion of immunoglobulins; or deficiencies of early complement components such as C1q, C2, or C4.[5,8] Accumulation of IgG to double-stranded DNA seems to be the most pathogenic, because it forms complexes of an intermediate size that become deposited in the glomerular basement membrane. In addition, anti-DNA antibody may also react directly with proteins such as α-actin, found in the basement membrane; this enhances activation of the complement cascade, which contributes to the kidney damage seen with this disease.[17]

Drug-induced lupus differs from the more chronic form of the disease in that symptoms usually disappear once the drug is discontinued. The most common drugs implicated are procainamide, hydralazine, chlorpromazine, isoniazid, quinidine, anticonvulsants such as methyldopa, and possibly oral contraceptives.[5,10] Typically, this is a milder form of the disease, usually manifested as fever, arthritis, or rashes; rarely are the kidneys involved.[5]

## Laboratory Diagnosis of Systemic Lupus Erythematosus

When SLE is suspected, the first test typically done is a screening test for **antinuclear antibodies (ANA).** **Fluorescent antinuclear antibody (FANA) testing** is the most widely used and accepted test, because it detects a wide range of antibodies and is positive in about 95 percent of patients with lupus.[5,17,18] This is an extremely sensitive test and relatively easy to perform, but it has low diagnostic specificity, because many of the antibodies are associated with other autoimmune diseases.[18] Mouse kidney or human epithelial HEp-2 cells are fixed to a slide and allowed to react with patient serum. After careful washing to remove all unreacted antibody, an antihuman immunoglobulin with a fluorescent tag or an enzyme label such as horseradish peroxidase is added. Approximately 2 percent of healthy individuals and up to 75 percent of elderly individuals test positive.[18,19] Conversely, up to 5 percent of SLE patients test negative, so this test cannot be used to absolutely rule out SLE. It is now common practice to screen with a 1:80 dilution (or 1:160 if the patient is over 65) to avoid low positive titers in the normal population.[18] Patients with SLE usually have high titers of high-affinity antibody against specific antigens. Profile testing for individual antibodies can be done as a follow-up. A diagram of the possible fluorescent patterns is shown in **Figure 14–2** (see also Color Plate 10). Some of the individual antinuclear antibodies and other categories of antibodies are discussed below.

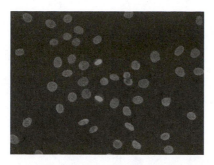

Homogeneous pattern

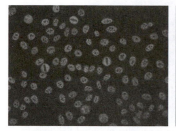

Speckled pattern

Nucleolar pattern

**FIGURE 14–2.** Patterns of immunofluorescent staining for antinuclear antibodies. Examples of predominant staining patterns obtained are homogeneous—staining of the entire nucleus; speckled pattern—staining throughout the nucleus; and nucleolar pattern—staining of the nucleolus. *(Courtesy of DiaSorin, Inc., with permission. Color Plate 11.)*

## Antinuclear Antibodies

### FANA Testing

Double-stranded DNA (ds-DNA) antibodies are the most specific for SLE, because they are mainly seen only in patients with lupus, and levels correlate with disease activity.[10,18] Although they are found in only 40 to 70 percent of patients, the presence of these antibodies is considered diagnostic for SLE, especially when they are found in combination with low levels of complement component C3.[20,21] Antibodies to ds-DNA typically produce a peripheral or a homogeneous staining pattern on indirect immunofluorescence (IIF).[18]

In testing for antibodies to ds-DNA, a purified antigen preparation that is free from single-stranded DNA (ss-DNA) must be used, as antibodies to ss-DNA occur in many individuals with other autoimmune or inflammatory diseases. One particularly sensitive assay for ds-DNA is an immunofluorescent test using *Crithidia luciliae*, a hemoflagellate, as the substrate. This trypanosome has circular ds-DNA in the kinetoplast. A positive test is indicated by a brightly stained kinetoplast with patient serum and an antibody conjugate. This test has a high degree of specificity, although it is less sensitive than other FANA tests.[18,20] Other assays that can be used to detect ds-DNA include immunodiffusion, radioimmunoassay (RIA), and enzyme immunoassay (EIA) tests.[20] EIA is now considered more sensitive than either

RIA or Crithidial testing, so it is the most widely used technique.[18,20]

A second major antibody found in lupus patients is *antihistone antibody*. Histone is a nucleoprotein that is a major constituent of chromatin. It can be detected in almost all patients with drug-induced lupus. About 70 percent of other patients with SLE have elevated levels of antihistone antibodies, but the titers are usually fairly low.[5] Presence of antihistone antibody alone or combined with antibody to ss-DNA supports the diagnosis of drug-induced lupus.[10,18] Antihistone antibodies are also found in rheumatoid arthritis (RA) and primary biliary cirrhosis, but the levels are usually lower. High levels of antihistone antibodies tend to be associated with the more active and severe forms of SLE.[10] Antihistone antibodies are typically detected by immunofluorescent assays, immunoblotting, and EIA. On IIF, either a homogeneous pattern is seen, representing fluorescence of the entire nucleus, or staining of the periphery occurs.[18]

Antibodies are also stimulated by DNA complexed to histone, known as *deoxyribonucleoprotein (DNP)*. Immunofluorescent patterns are similar to those discussed previously. Latex particles coated with DNP are used in a simple slide agglutination test for SLE.

Antibody to a preparation of extractable nuclear antigen was first described in a patient named Smith, hence the name *anti-Sm antibody*. Extractable nuclear antigens represent a family of small nuclear proteins that are associated with uridine-rich RNA. The anti-Sm antibody is specific for lupus, because it is not found in other autoimmune diseases. However, it is found in only 7 to 25 percent of patients with this disease.[10,21] This antibody produces a coarsely speckled pattern of nuclear fluorescence on IIF. Titers do not correlate with disease activity.[21] It can also be measured by immunodiffusion, immunoblotting, immunoprecipitation, and EIA.[18]

SS-A/Ro and SS-B/La antigens also belong to the family of extractable nuclear antigens. SS-A/Ro antigen is a RNA complexed to one of two proteins with molecular weights of 60 kD or 52 kD. Antibody to it appears in approximately 10 to 50 percent of patients with SLE.[10] This antibody is most often found in patients who have cutaneous manifestations of SLE, especially photosensitivity dermatitis.[10] Anti-Ro/SSA has been found to bind to cell surface antigens on neutrophils and can cause a mild neutropenia, often seen in patients with SLE.[22] SS-B/La antigen is a phosphoprotein that appears to be bound to products of RNA III polymerase.[10] Anti-SS-B/La is found in only 10 to 20 percent of patients with SLE, and all of these have anti-SS-A/Ro.[21] Both SS-A/Ro and SS-B/La antibodies are highly prevalent in patients with other autoimmune diseases, notably scleroderma and Sjögren's syndrome.[5] To detect the presence of these antibodies on IIF, human tissue culture cells such as HEp-2 (human epithelial) must be used, because SS-A/Ro and SS-B/La antigens are not found in mouse or rat liver and kidney. A finely speckled pattern is evident. These can also be detected by immunoprecipitation, immunoblotting, and EIA.[18]

An antibody that produces a coarsely speckled IIF pattern is *anti-nRNP antibody*. Ribonucleoprotein (RNP) is protein complexed to a particular type of nuclear RNA called *U1-nRNP* (*U* for "uridine-rich"). Although it is detected in 20 to 40 percent of patients with SLE, it is also found at a high titer in individuals with mixed connective tissue disease, systemic sclerosis, Sjögren's syndrome, and other autoimmune diseases.[10,18] Anti-nRNP can be measured by immunoblotting, immunoprecipitation, EIA, and IIF.[21,22]

Staining of the nucleolus in IIF may indicate antibody to fibrillarin, a dense component of the nucleolus. This is indicated by clumpy nucleolar fluorescence.[18] This pattern is common in systemic sclerosis.[18,21] Homogeneous staining of the nucleolus is associated with myositis and systemic sclerosis.[18]

### Other Assays for ANA

ANAs can also be detected by immunodiffusion. Typically, this method is used to determine the immunologic specificity of a positive FANA test. Such testing is valuable in identifying specific disease states and in ruling out those normal patients who exhibit a positive FANA test. Ouchterlony double diffusion detects antibody to several of the small nuclear ribonucleoproteins, or extractable nuclear antigens (ENA). These include antibodies to the following antigens: Sm, nRNP, SS-A/Ro, SS-B/La, Scl-70 (DNA topoisomerase I), and Jo-1 (antigens found in dermatopolymyositis).[21] **Table 14–2** shows the source of these antigens and associations with specific diseases. A positive reaction is indicated by immunoprecipitation lines of serological identity **(Fig. 14–3)**. (Refer to Chapter 8 for a description of the principles of Ouchterlony immunodiffusion.) Although this type of testing is not as sensitive as some other techniques, it is highly specific.[21]

Immunoblotting techniques separate out antigens by means of polyacrylamide gel electrophoresis. The pattern is then electrotransferred to a nitrocellulose sheet, which is incubated with dilutions of patient serum. Either radiolabeled or enzyme labeled antibody conjugates are then used to visualize individual bands. This technique is reliable, sensitive, and specific, and it should be considered the gold standard for characterization of specific antibodies.[10,21]

EIA has also come into wider use for detection of anti–ds-DNA, antihistone antibodies, and anti–SS-A and anti–SS-B. It is particularly good for detection of the latter two antibodies.[22,23] EIA testing is quantitative, is less subjective, and lends itself well to automation.[22,23] It is more sensitive than immunodiffusion, but the specificity is lower.[21] In addition, it has proven to be more sensitive than double immunodiffusion for the identification of extractable nuclear antigens.[24] Despite advances in EIA technology however, IIF is still considered the benchmark in identification of most autoantibodies associated with lupus.[18,22]

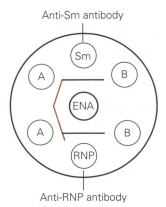

**FIGURE 14–3.** Extractable nuclear antibody (ENA) immunodiffusion pattern. A mixture of extractable nuclear antigens, including RNP, Sm, and other soluble nuclear antigens, is placed in a central well in an agarose gel. Sm antibody and RNP antibody are run as positive controls, and patient samples are placed between the controls. The pattern of precipitin lines formed indicates the antibodies present in patient serum. The arc of serological identity formed between Sm and patient A indicates that serum A contains anti-Sm antibodies. The arc of partial identity formed between serum A and RNP occurs because RNP is always found complexed to Sm antigen. RNP antibodies are not present. Serum B contains neither Sm nor RNP antibody.

### Antiphospholipid Antibodies

Antiphospholipid antibodies are a heterogeneous group of antibodies that bind to phospholipid alone or are complexed with protein. They can affect every organ in the body, but they are especially associated with deep-vein and arterial thrombosis and with morbidity in pregnancy.[25,26] They have been found in up to 60 percent of patients with lupus, but they are associated with several other disease states.[27] They can be identified by causing false-positive results for syphilis.

The lupus anticoagulant, one of the several types of antiphospholipid antibodies, was so named because it produces prolonged activated partial thromboplastin time (aPT) and prothrombin time (PTT). Ironically, patients with this antibody have an increased risk of clotting and spontaneous abortion. Platelet function may also be affected. In addition to determining the aPT and PPT, there are several EIAs for antiphospholipid antibodies that are sensitive and relatively simple to perform.[25–27] If these antibodies are suspected, factor assays may also need to be performed to rule out any factor deficiencies or factor-specific inhibitors.

### Treatment

If fever or arthritis is the primary symptom, a high dose of aspirin or other anti-inflammatory drug may bring relief. For skin manifestations, antimalarials such as hydroxychloroquine or chloroquine and topical steroids are often prescribed.[5] Systemic corticosteroids are used for acute fulminant lupus, lupus nephritis, or central nervous system complications, because these suppress the immune response and lower antibody titers.[5] Other drugs used include cyclophosphamide, azathioprine, methotrexate, and chlorambucil, but all of these may have serious side effects such as bone marrow suppression, and they must be monitored closely. A new approach for patients whose symptoms cannot be controlled by other means involves autologous stem cell harvesting and reinfusion after the patient undergoes intensive chemotherapy.[28] Results indicate that long-term remission may be possible using this method. Overall, the present 5-year survival rate approaches 90 percent.[5]

## RHEUMATOID ARTHRITIS

**Rheumatoid arthritis (RA)** is another example of a systemic autoimmune disorder. It affects approximately 1 percent of the population in the Western world.[29–31] Women are three times as likely to be affected as men. Typically it strikes individuals between the ages of 35 and 50, although it may occur at any age.[29] RA can be characterized as a chronic, symmetric, and erosive arthritis of the peripheral joints that can also affect multiple organs such as the heart and the lungs.[10,30] In addition to a decline in functional ability, there is a reduced life expectancy.[32,33] Progress of the disease varies, because there may be spontaneous remissions or an increasingly active disease in some individuals that rapidly progresses to joint deformity and disability.[34]

As in SLE, there appears to be an association of RA with certain MHC class II genes. These genes code for the beta chain, one of the two chains that make up the HLA class II antigens (see Chapter 3). The strongest association appears with certain DR4 alleles. These occur in 70 percent of patients with RA.[29] All of the alleles involved appear to code for a similar amino acid sequence at positions 67 to 74 in the β chain.[29] This "shared epitope" on the HLA class II β chain may act to facilitate antigen presentation to Th cells and to B cells.

### Clinical Signs

Diagnosis of RA is based on the 1987 criteria established by the American College of Rheumatology.[35] Key symptoms are morning stiffness around the joints lasting at least 1 hour; swelling of the soft tissue around three or more joints; swelling of the proximal interphalangeal, metacarpophalangeal, or wrist joints; symmetric arthritis; subcutaneous nodules; a positive test for rheumatoid factor (RF); and radiographic evidence of erosions in the joints of the hands, the wrists, or both. At least four of these must be present for 6 weeks or more for the diagnosis to be made.

Typically the patient experiences nonspecific symptoms such as malaise, fatigue, fever, weight loss, and transient joint pain that begins in the small joints of the hands and feet. Morning stiffness and joint pain usually improve during the day. Joint involvement progresses to the larger joints in a symmetric fashion, often affecting the knees, hips, elbows, shoulders, and cervical spine. The joint pain experienced leads to muscle spasm, which, because of the consequent

limitation of motion, results in permanent joint deformity. About 20 percent of patients have nodules over the bones. Nodules can also be found in the myocardium, pericardium, heart valves, pleura, lungs, spleen, and larynx. Other systemic symptoms may include anemia, formation of subcutaneous nodules, pericarditis, lymphadenopathy, splenomegaly, interstitial lung disease, or vasculitis. Felty's syndrome is a combination of several of these symptoms: chronic RA coupled with neutropenia, splenomegaly, and possibly thrombocytopenia.[29]

For many years, there has been a search for an infectious agent or agents that may be involved in the etiology of RA. Numerous agents, including *Mycoplasma*, rubella, cytomegalovirus, EBV, and parvovirus, have been proposed as possible triggering antigens.[29] In fact, an increased titer of antibody to EB and some other viruses has been found in patients with RA, but a causal relationship has not been established.[30]

### Immunologic Findings

The earliest lesions in rheumatoid joints show an increase in cells lining the synovium and an infiltration of mononuclear cells, mostly CD4+ T lymphocytes.[29] CD8+ T cells are scattered throughout, as are B cells and antibody-producing plasma cells. Macrophages and neutrophils are attracted to the area, and this results in the formation of an organized mass of cells called a *pannus*, which grows into the joint space and invades the cartilage.[10,34]

The balance between proinflammatory and anti-inflammatory cytokines appears to be tipped toward continual inflammation. Proinflammatory cytokines found in synovial fluid that contribute to inflammation are interleukin-1 (IL-1), interleukin-6 (IL-6), interleukin-8 (IL-8), interleukin-15 (IL-15), interleukin-18 (IL-18), and tumor necrosis factor-alpha (TNF-α).[34,36] (See Chapter 5 for a complete discussion of cytokines). TNF-α plays a key role in the inflammatory process by inducing continual secretion of IL-1, IL-6, and Il-8. In addition, TNF-α facilitates the transport of white blood cells to the affected areas.[34] Collagenase and other tissue-degrading enzymes are also released from synoviocytes and chondrocytes that line the joint cavity. The end result is destruction of connective tissue, cartilage, and bone.

It is not known what role autoantibodies play in the initiation of the inflammatory response. Approximately 75 percent of patients with RA have an antibody that has been called the **rheumatoid factor (RF)**.[29,30,34] It is most often of the IgM class and is directed against the Fc portion of IgG. However, this antibody is not specific for RA, as it is found in 5 percent of healthy individuals and in 10 to 20 percent of those over the age of 65.

In RA, IgM antibodies combine with IgG, and these immune complexes become deposited in the joints, resulting in a type III (or immune complex) hypersensitivity reaction. The complement protein C1 binds to the immune complexes, activating the classical complement cascade.

During this process, C3a and C5a are generated, which act as chemotactic factors for neutrophils and macrophages. The continual presence of macrophages leads to the chronic inflammation usually observed which damages the synovium itself.

Other autoantibodies found include antikeratin antibody, antiperinuclear antibody, antifilaggrin, and anti-Sa antibody. All of these antibodies are directed against citrullinated proteins, which are generated by modification of protein-bound arginine by the enzyme peptidylarginine deiminase.[30,37] This enzyme is associated with granulocytes, monocytes, and macrophages, as well as other types of cells. Death of granulocytes and macrophages triggers production of citrullinated proteins, and overexpression of these antigens may provoke an immune response.[37] This family of antibodies is detected using cyclic citrullinated peptides (CCP); hence the antibodies are called *anti-CCP*. Anti-CCP is now the lead marker for detection of RA, because it is much more specific than RF.[38]

In addition, low titers of antinuclear antibodies are present in about 40 percent of patients. The pattern most identified is the speckled pattern directed against ribonucleoprotein. The significance of this group of autoantibodies remains unclear, because they do not appear to be directly related to pathogenesis.

## Laboratory Diagnosis of Rheumatoid Arthritis

Diagnosis of RA is made on the basis of a combination of clinical manifestations, radiographic findings, and laboratory testing. RF is the antibody that is most often tested for to aid in making the initial diagnosis. Two types of agglutination tests for RF have been developed: one using sheep red blood cells coated with IgG and the other using latex particles coated with the same antigen. Because the latex test has a greater sensitivity, it is the predominant agglutination test used. Agglutination tests, however, detect only the IgM isotype, found in approximately 75 percent of patients. Thus, a negative result does not rule out the presence of RA. Conversely, a positive test result is not specific for RA, because RF can be found in other diseases such as syphilis, SLE, chronic active hepatitis, tuberculosis, leprosy, infectious mononucleosis, malaria, and Sjörgren's syndrome.[29,30]

Testing for two other antibody classes of RF, IgG or IgA, tends to be more specific. These two isotypes are rarely found in other disease states, which may help in making a differential diagnosis. The elevation of IgA early in the disease appears to be associated with a poorer prognosis, such as development of bone erosions and systemic manifestations, so this can be used to predict the disease outcome.[30] Testing for IgG and IgA isotypes and IgM can be performed using EIA techniques. Nephelometric assays can also test for the presence of all three isotypes. These are based on increases in light scattering as immune complexes accumulate, and the sensitivity is better than manual agglutination methods. Both EIA and nephelometric methods have greater precision and sensitivity, and because they are automated, they have largely replaced manual methods for detecting RF.[30]

However, since RF testing is not a specific indicator of RA, research led to the development of the anti-CCP assay. Second-generation anti-CCP EIA assays have achieved a sensitivity of 74 percent and a specificity of 96 percent, making it a more reliable indicator of RA than the RF test.[30,38] Approximately 35 to 40 percent of RF-negative patients are positive for anti-CCP, and studies have found that presence of anti-CCP precedes the onset of RA by several years.[31,37] A new rapid anti-CCP2 test on the market appears to be valid and reliable and may help to simplify testing.[39] Anti-CCP together with IgA RF testing appear to be the best predictors for future development of RA.[30,37] Hence, the combination of anti-CCP and RF testing provide useful information in the early and accurate diagnosis of RA.

Once the diagnosis is made, however, the most helpful tests used to follow progress of the disease are general indicators of inflammation, such as measurement of erythrocyte sedimentation rate, C-reactive protein (CRP), and complement components.[34] Typically, CRP and sedimentation rates are elevated, and the level of complement components is normal or increased, indicating increased synthesis. CRP levels correlate well with disease activity, because levels reflect the increase in proinflammatory cytokines.[34] Although not specific, following CRP levels reflects an increase in the inflammatory response and is a more sensitive measure of disease activity than is a change in RF levels.

## Treatment

Traditional therapy for RA has included anti-inflammatory drugs such as salicylates and ibuprofen to control local swelling and pain. The discovery that joint destruction occurs early on during the disease has prompted more aggressive treatment. Disease-modifying antirheumatic drugs (DMARDS)—such as methotrexate, hydroxychloroquine, sulfasalazine, leflunomide, and penicillamine[32,40,41]—are now prescribed if disease activity persists after 4 to 6 weeks of treatment with nonsteroidal anti-inflammatory drugs.[32,40] Corticosteroids such as prednisone cannot be used long-term, but they are given in short oral courses for disease flare-ups. These agents appear to halt the inflammatory response and slow the progression of joint erosion.

A recent development involves treatment with biological agents that block the activity of TNF-α. Agents that act against TNF-α are classified into two categories: (1) monoclonal antibody to TNF-α (infliximab and adalimumab) and (2) TNF-α receptors fused to an IgG molecule (etanercept). All three specifically target and neutralize TNF-α, and they have shown very promising results in halting joint damage without producing major side effects.[40,42–44] Any of the three in combination with methotrexate are very effective in preventing radiological damage.[34]

A new agent, rituximab, specifically targets the CD20 antigen on B cells. Reducing the B-cell population prevents further antibody formation, and this has had a modifying effect on the disease.[45] However, more research is needed to determine possible long-term side effects.

# AUTOIMMUNE THYROID DISEASES

**Autoimmune thyroid diseases (AITDs)** encompass several different clinical conditions, the most notable of which are Hashimoto's thyroiditis and Graves' disease. They represent examples of organic-specific autoimmune diseases. Although these conditions have distinctly different symptoms, they do share some antibodies in common, and both interfere with thyroid function. The thyroid gland is located in the anterior region of the neck and is normally between 12 and 20 grams in size. It consists of units called *follicles* that are spherical in shape and lined with cuboidal epithelial cells. Follicles are filled with material called *colloid*. The primary constituent of colloid is thyroglobulin, a large iodinated glycoprotein, which is the precursor of the thyroid hormones triiodothyronine (T3) and thyroxine (T4).

Under normal conditions, thyrotropin-releasing hormone (TRH) is secreted by the hypothalamus to initiate the process that eventually causes release of hormones from the thyroid. TRH acts on the pituitary to induce release of **thyroid-stimulating hormone (TSH).** TSH, in turn, binds to receptors on the cell membrane of the thyroid gland, causing thyroglobulin to be broken down into secretable T3 and T4. Production of autoantibodies interferes with this process and causes under- or overactivity of the thyroid. It is believed that the autoimmune response to the thyroid seen in these diseases is based on a combination of genetic susceptibility genes coupled with environmental triggers.[46] In the case of Hashimoto's disease, one environmental trigger is a high iodine intake.

## Genetic Predisposition

A genetic predisposition has been postulated for both Hashimoto's thyroiditis and Graves' disease, because the condition is more common in families in which another member has autoimmune thyroid disease. Genes associated with a predisposition to thyroid autoimmunity can be divided into two groups: immune-modulating genes and thyroid-specific genes. The first group includes the following: HLA antigens, cytotoxic T lymphocyte associated factor-4 (CTLA-4), and protein tyrosine phosphatase-22 (PTPN22). The second group includes the thyroglobulin gene and the thyroid-stimulating hormone receptor (TSHR) genes.

The first group of genes enhances the likelihood of an autoimmune response in several different ways. The HLA genes code for the HLA antigens that are responsible for presenting peptides to T cells to initiate an immune response (see Chapter 3). The association of HLA DR3 with Graves' disease is quite strong. It has been found that in the DRβ1 region, an arginine substitution at position number 74 of the beta chain allows for self-antigens to be recognized.[46,47] Association of Hashimoto's thyroiditis with inheritance of HLA antigens DR3, DR4, DR5, and DQw7 (DQb1*0301) has been reported, but this is not consistent among different ethnic populations.[46,48] A unique feature of both Graves' and Hashimoto's diseases is that HLA-DR antigens are expressed on the surface of thyroid epithelial cells, perhaps increasing the autoimmune response.

The CTLA-4 gene codes for a receptor found on T cells, which is responsible for down-regulation of the T-cell-mediated immune response. Polymorphisms in this gene reduce suppression of T cells and increase the likelihood of autoantibody production.[47,49,50] PTPN22 is also found on the surface of T cells and is involved in inhibiting T-cell activation. It is thought that variants in this receptor are responsible for lower T-cell signaling, allowing self-reactive T cells to survive in the thymus and be released to peripheral lymph nodes.[49] This gene is implicated in both Hashimoto's and Graves' disease.

Lastly, mutations in the thyroglobulin gene may allow for interaction with HLA-DR antigens, resulting in antithyroglobulin antibodies, which can be found in Graves' and Hashimoto's diseases.[49] Additionally, in Graves' disease, modifications in the TSHR gene may contribute to the immune system recognizing the receptor, with antibody production resulting.

## Clinical Signs and Immunologic Findings for Hashimoto's Thyroiditis

**Hashimoto's thyroiditis,** also known as *chronic autoimmune thyroiditis*, is most often seen in middle-aged women, although it may occur anywhere from childhood up to about 70 years of age, with the median age of diagnosis being 60.[10,51,52] Women are 5 to 10 times more likely to develop the disease.[53] Patients develop a combination of goiter (or enlarged thyroid), hypothyroidism, and thyroid autoantibodies. The goiter is irregular and rubbery, and immune destruction of the thyroid gland occurs. Symptoms of hypothyroidism include dry skin, decreased sweating, puffy face with edematous eyelids, pallor with a yellow tinge, weight gain, and dry and brittle hair.[51]

The thyroid shows hyperplasia with an increased number of lymphocytes. Cellular types present include activated T and B cells (with T cells predominating), macrophages, and plasma cells. The immune response results in the development of germinal centers that almost completely replace the normal glandular architecture of the thyroid and progressively destroy the thyroid gland.[51] Antibodies to thyroglobulin predominate, progressively destroying thyroglobulin and producing the symptoms associated with hypothyroidism.

## Clinical Signs and Immunologic Findings for Graves' Disease

**Graves' disease,** in contrast to Hashimoto's thyroiditis, is characterized by hyperthyroidism. It is, in fact, the most common cause of hyperthyroidism, affecting approximately 0.5 percent of the population.[54] It is also the most prevalent autoimmune disorder in the United States today.[54] Women exhibit greater susceptibility by a margin of about 10 to 1, and they most often present with the disease between the ages of 20 and 50.[51,52]

The disease is manifested as **thyrotoxicosis,** with a diffusely enlarged goiter that is soft instead of rubbery. Clinical symptoms include nervousness, insomnia, depression, weight loss, heat intolerance, sweating, rapid heartbeat, palpitations, breathlessness, fatigue, cardiac dysrhythmias, and restlessness.[51] Another sign present in approximately 35 percent of patients is exophthalmus, in which hypertrophy of the eye muscles and increased connective tissue in the orbit cause the eyeball to bulge out so that the patient has a large-eyed staring expression **(Fig. 14–4).**[55,56] There is evidence that orbital fibroblasts express TSH receptor-like proteins that are affected by thyroid-stimulating immunoglobulin just as the thyroid is.[55,57] Thus, Graves' disease is now seen as a multiorgan auto-immune disorder, causing hyperthyroidism, ophthalmopathy, and localized edema in the lower legs. The thyroid shows uniform hyperplasia with a patchy lymphocytic infiltration. The follicles have little colloid but are filled with hyperplastic epithelium. A large number of these cells express HLA-DR antigens on their surface in response to interferon (IFN)-λ produced by infiltrating T cells.[54] This allows presentation of self-antigens such as the thyrotropin receptor to activated T cells. B cells, in turn, are stimulated to produce antibody.

The major antibodies found in Graves' disease include **thyroid-stimulating hormone receptor antibody (TSHRab)** and antibodies to thyroid peroxidase. When antigen–antibody combination occurs, it mimics the normal action of TSH and results in receptor stimulation, with the release of thyroid hormones to produce the symptoms of hyperthyroidism. These have been shown to stimulate production of thyroid hormones by increasing cyclic adenosine monophosphate (AMP) levels after binding to receptors.[51,52,58] Thyroid peroxidase antibodies are actually found in both conditions.

An additional autoantibody found in numerous patients is a thyrotropin receptor–blocking antibody that may coexist with thyroid-stimulating antibody.[52,57,58] Depending on the relative activity of blocking and stimulating autoantibodies, patient symptoms may vary from hyperthyroidism to euthyroidism to hypothyroidism.[57] This may confound patient diagnosis.

## Laboratory Testing for Autoimmune Thyroid Diseases

The three major autoantibodies present are antibodies to thyroglobulin, thyroid peroxidase, and TSH receptors. Antibodies to thyroglobulin can be detected in 90 percent of patients with Hashimoto's thyroiditis.[52] Healthy individuals may have a low titer of antithyroglobulin antibody, but in patients with Hashimoto's thyroiditis, the titer is considerably higher, so differentiation can be made in this manner.

Antibodies to thyroglobulin can be demonstrated by indirect immunofluorescent assays, passive agglutination, and EIA.[52,58] Passive hemagglutination using tanned red blood cells is the most commonly used test. Indirect immunofluorescent testing is less sensitive than passive hemagglutination, but it can detect nonagglutinating antibody.[58] Indirect immunofluorescent assays use methanol-fixed monkey cryostat tissue sections as substrate.[52] Thyroglobulin antibodies will create a floccular or puffy staining pattern.

Since antithyroglobulin antibodies are not found in all patients, a negative test result does not necessarily rule out Hashimoto's disease. Other antibodies that may be present include colloid antibody (CA2) and TSH-binding inhibitory immunoglobulin. Antibody activity contributes to the destruction of thyroid cells. Antibody to CA2 produces a diffuse or ground-glass appearance.

Antibodies to thyroid peroxidase (TPO) are directed against a 105 kD membrane enzyme that catalyzes tyrosine iodination. They are found in approximately 90 to 95 percent of patients with the disease.[51] They seem to correlate most closely with disease activity. Antibodies to peroxidase are most commonly measured by EIA, although IIF and particle agglutination assays are also used.[48,52] Peroxidase antibodies produce staining of the cytoplasm and not the nucleus of thyroid cells. These antibodies can be found in approximately 90 percent of patients with Hashimoto's disease and 80 percent of patients with Graves' disease, so the two cannot be distinguished on the basis of this test.[53,58]

The third major autoantibody, anti-TSHR antibody, is typically associated with Graves' disease. However, because testing is difficult and expensive, elevation of the thyroid hormones and free triiodothyronine (T3) and thyroxine (T4) is checked for first if this disease is suspected. In addition, TSH levels can be determined and are low because of antibody stimulation of the thyroid. Increased uptake of radioactive iodine also helps to confirm the diagnosis.[59]

Measurement of thyroid receptor antibodies is done only when results of these assays are unclear. Tests for TSHR antibodies are of two types: bioassays and binding assays. Bioassays require tissue culture and thus are difficult to perform.[48,54,58] Binding assays are based on competition between radiolabeled TSH and patient autoantibodies for binding to thyrotropin receptors. Approximately 80 percent of

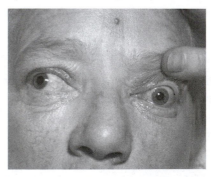

**FIGURE 14–4.** Exophthalmus indicative of Graves' disease. *(Courtesy of CDC/Dr. Sellers/Emory University.)*

patients with Graves' hyperthyroidism test positive by this method.[53,54] This may be due in part to the lack of sensitivity of these assays.[48]

A different type of anti-TSHR antibodies can be found in Hashimoto's thyroiditis. These antibodies are likely directed against a different epitope than the above antibodies, as they serve to block the receptors so that the TSH hormone cannot bind.[48]

## Treatment for Autoimmune Thyroid Diseases

Treatment for Hashimoto's disease consists of thyroid hormone replacement therapy. TSH levels should be monitored throughout treatment.[51] Several different protocols are used in the treatment of Graves' disease. In the United States, the first line of treatment involves radioactive iodine, which emits beta particles that are locally destructive within an area of a few millimeters. This is given for 1 to 2 years, and it results in a 30 to 50 percent long-term remission rate.[57] Some patients, however, become hypothyroidal within 5 years, so continued monitoring is essential. In Europe, the patient is first placed on antithyroid medications such as methimazole, carbimazole, or propylthiouracil with beta blockers as adjuvant therapy.[51,57] Surgery to remove part of the thyroid may also be considered as an alternative.

## TYPE I DIABETES MELLITUS

Autoimmune diabetes mellitus, now termed type IA diabetes, is a chronic autoimmune disease that occurs in a genetically susceptible individual as a result of environmental factors.[60] Approximately 10 percent of patients with diabetes mellitus have the immune-mediated form of the disease.[58] It is characterized by insufficient insulin production caused by selective destruction of the beta cells of the pancreas. Beta cells are located in the pancreas in clusters called the *islets of Langerhans*. Unlike other autoimmune endocrine diseases, hormone replacement cannot be given orally, and chronic vascular complications result in major morbidity and mortality.

Family studies indicate that there is an inherited genetic susceptibility to the disease, probably attributable to multiple genes. Approximately 90 percent of white diabetics carry the HLA-DR3 or DR4 gene.[61] There appears to be an increased risk when both of these genes are present. However, recent research indicates that the true susceptibility genes for **type I diabetes mellitus** may occur in the HLA-DQ region, especially in the coding of the DQβ chain. As discussed in Chapter 3, HLA antigens are made up of two separate protein chains, α and β. Both of these chains are involved in antigen recognition. Within the β chain, substitutions for the amino acid 57, aspartic acid, are associated with increasing risk for diabetes. This amino acid position is adjacent to the antigen-binding groove and may affect the structure and function of the binding site.[62]

This correlation is strongest with haplotypes DQA1*0301/DQB1*0302 and DQA1*0501/DQB1*0201.[61,63] About 90 percent of the Caucasian population with type I diabetes mellitus have DQB1*0302 and/or DQB1*0201 compared with less than 40 percent in the normal population.[63]

Environmental influences include the possibility of viral infections and early exposure to cow's milk.[61] Studies have attempted to link viruses, especially rubella virus, cytomegalovirus, and Coxsackie B4 virus with diabetes, but most research is inconclusive. Antibody production could possibly be initiated as a result of molecular mimicry, with a virus as the stimulating antigen triggering antibody production against a self-antigen.

## Immunopathology

Progressive inflammation of the islets of Langerhans in the pancreas leads to fibrosis and destruction of most beta cells. The subclinical period may last for years, and only when 80 percent or more of the beta cells are destroyed does hyperglycemia become evident. Immunohistochemical staining of inflamed islets shows a preponderance of CD8+ lymphocytes, along with plasma cells and macrophages.[61] B cells themselves may act as antigen-presenting cells, stimulating activation of CD4+ lymphocytes.[64] A shift to a Th1 response causes production of certain cytokines, including TNF-α, IFN-λ, and IL-1. The generalized inflammation that results is responsible for the destruction of beta cells. Although islet autoantibodies trigger the immune response, it is not known what role they play in cell destruction. There is increasing evidence that autoimmunity to insulin itself may be central to disease pathogenesis.[64] Cell death, however, is likely caused by apoptosis and attack by cytotoxic lymphocytes.

It is apparent that autoantibody production precedes the development of type IA diabetes mellitus by up to several years. Autoantibodies are present in prediabetic individuals (i.e., those who are being monitored because they have a high risk of developing diabetes) and in newly diagnosed patients.[58] Antibody production diminishes with time, however. Among the antibodies found are antibodies to two tyrosine phosphatase-like transmembrane proteins called *insulinoma antigen 2* (IA-2 or ICA 512) and IA-2βA (phogrin); anti-insulin antibodies; antibodies to the enzyme GAD; and antibodies to various other islet cell proteins, called *islet cell antibodies (ICAs)*.[52,58,65]

## Laboratory Testing

Although type I diabetes mellitus is usually diagnosed by the prime characteristic of hyperglycemia, it may be useful to have serological tests to screen for diabetes before beta-cell destruction occurs to the extent necessary to cause symptoms. Antibodies to islet cells have traditionally been detected by IIF using frozen sections of human pancreas.[52] ICAs have been reported in the sera of greater than 80 percent of patients newly diagnosed with type I diabetes mellitus.[52,61] However, such assays are rather cumbersome to perform, and current formats are available using radioimmunobinding assays.[58] Antibodies to insulin can be detected using RIA or EIA methods. RIA and EIA are also used to detect anti-GAD antibodies and anti–IA-2 antibodies.[58] Combined screening for IA-2A, ICA, and GAD antibodies appears to have the most sensitivity and best positive predictive value for type IA diabetes mellitus in high-risk populations.[52,58]

## Treatment

The use of injected insulin has been the mainstay of therapy for diabetes. However, new trials center around the use of immunosuppressive agents. Cyclosporin A, azathioprine, and prednisone have all been used to inhibit the immune response. All have potentially toxic side effects. Limited trials in humans using a small peptide self-antigen called a *heat shock protein* for immunization indicate that beta-cell destruction can be halted in this manner.[66] Research using anti-CD20 (rituximab) to cause B-cell depletion has been conducted and has the potential to decrease antibody production.[67] Growth factors or transplantation of beta islet cells may also be of use in the future.

## OTHER DISEASES

Other organ-specific diseases that appear to have an autoimmune etiology include multiple sclerosis (MS), myasthenia gravis (MG), and Goodpasture's syndrome. MS and MG are disorders of the nervous system, while Goodpasture's syndrome is responsible for glomerulonephritis. Each of these is discussed briefly. **Table 14–3** lists additional diseases for which there appears to be an autoimmune cause.

## Multiple Sclerosis

**Multiple sclerosis (MS)** is an inflammatory autoimmune disorder of the central nervous system, affecting approximately 350,000 Americans and 1.1 million individuals worldwide.[68,69] It is characterized by the formation of lesions called *plaques* in the white matter of the brain and spinal cord, resulting in the progressive destruction of the myelin sheath of axons. Plaques vary in size from 1 or 2 mm up to several centimeters.[68] As is the case for most other autoimmune diseases, a combination of genetic and environmental factors is responsible for development of this condition. Although there are probably several independent loci, MS is most closely associated with inheritance of a particular HLA molecule coding for the beta chain of DR, namely DRB1*1501.[70] It has been theorized that the inflammatory response is triggered by molecular mimicry, in which viral or other foreign peptides are presented in the groove of specific HLA class II molecules to T cells. Once initiated, the immune response becomes directed against self-antigens that are indistinguishable from the original foreign antigen.[69] Some studies indicate that patients with MS have four times the blood concentration of antibody to EBV as was found in a control population.[71] Other viruses possibly implicated are measles, herpes simplex, varicella, rubella, influenza C, human herpes virus-6, and some parainfluenza viruses.[68] There appears to be an additional genetic link to polymorphisms in the gene coding for the interleukin-7 receptor.[72] IL-7 may be involved in the generation of autoreactive T cells in this disease.

Damage to the tissue of the central nervous system can cause visual disturbances, weakness or diminished dexterity in one or more limbs, locomotor incoordination, dizziness,

| Table 14–3. | Other Autoimmune Diseases | |
|---|---|---|
| **DISEASE** | **ORGAN OR TISSUE** | **IMMUNOLOGIC MANIFESTATIONS** |
| Addison's disease | Adrenal glands | Antibody to adrenal cells |
| Autoimmune hemolytic anemia | Red blood cells | Antibody to red blood cells |
| Autoimmune thrombocytopenic purpura | Platelets | Antiplatelet antibody |
| Crohn's disease | Intestines | Inflammatory infiltrate of T and B cells: mechanism unknown |
| Disseminated encephalomyelitis | Central nervous system | Sensitized T cells |
| Pernicious anemia | Stomach | Parietal cell antibody, intrinsic factor antibody |
| Poststreptococcal glomerulonephritis | Kidney | Streptococcal antibodies that cross-react with kidney tissue |
| Rheumatic fever | Heart | Streptococcal antibodies that cross-react with heart tissue |
| Scleroderma | Connective tissue | Antinuclear antibodies: anti-Scl-70, anticentromere antibody |
| Sjögren's syndrome | Eyes, mouth | Antinuclear antibodies, RA factor antisalivary duct antibodies, antilacrimal gland antibodies |
| Sarcoidosis | Multisystem granulomas, pulmonary manifestations | Activation of T lymphocytes |

facial palsy, and numerous sensory abnormalities such as tingling or "pins and needles" that run down the spine or extremities and flashes of light seen on eye movement.[69] The disease is most often seen in young and middle-aged adults between the ages of 20 and 40, and it is twice as common in women as in men.[68] Typically, 50 to 70 percent of patients alternate between remissions and relapses for many years, while the remainder follow a chronic progressive course.[52]

Within the plaques, T cells and macrophages predominate, and they are believed to orchestrate demyelination.[68] Antibody binds to the myelin membrane and may initiate the immune response, stimulating macrophages and specialized phagocytes called *microglial cells*.[69] The cascade of immunologic events results in acute inflammation, injury to axons and glia, structural repair with recovery of some function, and then postinflammatory neurodegeneration.[69] Activated T cells must penetrate into the central nervous system to begin the response. They may do so by inducing changes in the endothelium that allows them to penetrate the blood–brain barrier, while vessel walls remain intact.[68] Cytokines IL-1, TNF-$\alpha$, and IFN-$\lambda$ have been thought to be central to the pathogenesis observed, thus implicating Th1 cells.[68] However, a Th2 response, characterized by production of interleukin-4 (IL-4), interleukin-5 (IL-5), and IL-10 may also contribute to pathogenesis.[68]

The two most common tests for diagnosis of MS are oligoclonal banding and the CSF IgG index. Immunoglobulin is increased in the spinal fluid in 75 to 90 percent of patients with MS, producing several distinct bands on protein electrophoresis that are not seen in the serum. These are called *oligoclonal bands*, and there may be as many as eight, but presence of at least four bands is indicative of MS.[73] Isoelectric focusing with immunoblotting is also used to identify these bands, and it is thought to be more sensitive than protein electrophoresis.[73] A measure of the IgG index, which compares the amount of IgG in spinal fluid to that of serum, may also be useful in making a diagnosis even though it is not specific for MS.

While there is not one specific antibody that is diagnostic for MS, a large percentage of patients produce antibody directed against a myelin basic protein peptide.[74] Other antibodies are directed against components of oligodendrocytes and against myelin membranes, but the majority of antibodies have yet to be identified.[69] Magnetic resonance imaging that shows damage at two or more individual sites in the central nervous system is also used to aid in diagnosis.

Many healthy individuals have antibodies that bind with low affinity, but antibody with high-affinity binding is found only in disease states. There is no one specific therapy, but newer treatment for relapsing-remitting MS centers around three drugs: IFN-$\beta$1a (Avonex, Rebif), IFN-$\beta$1b (Betaseron), and glatiramer acetate.[68,69] These are believed to work by causing down-regulation of MHC molecules on antigen-presenting cells and down-regulating production of proinflammatory cytokines.[68] Acute exacerbations are treated with methylprednisolone, but this cannot be used on a long-term basis. Other immunosuppressive drugs that appear to lessen the severity of symptoms include azathioprine, methotrexate, and cyclophosphamide.[75]

## Myasthenia Gravis

**Myasthenia gravis (MG)** is an autoimmune disease that affects the neuromuscular junction. It is characterized by weakness and fatigability of skeletal muscles. It occurs in 20 people per 100,000 annually, and the incidence appears to be increasing, especially in individuals over the age of 60.[76–78] Antibody-mediated damage to the acetylcholine receptors in skeletal muscle leads to this progressive muscle weakness. Early signs are drooping of the eyelids and the inability to retract the corners of the mouth, often resulting in a snarling appearance.[76,77,79] Other symptoms may include difficulty in speaking, chewing, and swallowing, and inability to maintain support of the trunk, the neck, or the head.[52] If respiratory muscle weakness occurs, it can be life-threatening.[77] Onset of symptoms can be acute, or they may develop and worsen over time.

MG is often associated with the presence of other autoimmune diseases, such as SLE, RA, pernicious anemia, and thyroiditis. Early onset disease, which is usually defined as occurring before the age of 40, appears to be linked to several HLA antigens, A1, B8, and DR3.[77,79] In this age group, the disease is seen more frequently in women and peaks in the third decade of life. Late-onset MG, presenting in patients older than 40, is linked to HLA antigens B7 and DR2 and is more likely to appear in men between the ages of 30 and 60.[76–78] Thymic hyperplasia is seen in 75 percent of patients, and this can lead to thymoma, a tumor of the thymus.

Approximately 80 to 85 percent of patients have antibody to ACH receptors, and this appears to be the main contributor to the pathogenesis of the disease.[52,76,78,79] Normally, ACH is released from nerve endings to generate an action potential that causes the muscle fiber to contract. It is believed that when the antibody combines with the receptor site, binding of ACH is blocked, and the receptors are destroyed because of the action of antibody and complement[79] **(Fig. 14–5)**. In the 15 percent of patients lacking this antibody, other antibodies are present, including antimuscle-specific kinase (MuSK).[77] Current research indicates that T regulatory cells may be impaired, allowing an immune response to occur that is characterized by Th1 cells producing inflammatory cytokines IL-2, IFN-$\gamma$, and TNF-$\alpha$.[79]

RIA procedures are used to detect antibody, based on assays that block the binding of receptors by anti-ACH receptor (ACHR) antibody. A radio-labeled snake venom called $\alpha$-bungarotoxin is used to irreversibly bind to ACHRs; precipitation of receptors caused by combination with antibody is then measured.[52]

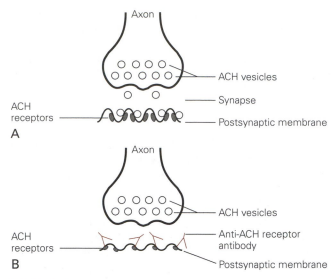

**FIGURE 14–5.** Mechanism of immunologic injury in MG. *(A)* Normal nerve impulse transmission. ACH is released from the axon and taken up by receptors on the postsynaptic membrane. *(B)* In MG, antibodies to the ACH receptors are formed, blocking transmission of nerve impulses.

Anticholinesterase agents are used as the main treatment therapy.[76] Thymectomy is beneficial to some patients, especially those younger than 60 with early onset disease, but there is some question about its overall benefits.[80] Corticosteroids such as azathioprine and cyclosporine are effective, as is etanercept, which inhibits the action of TNF-α.[79]

## Goodpasture's Syndrome

Goodpasture's syndrome is characterized by the presence of autoantibody to glomerular, renal tubular, and alveolar basement membranes, resulting primarily in injury to the glomerulus that can rapidly progress to renal failure. This rare disorder occurs with an annual incidence of approximately 0.5 per million.[81] Between 50 and 70 percent of patients also exhibit pulmonary hemorrhage resulting from interaction of antibody with basement membranes found in lung tissue. In contrast with other autoimmune diseases, Goodpasture's syndrome is more likely to occur in young males between the ages of 18 and 35.[81–83] Often it follows a viral infection. The mortality rate may be as high as 50 percent.[83]

Severe necrosis of the glomerulus is triggered by an antibody that has specificity for the noncollagenous region of the alpha 3 chain of type IV collagen.[81,82,84] This autoantibody reacts with collagen in the glomerular or alveolar basement membranes. Immune deposits accumulate, and complement fixation causes injury because of the release of oxygen species and proteolytic enzymes. These immune reactants progressively destroy the renal tubular, glomerular, and pulmonary alveolar basement membranes. Signs of renal involvement include gross or microscopic hematuria,

proteinuria, a decreased 24-hour creatinine clearance, and an increase in blood urea and serum creatinine levels. Pulmonary symptoms include hemorrhage, dyspnea, weakness, fatigue, and cough.

This syndrome differs from glomerulonephritis as a result of the nonspecific accumulation of circulating immune complexes found in other autoimmune diseases, because specific antibasement antibodies can be demonstrated by formation of a smooth, linear ribbonlike pattern on direct immunofluorescent assay of glomerular basement membrane from patients with the disease.[81] Greater than 90 percent of patients with Goodpasture's nephritis test positive for presence of this antibody. Although little is known about the circumstances that trigger the autoimmune response, 80 percent of those affected carry the HLA-DR15 or DR4 alleles, indicating a genetic predisposition. This is the case in most other autoimmune diseases.

Circulating antibodies can be detected by RIA, EIA, and IIF assay. The IIF assay, long held as the standard, uses frozen kidney sections that are incubated with patient serum and then overlaid with a fluorescein-labeled anti-IgG. It is often hard to interpret and has a high percentage of false-positive and false-negative results.[84] A Western blot technique has been developed, which separates out basement membrane antigens by polyacrylamide gel electrophoresis followed by transfer to nitrocellulose paper for immunoblotting. This is often used as a confirmatory test, because it appears to be the most sensitive and the most specific immunoassay.[84] An EIA technique, which uses the alpha 3 subunit to detect antibody, has also been developed, but it is less sensitive than the Western blot.[84] About 20 percent of patients also have low titers of ANAs, which usually exhibit the perinuclear staining pattern.

Current treatment strategies focus on removal of circulating antibodies by plasmapheresis or dialysis, or use of immunosuppressive agents such as glucocorticoids, cyclophosphamide, and azathioprine.[81] The sooner therapy is initiated, the more likely it is that renal failure can be prevented.

## SUMMARY

Autoimmune diseases result from a loss of self-tolerance, a delicate balance set up in the body to restrict the activity of T and B lymphocytes. Self-tolerance is maintained in two major ways: (1) by deleting potentially reactive B and T cells as they mature in the bone marrow and thymus, respectively, and (2) by peripheral tolerance, which occurs in the secondary lymphoid organs. Peripheral tolerance depends on the actions of T regulatory cells, which help to curtail a response to self-antigens. However, sometimes a combination of genetic and environmental factors work together to allow reactions to self-antigens to occur. Self-antigens become recognized in conjunction with certain MHC antigens, and it is here that genetic factors come into play. The shape of particular class II MHC molecules allows recognition to take place. Molecular mimicry in which foreign viral or bacterial agents resemble self-antigens may trigger antibodies that in turn react with self-antigens. Such agents may also act as polyclonal activators, turning on several clones of B cells. Each clone of B cells can manufacture a different type of antibody. Thus, environmental factors also play a role.

Autoimmune diseases can be classified as organ-specific or systemic, depending on whether tissue destruction is localized or affects multiple organs. SLE and RA are examples of systemic diseases, while Hashimoto's thyroiditis, Graves' disease, type I diabetes mellitus, MS, MG, and Goodpasture's syndrome are considered organ-specific diseases.

SLE is a chronic inflammatory disease characterized by joint involvement, an erythematous rash that appears on exposure to sunlight, and deposition of immune complexes in the kidney to cause glomerulonephritis. Autoantibodies include anti–ds-DNA, anti-DNP, antihistone, anti-Sm, anti-nRNP, anticytoplasmic, antinucleolar, and antiphospholipid antibodies. Each of these exhibits specific staining patterns in the fluorescent antibody screening test for this disease.

RA affects the synovial lining of joints; necrotic areas are surrounded by granulation tissue that eventually leads to joint disintegration. The main immunologic finding is the presence of an antibody called RF. This is typically a 19S antibody directed against IgG. Several other autoantibodies contribute to the inflammation observed in the joints, including an autoantibody called anti-CCP, directed against cyclic citrullinated proteins. Diagnosis of RA is made on the basis of clinical manifestations, a positive RF test result, and a positive anti-CCP test.

Hashimoto's thyroiditis is an organ-specific condition that affects the thyroid gland and causes it to be enlarged and rubbery. Lymphocyte infiltration in the thyroid with the presence of antithyroglobulin antibody leads to gradual thyroid destruction. Clinical symptoms are consistent with hypothyroidism. Laboratory assays focus on detection of two major antibodies, antithyroglobulin and antiperoxidase, which are measured by RIA, IIF, and agglutination.

The hyperthyroidism that is evident in Graves' disease produces symptoms such as nervousness, insomnia, weight loss, heat intolerance, sweating, rapid heartbeat, cardiac dysrhythmias, and bulging eyeballs. Thyroid stimulating hormone receptor antibodies (TSHRab) bind to receptors, causing continuous release of thyroid hormones. Elevated levels of thyroid hormones are the key laboratory findings, and testing for autoantibodies is done only when results of hormone assays are unclear.

While there are a number of causes of diabetes, type IA diabetes mellitus has an autoimmune origin. Genetic susceptibility appears to lie within the DQ region of the MHC group. Viral infections may provide the trigger for the autoimmune response. The progressive destruction of beta cells in the pancreas results in a lack of insulin production and symptoms of hyperglycemia. Antibodies to two transmembrane proteins, ICA 512 and IA-2βA; to the enzyme GAD; and to insulin can be detected by means of RIA or EIA. These can be important predictors of disease in high-risk populations.

MS is characterized by visual disturbances, weakness in the extremities, locomotor incoordination, and sensory abnormalities. T cells initiate a chain of events that include both antibody and cytokine production that progressively destroys the myelin sheath of axons and damages oligodendrocytes, causing lesions called plaques. Antibodies directed against myelin basic protein and against myelin oligodendrocyte glycoprotein are produced, but these are not diagnostic, because they are not present in all cases of disease. Protein electrophoresis of cerebrospinal fluid that shows two or more bands not present in serum is helpful in making a diagnosis. The IgG index, a measure of the ratio of antibody in the spinal fluid to that in the serum, may also be useful.

Another disease affecting the nervous system is MG. Extreme muscle weakness results from the presence of antibody to ACH receptors. By combining with the receptor site, antibody blocks the binding of ACH, and the receptors are destroyed as a result of complement activation. RIA procedures can be used to detect antibody, based on binding assays with ACH receptors.

Goodpasture's syndrome is characterized by severe necrosis of the glomerulus triggered by an antibody that reacts with glycoprotein in the glomerular basement membrane. The result is glomerulonephritis, in which immune deposits accumulate and complement fixation causes injury to the tissue, eventually producing renal failure. This antibody can also react with basement membrane in lung tissue, producing pulmonary hemorrhage. Antibasement antibody is usually detected by IIF, RIA, or EIA.

These examples represent a sampling of the autoimmune diseases for which some of the responsible immunologic mechanisms have been discovered. There is a common thread in all of the diseases covered in this chapter: They are the result of a combination of genetic and environmental factors. It appears that the MHC antigens recognized by T cells are a key factor in whether a response will be mounted to a particular self-antigen. Small changes in amino acid sequences change the shape of the receptor and allow self-antigen to be recognized. Environmental factors, probably in the nature of viral or bacterial infections, trigger an inflammatory response that polyclonally activates T and B cells. As more is learned about the mechanisms that trigger autoimmune responses, it may be possible to specifically turn off those responses without affecting the rest of the immune system.

# CASE STUDIES

A 25-year-old female consulted her physician because she had been experiencing symptoms of weight loss, joint pain in the hands, and extreme fatigue. Her laboratory results were as follows: RA slide test positive at 1:10; ANA slide test positive at 1:40; red blood cell count $3.5 \times 10^{12}$ per L (normal is 4.1 to $5.1 \times 10^{12}$ per L); white blood cell count $5.8 \times 10^9$ per L (normal is 4.5 to $11 \times 10^9$ per L).

## Questions

a. What is a possible explanation for positive results on both the RA test and the ANA test?

b. What is the most likely cause of the decreased red blood cell count?

c. What further testing would help the physician distinguish between RA and SLE?

A 40-year-old female went to her doctor because she was feeling tired all the time. She had gained about 10 pounds in the last few months and exhibited some facial puffiness. Her thyroid gland was enlarged and rubbery. Laboratory results indicated a normal red and white blood cell count, but her T4 level was decreased, and an assay for antithyroglobulin antibody was positive.

## Questions

a. What do these results likely indicate?

b. What effect do antithyroglobulin antibodies have on thyroid function?

c. How can this condition be differentiated from Graves' disease?

# EXERCISE

## RAPID SLIDE TEST FOR ANTINUCLEOPROTEIN ANTIBODY FOUND IN SYSTEMIC LUPUS ERYTHEMATOSUS

### Principle

Antibodies to DNP, a histone associated with DNA, are found in over 90 percent of patients with SLE. They are the most common antinuclear antibodies encountered in lupus. Although they are not specific for lupus, testing for their presence is a helpful screening procedure. In this test system, latex particles are coated with DNP extracted from calf thymus. When combined with patient serum containing antibody to DNP, visible agglutination occurs.

### Specimen Collection

Collect blood by venipuncture, using aseptic technique and avoiding hemolysis. Hemolyzed or contaminated serum may give erroneous results and should not be used. Allow the blood to clot for at least 10 minutes at room temperature. Serum should be removed and refrigerated if not tested immediately. Specimens can be kept at 2°C to 8°C for up to 72 hours. If longer storage is required, the sample may be frozen and tested at a later time. Avoid repeated freezing and thawing. Plasma should not be used for this procedure.

### Reagents, Materials, and Equipment

Reagent test kit such as Seradyn SLE or Immunoscan SLE, which contains the following:

SLE test reagent-latex particles coated with DNP

SLE positive control

SLE negative control

Glass agglutination slide

Capillary pipettes

Applicator sticks

Other materials required but not provided:

Serological pipettes or automatic pipettes and tips

Timer

Physiological saline (0.85 or 0.9 percent sodium chloride)

Disposable test tubes (12 × 75 mm)

Test tube rack

CAUTION: The reagent test kit contains sodium azide. Azides are reported to react with lead to form compounds that may detonate on percussion. When disposing of solutions containing sodium azide, flush with large volumes of water to minimize the buildup of metal azide compounds.

Sera used for controls were negative when tested for hepatitis B surface antigen and HIV by FDA-required test. However, the controls should be handled with the same precautions as those used in handling human sera.

### Procedure*

#### Qualitative Test

1. Bring all reagents and test samples to room temperature before use.
2. Gently mix the SLE test reagent to disperse and suspend the latex particles in the buffer. Avoid vigorous shaking.
3. Thoroughly clean a glass slide before use. The slide should be washed with detergent, rinsed with deionized water, and dried with a lint-free tissue.
4. Using a capillary pipette provided, place 1 drop (50 μL) of patient specimen in one section of the glass slide. Hold the capillary perpendicular to the slide to deliver a full drop of specimen.
5. Place 1 drop of positive control in the left section of the slide and 1 drop of negative control in the right section by inverting the appropriate dropper vial and squeezing out 1 drop onto the test slide.
6. Using the dropper, add 1 drop of the SLE reagent to each of the divisions containing specimen and controls.
7. Mix each section with a disposable applicator stick, spreading each mixture over the entire section. Use a clean applicator stick for each section.
8. Tilt the slide slowly back and forth for 3 minutes. Read immediately for agglutination under direct light.
9. Positive specimens should be diluted and retested.

#### Quantitative Test

1. Bring all reagents and test samples to room temperature before use.
2. Using physiological saline, dilute specimens 1:2, 1:4, 1:8, 1:16, 1:32, or as needed.
3. Gently mix the SLE test reagent to disperse and suspend the latex particles in the buffer. Avoid vigorous shaking.
4. Using a capillary pipette provided, place 1 drop (50 μL) of each dilution on successive fields of the reaction slide. Hold the capillary perpendicular to the slide to deliver a full drop of specimen each time.
5. Place 1 drop of positive control in the left section of the slide and 1 drop of negative control in the right section by inverting the appropriate dropper vial and squeezing out 1 drop onto the test slide.
6. Mix each section with a disposable applicator stick, spreading each mixture over the entire section. Use a clean applicator stick for each section.

* Adapted from the package insert from Seradyn Seratest for SLE, Remel, Lenexa, KS 66215.

7. Tilt the slide slowly back and forth for 3 minutes. Read immediately for agglutination under direct light.

## Results and Interpretation

The negative control should give a smooth or slightly granular suspension with no agglutination, while the positive control should form a visible agglutination reaction distinctly different from the slight granularity observed with the negative control. This test will be positive for over 90 percent of patients with untreated SLE. However, it may also be positive with other diseases such as RA, scleroderma, chronic liver disease, and progressive systemic sclerosis. Antinuclear antibodies can also be found in about 10 percent of the normal healthy population, but typically the titer is too low in individuals under the age of 60 to produce a positive agglutination test. A positive reaction in this test indicates that the level of antinuclear antibody is in the range commonly found in SLE. This is a screening test, and clinical manifestations and laboratory results must be taken into account when a diagnosis is made.

# EXERCISE

## SLIDE AGGLUTINATION TEST FOR THE DETECTION OF RHEUMATOID FACTOR

### Principle

RF is an IgM antibody directed against IgG. It is found in 70 to 80 percent of patients with RA. Passive agglutination can be employed to test for the presence of the antibody, using a carrier particle such as sheep erythrocytes sensitized with IgG. When patient serum containing RF is mixed with the sensitized reagent cells, visible agglutination occurs.

### Specimen Collection

Collect blood by venipuncture, using aseptic technique and avoiding hemolysis. Allow the blood to clot for at least 10 minutes at room temperature. Loosen the clot with a wooden applicator stick, and centrifuge at 1000 g for 10 minutes or until the supernatant is free of cells. Serum should be removed and tested immediately. Specimens may be kept refrigerated for up to 24 hours. For longer storage, freeze specimens at –20°C. Avoid repeated freezing and thawing. Plasma should not be used.

### Reagents, Materials, and Equipment

Reagent test kit such as Rheumaton Kit, which contains the following:

Stabilized sheep erythrocytes sensitized with rabbit gamma globulin

Positive control

Negative control

Calibrated capillary tubes with rubber bulbs

Glass slide

Other materials needed:

Disposable stirrers

Distilled water or isotonic saline

Test tubes, 12 × 75 mm

Centrifuge capable of 1000 g

Serological pipettes or automatic pipettes and tips

Timer

> **CAUTION:** The reagent test kit contains sodium azide. Azides are reported to react with lead to form compounds that may detonate on percussion. When disposing of solutions containing sodium azide, flush with large volumes of water to minimize the buildup of metal azide compounds.
>
> Sera used for controls were negative when tested for hepatitis B surface antigen and HIV by FDA-required test. However, the controls should be handled with the same precautions as those used in handling human sera.

### PROCEDURE*

1. Bring all reagents and test samples to room temperature before use.
2. Fill a capillary to the mark with patient serum, and empty it into the center of the middle section of the slide.
3. Place 1 drop of positive control in the left section of the slide and 1 drop of negative control in the right section.
4. Add 1 drop of well-shaken reagent to each section of the slide.
5. Mix with a disposable stirrer, spreading each mixture over the entire section. Use a clean disposable stirrer for each mixture.
6. Rock the slide gently with a rotary motion for 2 minutes and immediately observe for agglutination. If the test is positive for agglutination, dilute the specimen 1:10 with distilled water or isotonic saline, and repeat the test.

### Quantitative Procedure

If a titer is desired, the following procedure can be used:

1. Label eight 12 × 75 mm test tubes 1 through 8 and place in a test tube rack.
2. Add 1.8 mL of saline to tube 1 and 1.0 mL of saline to tubes 2 through 8.
3. Add 0.2 mL of specimen to tube 1, mix, and transfer 1.0 mL of this mixture to tube 2. Mix the contents of tube 2 and transfer 1.0 mL of this mixture to tube 3. Continue serially diluting in this manner through tube 8. Starting with a 1:10 dilution in the first tube, the dilution in the final tube will be 1:1280.
4. Test each dilution as described in the qualitative procedure. The last dilution to show positive agglutination is reported as the titer.

### Results and Interpretation

Positive specimens show readily visible agglutination, while negative specimens show no agglutination or a finely granular pattern. If agglutination is positive in only the undiluted specimen, this represents a very low titer that might be present in a variety of other diseases. Some of these other diseases are SLE; endocarditis; tuberculosis; syphilis; viral infections; and diseases of the liver, lung, or kidney. In addition, low titer can be found in approximately 1 percent of healthy individuals. Thus, a positive test is not specific for RA.

Conversely, a negative test does not rule out RA, because approximately 25 percent of patients with the disease test negative for RF. The results of this simple screening test for RA must be interpreted in the light of clinical symptoms.

---

* Adapted from the package insert for the Rheumaton Test with permission from Inverness Medical, Waltham, MA.

# REVIEW QUESTIONS

1. All of the following may contribute to autoimmunity *except*

   a. clonal deletion of self-reactive T cells.
   b. molecular mimicry.
   c. new expression of class II MHC antigens.
   d. polyclonal activation of B cells.

2. Which of the following would be considered an organ-specific autoimmune disease?

   a. SLE
   b. RA
   c. Hashimoto's thyroiditis
   d. Goodpasture's syndrome

3. SLE can be distinguished from RA on the basis of which of the following?

   a. Joint pain
   b. Presence of antinuclear antibodies
   c. Immune complex formation with activation of complement
   d. Presence of anti-ds DNA antibodies

4. Which of the following would support a diagnosis of drug-induced lupus?

   a. Antihistone antibodies
   b. Antibodies to Smith antigen
   c. Presence of RF
   d. Antibodies to SS-A and SS-B antigens

5. A homogeneous pattern of staining of the nucleus on IIF may be caused by which of the following antibodies?

   a. Anti-Sm antibody
   b. Anti-SSA/Ro antibody
   c. Antihistone antibody
   d. Anti–double-stranded DNA

6. Which of the following is characteristic of RA?

   a. Association with certain HLA-DR genes
   b. Joint involvement that is symmetric
   c. Presence of antibody against IgG
   d. All of the above

7. Which of the following best describes the slide agglutination test for RF?

   a. It is specific for RA.
   b. A negative test rules out the possibility of RA.
   c. It is a sensitive screening tool.
   d. It detects IgG made against IgM.

8. Hashimoto's thyroiditis can best be differentiated from Graves' disease on the basis of which of the following?

   a. Decrease in thyroid hormone levels
   b. Presence of thyroid peroxidase antibodies
   c. Enlargement of the thyroid
   d. Presence of lymphocytes in the thyroid

9. Which of the following would be considered a significant finding in Graves' disease?

   a. Increased TSH levels
   b. Antibody to TSHR
   c. Decreased T3 and T4
   d. Antithyroglobulin antibody

10. Immunologic findings in type I diabetes mellitus include all of the following *except*

    a. presence of CD8 T cells in the islets of Langerhans.
    b. antibody to colloid.
    c. antibody to insulin.
    d. antibody to GAD.

11. Destruction of the myelin sheath of axons caused by the presence of antibody is characteristic of which disease?

    a. MS
    b. MG
    c. Graves' disease
    d. Goodpasture's syndrome

12. Blood was drawn from a 25-year-old woman with suspected SLE. A FANA screen was performed, and a speckled pattern resulted. Which of the following actions should be taken next?

    a. Report out as diagnostic for SLE
    b. Report out as drug-induced lupus
    c. Perform an antibody profile
    d. Repeat the test

# References

1. Kindt, TJ, Goldsby, RA, and Osborne, BA. Kuby Immunology, ed. 6. WH Freeman, New York, 2007, pp. 401–424.
2. Anolik, JH. B cell biology and dysfunction in SLE. Bull NYU Hosp Jt Dis 665:182–186, 2007.
3. Whitacre, CC, Blankenhorn, E, and Brinley, Jr, FJ, et al. Sex differences in autoimmune disease: Focus on multiple sclerosis. Science Magazine. Available at http://www.sciencemag.org/feature/data/983519.shl. Accessed July 20, 2002.
4. Ruiz-Irastorza, G, Khamashta, MA, and Castellino, G, et al. Systemic lupus erythematosus. Lancet 357:1027–1032, 2001.
5. Hahn, BH. Systemic lupus erythematosus. In Kasper, DL, Braunwald, E, Fauci, AE, Hauser, SL, et al. (eds): Harrison's Principles of Internal Medicine, ed. 16. McGraw-Hill, New York, 2005, pp. 1960–1967.
6. Campbell, R Jr, Cooper, GS, and Gilkeson, GS. Two aspects of the clinical and humanistic burden of systemic lupus erythematosus: Mortality risk and quality of life early in the course of disease. Arthritis Rheum 59:458–464, 2008.
7. Gergely, P, Isaak, A, Szekeres, Z, Prechl, J, et al. Altered expression of Fcγ and complement receptors on B cells in systemic lupus erythematosus. Ann NY Acad Sci 1108:183–192, 2007.
8. Tsokos, GC. Systemic lupus erythematosus. A disease with a complex pathogenesis. Lancet 358:ps65, 2001.
9. Heinlen, LD, McClain, MT, Merrill, J, Akbarali, YW, et al. Clinical criteria for systemic lupus erythematosus precede diagnosis, and associated autoantibodies are present before clinical symptoms. Arthritis Rheum 56: 2344–2351, 2007.
10. Von Mühlen, CA, and Nakamura, RM. Clinical and laboratory evaluation of systemic rheumatic diseases. In McPherson, RA, and Pincus, MR (eds): Henry's Clinical Diagnosis and Management by Laboratory Methods, ed. 21. Saunders Elsevier, Philadelphia, 2007, pp. 916–932.
11. Mak, TW, and Sanders, ME. The Immune Response: Basic and Clinical Principles. Elsevier, Burlington, MA, 2006, pp. 964–1023.
12. Kimberly, RP. Prospects for autoimmune disease: Research advances in systemic lupus erythematosus. JAMA 285:650–652, 2001.
13. Parietti, V, Chifflot, H, Muller, S, and Monneaux, F. Regulatory T cells and systemic lupus erythematosus. Ann NY Acad Sci 1108:64–75, 2007.
14. Csiszar, A, Nagy, G, and Gergely, P, et al. Increased interferon-gamma (IFN-gamma), IL-10 and decreased IL-4 mRNA expression in peripheral blood mononuclear cells (PBMC) from patients with systemic lupus erythematosus. Clin Exp Immunol 122:464–470, 2000.
15. Tyrrell-Price, J, Lydyard, PM, and Isenberg, DA. The effect of interleukin-10 and of interleukin-12 on the in vitro production of anti-double-stranded DNA antibodies from patients with systemic lupus erythematosus. Clin Exp Immunol 124:118–125, 2001.
16. Bussolati, B, Rollino, C, and Mariano, F, et al. IL-10 stimulates production of platelet-activating factor by monocytes of patients with active systemic lupus erythematosus (SLE). Clin Exp Immunol 122:471–476, 2000.
17. Isenberg, DA, Manson, JJ, Ehrenstein, MR, and Rahman, A. Fifty years of anti-ds DNA antibodies: Are we approaching journey's end? Rheumatology 46:1052–1056, 2007.
18. Bradwell, AR, Hughes, RG, and Karim, AR. Immunofluorescent antinuclear antibody tests. In Detrick, B, Hamilton, RG, and Folds, JD, et al. (eds): Manual of Molecular and Clinical
Laboratory Immunology, ed. 7. ASM Press, Washington, DC, 2006, pp. 995–1006.
19. Ulvestad, E, Kanestrom, A, and Madland, TM, et al. Evaluation of diagnostic tests for antinuclear antibodies in rheumatological practice. Scand J Immunol 52:309–315, 2000.
20. Tran, TT, and Pisetsky, DS. Detection of anti-DNA autoantibodies. In Detrick, B, Hamilton, RG, and Folds, JD, et al. (eds): Manual of Molecular and Clinical Laboratory Immunology, ed. 7. ASM Press, Washington, DC, 2006, pp. 1027–1032.
21. Reeves, WH, Satoh, M, Lyons, R, Nichols, C, et al. Detection of autoantibodies against proteins and ribonucleoproteins by double immunodiffusion and immunoprecipitation. In Detrick, B, Hamilton, RG, and Folds, JD, et al. (eds): Manual of Molecular and Clinical Laboratory Immunology, ed. 7. ASM Press, Washington, DC, 2006, pp. 1007–1018.
22. Chan, EKL, Burlingame, RW, and Fritzler, MJ. Detection of autoantibodies by using immobilized natural and recombinant antigens. In Detrick, B, Hamilton, RG, and Folds, JD, et al. (eds): Manual of Molecular and Clinical Laboratory Immunology, ed. 7. ASM Press, Washington, DC, 2006, pp. 1019–1026.
23. Blomberg, S, Ronnblom, L, and Wallgren, AC, et al. Anti-SSA/Ro antibody determination by enzyme-linked immunosorbent assay as a supplement to standard immunofluorescence in antinuclear antibody screening. Scand J Immunol 51:612–617, 2000.
24. Orton, SM, Peace-Brewer, A, Schmitz, JL, Freeman, K, et al. Practical evaluation of methods for detection and specificity of autoantigens to extractable nuclear antigens. Clin Diagn Lab Immunol 11:297–301, 2004.
25. Schmitz, JL. Laboratory testing for antibodies associated with antiphospholipid antibody syndrome. In Detrick, B, Hamilton, RG, and Folds, JD, et al. (eds): Manual of Molecular and Clinical Laboratory Immunology, ed. 7. ASM Press, Washington, DC, 2006, pp. 1046–1052.
26. Vlachoyiannopoulos, PG, Samarkos, M, Sikara, M, and Tsiligros, P. Antiphospholipid antibodies: Laboratory and pathogenetic aspects. Crit Rev Clinl Lab Sci 44:271–338, 2007.
27. Marlar, RA, Fink, LM, and Miller, JL. Laboratory approach to thrombotic risk. In McPherson, RA, and Pincus, MR (eds): Henry's Clinical Diagnosis and Management by Laboratory Methods, ed. 21. Saunders Elsevier, Philadelphia, 2007, pp. 770–777.
28. Traynor, AE, Schroeder, J, and Rosa, RM, et al. Treatment of severe systemic lupus erythematosus with high-dose chemotherapy and haemopoietic stem-cell transplantation: A phase I study. Lancet 356:701–707, 2000.
29. Lipsky, PE. Rheumatoid arthritis. In Kasper, DL, Braunwald, E, Fauci, AE, Hauser, SL, et al. (eds): Harrison's Principles of Internal Medicine, ed. 16. McGraw-Hill, New York, 2005, pp. 1968–1976.
30. Narain, S, Kosboth, M, and Hahn, P. Autoantibody testing in rheumatoid arthritis. In Detrick, B, Hamilton, RG, and Folds, JD, et al. (eds): Manual of Molecular and Clinical Laboratory Immunology, ed. 7. ASM Press, Washington, DC, 2006, pp. 1033–1045.
31. Oliver, S. Best practice in the treatment of patients with rheumatoid arthritis. Nurs Stand 21:47–56, 2007.
32. Hill, J. The what, whys and wherefores of rheumatoid arthritis. Nurs Res Care 10:123–126, 2008.

33. Wolfe, F, Freundlich, B, and Straus, WL. Increase in cardio-vascular and cerebrovascular disease prevalence in rheumatoid arthritis. J Rheumatol 30:36–40, 2003.

34. Emery, P, McInnes, IB, van Vollerhoven, R, and Kraan, MC. Clinical identification and treatment of a rapidly progressing disease state in patients with rheumatoid arthritis. Rheumatology 47:392–398, 2008.

35. Arnett, FC, Edworthy, SM, and Bloch, DA, et al. The American Rheumatism Association 1987 revised criteria for the classification of rheumatoid arthritis. Arthritis Rheum 31:315, 1988.

36. Koopman, WJ. Prospects for autoimmune disease: Research advances in rheumatoid arthritis. JAMA 285:648–650, 2001.

37. Lee, AN, Beck, CE, and Hall, M. Rheumatoid factor and anti-CCP autoantibodies in rheumatoid arthritis: A review. Clin Lab Sci 21:15–18, 2008.

38. Wild, N, Johann, K, Grunert, VP, Schmitt, RI, et al. Diagnosis of rheumatoid arthritis: Multivariate analysis of biomarkers. Biomarkers 13:88–105, 2008.

39. Snijders, GF, Broeder, AA, Bevers, K, Jeurissen, ME et al. Measurement characteristics of a new rapid anti-CCP2 test compared to the anti-CCP2 ELISA. Scand J Rheumatol 37:151–154, 2008.

40. Lee, DM, and Weinblatt, ME. Rheumatoid arthritis. Lancet 358:903–911, 2001.

41. Wessels, JAM, Huizinga, TWJ, and Guchelaar. Recent insights in the pharmacological actions of methotrexate in the treatment of rheumatoid arthritis. Rheumatology 47:249–255, 2008.

42. Furst, DE, Keystone, EC, and Breedveld, FC, et al. Updated consensus statement on tumour necrosis factor blocking agents for the treatment of rheumatoid arthritis and other rheumatic diseases. Ann Rheum Dis 60 (suppl III):2–5, 2001.

43. Moreland, LW, Cohen, SB, and Baumgartner, SW, et al. Long-term safety and efficacy of etanercept in patients with rheumatoid arthritis. J Rheumatol 28:1238–1244, 2001.

44. Day, R. Adverse reactions to TNF-alpha inhibitors in rheumatoid arthritis. Lancet 359:540–541, 2002.

45. Dorner, T, and Lipsky, PE. B-cell targeting: A novel approach to immune intervention today and tomorrow. Expert Opin Biol Ther 7:1287–1299, 2007.

46. Jacobson, EM, Huber, A, and Tomer, Y. The HLA gene complex in thyroid autoimmunity: From epidemiology to etiology. J Autoimmun 30:58–62, 2008.

47. Ban, Y, and Tomer, Y. The contribution of immune regulatory and thyroid specific genes to the etiology of Graves' and Hashimoto's diseases. Autoimmunity 36:367–379, 2003.

48. Sinclair, D. Clinical and laboratory aspects of thyroid autoantibodies. Ann Clin Biochem 43:173–183, 2006.

49. Jacobson, EM, and Tomer, Y. The genetic basis of thyroid autoimmunity. Thyroid 17:949–961, 2007.

50. Zeitlin, AA, Simmonds, MJ, and Gough, SCL. Genetic developments in autoimmune thyroid disease: An evolutionary process. Clinl Endocrinol 68:671–682, 2008.

51. Jameson, JL, and Weetman, AP. Disorders of the thyroid gland. In Kasper, DL, Braunwald, E, Fauci, AE, Hauser, SL et al. (eds): Harrison's Principles of Internal Medicine, ed. 16. McGraw-Hill, New York, 2005, pp. 2104–2126.

52. Bylund, DJ, and Nakamura, RM. Organ-specific autoimmune diseases. In McPherson, RA, and Pincus, MR (eds): Henry's Clinical Diagnosis and Management by Laboratory Methods, ed. 21. Saunders Elsevier, Philadelphia, 2007, pp. 945–960.

53. Weetman, AP. Autoimmune thyroid disease. Autoimmunity 37:337–340, 2004.

54. Weetman, AP. Graves' disease. N Engl J Med 343:1236–1248, 2000.

55. Rocchi, R. Critical issues on Graves' ophthalmopathy. MLO 10–15, May 2006.

56. Gopinath, B, Musselman, R, Beard, N, El-Kaissi, Tani, J, et al. Antibodies targeting the calcium binding skeletal muscle protein calsequestrin are specific markers of ophthalmopathy and sensitive indicators of ocular myopathy in patients with Graves' disease. Clin Exp Immunol 145:56–62, 2006.

57. McKenna, TJ. Graves' disease. Lancet 357:1793–1796, 2001.

58. Burek, CL, Bigazzi, PE, and Rose NR, et al. Endocrinopathies. In Detrick, B, Hamilton, RG, and Folds, JD, et al. (eds): Manual of Molecular and Clinical Laboratory Immunology, ed. 7. ASM Press, Washington, DC, 2006, pp. 1062–1077.

59. Maugendre, D, and Massart, C. Clinical value of a new TSH binding inhibitory activity assay using human TSH receptors in the follow-up of antithyroid drug treated Graves' disease. Comparison with thyroid stimulating antibody bioassay. Clin Endocrinol 54:89–96, 2001.

60. Nakamura, RM. Human autoimmune diseases: Progress in clinical laboratory tests. MLO 32:32–45, 2000.

61. Powers, AC. Diabetes mellitus. In Kasper, DL, Braunwald, E, Fauci, AE, Hauser, SL, et al. (eds): Harrison's Principles of Internal Medicine, ed. 16. McGraw-Hill, New York, 2005, pp. 2152–2179.

62. Sanjeevi, CB, Lybrand, TP, and DeWeese, C, et al. Polymorphic amino acid variations in HLA-DQ are associated with systematic physical property changes and occurrence of IDDM. Members of the Swedish Childhood Diabetes Study. Diabetes 44:125–131, 1995.

63. Cerna, M. Genetics of autoimmune diabetes mellitus. Wien Med Wochenschr 158:2–12, 2008.

64. Zhang, L, Nakayama, M, and Eisenbarth, GS. Insulin as an autoantigen in NOD/human diabetes. Curr Opin Immunol 20:111–118, 2008.

65. Taplin, CE, and Barker, JM. Autoantibodies in type 1 diabetes. Autoimmunity 41:11–18, 2008

66. Raz, I, Elias, D, and Avron, A, et al. Beta-cell function in new-onset type 1 diabetes and immunomodulation with a heat-shock protein peptide (DiaPep277): A randomised, double-blind, phase II trial. Lancet 358:1749–1753, 2001.

67. Bour-Jordan, H, and Bluestone, JA. B cell depletion: A novel therapy for autoimmune diabetes? J Clin Invest 117:3642–3645, 2007.

68. Hauser, SL, and Goodin, DE. Multiple sclerosis and other demyelinating diseases. In Kasper, DL, Braunwald, E, Fauci, AE, Hauser, SL, et al. (eds): Harrison's Principles of Internal Medicine, ed. 16. McGraw-Hill, New York, 2005, pp. 2461–2470.

69. Compston, A, and Coles, A. Multiple sclerosis. Lancet 359:1221–1231, 2002.

70. Baranzini, SE, Oksenberg, JR, and Hauser, SL. New insights into the genetics of multiple sclerosis. J Rehabil Res Dev 39:201–209, 2002.

71. Ascherio, A, Munger, KL, and Lennette, ET, et al. Epstein-Barr virus antibodies and risk of multiple sclerosis: A prospective study. JAMA 286:3083–3088, 2001.

72. Hafler, DA, Compston, A, Sawcer, S, Lander, ES, et al. Risk alleles for multiple sclerosis identified by a genomewide study. N Engl J Med 357:851–862, 2007.

73. Katzmann, JA, and Kyle, RA. Immunochemical characteristics of immunoglobulins in serum, urine, and cerebrospinal fluid. In Detrick, B, Hamilton, RG, and Folds, JD, et al. (eds): Manual of Molecular and Clinical Laboratory Immunology, ed. 7. ASM Press, Washington, DC, 2006, pp. 88–100.

74. Prat, E, and Martin, R. The immunopathogenesis of multiple sclerosis. J Rehabil Res Dev 39:187–199, 2002.

75. Tullman, MJ, Lublin, FD, and Miller, AE. Immunotherapy of multiple sclerosis—Current practice and future directions. J Rehabil Res Dev 39:273–285, 2002.

76. Drachman, DB. Myasthenia gravis and other diseases of the neuromuscular junction. In Kasper, DL, Braunwald, E, Fauci, AE, Hauser, SL, et al. (eds): Harrison's Principles of Internal Medicine, ed. 16. McGraw-Hill, New York, 2005, pp. 2518–2523.

77. Vincent, A, Palace, J, and Hilton-Jones, D. Myasthenia gravis. Lancet 357:2122–2128, 2001.

78. Flachenecker, P. Epidemiology of neuroimmunological diseases. J Neur 253(Suppl 5): V2–V8, 2006.

79. Conti-Fine, BM, Milani, M, and Kaminski, HJ. Myasthenia gravis: Past, present, and future. J Clin Invest 116:2843–2854, 2006.

80. Werneck, LC, Cunha, FM, and Scola, RH. Myasthenia gravis: A retrospective study comparing thymectomy to conservative treatment. Acta Neurol Scand 101:41–46, 2000.

81. Winters, JL, and Pineda, AA. Hemapheresis. In McPherson, RA, and Pincus, MR (eds): Henry's Clinical Diagnosis and Management by Laboratory Methods, ed. 21. Saunders Elsevier, Philadelphia, 2007, pp. 685–715.

82. Brady, HR, O'Meara, YM, and Brenner, BM. Glomerular diseases. In Kasper, DL, Braunwald, E, Fauci, AE, Hauser, SL, et al. (eds): Harrison's Principles of Internal Medicine, ed. 16. McGraw-Hill, New York, 2005, pp. 1674–1693.

83. Salama, AD, Levy, JB, and Lightstone, L, et al. Goodpasture's disease. Lancet 358:917–920, 2001.

84. Collins, AB, and Colvin, RB. Kidney and lung disease mediated by anti-glomerular basement membrane antibodies: Detection by western blot analysis. In Detrick, B, Hamilton, RG, and Folds, JD, et al. (eds): Manual of Molecular and Clinical Laboratory Immunology, ed. 7. ASM Press, Washington, DC, 2006, pp. 1110–1115.

# 15 Immunoproliferative Diseases

*Donald C. Lehman, EdD, and Maureane Hoffman, MD, PhD*

## LEARNING OBJECTIVES

*After finishing this chapter, the reader will be able to:*

1. Contrast leukemias and lymphomas.
2. Compare the different hypotheses explaining the transformation of normal cells into malignant cells.
3. Discuss the clonal hypothesis of malignancy.
4. Describe how surface (CD) antigens reflect the differentiation of hematopoietic cells.
5. Discuss the evidence linking Epstein-Barr virus to Hodgkin's lymphoma.
6. Describe how uncontrolled proliferation of lymphoid cells and overproduction of antibody can lead to clinical manifestations.
7. Differentiate multiple myeloma from Waldenström's macroglobulinemia.
8. Discuss how laboratory tests can be used to diagnose and follow the progression of immunoproliferative disorders.
9. Describe how laboratory tests are used to diagnose and classify leukemias and lymphomas.
10. Compare the laboratory results seen for monoclonal gammopathy and polyclonal increase in immunoglobulins.

## KEY TERMS

- Aneuploidy
- Cold agglutinin
- Cryoglobulins
- Hairy cell leukemia
- Hodgkin's lymphoma (HL)
- Non-Hodgkin's lymphoma (NHL)
- Leukemia
- Lymphoma
- Monoclonal gammopathy
- Multiple myeloma
- Oncogene
- Paraprotein (M protein)
- Plasma cell dyscrasias
- Waldenström's macroglobulinemia

## CHAPTER OUTLINE

This chapter focuses on malignancies of the immune system, particularly cells of lymphoid lineage. The lymphoid malignancies are broadly classified as leukemias and lymphomas. In **leukemias,** the malignant cells are primarily present in the bone marrow and peripheral blood. In **lymphomas,** the malignant cells arise in lymphoid tissues, such as lymph nodes, tonsils, or spleen. There can be an overlap between the sites affected by leukemias and lymphomas, especially when the malignancy is far advanced. However, it is generally most useful to classify the malignancy according to the site where it first arose, rather than the sites it can ultimately involve.

The **plasma cell dyscrasias** (disorders) primarily include multiple myeloma and Waldenström's macroglobulinemia. These commonly involve the bone marrow, lymphoid organs, and other nonlymphoid sites. They are considered biologically distinct and not classified as either leukemias or lymphomas. However, plasma cells may be found in the blood late in the course of myeloma. This phenomenon is sometimes referred to as *plasma cell leukemia.*

The chapter will also cover the diagnosis and monitoring of lymphoid malignancies by the clinical laboratory. This chapter is not intended as a comprehensive treatment of hematopoietic malignancy but rather as an introduction to the malignancies most commonly evaluated by the clinical laboratory. Benign hyperactivity or inappropriate activity of the immune system (autoimmunity) is discussed in Chapter 14.

## CONCEPTS OF MALIGNANT TRANSFORMATION

Malignancy is characterized by an excess accumulation of cells. In some cases this is because of rapid proliferation of the cells (i.e., excess production). In other cases, the cells proliferate at a normal rate but fail to undergo apoptosis (programmed cell death). Cells of the immune system, especially lymphoid cells, normally respond to a stimulus by proliferating. Thus, malignancy may reflect an initially normal process in which regulatory steps have failed. In addition to a failure of growth regulation, the mutations can result in arrest of maturation. The malignant cells do not develop into properly functioning mature cells but are "stuck" at some earlier stage of differentiation. Malignancies are generally multifactorial in onset. Malignant transformation may require altered or abnormal genes (mutations); however, this alone is often insufficient. The failure of cellular regulation may be triggered by a viral infection or other proliferative stimulus.

The cells of the immune system are at great risk for malignant transformation, because the features that characterize the development of malignancy are also a normal part of the immune response: an antigenic stimulus results in proliferation of lymphoid cells and a high rate of mutation during gene rearrangement and affinity maturation.

Malignant and premalignant proliferation of cells can occur at any stage in the differentiation of the lymphoid lineages. Despite suffering from abnormal regulation, the malignant cells generally retain some or all of the morphological and functional characteristics of their normal counterpart—for example, their characteristic cell surface antigens or secretion of immunoglobulin. These characteristics are used to classify lymphoid malignancies.

Based largely on animal experiments, a dysregulative theory of lymphoma was developed several years ago. The concept of this theory was that lymphomas arise when persistent immunostimulation coincides with an immune deficiency. The persistent stimulation provokes continuous proliferation and mutations in lymphoid precursors. The immune deficiency can play two roles. First, the presence of an ineffective immune response can permit persistent stimulation by failing to clear an infection. Second, the immune system is responsible for surveillance against malignancy. The immune system attacks and removes those cells that escape proper regulation. It is reported that patients with an immunodeficiency have a higher rate of malignancy, especially malignancies linked to a viral etiology, than individuals with a normally functioning immune system.

The immune system is naturally diverse and heterogeneous in preparation for its encounters with a wide range of potential pathogens. However, malignancies are thought to arise from the excessive proliferation of a single genetically identical line, or clone, of cells—that is, all the malignant cells arise from a single mutant parent cell. This is referred to as the *clonal hypothesis of malignancy.* The mutation gives the affected cell a survival advantage. It either proliferates uncontrollably or fails to die appropriately, thus producing a large number of similarly malignant offspring.

Normal immune responses are polyclonal (i.e., cells with different features such as antigen specificity all proliferate in response to an immune stimulus). Therefore, malignancy can often be diagnosed when a population of cells is found to be more uniform than normal. For example, because each plasma cell produces only one type of immunoglobulin, the persistent presence of a large amount of a single type of immunoglobulin with a single idiotype suggests malignancy. *Idiotype* refers to the antigen specificity of the immunoglobulin. By contrast, an increase in the amount of total immunoglobulin, without an increase in any one specific class, is characteristic of benign reactive immunoproliferation. Similarly, it is nearly always diagnostic of malignancy when the lymphocytic cells in the bloodstream, bone marrow, or lymphoid tissues consist primarily of a uniform population of cells.

Many of the genes involved in regulating cell growth and proliferation were originally identified, because they are the normal cellular counterparts of viral products that stimulate host-cell proliferation and eventual malignant transformation. These viral products are called viral **oncogenes,** and the corresponding host genes are called *proto-oncogenes.* One such proto-oncogene, c-Myc, plays an important role in regulating cell growth. C-Myc levels rise early in the process of normal lymphocyte activation, and a fall in c-Myc levels is linked to a return to a nonproliferative state. A failure in regulation of c-Myc levels is seen in some malignancies of lymphocytic cells.[1] One example is Burkitt's lymphoma, a B-cell malignancy associated with Epstein-Barr virus (EBV) infection. In this case, a gene translocation involving the c-Myc locus and the immunoglobulin μ heavy chain alters regulation of c-Myc levels. The high c-Myc levels drive the affected cells to continually proliferate.

Most cases of follicular lymphoma have a t(14;18) gene translocation.[2] This results in a rearranged and constitutively overexpressed gene called *bcl-2*. The bcl-2 gene induces production of an inner mitochondrial membrane protein that blocks apoptosis. Therefore, the cells affected by this translocation do not die normally. Even though the malignant clone may not be proliferating at an excessive rate, an excessive number of the cells accumulate, because their survival is enhanced compared to normal cells. Many cases of small noncleaved cell lymphomas, including Burkitt's lymphoma, also have a gene translocation—the c-Myc gene, t(8;14). Most mantle cell lymphomas rearrange the bcl-1 gene, t(11;14).

The specific mutation(s) leading to malignant transformation are not known for most malignancies. However, more are being identified every day. This knowledge suggests that we may someday be able to treat malignancies by administering drugs that specifically target the abnormal protein produced by the mutant gene in a specific malignancy.

## LYMPHOMAS

The lymphomas are divided into **Hodgkin's lymphoma (HL)** and **non-Hodgkin's lymphoma (NHL).** The classification of NHL has frustrated pathologists and clinicians alike for decades. Many classification schemes have been proposed, the oldest of which is the Rappaport classification, which was developed before a difference in B cells and T cells was known. The classification scheme is based solely on morphological features by light microscopy. From this scheme comes the following terms that are still encountered occasionally today: *well-differentiated lymphocytic lymphoma (WDLL)* (small lymphocytic lymphoma), *poorly differentiated lymphocytic lymphoma (PDDL)* (follicular center cell lymphoma with primarily small-cleaved cells), and *histiocytic lymphoma* (large-cell lymphoma).

By the 1980s, several different schemes were in use to classify lymphomas. Investigators at the National Cancer Institute reviewed existing lymphoma classification schemes. None of them clearly emerged as superior. Therefore, they developed the Working Formulation Classification Scheme, which ultimately became the standard. It, too, was based on the lymph node architecture and the cytology of the malignant cells by light microscopy. It also did not consider the B- or T-cell lineage. The scheme classified the lymphomas into low-, intermediate-, and high-grade processes, based on the aggressiveness of the untreated lymphoma.

In the 1990s, most investigators and clinicians were using immunologic, cytogenetic, and molecular techniques to assist in lymphoma classification. Advances in understanding basic lymphocyte biology led to major rethinking of the use of a classification scheme based solely on morphology. In 1994, the International Lymphoma Study Group proposed the Revised European-American Lymphoma (REAL) classification. This list set forth the diagnostic features of lymphomas that the group members considered to be widely recognized and clearly diagnosable by contemporary techniques.[3]

The REAL approach represented a new paradigm in lymphoma classification. The recognized lymphomas are distinct biological entities defined by clinicopathologic and immunogenetic features. The classification is based on the principle that a classification is a list of "real" disease entities, which are defined by a combination of cell origins, morphology, immunophenotype, genetic features, and clinical features. The relative importance of each of these features varies among diseases, and there is no one "gold standard." In some tumors, morphology is paramount; in others, it is immunophenotype, a specific genetic abnormality, or clinical features. The REAL scheme divides NHL into neoplasms of precursor cells and neoplasms of mature cells of B, T, or natural killer (NK) cell lineage. An individual entity can exhibit a range of morphological appearances and a range of clinical behaviors. The REAL classification was validated by a major multi-institutional study involving 1378 cases, showing that it is both reproducible and clinically relevant.[4] This REAL scheme is the basis for the classification scheme adopted by the World Health Organization (WHO).[5] The REAL classification scheme is detailed in **Tables 15–1 and 15–2.**

## HODGKIN'S LYMPHOMA

Hodgkin's lymphoma (HL) is a highly treatable and often curable lymphoma that occurs both in young adults and in the elderly.[6] It is characterized by the presence of Reed-Sternberg (RS) cells in affected lymph nodes and lymphoid organs. RS cells are typically large with a bilobed nucleus and two prominent nucleoli. This gives the cell an owl's-eyes appearance. Variants of RS cells do not have this typical appearance. Although the origin of the RS cells has long been a matter of debate, a consensus has now been reached that the malignant RS cells are generally of B-cell lineage.

| Table 15-1. Hodgkin's Lymphoma |
| --- |
| I. Nodular lymphocyte predominant Hodgkin's lymphoma |
| II. Classic Hodgkin's lymphoma |
| • Nodular sclerosis Hodgkin's lymphoma |
| • Lymphocyte-rich Hodgkin's lymphoma |
| • Mixed cellularity Hodgkin's lymphoma |
| • Lymphocyte depleted Hodgkin's lymphoma |

## Table 15–2.   Non-Hodgkin Lymphomas

### B-Cell Neoplasms

I. Precursor B-cell neoplasm
- Precursor B lymphoblastic leukemia/lymphoma

II. Mature (peripheral) B-cell neoplasms
- B-cell chronic lymphocytic leukemia/small
- B-cell prolymphocytic leukemia lymphocytic lymphoma
- Lymphoplasmacytic lymphoma
- Burkitt's lymphoma
- Hairy cell leukemia
- Plasma cell myeloma/plasmacytoma
- Extranodal marginal zone B-cell lymphoma of mucosa-associated lymphoid tissue
- Nodal marginal zone lymphoma
- Follicle center lymphoma
- Mantle cell lymphoma
- Diffuse large-cell B-cell lymphoma
- Splenic marginal zone B-cell lymphoma

### T-Cell and NK-Cell Neoplasms

I. Precursor T-cell neoplasm
- Precursor T lymphoblastic lymphoma/leukemia

II. Mature (peripheral) T-cell and NK-cell neoplasms
- T-cell prolymphocytic leukemia
- T-cell granular lymphocytic leukemia
- Aggressive NK-cell leukemia
- Adult T-cell lymphoma/leukemia (Human T lymphotropic virus 1)
- Extranodal NK/T-cell lymphoma, nasal type
- Enteropathy-type T-cell lymphoma
- Hepatosplenic gamma-delta T-cell lymphoma
- Subcutaneous panniculitis-like T-cell lymphoma
- Sezary's syndrome
- Anaplastic large-cell lymphoma, T/null cell, primary cutaneous type
- Peripheral T-cell lymphoma, not otherwise characterized
- Angioimmunoblastic T-cell lymphoma
- Anaplastic large-cell lymphoma, T/null cell, primary systemic type

NK = Natural killer

The REAL/WHO classification recognizes a basic distinction between nodular lymphocyte predominant HL (NLP-HL) and classic HL, reflecting the differences in clinical presentation, morphology, phenotype, and molecular features. Classic HL is subdivided into four types: lymphocyte-rich, nodular sclerosis, mixed cellularity, and lymphocyte depleted. RS cells in all subtypes of classic HL have a similar immunophenotype. They are all CD30 positive, and about 80 percent of the cases are CD15 positive. Expression of the B-cell marker CD20 is weak or absent. Most of the cells in affected lymph nodes are reactive and appear to represent a host immune response to the malignant cells. The more intense the immune response, the better the prognosis. RS cells of NLP-HL have a different morphology compared to those found in classic HL; they are referred to as *lymphocytic* and *histiocytic cells*. These cells rarely express CD30 or CD15 but instead express the B-cell antigens CD19 and CD20, which are typically absent on Reed-Sternberg cells of classic HL.

The lymphocyte-rich form represents about 5 percent of the cases of HL and tends to occur in slightly older individuals. Nodular sclerosis HL is the most common subtype, representing about 70 percent of cases and having the best prognosis. It is characterized by infiltration of a mixture of normal macrophages, lymphocytes, and granulocytes in affected tissues along with small numbers of RS cells. There is also marked fibrosis, dividing affected lymph nodes into nodules. Mixed cellularity HL also has a mixed infiltrate of normal cells but with less fibrosis and greater numbers of RS cells. It accounts for about 25 percent of cases. Lymphocyte-depleted HL has diffuse fibrosis, few infiltrating normal cells, the greatest number of RS cells, and the worst prognosis than the other HL subtypes.

Epidemiological studies suggest that HL has an infectious etiology. Patients with HL have elevated levels of antibody to Epstein-Barr virus (EBV), the causative agent of infectious mononucleosis. In addition, histochemical stains demonstrate EBV in approximately 40 percent of all HLs and about 75 percent of the cases of mixed-cellularity classic HL. This indicates a role in tumorigenesis and the potential for EBV-targeted therapy.[7]

Detection of EBV-encoded RNAs (EBER1 and EBER2) is a sensitive method to determine the presence of EBV in RS cells.[8] This RNA assay is the most sensitive method for detecting EBV latent infections in clinical specimens. History of infectious mononucleosis is associated with an increased risk of HL, particularly in EBV-positive HL in younger adults, while no increase of risk between infectious mononucleosis and EBV-negative HL was found.[9] This suggests more than one cause of HL. While the specific mechanism of tumorigenesis is unknown, EBV is known to preferentially infect B cells. In addition, viral proteins can induce activation of key signaling pathways, producing phenotypic changes seen in EBV-infected B cells.

## NON-HODGKIN'S LYMPHOMA

NHL includes a wide range of neoplasms. Overall, B-cell lymphomas represent the majority (about 85 percent in the United States) of NHL cases. The most common is diffuse large B-cell lymphoma, which accounts for 30 to 40 percent of NHL. The next most common type is follicular lymphoma, characterized by a much more aggressive course than diffuse large B-cell lymphoma. Marginal-zone B cell (including those of mucus-associated lymphoid tissue [MALT]), peripheral T cell, small B lymphocytic, and mantle cell lymphoma each constitute between 5 and 10 percent of all lymphoma cases. Some of these lymphomas tend to be slowly progressive and compatible with long-term survival, while others are typically highly aggressive and rapidly fatal if not treated. The various B-cell lymphoma types can be divided into three broad groups for prognostic purposes: (1) the low-risk group includes chronic lymphocytic leukemia/lymphoma, follicular lymphomas, and MALT lymphomas; (2) the intermediate-risk group includes diffuse large B-cell lymphoma and Burkitt's lymphoma; and (3) the high-risk group includes mantle cell lymphoma and lymphoblastic lymphoma. MALT lymphoma is often associated with autoimmune conditions such as Sjörgren syndrome and Hashimoto thyroiditis or certain infections (e.g., *Helicobacter pylori* and hepatitis C virus).

In the stepwise process of oncogenesis, a lymphoma may progressively develop a more aggressive phenotype over the course of the disease, a process referred to as *lymphoma progression*. Changes in lymphoma morphology frequently indicate alterations in the clinical and biological behavior of the disease.[10] Three characteristics usually identify lymphomas as having a B-cell origin: (1) surface immunoglobulin, which is found on no other cell type; (2) other cell surface proteins such as CD19 and CD20 that are both sensitive and specific for B cells; and (3) rearranged immunoglobulin genes. In almost all cases, both the surface immunoglobulin and the rearranged immunoglobulin genes have features of clonality.

Some lymphomas, such as small lymphocytic lymphoma, originate from small lymphocytes that are quietly awaiting their first encounter with an immunogen. These lymphomas are indolent but inexorable diseases that are compatible with survival for up to a decade. They progress to prolymphocytic leukemia in 10 to 30 percent of cases and to large-cell lymphoma or other aggressive lymphoid malignancies in 10 to 15 percent of cases.

Other B-cell lymphomas, such as diffuse large-cell lymphoma or lymphoblastic lymphoma, derive from rapidly dividing cells. Lymphoid cells undergo proliferation at two stages in their development: an early cycle as they first emerge from the bone marrow and a later cycle in response to immunogen exposure. Thus, rapidly proliferative lymphomas can correspond to either early or late stages of normal development. These lymphomas behave aggressively, and if untreated, they may kill their victims in less than a year.

The T-cell lymphomas are more difficult to characterize than B-cell lymphomas, because in cases that are morphologically not clearly malignant, no easy way exists to assay their clonality in a similar way to testing for monotypic light-chain expression in B-cell cases. Also, a number of T-cell syndromes progress stealthily from atypical but nonclonal proliferations into clonal malignancies. In cases that are not clearly malignant based on their morphology, two ancillary methods of establishing clonality are available. The first is to use molecular techniques to detect a clonal rearrangement of the T-cell receptor gene. In benign populations, each cell exhibits a slightly different rearrangement, but in malignant proliferations, the population of cells uniformly expresses the same rearrangement. A second method is to demonstrate by flow cytometry that the suspicious

population of T cells uniformly fails to express an antigen that is normally expressed on all T cells.

## LYMPHOBLASTIC LEUKEMIAS

Leukemias are generally classified as either acute or chronic. Chronic leukemias are usually slowly progressive and compatible with extended survival. However, they are generally not curable with chemotherapy. By contrast, acute leukemias are generally much more rapidly progressive but have a higher response rate to therapy.

### Acute Lymphoblastic Leukemia

Acute lymphoblastic leukemia (ALL) is characterized by the presence of very poorly differentiated precursor cells (blast cells) in the bone marrow and peripheral blood. These cells can also infiltrate soft tissues, leading to organ dysfunction. ALL is usually seen in children, between 2 and 10 years of age, and is the most common form of leukemia in this age group. ALL is a treatable disease, with a remission rate of 90 percent and a cure rate of 60 to 70 percent in children. The remission and cure rates are lower in adults with ALL. Immunologically, ALL is divided into four types: CALLa (CD10)-expressing immature B cell ALL, pre-B cell ALL without CALLa (CD10), T-cell ALL, and B-cell ALL. CALLa (CD10)-expressing immature B cell ALL is the most common ALL, while pre-B cell is the second most common. B cell ALL is rare.

### Chronic Lymphoid Leukemia/Lymphoma

The chronic lymphocytic leukemias/lymphomas are a group of diseases almost exclusively of B-cell origin. They include chronic lymphocytic leukemia (CLL), small lymphocytic lymphoma (SLL), prolymphocytic leukemia, and hairy cell leukemia.

The World Health Organization (WHO) considers CLL/SLL a single disease with different clinical presentations. Both reveal B-cell marker CD19 but weakly express CD20. CLL is a common hematopoietic malignancy that involves the expansion of a clone of B cells that have the appearance of small mature lymphocytes. In about 5 percent of cases, the malignant clone is T-cell derived. The cytologically normal lymphocytes accumulate in the bone marrow and blood as well as in the spleen, lymph nodes, and other organs. CLL primarily occurs in patients over 45 years of age with a two-to-one male predominance. Patients usually present with an increase in the blood lymphocyte count, which may be an incidental finding on a routine physical examination. As the malignant lymphocytes continue to increase in number, replacement of normal elements in the bone marrow leads to anemia and thrombocytopenia. Lymph node enlargement is prominent early in the disease. CLL is compatible with a long survival. Palliative therapy—treatment that helps control or reduce symptoms but is not curative—is used.

## Hairy Cell Leukemia

**Hairy cell leukemia** is a rare, slowly progressive disease characterized by infiltration of the bone marrow and spleen by leukemic cells, without involvement of lymph nodes. It has a four-to-one male predominance and is seen in individuals over 20 years of age. Patients usually present with cytopenias because of bone marrow infiltration, but the blood lymphocyte count is usually not very high. However, the splenomegaly may be striking. The malignant lymphocytes are round with a "bland" cytological appearance. They often have irregular "hairy" cytoplasmic projections from their surfaces, most easily visible on a wet-mount preparation. The malignant cells strongly express B-cell markers CD19, CD20, and CD22. They characteristically contain tartrate-resistant acid phosphatase in their cytoplasm, which can be identified by histochemical staining.

## PLASMA CELL DYSCRASIAS

The plasma cell dyscrasias include several related syndromes: multiple myeloma, Waldenström's macroglobulinemia, and the premalignant conditions monoclonal gammopathy of undetermined significance (MGUS) and smoldering multiple myeloma (SMM). These conditions are characterized by the overproduction of a single immunoglobulin component called a myeloma protein (M protein), or **paraprotein**, by a clone of plasma cells. M protein is rarely associated with other lymphoproliferative disorders, such as non-Hodgkin lymphoma or primary amyloidosis. Laboratory evaluation is important in the diagnosis and differentiation of these conditions. Diagnosis and monitoring of the plasma cell dyscrasias depend heavily on detecting and quantitating the M protein.

## Multiple Myeloma

**Multiple myeloma** is a malignancy of mature plasma cells that accounts for about 10 percent of all hematologic cancers. It is the most serious and common of the plasma cell dyscrasias. It is usually diagnosed in persons between 40 and 70 years of age with a peak age of 67 years. Men are slightly more likely than women to develop multiple myeloma. The American Cancer Society estimates there are about 20,000 new cases of multiple myeloma diagnosed each year in the United States, along with about 11,000 deaths.[11] Patients progress from asymptomatic MGUS to SMM to the symptomatic disease multiple myeloma. Between 20 to 25 percent of individuals with MGUS will progress to multiple myeloma. Patients with multiple myeloma typically have excess plasma cells in the bone marrow, a monoclonal immunoglobulin component in the plasma and/or urine, and lytic bone lesions. The plasma cells infiltrating the bone marrow may be morphologically normal or may show atypical or bizarre cytological features. Malignant plasma cells phenotypically express CD38, CD56, and CD138. Approximately 20 percent of myeloma cells express CD20.

The immunoglobulin produced by the malignant clone can be of any type, with IgG being the most common (50 percent), followed by IgA, IgM, and light chains only. Very often the production of heavy and light chains by the malignant plasma cells are not well synchronized, and an excess of light chains may be produced. In about 10 percent of cases, the myeloma cells exclusively produce light chains. The light chains are rapidly excreted in the urine. *Bence Jones protein* is the name given to free immunoglobulin light chains (κ or λ) excreted in the urine. Rarely do myelomas produce IgD, IgE, or heavy chains only. Very rarely, two or more distinct M proteins are produced, or a clinically typical myeloma may produce no secretory product. The level of normal immunoglobulin is often decreased in proportion to the amount of abnormal immunoglobulin (M protein) present in the serum.

The clinical manifestations of multiple myeloma are primarily hematologic, skeletal, and immunologic. Hematologic problems are often related to the failure of the bone marrow to produce a normal number of hematopoietic cells, because myeloma cells progressively replace them. This leads to anemia, thrombocytopenia, and neutropenia. High levels of M protein can interfere with coagulation factors, leading to abnormal platelet aggregation and abnormal platelet function. This, coupled with thrombocytopenia, makes hemorrhaging, bruising, and purpura a common complication of multiple myeloma.

Multiple myeloma tends to preferentially involve bone and forms multiple lytic lesions, often leading to bone pain and pathological fractures. Bone pain, usually involving the spine or chest, is the most common presenting symptom of multiple myeloma. Hypercalcemia is very common, because the myeloma promotes bone resorption. In advanced disease, the hypercalcemia itself can reach life-threatening levels.

When immunoglobulin levels in the blood are sufficiently high, the presence of rouleaux may be seen on examination of the peripheral blood smear. The excess production of the abnormal immunoglobulin is accompanied by a progressive decrease in the normal immunoglobulins. This leads to a deficiency of normal antibody responses and a higher incidence of infectious diseases. Hyperviscosity can develop when the level of M protein in the plasma is high. Because viscosity depends on the size of the molecule in solution, and IgM is the largest of the immunoglobulins, hyperviscosity is most often seen with IgM-producing tumors. Hyperviscosity syndrome is also sometimes seen with an IgG3-producing myeloma, because IgG3 is the largest of the IgG subclasses.

The type and severity of clinical manifestations depend on the type of immunoglobulin component produced. Up to 15 percent of patients with multiple myeloma develop light-chain deposition disease or amyloidosis. These are two related disorders in which free light chains or fragments of immunoglobulin are deposited in the tissues. Amyloid fibers stain with the dye Congo red and show apple-green birefringence when viewed under a polarizing microscope. Light chains can be identified in tissue sections by immunofluorescence or immunohistochemical staining with specific antibodies. The deposition of antibody-derived material results in organ dysfunction. The kidneys are most often affected, but every tissue in the body can develop the deposition of amyloid. Cardiomyopathy, peripheral neuropathy, hepatosplenomegaly, and ecchymoses are the most common manifestations.

Patients with myeloma can develop either acute or chronic renal failure. As many as two-thirds of patients with multiple myeloma exhibit some degree of renal insufficiency. Patients with myelomas that produce light chains or IgD are much more likely to develop renal failure than those with other types. Renal insufficiency, due to Bence Jones proteins, is seen in about 50 percent of patients. After infection, this is the second leading cause of death. Bence Jones proteins are thought to be directly toxic to tubular epithelial cells and can damage the kidneys by precipitating in the tubules, causing intrarenal obstruction. The median survival for patients with multiple myeloma is approximately 3 years. Prognosis is generally best with IgM disease and worse with IgG disease. Evidence of a deletion in chromosome 13 has a significant negative impact on outcome.[12,13]

Criteria for the diagnosis of multiple myeloma include plasma cells comprising greater than 10 percent of bone marrow cells or a plasmacytoma (a solid tumor mass of plasma cells), plus either serum M protein greater than 3g/dL, urinary M protein, or osteolytic bone lesions. Serum M proteins can be detected by serum protein electrophoresis and by serum immunofixation. It is important to differentiate among monoclonal free light chains, heavy chains, and gamma globulins. Patients with monoclonal gammopathy can have MGUS, SMM, multiple myeloma, or one of several other clonal expansions of plasma cells or B cells.

An important feature supporting the diagnosis of multiple myeloma is the presence of Bence Jones protein in the urine. About 60 to 70 percent of the patients with myeloma excrete Bence Jones protein in the urine, which can be detected by specific techniques, such as immunoelectrophoresis, or nonspecific techniques, such as heat precipitation (see Exercise: Detection of Urinary Bence Jones Proteins at the end of the chapter).

## Waldenström's Macroglobulinemia

**Waldenström's macroglobulinemia** is a malignant proliferation of IgM-producing lymphocytes and corresponds to lymphoplasmacytoid lymphoma as defined by the WHO. The malignant cells are more immature than plasma cells and have a microscopic appearance somewhere between that of small lymphocytes and plasma cells. These cells produce the pan-B-cell markers CD19, CD20, CD22, and FMC7. In most cases, CD10 and CD23 are not expressed.[14] These plasmacytoid lymphocytes infiltrate the bone marrow, spleen, and lymph nodes. The median age of affected patients is 65 years; Waldenström's macroglobulinemia is

about 10 to 20 percent as common as multiple myeloma, and the etiology of this disease is unknown. However, because of familial clustering of Waldenström's macroglobulinemia and other B-cell disorders (e.g., non-Hodgkin lymphoma), genetic factors are thought to be involved.[15,16]

The clinical signs and symptoms of Waldenström's macroglobulinemia are due to infiltration of the malignant cells into bone marrow, the spleen, and lymph nodes with the overproduction of monoclonal IgM. Symptoms often include weakness, fatigue, anemia, bleeding, and hyperviscosity. Bleeding can be due to a combination of thrombocytopenia and interference of platelet function by monoclonal IgM. The monoclonal IgM can accumulate in any tissue, forming deposits that lead to inflammation and tissue damage. Lytic bone lesions, hypercalcemia, and renal tubular abnormalities are rare. The median length of survival for patients with Waldenström's macroglobulinemia is longer than with multiple myeloma—5 years versus 3 years.

All individuals with Waldenström's macroglobulinemia have elevated serum monoclonal protein that migrates in the gamma region. However, the concentration varies widely, and it is not possible to define a concentration that differentiates this disease from other B-cell lymphoproliferative disorders. Serum protein electrophoresis should be used to evaluate the amount of the monoclonal protein, and the concentration of IgM should be confirmed by immunofixation. In 70 to 80 percent of the patients, the light chain is κ. While Bence Jones proteinuria is often present, protein concentrations rarely exceed 1.0 g/day. Serum $\beta_2$-microglobulin levels are generally over the reference range's upper limit of 3.0 mg/L.

In 10 to 20 percent of patients, the IgM paraproteins behave as **cryoglobulins**. Cryoglobulins precipitate at cold temperatures and can occlude small vessels in the extremities in cold weather. Occlusion of small vessels can lead to the development of skin sores or even necrosis of portions of the fingers or toes. Some of the clinical symptoms are due to autoantibody activity of the monoclonal IgM antibody. Some IgM paraproteins have specificity for i or I antigens and will agglutinate red blood cells in the cold (**cold agglutinins**). Cryoglobulins can be detected when a blood or plasma sample is refrigerated in the clinical laboratory. The precipitate that forms at low temperature dissolves upon warming.

Approximately 20 percent of the patients with Waldenström's macroglobulinemia will present with peripheral neuropathy.[17] It appears that the monoclonal IgM is directed against glycoproteins or glycolipids of the peripheral nerves. In addition, IgM can be demonstrated against polyclonal IgG. This results in immune complex disease characterized by vasculitis, affecting small vessels of the skin, kidneys, liver, and peripheral nerves.

## ROLE OF THE LABORATORY IN EVALUATING IMMUNOPROLIFERATIVE DISEASES

The laboratory is involved in three major ways in evaluating lymphoproliferative disorders. First, it can assess the immunophenotype of hematopoietic cells in the blood, bone marrow, or lymphoid tissues by flow cytometry. This is done by detecting the antigens on the surface of the cells that are characteristic of a specific lineage and stage of differentiation. This technology serves as an excellent complement to microscope-based traditional diagnostic methods and adds distinctive, discriminatory capabilities that are unmatched by any other diagnostic technique. Applications include detection of clonal cells in B-cell lymphoma, the recognition of antigenic expression anomalies in B- or T-cell malignancies, the identification of malignant plasma cells, and the rapid measurement of cell cycle fractions.

The second and probably most straightforward role of the laboratory is in evaluating the amount and characteristics of immunoglobulins. Because the B-cell lineage develops into plasma cells that produce antibody, malignancies of certain B cells are associated with excessive or abnormal antibody production. The amount and characteristics of plasma or urine immunoglobulin can be used to diagnose and evaluate the plasma cell dyscrasias.

Third, the laboratory is increasingly involved in the assessment of genetic and chromosomal abnormalities in hematopoietic malignancies. Although this is mostly done in large referral centers or reference laboratories, genetic techniques are moving progressively closer to routine practice. The polymerase chain reaction can be used to detect sequences (mutations) within genes that have been linked to particular diseases. Cytogenetic studies are useful to detect chromosomal abnormalities (e.g., translocations).

## Immunophenotyping by Flow Cytometry

Analysis of cell surface marker expression is commonly used in the diagnosis and classification of leukemias and lymphomas.[18] Because the malignant cells express markers that often correspond to those of their normal precursors, insight into the lineage of origin and stage of maturation can often be determined by this technique.

Researchers in several laboratories have identified many lymphoid surface antigens and developed antibodies to them. Not surprisingly, antibodies from different laboratories and bearing different names were often found to detect the same antigen/molecule. At that point, the antigen would be assigned a cluster of differentiation (CD), or cluster designation number, meaning that a known cluster of antibodies recognized this antigen.

The presence of CD antigens on the surface of hematopoietic cells is often detected by flow cytometry. **Tables 15-3 and 15-4** list a few of the important cell markers often detected by flow cytometry (see also Chapter 12). Samples of potentially neoplastic cells are incubated with antibody preparations specific for relevant antigens. In many cases, the antibodies contain a fluorescent label. Thus, cells that express a particular antigen are bound by the antibody and become fluorescent. This allows the antigenic profile, or phenotype, of the cell population to be determined.

| Table 15-3. | CD Makers Important in Flow Cytometry, Listed by Cell Type |
|---|---|
| **CELL TYPE** | **CD MARKER** |
| All lymphoid cells | CD45, also called leukocyte common antigen |
| B cells | Almost all B cells express CD19, CD20, and CD22. B-cell lymphomas are sometimes reactive for CD5 and CD43, which are otherwise found on T cells. |
| T cells | Almost all T cells express CD2, CD3, CD5, and CD7. Most T cells are also positive for either CD4 (helper cells) or CD8 (suppressor or cytotoxic T cells). |
| Natural killer cells | Usually express CD16, CD56, or CD57 |

| Table 15-4. | CD Markers Important in Flow Cytometry, Listed by CD Marker |
|---|---|
| **CD MARKERS** | **CELL SPECIFICITY** |
| CD2 | T cell |
| CD3 | T cell |
| CD4 | T helper cell |
| CD5 | T cell and CLL |
| CD7 | T cell |
| CD8 | T suppressor cell |
| CD10 | Burkitt's and follicular lymphoma |
| CD11b | Myeloid cell |
| CD11c | Monocyte and HCL |
| CD13 | Myeloid cell |
| CD14 | Monocyte |
| CD15 | Myeloid/monocytic cells |
| CD16 | Natural killer cell |
| CD19 | B cell |
| CD20 | B cell |
| CD22 | B cell and HCL |
| CD23 | B cell and CLL |
| CD38 | Plasma cell and prognostic indicator for CLL |
| CD45 | All white blood cells |
| CD56 | Natural killer and abnormal plasma cells |
| CD103 | HCL |

CLL = chronic lymphocytic leukemia; HCL = hairy cell leukemia

Flow cytometry is ideal for fluids in which cells are naturally suspended, but it is also useful in lymphoid tissues, from which single-cell suspensions can be easily made. The advantages of flow cytometry are largely based on its ability to very rapidly and simultaneously analyze, even in small samples, multiple-cell properties, including size, granularity, and surface and intracellular antigens. The quantitative nature of the data produced, both with regard to cell population distributions and to expression of individual cell antigens, offers objective criteria for interpretation of results.

## Evaluation of Immunoglobulins

As discussed in Chapter 4, the basic immunoglobulin unit consists of two identical heavy chains and two identical light chains, covalently linked by disulfide bonds. The structure of the heavy chain defines the class of the antibody (e.g., $\gamma$ heavy chain and IgG, $\mu$ heavy chain and IgM, etc.). The two types of light chains ($\kappa$ and $\lambda$) can each occur in combination with any of the types of heavy chains. The heavy and light chains each contain constant and variable regions. The constant regions contain the sites of immunoglobulin binding to cellular receptors and sites involved in complement fixation. The variable regions are responsible for the antigen specificity of the antibody. The immunoglobulins in plasma are heterogeneous in structure, because they recognize a variety of different antigens. The variability in their amino acid sequences means that they also vary slightly in their physical characteristics, such as molecular weight and charge.

B cells differentiate into antibody-producing plasma cells by maturation through several stages. Each B cell recognizes only a single antigenic site or epitope. An early B-cell precursor is stimulated to proliferate and mature when it encounters an immunogen that it recognizes. When a foreign molecule enters the body, the many different epitopes on it each stimulate a B-cell response, leading to the production of an array of different antibodies. However, in a malignant disorder, the clonal proliferation of transformed plasma cells leads to overproduction of a single immunoglobulin. This is called a **monoclonal gammopathy.**

Quantitative measurement of serum or urine immunoglobulins is used in the diagnosis of some lymphoproliferative disorders. However, the evaluation of a patient for the possibility of a monoclonal gammopathy requires both qualitative and quantitative analysis of immunoglobulins.[19] The initial tests used to screen for the presence of a monoclonal gammopathy are serum immunoglobulin levels and serum protein electrophoresis. A high clinical index of suspicion, abnormal results on immunoglobulin levels, or findings suggestive of a monoclonal component on serum protein electrophoresis will prompt additional testing.

## Serum Protein Electrophoresis

Serum protein electrophoresis (SPE) is a technique in which serum proteins are separated on the basis of their size and electrical charge, as discussed in Chapter 4. SPE results in four regions: albumin, and alpha, beta, and gamma globulins. IgG, IgM, IgD, and IgE migrate in the gamma globulin region, while IgA migrates as a broad band in the beta and gamma regions. **Figure 15–1**, panel A, shows a stylized drawing of the protein distribution in normal serum. As can be seen, immunoglobulins normally show a range of mobilities.

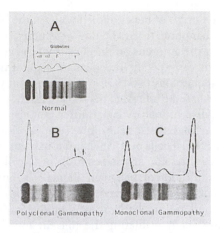

**FIGURE 15–1.** Serum protein electrophoresis of normal and abnormal samples. The lower portion of each panel is a representation of a stained agarose electrophoresis gel. The intensity of staining corresponds to the amount of protein in each region of the gel. In the upper portion of each panel is a densitometer tracing of a gel similar to the one beneath it. In the upper panel showing a normal serum sample, the largest peak is albumin. The globulin regions are as indicated.

The SPE pattern for a polyclonal increase in serum immunoglobulins and a monoclonal gammopathy are shown in panels B and C, respectively. Polyclonal increases in serum immunoglobulins are seen in a variety of disorders, including infections, autoimmune disorders, liver disease, and some immunodeficiency states (e.g., hyper-IgM syndrome).

Additional evaluation of serum immunoglobulin is performed if the SPE shows a monoclonal component, if there is a significant quantitative abnormality of serum immunoglobulins, or if the clinical picture strongly suggests a plasma cell dyscrasia. Myeloma in which only light chains are produced may not be detected on SPE, because the light chains are rapidly cleared in the urine. Therefore, additional studies on a random or 24-hour urine sample may be indicated even in the presence of a normal SPE.

## Immunofixation Electrophoresis

The next step in evaluating a monoclonal gammopathy is typically either immunoelectrophoresis (IEP) or immunofixation electrophoresis (IFE). IEP is not very sensitive, and the turnaround time is lengthy (about 18 hours). Due to these limitations, IEP has generally been replaced by IFE. In IFE, serum samples are electrophoresed, just as for SPE, and then specific antibody is applied directly to the separating gel. The antibodies and antigens diffuse toward each other, and the antibody–antigen complexes formed are visualized by staining. Areas of diffuse staining indicate polyclonal immunoglobulins, while monoclonal bands produce narrow, intensely stained bands **(Fig. 15–2).** IFE is much faster (about 1 hour) than IEP, has much greater sensitivity, and is the most accurate assay for typing paraproteins. However, IFE is also labor intensive and expensive.

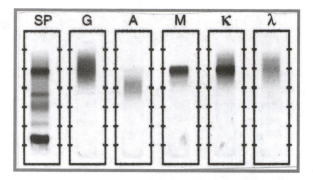

**FIGURE 15–2.** Agarose gel immunofixation electrophoresis of serum. The same patient sample is placed on all six lanes and electrophoresed. Following electrophoresis, antisera are added to each lane as follows: lane 1—antitotal serum protein; lane 2—anti-IgG; lane 3—anti-IgA; lane 4—anti-IgM; lane 5—anti-κ; and lane 6—anti-λ. The patient is exhibiting a monoclonal IgM κ immunoglobulin. *(Courtesy of Helena Laboratories, Beaumont, TX.) See Color Plate 12.*

## Evaluation of Genetic and Chromosomal Abnormalities

The majority of B-cell lymphomas and some T-cell lymphomas are characterized by specific chromosome translocations. Often these translocations can be detected by cytogenetic techniques. Like most cells, malignant lymphoid cells can be made to proliferate in vitro, and their metaphase chromosomes can be examined for grossly visible abnormalities that correspond to characteristic translocations. Many of the translocations involve the immunoglobulin or T-cell receptor loci with various partner chromosomes and lead to abnormal proto-oncogene expression. Other characteristic translocations result in the production of a novel fusion protein. The detection of translocations is of particular value in diagnosis of disease. **Aneuploidy** (abnormal number of chromosomes) and deletion of specific chromosome regions are common secondary chromosome events that are rarely specific to a particular type of lymphoma but provide valuable prognostic information.

Traditional cytogenetic evaluation has been expanded by a technique known as *fluorescence in situ hybridization (FISH)*. FISH is used to directly identify a specific region of DNA in a cell. It involves the preparation of short sequences of single-stranded DNA, called *probes*, which are complementary to the DNA sequences of interest. These probes bind to the complementary chromosomal DNA and, because they contain a fluorescent label, allow one to see the location of those sequences of DNA. Probes can be used on chromosomes, interphase nuclei, or tissue biopsies. FISH is rapid and

quite sensitive and does not require cell culture. However, it only provides information about the specific probe being tested.

Lymphoid malignancies can also be evaluated by molecular genetic techniques. These methods are usually geared toward finding clonal rearrangements of the immunoglobulin gene in B-cell malignancies or of the T-cell receptor gene in T-cell malignancies. These rearrangements are too subtle to be detected by conventional cytogenetics.

As a result of the Human Genome Project completed in 2003, approximately 20,000 genes have been identified.[20] It is estimated that the human genome contains 20,000 to 25,000 genes; however, it will probably take several years before an accurate gene count can be established. Most of these genes are only partially characterized, and the functions of the vast majority are still unknown. It is likely that many genes that might be useful for diagnosis or prognostication of human malignancies have yet to be recognized.

The advent of complementary DNA (cDNA) microarray technology now allows the efficient measurement of expression for almost every gene in the human genome in a single overnight hybridization experiment. This genomic scale approach has begun to reveal novel molecular-based subclasses of many malignancies, including lymphoma and leukemia.[21] Molecular techniques, including nucleic acid amplification, have found their way into routine clinical practice.

## SUMMARY

Malignancies of lymphocytes, both lymphomas and leukemias, are commonly encountered in clinical practice. The classification of these disorders depends on the identification of their cell of origin. The B- or T-cell derivation of a lymphoid malignancy is often determined in the laboratory by flow cytometry. Some B-cell disorders result in abnormal immunoglobulin secretion. Multiple myeloma is a malignancy of plasma cells characterized by production of a monoclonal immunoglobulin or paraprotein (M protein). The paraprotein may be of any immunoglobulin class or may be an immunoglobulin heavy or light chain. Waldenström's macroglobulinemia is a malignancy of plasmacytoid lymphocytes that produces an IgM paraprotein. Identification and quantification of the paraprotein are central to the diagnosis and monitoring of these conditions. SPE is used to detect the presence of a paraprotein, which is then characterized by immunoelectrophoresis or immunofixation electrophoresis. Evaluation of genetic and chromosomal abnormalities is a rapidly evolving area of laboratory practice.

# CASE STUDY

A 63-year-old male visits his primary care physician complaining of fatigue and shortness of breath, upper back pain, and a cough that has become productive the last 2 days. The patient was febrile and appeared acutely ill. A chest X-ray revealed pneumonia, and the following significant laboratory results were found: red blood cell count of $4.1 \times 10^{12}$/L (reference range 4.6 to 6.0 $\times$ $10^{12}$/L), hemoglobin 13 g/dL (reference range 14.0 to 18.0 g/dL), white blood cell count $4.8 \times 10^{9}$/L (reference range 4.5 to 11.0 $\times$ $10^{9}$/L), and an erythrocyte sedimentation rate of 12 mm/hr (reference range 0 to 9 mm/hr). Based on these results, the physician ordered serum immunoglobulin levels. The following results were reported: IgG 3250 mg/dL (reference range 600 to 1500 mg/dL), IgM 48 mg/dL (reference range 75 to 150 mg/dL), and IgA 102 mg/dL (reference range 150 to 250 mg/dL).

## Questions

a. What disease(s) should you suspect, and what additional tests could help confirm the diagnosis?

# EXERCISE

## DETECTION OF URINARY BENCE JONES PROTEINS

### Principle

Reagent test strips used to screen for proteinuria are generally not sensitive to immunoglobulin or free light chains. Therefore, other techniques are required to detect Bence Jones proteins in the urine. One method exploits the unique heat solubility properties of these proteins. Bence Jones proteins precipitate at temperatures between 40°C and 60°C and redissolve again around 100°C. This approach can generally detect levels of protein down to about 30 mg/dL.

### Specimen Collection

A 24-hour or random urine specimen is collected into a clean container. The sample may be stored in a refrigerator to prevent bacterial growth.

### Reagents, Materials, and Equipment

Acetate buffer, 2 mol/L, pH 4.9

Test tubes

Boiling water bath

NOTE: For acetate buffer, add 4.1 mL of glacial acetic acid to 17.5 g of sodium acetate trihydrate and then add water to give a total volume of 100 mL.

### Procedure

1. Place 4 mL of clear urine in a test tube. Add 1 mL of acetate buffer and mix.

2. Heat for 15 minutes at 56 °C in a water bath or heating block. The development of turbidity is indicative of Bence Jones proteins.

3. If the sample has become turbid, transfer the test tube to a boiling water bath for 3 minutes. The turbidity should decrease if it is due to the presence of Bence Jones proteins, which redissolve at 100°C.

4. If the turbidity of the sample increases after boiling, it is because of albumin and globulins. Filter the test sample immediately on removing from the boiling water bath. If Bence Jones proteins are present, the sample will become cloudy as it cools, then clear again as it reaches room temperature. If the precipitate is quite heavy at 56°C, it may not dissolve easily on boiling. It is best to repeat the test with a diluted urine specimen.

### Comments

This is simply a screening test for detection of Bence Jones proteinuria. The best method of detecting Bence Jones proteins is protein electrophoresis followed by immunofixation electrophoresis. See the exercise in Chapter 16.

# REVIEW QUESTIONS

1. In general, a myeloma secreting which type of M protein is most likely to cause renal failure?

    a. IgG
    b. IgM
    c. κ light chains
    d. μ heavy chains

2. Which of the following would be the best indicator of a malignant clone?

    a. Overall increase in antibody production
    b. Increase in IgG and IgM only
    c. Increase in antibody directed against a specific epitope
    d. Decrease in overall antibody production

3. All of the following are features of malignancy *except*

    a. excess apoptosis.
    b. rapid proliferation.
    c. clonal proliferation.
    d. chromosomal mutations.

4. All of the following features are commonly used to classify lymphoid neoplasms *except*

    a. Cell of origin
    b. Presence of gene translocations
    c. Exposure of the patient to carcinogens
    d. Morphology/cytology of the malignant cells

5. Hodgkin's lymphoma is characterized by

    a. proliferation of T cells.
    b. excess immunoglobulin production.
    c. an incurable, rapidly progressive course.
    d. the presence of Reed-Sternberg cells in lymph nodes.

6. Chronic leukemias are characterized as

    a. usually being of B-cell origin.
    b. being curable with chemotherapy.
    c. usually occurring in children.
    d. following a rapidly progressive course.

7. Which best describes acute leukemias?

    a. Usually of B-cell origin
    b. Usually occurring in children
    c. Poor response to chemotherapy
    d. Cells are well differentiated

8. Flow cytometry results on a patient reveal a lack of cells with CD2 and CD3. What does this indicate?

    a. Lack of B cells
    b. Lack of T cells
    c. Lack of monocytes
    d. Lack of natural killer cells

9. Which of the following is true of Waldenström's macroglobulinemia but not multiple myeloma?

    a. Hyperviscosity syndrome is often present.
    b. A single protein-producing clone is elevated.
    c. The cancerous cell is a preplasma cell.
    d. Bence Jones proteins are present in the urine.

# References

1. Potter, M. Pathogenetic mechanisms in B-cell non-Hodgkin's lymphomas in humans. Cancer Res 52:5522s, 1992.
2. Falini, B, and Mason, DY. Proteins encoded by genes involved in chromosomal alterations in lymphoma and leukemia: Clinical value of their detection by immunocytochemistry. Blood 99(2):409–426, 2002.
3. Harris, NH, Jaffe, ES, Stein, H, et al. A revised European-American classification of lymphoid neoplasms: A proposal from International Study Group. Blood 87:1361, 1994.
4. The non-Hodgkin's Lymphoma Classification Project: A clinical evaluation of the International Lymphoma Study Group classification of non-Hodgkin's lymphoma. Blood 89(11): 3909–3918, 1997.
5. Harris, ML, Jaffe, ES, Diebold, J, et al. The World Health Organization classification of hematological malignancies. Report of the Clinical Advisory Committee meeting, Airline House, Virginia, November 1997. Mod Pathol 13:193, 2000.
6. Pileri, SA, Ascani, S, Leoncini, L, et al. Hodgkin's lymphoma: The pathologist's viewpoint. J Clin Pathol 55(3):162–176, 2002.
7. Jaffett, RF. Viruses and Hodgkin's lymphoma. Ann Oncol 13(Suppl 1):23–29, 2002.
8. Kapatai, G, and Murray, P. Contribution of the Epstein-Barr virus to the molecular pathogenesis of Hodgkin lymphoma. J Clin Pathol 60:1342–1349, 2007.
9. Hjalgrim H, Smedby KE, Rostgaard K, et al. Infectious mononucleosis, childhood social environment, and risk of Hodgkin lymphoma. Cancer Res 67(5):2382–2388, 2007.
10. Muller-Hermelink, HK, Zettl, A, Pfeifer, W, et al. Pathology of lymphoma progression. Histopathology 38(4):285–306, 2001.
11. American Cancer Society. Cancer Facts and Figures 2008. Atlanta: American Cancer Society, 2008. Available online at http://www.cancer.org/downloads/STT/2008CAFFfinalsecured.pdf. Accessed July 10, 2008.
12. Chiecchio, L, Protheroe, RKM, Ibrahim, AH, et al. Deletion of chromosome 13 detected by conventional cytogenetics is a critical prognostic factor in myeloma. Leukemia 20:1610–1617, 2006.
13. Chng, WJ, Santanna-Davilia, R, Van Wier, SA, et al. Prognostic factors for hyperdiploid-myeloma: Effects of chromosome 13 deletions and IgH translocations. Leukemia 20:807–813, 2006.
14. Owen, RG, Barrans, SL, Richards, SJ, et al. Waldenström's macroglobulinemia. Development of diagnostic criteria and identification of prognostic factors. Am J Clin Pathol 116: 420–428, 2001.
15. McMaster, M. Familial Waldenström's macroglobulinemia. Semin Oncol 30:146–152, 2003.
16. Treon, SP, Hunter, ZR, Aggarwal, A, et al. Characterization of familial Waldenström's macroglobulinemia. Annals Oncol 17:488–494, 2005.
17. Vital, A. Paraproteinemic neuropathies. Bran Pathol 11:399–407, 2001.
18. Stetler-Stevenson, M, and Braylan, RC. Flow cytometric analysis of lymphomas and lymphoproliferative disorders. Semin Hematol 38(2):111–123, 2001.
19. Guinan, JEC, Kenny, DF, and Gatenby, PA. Detection and typing of paraproteins: Comparison of different methods in a routine diagnostic laboratory. Pathology 21:35, 1989.
20. Human Genome Project. Available at http://www.ornl.gov/sci/techresources/Human_Genome/home.shtml. Accessed July 12, 2008.
21. Rosenwald, A, and Staudt, LM. Clinical translation of gene expression profiling in lymphomas and leukemias. Semin Oncol 29(3):258–263, 2002.

# 16 Immunodeficiency Diseases

*Thomas S. Alexander, PhD, D(ABMLI)*
*and Maureane Hoffman, MD, PhD*

## LEARNING OBJECTIVES

*After finishing this chapter, the reader will be able to:*

1. Recall the organization and development of the cellular and humoral arms of the immune system.
2. Explain how a defect in the B-cell, T-cell, myeloid, or complement systems can lead to typical clinical manifestations.
3. Discuss how laboratory tests can be used to diagnose and monitor the different types of congenital immunodeficiency syndromes.
4. Distinguish common variable immunodeficiency from Bruton's X-linked agammaglobulinemia.
5. Discuss the manifestations of the DiGeorge anomaly, purine-nucleoside phosphorylase (PNP) deficiency, severe combined immunodeficiency (SCID), Wiskott-Aldrich syndrome (WAS), and ataxia-telangiectasia (AT).
6. Recognize the association between immunodeficiency states and the risk of developing malignancy.
7. Explain how the loss of neutrophil function affects host defenses.
8. Describe the basics of performing and interpreting immunofixation electrophoresis

## KEY TERMS

___ Ataxia-telangiectasia (AT)

___ Bruton's agammaglobulinemia

___ Chronic granulomatous disease (CGD)

___ Common variable immunodeficiency (CVI)

___ DiGeorge anomaly

___ Oxidative burst

___ Purine nucleoside phosphorylase (PNP) deficiency

___ Severe combined immunodeficiency (SCID)

___ Transient hypogamma-globulinemia

___ Wiskott-Aldrich syndrome (WAS)

## CHAPTER OUTLINE

The immune system is a diverse and complicated network of many biochemical and cellular components. The antigen-specific, or acquired immunity, arm includes the T-cell system (cellular immunity, T cells, and their cytokines); and the B-cell system (humoral immunity, B cells, and immunoglobulins). The innate immunity arm includes the phagocytic system (mononuclear phagocytes, dendritic cells, and granulocytes); and the complement system. A simplified rendition of the organization of cellular components of the immune system is shown in **Figure 16–1**. The organization, development, and function of the immune system have been discussed in greater detail in Chapters 2, 4, and 5. This chapter focuses on primary, or inherited, dysfunctions of the immune system. The material will emphasize the antigen-specific arm of the immune system and the means by which dysfunctional states can be diagnosed and monitored by the clinical laboratory. Deficiencies in the innate immune system will be covered in less detail. This chapter is not intended as a comprehensive treatment of abnormalities of the immune system, but rather as an introduction to the conditions most commonly evaluated in the clinical laboratory.

# IMMUNODEFICIENCY DISEASES

## General Observations

The components of the immune system play unique but overlapping roles in the host-defense process. Therefore,

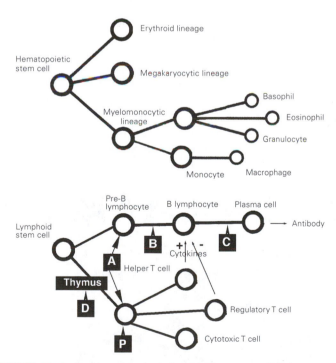

**FIGURE 16–1.** Developmental relationships between cellular components of the immune system. The letters indicate the stages at which a defect occurs in some of the congenital immunodeficiency syndromes. *A*, adenosine deaminase deficiency; *B*, Bruton's agammaglobulinemia; *C*, common variable immunodeficiency; *D*, DiGeorge anomaly; and *P*, PNP deficiency.

defects in any one of the cellular or soluble components result in distinct clinical manifestations. However, because the components of the immune system interact extensively through many regulatory and effector loops, a defect in one arm of the system may affect other aspects of immune function as well. In many cases, it appears that deficiency of one component of the system is accompanied by hyperactivity of other components. This may be because persistent infections continuously stimulate the remaining immune cells, or this is a compensatory mechanism to correct for the deficient immune function. In addition, the deficient component may normally exert regulatory control over other components of the immune system—control that is lacking in the deficiency state. For instance, as illustrated in Figure 16–1, T-cell subsets each secrete cytokines that regulate the development of B cells into plasma cells. A defect in T-cell function removes or unbalances this regulatory loop. Whatever the mechanism, many partial immunodeficiency states are associated with allergic or autoimmune manifestations.

With the exception of IgA deficiency, primary immunodeficiency syndromes are rare, with a combined incidence of about 2 in 10,000 live births.[1,2] Several of the most important immunodeficiency syndromes show X-linked inheritance and, therefore, affect primarily males. Others show autosomal recessive inheritance. Despite the rarity of primary immunodeficiency syndromes, it is important to consider this possibility in children with recurrent infections, because early detection and treatment can help prevent the development of serious, long-term tissue damage or overwhelming sepsis. Early diagnosis can also provide the opportunity for appropriate genetic counseling, carrier detection, and prenatal diagnosis for other family members.[3]

More than 120 different congenital forms of immunodeficiency have been reported, including defects in lymphoid cells, phagocytic cells, and complement proteins.[1] The molecular mechanisms have been determined for many of these deficiencies. The clinical symptoms associated with immune deficiencies range from very mild or subclinical to severe recurrent infections or failure to thrive. The types of infection or symptoms can give important clues to the specific immunodeficiency present. In general, defects in humoral immunity (antibody production) result in pyogenic bacterial infections, particularly of the upper and lower respiratory tract. Recurrent sinusitis and otitis media are common. The clinical course of infections with viral agents is not significantly different from that in normal hosts, with the exception of hepatitis B, which may have a fulminant course in agammaglobulinemic patients. Defects in T-cell-mediated immunity result in recurrent infections with intracellular pathogens such as viruses, fungi, and intracellular bacteria, and patients with these defects almost always develop mucocutaneous candidiasis. They are also prone to disseminated viral infections, especially with latent viruses such as herpes simplex, varicella zoster, and cytomegalovirus. T cells also play a crucial role in tumor surveillance. Age-adjusted rates of malignancy in patients with immunodeficiency disease are 10 to 200 times greater than the expected rates.[1] Most of the malignancies are lymphoid and may be related to persistent stimulation of the remaining immune cells, coupled with defective immune regulation.

The phagocytic system is part of the innate, antigen-nonspecific immune response and includes neutrophils and mononuclear phagocytes. Neutrophils are the first line of defense against invading organisms and are important effector cells in antibody-mediated killing. Defects in neutrophil function are usually reflected in recurrent pyogenic bacterial infections or impaired wound healing. Macrophages within the liver and spleen are in contact with the blood and are responsible for clearing circulating microorganisms. Splenectomy is associated with an increased risk of overwhelming bacterial infection accompanied by septicemia. Macrophages are present in all tissues and also play an important role in processing and presenting antigens to T cells in combination with class II major histocompatibility complex (MHC) molecules to initiate a specific immune response.

The complement system, as discussed in Chapter 6, is activated to produce biologically active molecules that enhance inflammation and promote lysis of cells and microorganisms. Deficiency of complement components results in recurrent bacterial infections and autoimmune-type manifestations. The severity of the syndrome varies with the particular complement component that is deficient. Specific defects of each component of the immune system are described in the following sections.

## Deficiencies of the B-Cell System (Agammaglobulinemias)

Immunoglobulins migrate in the "gamma region" of the serum protein electrophoretic profile (discussed in Chapter 4). Therefore, deficiencies of immunoglobulins have been termed *agammaglobulinemias*. The mechanisms of the agammaglobulinemias include genetic defects in B-cell maturation or mutations leading to defective interactions between B and T cells. A wide range of immunoglobulin deficiency states have been reported and involve virtually all combinations of immunoglobulins and all degrees of severity. In some cases, only a single isotype of one immunoglobulin class is deficient, while all the other isotypes are normal. Only the more common and well-characterized syndromes are described here and are summarized in **Table 16–1**.

In evaluating immunoglobulin deficiency states, it is important to remember that blood levels of immunoglobulins change with age. The blood level of IgG at birth is about the same as the adult level, reflecting transfer of maternal IgG across the placenta. The IgG level drops over the first 2 or 3 months of life as maternal antibody is catabolized. Levels of IgA and IgM are very low at birth. The concentrations of all immunoglobulins gradually rise when the infant begins to produce antibodies at a few months of age, in response to environmental stimuli. IgM reaches normal adult levels first, around 1 year of age, followed by IgG at about 5 to 6 years of age. In some normal children, IgA levels do not reach normal adult values until adolescence. Therefore, it is important to compare a child's immunoglobulin levels to age-matched reference ranges.

### Transient Hypogammaglobulinemia of Infancy

All infants experience low levels of immunoglobulins at approximately 5 to 6 months of age, but in some babies, the low levels persist for a longer time. Because these children do not begin synthesizing immunoglobulin promptly, they can experience severe pyogenic sinopulmonary and skin infections as protective maternal IgG is cleared. Cell-mediated immunity is normal, and there may be normal levels of IgA and IgM.[4] IgG appears to be the most affected, dropping to at least two standard deviations (SD) below the age-adjusted mean with or without a depression of IgM and IgA.[4] Immunoglobulin levels usually normalize spontaneously, often by 9 to 15 months of age. The mechanism of this **transient hypogammaglobulinemia** is not known. These

| Table 16–1. | Characteristics of Selected Defects of the B-Cell System | | |
|---|---|---|---|
| **CONDITION** | **DEFICIENCY** | **LEVEL OF DEFECT** | **PRESENTATION** |
| Transient hypogammaglobulinemia of infancy | All antibodies, especially IgG | Slow development of helper function in some patients | 2–6 months; resolves by 2 years |
| IgA deficiency | IgA; some with reduced IgG2 also | IgA–B cell differentiation | Often asymptomatic |
| X-linked agammaglobulinemia | All antibody isotypes reduced | Pre-B cell differentiation | Infancy |
| Common variable immunodeficiency | Reduced antibody; many different combinations | B cell; excess T suppression | Usually 20–30 years of age |
| Isolated IgG subclass deficiency | Reduced IgG1, IgG2, IgG3, or IgG4 | Defect of isotype differentiation | Variable with the class and degree of deficiency |
| Immunodeficiency with hyperimmunoglobulin M | Reduced IgG, IgA, IgE, with elevated IgM | B-cell switching | Infancy |

patients have normal numbers of circulating CD19 positive B cells. This condition does not appear to be X-linked, although it is more common in males. The cause may be related to a delayed maturation of one or more components of the immune system, possibly T helper cells.[4]

## X-Linked Bruton's Agammaglobulinemia

**Bruton's agammaglobulinemia,** first described in 1952, is X chromosome–linked, so this syndrome affects males almost exclusively. Patients with X-linked agammaglobulinemia lack circulating mature CD19 positive B cells and exhibit a deficiency or lack of immunoglobulins of all classes.[4,5] Furthermore, they have no plasma cells in their lymphoid tissues, but they do have pre-B cells in their bone marrow.[6] Because of the lack of B cells, the tonsils and adenoids are small or entirely absent, and lymph nodes lack normal germinal centers. T cells are normal in number and function. About half of the patients have a family history of the syndrome. They develop recurrent bacterial infections beginning in infancy, as maternal antibody is cleared. They most commonly develop sinopulmonary infections caused by encapsulated organisms such as streptococci, meningococci, and *Haemophilus influenzae*. Other infections seen include bacterial otitis media, bronchitis, pneumonia, meningitis, and dermatitis.[4] Some patients also have a susceptibility to certain types of viral infections, including vaccine-associated poliomyelitis. In general, live virus vaccines should be avoided in immunodeficient patients.

X-linked hypogammaglobulinemia results from arrested differentiation at the pre-B cell stage, leading to a complete absence of B cells and plasma cells. The underlying genetic mechanism is a deficiency of an enzyme called the *Bruton tyrosine kinase (Btk)* in B-cell progenitor cells.[6] Lack of the enzyme apparently causes a failure of Vh gene rearrangement. As discussed in Chapter 4, during B-cell maturation, there is a rearrangement of V, D, and J segments to create functioning genes that code for immunoglobulin heavy and light chains. The syndrome can be effectively treated by administering intramuscular or intravenous immunoglobulin preparations and vigorous antimicrobial treatment of infections. The syndrome can be differentiated from transient hypogammaglobulinemia of infancy by the absence of CD19 positive B cells in the peripheral blood, by the abnormal histology of lymphoid tissues, and by its persistence beyond 2 years of age.

Recently, it has been found that patients with a similar clinical presentation to Bruton's appear to have a genetic defect that is inherited in an autosomal recessive manner.[4,7]

## IgA Deficiency

Selective IgA deficiency is the most common congenital immunodeficiency, occurring in about 1 in 500 persons of American-European descent.[4] Most patients with a deficiency of IgA are asymptomatic. Those with symptoms usually have infections of the respiratory and gastrointestinal tract and an increased tendency to autoimmune diseases such as systemic lupus erythematosus, rheumatoid arthritis,

celiac disease, and thyroiditis. Allergic disorders and malignancy are also more common.[5] About 20 percent of the IgA-deficient patients who develop infections also have an IgG2 subclass deficiency. If the serum IgA is less than 5 mg/mL, the deficiency is considered severe. If the IgA level is two standard deviations below the age-adjusted mean but greater than 5 mg/mL, the deficiency is partial. Although the genetic defect has not been established, it is hypothesized that lack of IgA is caused by impaired differentiation of lymphocytes to become IgA-producing plasma cells.[4]

Anti-IgA antibodies are produced by 30 to 40 percent of patients with severe IgA deficiency. These antibodies can cause anaphylactic reactions when blood products containing IgA are transfused.[5] Because many patients with severe IgA deficiency have no other symptoms, the IgA deficiency may not be detected until the patient experiences a transfusion reaction resulting from the presence of anti-IgA antibodies. Products for transfusion to known IgA-deficient patients should be collected from IgA-deficient donors, or cellular products should be washed to remove as much donor plasma as possible.

Most gamma globulin preparations contain significant amounts of IgA. However, replacement IgA therapy is not useful, because the half-life of IgA is short (around 7 days), and intravenously or intramuscularly administered IgA is not transported to its normal site of secretion at mucosal surfaces. Furthermore, administration of IgA-containing products can induce the development of anti-IgA antibodies or provoke anaphylaxis in patients who already have antibodies.

## Common Variable Immunodeficiency

**Common variable immunodeficiency (CVI)** is a heterogeneous group of disorders with a prevalence of about 1 in 25,000.[8] While this is a low incidence, it does make CVI the most common primary immune deficiency with a severe clinical syndrome.[5] Patients usually begin to have symptoms in their 20s and 30s, but age at onset ranges from 7 to 71 years of age. The disorder can be congenital or acquired, familial or sporadic, and it occurs with equal frequency in men and women. CVI is characterized by hypogammaglobulinemia that leads to recurrent bacterial infections, particularly sinusitis and pneumonia. In addition, up to 20 percent of CVI patients develop herpes zoster (shingles), a much higher incidence than in immunologically normal young adults. There is usually a deficiency of both IgA and IgG, but selective IgG deficiency may occur. CVI is often associated with a spruelike syndrome characterized by malabsorption and diarrhea. CVI is also associated with an increased risk of lymphoproliferative disorders, gastric carcinomas, and autoimmune disorders.[5] The most common autoimmune manifestations of CVI are immune thrombocytopenia and autoimmune hemolytic anemia. Other symptoms may include lymphadenopathy, splenomegaly, and intestinal hyperplasia.[5]

CVI is diagnosed when patients with recurrent bacterial infections demonstrate a low serum IgG level. Additionally, blood group isohemagglutinins, or naturally occurring antibodies, are typically absent or low. In contrast to X-linked agammaglobulinemia, most patients with CVI have normal numbers of mature B cells. However, these B cells do not differentiate normally into immunoglobulin-producing plasma cells. Three major types of cellular defects have been found in CVI patients. In some cases, T cells or their products appear to suppress differentiation of B cells into plasma cells. Secondly, T cells may fail to provide adequate help to support terminal differentiation of B cells. Finally, there appears to be a primary defect in the B-cell line in some patients. CVI is often a diagnosis of exclusion, where an immunodeficiency is present with no specific genetic defect defined.[7]

CVI can usually be effectively treated with intramuscular or intravenous immunoglobulin preparations.[9] However, because of their low levels of secretory IgA, patients are still susceptible to respiratory and gastrointestinal infections, and the clinician should be vigilant for these infections and treat them vigorously with antibiotics.

## Isolated IgG Subclass Deficiency

There are four subclasses of IgG in the human. IgG subclass deficiencies, initially described in 1970, are conditions where the level of one or more of the IgG subclasses is more than two standard deviations below the mean age-appropriate level.[4] About 70 percent of the total IgG is normally IgG1, 20 percent IgG2, 6 percent IgG3, and 4 percent IgG4. Therefore, a deficiency of a single subclass may not result in a total IgG level below the normal range. In patients with recurrent infections, levels of the different subclasses should be measured if the total IgG level is normal but the clinical picture suggests immunoglobulin deficiency.[4]

Most IgG antibodies directed against protein antigens are of the IgG1 and IgG3 subclasses, while most IgG antibodies against carbohydrate antigens are IgG2 or IgG4. Thus, deficiencies involving IgG1 or IgG3 lead to a reduced response capability to protein antigens such as toxins, while selective deficiencies of IgG2 can result in impaired responses to polysaccharide antigens, which cause recurrent infections with polysaccharide-encapsulated bacteria such as *Streptococcus pneumoniae* and *Haemophilus influenzae*.[4] A variety of genetic defects have been associated with IgG subclass deficiency. These include heavy chain gene deletions and transcriptional defects. The most common subclass deficiency is IgG4, with IgG1 deficiency being the least common, although IgG4 subclass deficiency may have the least clinical significance.[4]

## Deficiencies of Cellular Immunity

Defects in cell-mediated immunity can result from abnormalities at many different stages of T-cell development. Many different molecular defects can result in a similar clinical picture (as in severe combined immunodeficiency [SCID]). In some cases, a primary defect in cell-mediated immunity can also have secondary effects on humoral immunity. This is because T cells provide helper functions that are necessary for normal B-cell development and differentiation. Some of the more common defects of cellular and combined cellular and humoral immunity are summarized in **Table 16–2**.

In general, defects in cellular immunity are more difficult to manage than defects in humoral immunity. When immunoglobulin production is deficient, replacement therapy is often very effective. However, there is usually no

| Table 16–2. | Characteristics of Selected Defects of the T-Cell System and Combined Defects | | |
|---|---|---|---|
| CONDITION | DEFICIENCY | LEVEL OF DEFECT | PRESENTATION |
| DiGeorge anomaly | T cells; some secondary effects on antibody production | Embryological development of the thymus | Neonatal, with hypocalcemia or cardiac defects if severe; incomplete forms may present later with infection |
| PNP deficiency | T cells; some secondary effects on antibody production | PNP, purine metabolism | Infancy |
| SCID | Both T and B cells | ADA, purine metabolism; HLA expression; RAG1/2; JAK3; common gamma chain receptor | Infancy |
| WAS | Reduced IgM and T-cell defect | CD43 expression | Usually infancy; mild variants occur |
| AT | Reduced IgG2, IgA, IgE, and T lymphocytes | DNA instability | Infancy |
| Reticular dysgenesis | All leukocytes | Stem cell defect | Neonatal |

PNP = purine nucleoside phosphorylase; SCID = severe combined immunodeficiency; ADA = adenosine deaminase; HLA = human leukocyte antigen; WAS = Wiskott-Aldrich syndrome; AT = ataxia-telangiectasia

soluble product that can be administered to treat a deficiency of cell-mediated immunity. Transplantation of immunologically intact cells, usually in the form of allogenic bone marrow transplantation, is often required to reconstitute immune function.

Patients with severe defects in cell-mediated immunity may develop graft-versus-host (GvH) disease. Transfused lymphocytes are normally destroyed by the recipient's T-cell system. However, a severe defect in the T-cell system allows the donor lymphocytes to survive, proliferate, and attack the recipient's tissues as foreign. GvH disease can occur in any individual with a severe defect in cell-mediated immunity (e.g., in bone marrow transplant recipients) and can be fatal. Irradiation of cell-containing blood products (platelet concentrates, packed red blood cells, and whole blood) before transfusion destroys the ability of the donor lymphocytes to proliferate and prevents development of GvH disease in immunodeficient recipients. It should be noted that a defect in humoral immunity does not predispose one to GvH disease.

GvH disease also occurs in patients who have received a bone marrow transplant as therapy for a congenital immune deficiency. The closer the match between the genetic constitution of the patient and the graft donor, the less severe the GvH disease is likely to be. Thus, although bone marrow transplantation can potentially cure the immune defect, it can also have serious, lifelong complications of its own.

## DiGeorge Anomaly

**DiGeorge anomaly** is a developmental abnormality of the third and fourth pharyngeal pouches that affects thymic development. Specifically, most patients show a deletion in chromosome 22, region q11,[10] although this anomaly is not required for diagnosis.[5] All organs derived from these embryonic structures can be affected. Associated abnormalities include mental retardation, absence of ossification of the hyoid bone, cardiac anomalies, abnormal facial development, and thymic hypoplasia.[5] The severity and extent of the developmental defect can be quite variable. Many patients with a partial DiGeorge anomaly have only a minimal thymic defect and are thus near normal immune function.[5] However, about 20 percent of children with a defect of the third and fourth pharyngeal pouches have a severe and persistent decrease in T-cell numbers.[11] These children tend to have severe, recurrent viral and fungal infections. Severely affected children usually present in the neonatal period with tetany (caused by hypocalcemia resulting from hypoparathyroidism) or manifestations of cardiac defects. The possibility of immune deficiency can be overlooked if the association between the presenting abnormality and a possible thymic defect is not recognized.

The immunodeficiency associated with the DiGeorge anomaly is a quantitative defect in thymocytes. Not enough mature T cells are made, but those that are present are functionally normal. The immunodeficiency of DiGeorge syndrome can be treated with fetal thymus transplantation. Bone marrow transplantation has also been successful in some patients, as has administration of thymic hormones.

## Purine Nucleoside Phosphorylase Deficiency

One immunodeficiency state for which a specific enzymatic basis has been defined is **purine nucleoside phosphorylase (PNP) deficiency.** PNP deficiency is a rare autosomal recessive trait.[11] The condition presents in infancy with recurrent or chronic pulmonary infections, oral or cutaneous candidiasis, diarrhea, skin infections, urinary tract infections, and failure to thrive. PNP deficiency affects an enzyme involved in the metabolism of purines. It produces a moderate to severe defect in cell-mediated immunity, with normal or only mildly impaired humoral immunity.[11] The number of T cells progressively decreases because of the accumulation of deoxyguanosine triphosphate, a toxic purine metabolite. The levels of immunoglobulins are generally normal or increased. About two-thirds of PNP-deficient patients also have neurological disorders, but no characteristic physical abnormalities have been described. Because of the relatively selective defect in cell-mediated immunity, PNP deficiency can be confused with neonatal HIV infection. The two conditions can usually be distinguished by specific tests for anti-HIV antibody (if the infant is old enough to be producing antibody) and by assays for PNP activity.

## Combined Deficiencies of Cellular and Humoral Immunity

Defects in both humoral (B cell) and cell-mediated (T cell) immunity can be caused by a defect that affects development of both types of lymphocytes or a defective interaction between the two limbs of the immune system. Because helper T cell functions are necessary for normal differentiation and antibody secretion by B cells, a severe defect of T-cell function will affect immunoglobulin levels as well. Combined deficiencies are referred to using a shorthand of $T^{+-}B^{+-}NK^{+-}$ with the superscript $^{+-}$ denoting whether or not each cell type is present in the deficiency.[5]

### Severe Combined Immunodeficiency

The most serious of the congenital immune deficiencies is **severe combined immunodeficiency (SCID).** It is actually a group of related diseases that all affect T- and B-cell function but with differing causes. X-linked SCID is the most common form of the disease, accounting for approximately 46 percent of the cases in the United States today.[2,12] This occurs with a frequency of about 1 in 50,000 births.[13] The abnormal gene involved codes for a protein chain called the *common gamma chain*, which is common to receptors for interleukins-2, 4, 7, 9, 15, and 21.[12] The gene is referred to as the *IL2RG gene* and is located on the X chromosome. Normal signaling cannot occur in cells with defective receptors, thus halting natural maturation.[2,13] This may result in either a

$T^-B^+NK^+$ or a $T^-B^+NK^-$ phenotype, depending on whether or not there is an additional defect in the JAK3 gene.[5] JAK3 is required for processing an interleukin binding signal from the cell membrane to the nucleus. In such cases, no antibody production or lymphocyte proliferative response follows an antigen or mitogen challenge.

A JAK3 deficiency may be found without the common gamma chain deletion. This results in an autosomal recessive form of SCID, affecting both males and females.[5] The lack of the intracellular kinase JAK3 means that lymphocytes are unable to transmit signals from interleukins-2 and 4.[2,11] These patients have a $T^-B^+NK^-$ phenotype, and symptoms are similar to the X-linked form of the disease.[5] The JAK3 gene is located on chromosome 19, region p12.

About 15 to 20 percent of the patients with SCID have an adenosine deaminase (ADA) deficiency, leading to a $T^-B^-NK^-$ phenotype.[5] The ADA gene is located on chromosome 1, region q21. Like PNP deficiency, ADA deficiency affects an enzyme involved in the metabolism of purines. In ADA deficiency, toxic metabolites of purines accumulate in lymphoid cells and impair proliferation of both B and T cells. As in PNP deficiency, there is a progressive decrease in lymphocyte numbers. Several different mutations have been found to lead to ADA deficiency, and the degree of immunodeficiency correlates with the degree of ADA deficiency. Patients with only mildly reduced ADA activity may have only a slight impairment of immune function.[5]

Other molecular defects have been identified as causes of SCID. Infants with a lack of both T and B cells but with functioning NK cells were found to have a mutation in a recombinase activating gene (RAG1 or RAG2).[12] These mutations cause a profound lymphocytopenia because of the inability of T and B cells to rearrange the DNA necessary to produce functional immunoglobulins or T-cell receptors.[11] This condition has been referred to as Ommen's syndrome.[6] Defective expression of human leukocyte antigen (HLA) class II antigens, normally found on B cells, leads to bare lymphocyte syndrome. HLA class II molecules are intimately involved in antigen presentation; thus, this defect profoundly impairs the immune response.[5,12] A newly identified molecular defect is a mutation in the gene encoding a common leukocyte protein called CD45. It is a transmembrane phosphatase that regulates signal transduction of T- and B-cell receptors.[11,12]

Patients with SCID generally present early in infancy with infection by nearly any type of organism. Oral candidal infections, pneumonia, and diarrhea are the most common manifestations. The receipt of live vaccines can cause severe illness. Unless immune reconstitution can be achieved by bone marrow transplantation or by specifically replacing a deficient enzyme, patients with SCID die before they reach 2 years of age.[12]

ADA deficiency is a special case, because it presents a good opportunity for enzyme replacement therapy or somatic cell gene therapy. Although the ADA is normally located within cells, its deficiency can be treated by maintaining high plasma levels of ADA. Red blood cell transfusion has been used in some patients to raise ADA to near normal levels. However, bovine ADA conjugated with polyethylene glycol (PEG) has a longer half-life than native ADA and can be used to raise the ADA level up to three times higher than normal. This treatment increases T-cell production and specific antibody responses. Side effects of ADA–PEG administration appear to be minimal. However, this therapy is very expensive (about $250,000/year) and is primarily used in patients for whom a suitable bone marrow donor cannot be found or for those who are too sick to undergo marrow transplantation.[14] Human cord blood stem cell transplantation has been used with moderate success.[15] Studies are currently under way to attempt to treat ADA deficiency by transfecting a normal ADA gene into patients' T cells or stem cells. These cells could then be reinfused into the patient. Theoretically, the gene therapy approach could be curative, but there are many obstacles to overcome.

## Wiskott–Aldrich Syndrome

**Wiskott-Aldrich syndrome (WAS)** is a rare X-linked recessive syndrome that probably affects six patients a year in the United States.[16] It is defined by the triad of immunodeficiency, eczema, and thrombocytopenia. WAS is usually lethal in childhood because of infection, hemorrhage, or malignancy. Milder variants have also been described, such as an X-linked form of thrombocytopenia.

The laboratory features of WAS include a decrease in platelet number and size with a prolonged bleeding time.[5] The bone marrow contains a normal or somewhat increased number of megakaryocytes. There are abnormalities in both the cellular and humoral arms of the immune system, related to a general defect in antigen processing. This is manifest as a severe deficiency of the naturally occurring antibodies to blood group antigens (isohemagglutinins). Patients with WAS can have a variety of different patterns of immunoglobulin levels, but they usually have low levels of IgM, normal levels of IgA and IgG, and increased levels of IgE.[5] Absence of isohemagglutinins (IgM antibodies against ABO blood group antigens) is the most consistent laboratory finding in WAS and is often used diagnostically. In addition, these patients have persistently increased levels of serum alpha-fetoprotein, which can also be a useful diagnostic feature.

The primary molecular defect in the syndrome appears to be an abnormality of the integral membrane protein CD43, which is involved in the regulation of protein glycosylation.[6] The gene responsible for the defect is called the WASp gene, and it is located on the X chromosome, region p11. Abnormalities cause defective actin polymerization and affect its signal transduction in lymphocytes and platelets.[6]

Platelets have a shortened half-life, and T lymphocytes are also affected, although B lymphocytes appear to function normally. Splenectomy can be very valuable in controlling the thrombocytopenia. Current treatment for this immunodeficiency is bone marrow transplantation or cord blood stem cells from an HLA-identical sibling.[9]

## Ataxia-Telangiectasia

**Ataxia-telangiectasia (AT)** is a rare autosomal recessive syndrome characterized by cerebellar ataxia and telangiectasias, especially on the earlobes and conjunctiva. Blood vessels in the sclera of the eyes may be dilated, and there may also be a reddish butterfly area on the face and ears. Ninety-five percent of patients exhibit increased levels of serum alpha-fetoprotein.[11] The incidence is between 1 in 10,000 to 1 in 100,000, although as much as 1 percent of the population is heterozygous for the gene.[17] Abnormal genes produce a combined defect of both humoral and cellular immunity.[5,17] Antibody response to antigens, especially polysaccharides, is blunted. The levels of IgG2, IgA, and IgE are often low or absent, although the pattern can be quite variable. In addition, the number of circulating T cells is often decreased. Death usually occurs in early adult life from either pulmonary disease or malignancy.[2]

Patients with AT have a defect in a gene that is apparently essential to the recombination process for genes in the immunoglobulin superfamily. The AT gene is located on chromosome 11, region q22. This abnormality results in a defective kinase involved in DNA repair and in cell cycle control.[13] Rearrangement of T-cell receptor and immunoglobulin genes does not occur normally.[11] Patients' lymphocytes often exhibit chromosomal breaks and other abnormalities involving the T-cell receptor genes in T cells and immunoglobulin genes in B cells. These are sites of high levels of chromosomal recombination, and errors that occur during gene rearrangements may not be repaired properly. The syndrome is associated with an even greater risk of lymphoid malignancy than other immunodeficiency syndromes, presumably because the failure to properly repair DNA damage leads to accumulation of mutations. The only effective therapy for AT is allogenic bone marrow transplantation.

## Defects of Neutrophil Function

Neutrophils play a crucial role in the immediate and non-specific response to invading organisms by reacting before specific antibody and cell-mediated immune responses can be mounted. In addition, neutrophils are even more effective at ingesting and killing organisms coated with specific antibody and thus continue to play an important role in host defense even after a specific immune response is established. To destroy invading organisms, neutrophils must adhere to vascular endothelial lining cells, migrate through the capillary wall to a site of infection, and ingest and kill the microbes. Defects affecting each of these steps have been described, each leading to an increased susceptibility to pyogenic infections.

## Chronic Granulomatous Disease

**Chronic granulomatous disease (CGD)** is a group of disorders inherited as either an X-linked or autosomal recessive gene that affects neutrophil microbicidal function. The X-linked disease accounts for 70 percent of the cases, and it tends to be more severe.[5] Symptoms of CGD include recurrent suppurative infections, pneumonia, osteomyelitis, draining adenopathy, liver abscesses, dermatitis, and hypergammaglobulinemia. Typically, catalase-positive organisms such as *Staphylococcus aureus*, *Burkholderia cepacia*, and *Chromobacterium violaceum* are involved, in addition to fungi such as *Aspergillus* and *Nocardia*.[5,17] Infections usually begin before 1 year of age, and the syndrome is often fatal in childhood.

CGD is the most common and best characterized of the neutrophil abnormalities. Several specific molecular defects have been described in this syndrome, all of which result in the inability of the patient's neutrophils to produce the reactive forms of oxygen necessary for normal bacterial killing. There are three different autosomal recessive genes involved, and all of these affect subunits of nicotinamide adenine dinucleotide phosphate (NADPH) oxidase.[18] Normally, neutrophil stimulation leads to the production of reactive oxygen molecules, such as hydrogen peroxide ($H_2O_2$), by NADPH oxidase on the plasma membrane. The plasma membrane enfolds an organism as it is phagocytized, and hydrogen peroxide is generated in close proximity to the target microbe. Neutrophil granules fuse with, and release their contents into, the forming phagosome. Hydrogen peroxide is then used by the granule enzyme myeloperoxidase to generate the potent microbicidal agent hypochlorous acid.[18]

The process of generating partially reduced forms of oxygen by stimulated neutrophils was first detected as an increase in oxygen consumption. Therefore, this response was originally termed the neutrophil "respiratory burst." A more correct term is **oxidative burst.** A genetic defect in any of the several components of the NADPH oxidase system can result in the CGD phenotype by making the neutrophil incapable of generating an oxidative burst.

CGD was historically diagnosed by measuring the ability of a patient's neutrophils to reduce the dye nitro-blue tetrazolium (NBT). NBT reduction is caused by the production of hydrogen peroxide and other reactive forms of oxygen. Reduction converts the nearly colorless NBT into a blue precipitate that can be assessed visually on a microscope slide.[18] More recently, a flow cytometric assay has been used. In this assay, neutrophils are labeled with dihydrorhodamine (DHR). DHR will fluoresce when it is reduced. The neutrophils are then activated using phorbol myristate acetate (PMA), which is mitogenic for neutrophils. The resultant oxidative burst will reduce the DHR, resulting in fluorescence that may be quantitated on a flow cytometer. Neutrophils from CGD patients will be unable to undergo the oxidative burst and will show less fluorescence than normal neutrophils.[18] This technique is more objective and quantitative than the traditional NBT technique.

Although therapy with granulocyte transfusions may resolve an acute infectious episode, it is impossible to provide enough granulocytes to treat the condition on a chronic basis. Administration of cytokines, such as interferon, may increase the oxidative burst activity in some patients. Continuous use of antibiotics can greatly reduce the occurrence of severe infections.[13] Bone marrow transplantation or use of peripheral blood stem cells may result in a permanent cure.[18]

## Other Microbicidal Defects

Several other recognized defects can result in impaired neutrophil microbicidal activity. Neutrophil glucose-6-phosphate dehydrogenase deficiency leads to an inability to generate enough NADPH to supply reducing equivalents to the NADPH oxidase system. This leads to a defect in hydrogen peroxide production and a clinical picture similar to that of CGD. Myeloperoxidase deficiency is relatively common, occurring in about 1 in 3000 persons in the United States. Deficient patients may have recurrent candidal infections. Defects of neutrophil secondary granules have also been described. However, the molecular nature of the defects is unknown.[9]

## Leukocyte Adhesion Deficiency

Even if microbicidal activity is normal, neutrophils cannot perform their functions properly if they fail to leave the vasculature and migrate to a site of incipient infection. Adhesion receptors on leukocytes and their counter-receptors on endothelial cells and extracellular matrix play important roles in these activities. In leukocyte adhesion deficiency (LAD), a protein (CD18) that is a component of adhesion receptors on neutrophils and monocytes (with CD11b or CD11c) and on T cells (with CD11a) is defective.[5,18] The CD18 deficiency is transmitted with autosomal recessive inheritance and has variable expression. This defect leads to abnormal adhesion, motility, aggregation, chemotaxis, and endocytosis by the affected leukocytes. The defects are clinically manifested as delayed wound healing, chronic skin infections, intestinal and respiratory tract infections, and periodontitis. A defect in CD18 can be diagnosed by detecting a decreased amount of the CD11/18 antigen on patient leukocytes by flow cytometry.[18]

The CD11/18 protein is not the only neutrophil molecule involved in adhesion, motility, and phagocytosis. Recently, another type of adhesion molecule deficiency (LAD II) has been characterized. A carbohydrate molecule involved in adhesive interactions, CD15s, or sialyl Lewis X, was found to be deficient.[18]

## Complement Deficiencies

Complement consists of a series of proteins that work in a cascade to assist in antibody destruction of cells, as described in Chapter 6. The complement system is also part of the innate immune system and can work as part of the inflammatory system to directly eliminate a potential pathogen. Deficiencies in each of the major complement components have been described, leading to various clinical sequelae.[19]

Deficiencies in the early complement components, C1q, 4, and 2, are usually associated with a lupuslike syndrome. Deficiency of C2 is believed to be the most common complement component deficiency. A C3 deficiency may also have a lupuslike clinical presentation but is more likely to involve

recurrent encapsulated organism infection. Deficiencies of the later components of complement (C5 through C9) are often associated with recurrent Neisserial infections. A deficiency of C1 esterase inhibitor has been found in patients with hereditary angioedema. Most complement deficiencies appear to be inherited in an autosomal recessive manner and are likely due to mutations as opposed to genetic deletions.[19]

## LABORATORY EVALUATION OF IMMUNE DYSFUNCTION

It is important in performing diagnostic testing for immunodeficiency that the results for a patient be compared with appropriate age-matched controls. In tests of cellular function, the patient's cells need to be tested in parallel with cells from a normal control. If an abnormal test result is obtained, it should be confirmed by repeat testing.

## Screening Tests

Screening tests used for the initial evaluation of suspected immunodeficiency states are summarized in **Table 16-3**. Most of these tests can be performed routinely in any hospital laboratory. The evaluation of possible immunodeficiency starts with a complete blood count and white blood cell differential, which may reveal a reduced lymphocyte count. Thrombocytopenia with small platelets can be detected in WAS.

Measurement of the levels of serum IgG, IgM, and IgA and levels of the subclasses of IgG are used to screen for defects in antibody production. Assay for isohemagglutinins is easily performed by the transfusion service. By the age of 2, a child should have naturally occurring IgM antibodies

| Table 16-3. | Screening Tests for Immunodeficiencies |
|---|---|
| **SUSPECTED DISORDER** | **TESTS** |
| All immunodeficiencies Humoral immunity | Complete blood cell count, white blood cell differential count Serum IgG, IgA, IgM levels, IgG subclass levels, isohemag-glutinin titers (IgM), IgG antibody response to protein and polysaccharide antigens |
| Cell-mediated immunity | Delayed hypersensitivity skin tests (i.e., candida, diphtheria, tetanus, PPD) Chest X-ray (thymus shadow) |
| Phagocyte defect | NBT test IgE level (hyper-IgE syndrome) |
| Complement | CH$_{50}$ (classical pathway) Serum C3 level |

PPD = Purified protein derivative; NBT = nitroblue tetrazolium.

against ABO blood group antigens. The absence of these antibodies suggests an abnormal IgM response.

An overall assessment of antibody-mediated immunity can be made by measuring antibody responses to antigens to which the population is exposed normally or following vaccination. This can be easily done by measuring the titer of the specific antibody produced in response to immunization with a commercial vaccine such as diphtheria/tetanus. In an unimmunized child, the development of tetanus or diphtheria antibodies is determined 2 weeks after immunization. In a previously immunized patient, the response to a booster injection can be evaluated, normally 4 to 6 weeks postvaccination. A wide range of other protein and polysaccharide antigens can also be used in these tests. This technique is often used to evaluate a possible IgG subclass deficiency. IgG1 and 3 isotypes normally respond to protein antigens, such as tetanus and diphtheria. IgG2 normally responds to polysaccharide antigens, such as those in the *Haemophilus influenza* and *Streptococcus pneumoniae* vaccines.[4]

Delayed-hypersensitivity-type skin reactions can be used to screen for defects in cell-mediated immunity. These tests are generally performed by the clinician and not by laboratory personnel. Delayed cutaneous hypersensitivity is a localized cell-mediated reaction to a specific antigen. The prototype is the tuberculin skin test. An antigen to which most of the population has been exposed, such as candida, mumps, or tetanus toxoid, is injected intradermally. The presence of induration 48 to 72 hours later indicates a cell-mediated immune response. A negative test is not always informative, because the patient may not have been previously exposed to the test antigen.

Screening for complement deficiencies usually begins with a CH50 assay.[19] This procedure determines the level of functional complement in an individual. Undetectable CH50 levels may indicate a deficiency of a specific component. Based upon the clinical history, individual component assays would be indicated. The laboratorian should be aware, however, that low CH50 levels may be due to complement consumption and do not, by themselves, indicate a complement deficiency.

Defects in neutrophil oxidative burst activity may be detected by a flow cytometric assay, as mentioned above. Neutrophils labeled with dihydrorhodamine (DHR) are stimulated to undergo an oxidative burst by exposure to a mitogen. The oxidative burst will reduce the DHR, causing it to fluoresce. The resultant fluorescence may be measured objectively by flow cytometry. Flow cytometry looking for the expression of the CD18 antigen may be used to diagnose LAD, type 1.

## Confirmatory Tests

If the screening tests detect an abnormality or if the clinical suspicion is high, more specialized testing will probably be necessary to precisely identify an immune abnormality.

Some of the tests used for confirming an immunodeficiency state are summarized in **Table 16–4**.

Enumeration of classes of lymphocytes in the peripheral blood is performed by flow cytometry. Even though types of lymphocytes cannot be distinguished morphologically, they exhibit different patterns of antigen or surface immunoglobulin expression that correlate with functional characteristics. For flow cytometric evaluation, antibodies to antigens specific for different types of lymphocytes are labeled with a fluorescent probe. These antigens are generally referred to by cluster of differentiation (CD) number. The antibodies are allowed to react with peripheral blood mononuclear cells. The flow cytometer is used to count the cells that are labeled with each fluorescent antibody. Lymphocytes can then be assigned to specific types based on antigen expression: B cells (CD19), T cells (CD3), T helper cells (CD3/CD4), cytotoxic T cells (CD3/CD8), and NK cells (CD16 and/or CD56). Flow cytometry is objective and quite reliable. It allows detection of those defects that result in a decrease in one or more types of lymphocytes. For example, an absence or profound decrease in the number of CD3 cells would be consistent with DiGeorge syndrome. An absence of CD19 positive B cells suggests Bruton's agammaglobulinemia.

Most of the genes associated with primary immune deficiencies have been identified and localized. Thus, genetic testing is available for many conditions, including the DiGeorge deletion, the Wiskott-Aldrich gene, and the IL2RG mutations. While genetic testing is useful to understand the pathology of the disease, it is often not

| Table 16–4. | Specialized Confirmatory Tests for Immunodeficiencies |
|---|---|
| **SUSPECTED DISORDER** | **TESTS** |
| Humoral immunity | B cell counts (total and IgM, IgD, IgG, IgA-bearing) <br> B cell proliferation in vitro <br> Histology of lymphoid tissues |
| Cell-mediated immunity | T cell counts (total and helper-supressor subsets) <br> T cell functions *in vitro* <br> Enzyme assays (ADA, PNP) |
| Phagocyte defect | Leukocyte adhesion molecule analysis (CD11a, CD11b, CD11c, CD18) <br> Phagocytosis and bacterial killing assays <br> Chemotaxis assay <br> Enzyme assays (myeloperoxidase, glucose-6-phosphate dehydrogenase, components of NADPH oxidase) |
| Complement | Other specific component assays |

NADPH = Nicotinamide adenine dinucleotide phosphate.

required for making a diagnosis. Genetic testing of family members of affected patients may be helpful in determining who may be at risk of developing the disease or passing it on to offspring.

T-cell function can be measured by assessing the ability of isolated T cells to proliferate in response to an antigenic stimulus or to nonspecific mitogens in culture. Classically, the T-cell response may be measured by quantitating the uptake of radioactive thymidine, a precursor of DNA. Increased thymidine uptake suggests cell division and activation. This assay requires experienced technologists, a radioactive materials license, and laboratory-determined reference ranges.

More recently, antigen- or mitogen-stimulated T-cell activation has been measured without the use of radioactive materials. As of August 2008, three such assays have been FDA cleared for diagnostic use. The QuantiFERON TB assay and the T-Spot assay measure an individual's response to *Mycobacterium tuberculosis* antigens. Following overnight whole blood activation with TB antigens, gamma interferon (secreted by activated Th1 cells) is quantitated by either an ELISA or ELISpot-type procedure. Either of these assays may be used as an in vitro assessment of exposure to *Mycobacterium tuberculosis*.

A second assay, Cylex ImmuKnow, uses the mitogen phytohemagglutinin (PHA) to activate T cells. Following incubation, ATP production is measured by a fluorescent immunoassay technique. Production of ATP is a general measurement of T-cell function and is often used to monitor individuals receiving immunosuppressant therapy. The assay may be used to determine overall T-cell functional capabilities in an individual suspected of a primary immune deficiency.

## Evaluation of Immunoglobulins

Quantitative measurement of serum or urine immunoglobulins is used in the workup of both immunodeficiency states and some lymphoproliferative disorders. Serum protein electrophoresis can be quantitative if the total serum protein is determined and the results are read using a densitometer.

### Serum Protein Electrophoresis

Serum protein electrophoresis (SPE) is a technique in which molecules are separated on the basis of their size and electrical charge. SPE allows reproducible separation of the major plasma proteins (see Chapter 4 for details). The serum protein electrophoretic profile is traditionally divided into five regions: albumin and alpha-1, alpha-2, beta, and gamma globulins. Some laboratories now use six regions, dividing the beta region into beta-1 (transferrin) and beta-2 (complement component C3) regions. IgG, IgM, IgD, and IgE migrate in the gamma globulin region, while IgA migrates as a broad band overlapping the beta and gamma regions. Immunoglobulins normally show a range of mobilities. Additional evaluation of serum immunoglobulin is performed if the SPE shows a monoclonal component or if there is a significant quantitative abnormality of serum immunoglobulins.

### Immunofixation Electrophoresis

Another method of characterizing immune deficiencies is immunofixation electrophoresis (IFE). In IFE, serum samples are electrophoresed, just as for SPE, and then specific antibody is applied directly to the separating gel. The antibody–antigen complexes form and are visualized by staining. Polyclonal immunoglobulins are indicated by areas of diffuse staining, while monoclonal bands produce narrow, intensely stained bands (refer to Fig. 15–2 in Chapter 15.). Lack of bands indicates immunodeficiencies of one or more immunoglobulin classes. IFE is labor-intensive and expensive, although it is fairly fast. For accurate interpretations, specific immunoglobulin isotype levels, determined by nephelometry, are necessary.

## Bone Marrow Biopsy

A bone marrow aspirate and biopsy is indicated in any evaluation of monoclonal gammopathy or immunodeficiency state. It is important in establishing the diagnosis of such disorders and for excluding other diseases. The bone marrow specimen will be analyzed microscopically and by flow cytometry. Cytogenetic analysis may also be performed to detect the specific genetic anomalies associated with the primary immune deficiency diseases.[6,12,20]

## SUMMARY

The immune system consists of a network of interconnected components. Defects in the development and regulation of individual portions of the immune system are recognized as causes of clinically distinct syndromes. Defects in antibody-mediated immunity lead to recurrent infections with pyogenic bacteria, particularly of the respiratory and intestinal tracts. Defects in T cell–mediated immunity generally lead to recurrent infections with intracellular pathogens. Primary defects in T-cell function can also lead to secondary abnormalities in antibody production and an increased risk of malignancy. Defects in phagocyte function generally lead to pyogenic bacterial infections, often of the skin. The clinical manifestations of these deficiency states have led to a better understanding of the normal roles of the different components of the immune system.

Immunodeficiency states run the gamut from quite mild to lethal. It is important to diagnose immunodeficiency states early in life, because effective therapies are available for many of them. Failure to begin therapy as soon as possible can result in permanent organ damage or death caused by infection. The diagnosis must be suspected clinically and is evaluated by serological analysis, first by screening tests measuring leukocyte counts and immunoglobulin levels, then by specialized laboratory testing. Prenatal diagnosis and carrier detection is possible for some familial immunodeficiency syndromes.

# CASE STUDIES

1. A 7-month-old male was diagnosed with bacterial meningitis. Previously he had been hospitalized with bacterial pneumonia. Laboratory testing results were as follows: red cell count: normal; white cell count: $22 \times 10^9$/L (normal is 5 to $24 \times 10^9$/L); differential: 70 percent neutrophils, 15 percent monocytes, 5 percent eosinophils, and 10 percent lymphocytes; and SPE: no gamma band present.

## Questions

a. What possible conditions do these results indicate?

b. How are these conditions inherited?

c. What type of further testing do you recommend?

2. A 3-year-old female appeared to be developmentally slow. She had several facial anomalies, including a small jaw and ears that were set farther back than usual. She seemed prone to infections, especially yeast infections. Laboratory testing results were as follows: red cell count was normal; white cell count was low normal; and a differential white cell count indicated a decrease in lymphocytes. Flow cytometry results demonstrated that the decrease in lymphocyte population was caused by low numbers of T cells. SPE showed a weak gamma band present.

## Questions

a. What immunodeficiency do you suspect?

b. Are the facial anomalies linked to the immunologic findings?

c. What kinds of treatment are possible?

3. A 37-year-old female presents with a history of recurrent upper respiratory infections. She states that she was always a sick child, usually with respiratory infections, but occasional diarrhea would also occur. She has received countless antibiotic regimens over the years. The physician orders a serum protein electrophoresis (SPE) and immunoglobulin levels. The SPE is read as a low gamma level with no monoclonal proteins detected. Levels of IgG, IgM, and IgA are below the reference ranges. The physician then orders an immunofixation assay (Fig. 16–2).

## Questions

a. Which pattern would be most representative of the expected pattern for this patient?

b. Explain why you chose this answer.

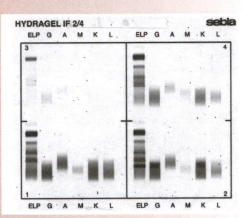

**FIGURE 16–2.** Four different patient immunofixation patterns. (See Color Plate 13.)

# EXERCISE

## IMMUNOFIXATION

### Principle

Immunofixation (IFE) is used to identify a monoclonal immunoglobulin. This assay is a combination of serum protein electrophoresis and immunoprecipitation. Serum proteins are separated by agarose gel electrophoresis. The gel is then overlayed with antibodies to specific immunoglobulin heavy and light chain isotypes, each on an individual electrophoresis pattern or lane. Following an incubation period, the gel is stained for antigen–antibody complexes. A monoclonal immunoglobulin will appear as a band in a lane reacting with a heavy chain antibody (e.g., gamma) and a light chain antibody (e.g., lambda). Normal polyclonal immunoglobulins appear as a diffuse region. Urine may be examined by this method for the presence of Bence Jones protein.

### Sample Preparation

Immunofixation is performed on both serum and urine. Plasma should not be used due to the presence of a fibrinogen. Fibrinogen appears as a gamma band, which can mimic a monoclonal immunoglobulin. A 24-hour urine specimen is recommended for Bence Jones protein analysis.

### Reagents, Materials, and Equipment

Instrument:

1. At least three companies make immunofixation electrophoresis equipment: Beckman-Coulter, Helena, and Sebia. Although there are some variations in the specific procedures among these companies, the basic format is the same, regardless of the equipment the company uses in a given laboratory. The guidelines given here will be based primarily on the Sebia procedure.

   a. Materials and reagents: electrophoresis chamber and power supply

   b. IFE agarose gels (options exist for gels to handle 1–9 IFE assays)

   c. Electrophoresis buffer

   d. Application tool

   e. Isotype-specific antisera

   f. Staining reagents

**Protocol:**

1. Ensure that the electrophoresis buffer chambers are filled with the appropriate buffer.

2. Allow the gels to reach room temperature.

3. Apply the specimen as directed.

   a. The gels contain six lanes for each specimen. One lane is used for a standard protein electrophoresis (SPE) reading. The other five lanes are used for immunoglobulin isotype analysis. Serum is normally diluted prior to application. Each manufacturer may have a specific dilution; however, Sebia recommends a 1:3 dilution for the SPE lane and the IgG lane and a 1:6 dilution for each additional isotype lane. This dilution may need to be adjusted based on the total protein concentration. Concentrated urine specimens are run undiluted in all lanes.

4. Place the gel on the electrophoresis instrument.

5. Apply power and electrophorese for the appropriate time. The Sebia automated system uses a 9-minute electrophoresis time.

6. Overlay each lane with an appropriate antisera. This step may be automated or performed manually.

   a. Three of the lanes are covered with anti–heavy chain antisera (antigamma, antialpha, and antimu).

   b. Two of the lanes are covered with anti–light chain antisera (antikappa and antilambda).

7. Following incubation (5 minutes in the Sebia system), the gel is washed, stained, and dried.

8. The patterns are read. A pathologist or clinical board–certified PhD (ABMLI or AACC) may sign out the interpretations.

### Interpretation

In normal serum, there are many immunoglobulins, each with its own specific amino acid sequence. Thus, each immunoglobulin molecule will migrate to a slightly different location during electrophoresis than the other immunoglobulins. Therefore, the stained regions in each isotype lane will have a diffuse appearance in a normal specimen. A monoclonal immunoglobulin will appear as a dense band in the same electrophoretic location in one of the heavy chains and in one of the light chains. For example, a matching band in the gamma lane and lambda lane indicates the presence of a monoclonal IgG lambda protein. Multiple monoclonal proteins may be seen in a specimen. Biclonal gammopathies with two monoclonal proteins have been described. IgA and IgM monoclonal proteins may appear as two or more bands due to the presence of monomers, dimers, trimers, and pentamers. Specimens with multiple IgA or IgM monoclonal bands may be reduced with 2-mercaptoethanol and repeated on an IFE gel. This reduction process will break apart the multimers into individual immunoglobulin molecules, and a single band should result.

One may see a matching monoclonal heavy and light chain band with an additional nonmatching light chain. This indicates the presence of free serum light chains. The presence of a light chain band with no associated heavy chain band may indicate either light chain disease or possibly an IgD or IgE monoclonal protein. A repeat IFE with antidelta and antiepsilon sera would be recommended in that case.

Immunoglobulin levels, determined by nephelometry, should be performed with an immunofixation. The IFE technique is not quantitative, and the immunoglobulin levels along with the IFE interpretation are useful in assisting the physician to arrive at the proper diagnosis.

Urine IFEs are performed to look for the presence of Bence Jones protein or free monoclonal light chains. It is essential to use antifree light chain antisera in the urine assay. A 24-hour specimen is preferred due to the low sensitivity of detecting Bence Jones proteins in random urine specimens. Urine specimens are routinely concentrated prior to being run in an IFE procedure.

# REVIEW QUESTIONS

1. For which immunodeficiency syndrome should patients receive irradiated blood products to protect against the development of GvH disease?

    a. Bruton's agammaglobulinemia
    b. Severe IgA deficiency
    c. SCID
    d. CGD

2. T-cell subset enumeration by flow cytometry would be most useful in making the diagnosis of which disorder?

    a. Bruton's agammaglobulinemia
    b. Severe IgA deficiency
    c. SCID
    d. Multiple myeloma

3. What clinical manifestations would be seen in a patient with myeloperoxidase deficiency?

    a. Defective T-cell function
    b. Inability to produce IgG
    c. Defective NK cell function
    d. Defective neutrophil function

4. Defects in which arm of the immune system are most commonly associated with severe illness after administration of live virus vaccines?

    a. Cell-mediated immunity
    b. Humoral immunity
    c. Complement
    d. Phagocytic cells

5. Which of the following statements applies to Bruton's X-linked agammaglobulinemia?

    a. It typically appears in females.
    b. There is a lack of circulating CD19 positive B cells.
    c. T cells are abnormal.
    d. There is a lack of pre-B cells in the bone marrow.

6. DiGeorge anomaly may be characterized by all of the following *except*

    a. autosomal recessive inheritance.
    b. cardiac abnormalities.
    c. parathyroid hypoplasia.
    d. decreased number of mature T cells.

7. A 3-year-old boy is hospitalized because of recurrent bouts of pneumonia. Laboratory tests are run, and the following findings are noted: prolonged bleeding time, decreased platelet count, increased level of serum alpha-fetoprotein, and a deficiency of naturally occurring isohemagglutinins. Based on these results, which is the most likely diagnosis?

    a. PNP deficiency
    b. Selective IgA deficiency
    c. SCID
    d. WAS

8. Which of the following is associated with AT?

    a. Inherited as an autosomal recessive
    b. Defect in both cellular and humoral immunity
    c. Chromosomal breaks in lymphocytes
    d. All of the above

# References

1. Primary immunodeficiency diseases. Report of a WHO scientific group. Immunodefic Rev 3:195–236, 1992.
2. Buckley, R. Primary immunodeficiency diseases due to defects in lymphocytes. N Engl J Med 343:1313–1324, 2000.
3. Puck, J. Prenatal diagnosis and genetic analysis of X-linked immunodeficiency disorders. Pediatr Res, 33(suppl):S29, 1993
4. Conley, ME. Primary antibody deficiency diseases. In Detrick, B, Hamilton, RG, and Folds, JD (eds): Manual of Molecular and Clinical Laboratory Immunology, ed. 7. ASM Press, Washington, D.C., pp. 906–913, 2006.
5. Fleisher, TA. Back to basics: Primary immune deficiencies: Window into the immune system. Pediatric Reviews. 27(10): 363–372, 2006.
6. Fischer, A. Human primary immunodeficiency diseases. Immunity 27:835–45, 2007.
7. Stiehm, RE. The four most common pediatric immunodeficiencies. Adv Exp Med and Biol 601:15–26, 2007.
8. Fischer, A. Primary immunodeficiency diseases: An experimental model for molecular medicine. Lancet 357:1863–1869, 2001.
9. Garcia, JM, et al. Update on the treatment of primary immunodeficiencies. Allergol Immunopath 35(5):184–192, 2007.
10. Taddei, I, Morishima, M, Huynh, T, and Lindsay, EA. Genetic factors are major determinants of phenotypic variability in a mouse model of the DiGeorge/del22q11 syndromes. PNAS 98(20):11428–11431, 2001.
11. Primary immunodeficiency diseases. Report of an IUIS Scientific Committee. International Union of Immunological Societies. Clin Exp Immunol 118(Suppl 1):1–28, 1999.
12. Roifman, CM. Approach to the diagnosis of severe combined immunodeficiency. In Detrick, B, Hamilton, RG, and Folds, JD (eds): Manual of Molecular and Clinical Laboratory Immunology, ed. 7. ASM Press, Washington, D.C., pp. 895–900, 2006.
13. Puck, JM. Primary immunodeficiency diseases. JAMA 278:1835–1841, 1997.
14. Hilman, B, and Sorensen, RU. Management options: SCIDS with adenosine deaminase deficiency. Ann Allergy 72, 1994.
15. Gennery, AR, and Cant, AJ. Cord blood stem cell transplantation in primary immune deficiencies. Curr Opin Allergy Clin Immunol 7:528–534, 2007.
16. Peacocke, M, and Siminovitch, KA. Wiskott-Aldrich syndrome: New molecular and biochemical insights. J Am Acad Dermatol 27, 1992.
17. Cooper, M, and Schroeder, HW, Jr. Primary immune deficiency diseases. In Braunwald, E, Fauci, AS, Kasper, DL, et al. (eds): Harrison's Principles of Internal Medicine, ed. 15, McGraw-Hill, New York, pp. 1843–1851, 2001.
18. Holland, SM. Neutropenia and neutrophil defects. In Detrick, B, Hamilton, RG, and Folds, JD (eds): Manual of Molecular and Clinical Laboratory Immunology, ed. 7. ASM Press, Washington, D.C., pp. 924–932, 2006.
19. Giclas, PC. Hereditary and acquired complement deficiencies. In Detrick, B, Hamilton, RG, and Folds, JD (eds): Manual of Molecular and Clinical Laboratory Immunology, ed. 7. ASM Press, Washington, D.C., pp. 914–923, 2006.
20. Verbsky, JW, and Grossman, WJ. Cellular and genetic basis of primary immune deficiencies. Pediatr Clin North Am 53:649–684, 2006.

# 17 Transplantation Immunology

*John L. Schmitz, Ph.D., D(ABMLI, ABHI)*

## LEARNING OBJECTIVES

*After finishing this chapter, the reader will be able to:*

1. List the histocompatibility systems relevant to clinical transplantation.
2. Discuss the mechanism of alloantigen recognition.
3. Distinguish allograft, autograft, xenograft, and syngeneic graft.
4. Discuss the mechanisms of graft rejection.
5. Identify risk factors for graft-versus-host (GvH) disease.
6. Discuss the major classes of immunosuppressive agents.
7. Discuss methods for HLA typing.
8. Discuss methods for detecting and identifying HLA antibodies.

## KEY TERMS

- ____ Accelerated rejection
- ____ Acute rejection
- ____ Acute GVHD
- ____ Allograft
- ____ Autograft
- ____ Chronic rejection
- ____ Complement-dependent cytotoxicity (CDC)
- ____ Crossmatch
- ____ Direct allorecognition
- ____ Graft-versus-host disease (GVHD)
- ____ Haplotypes
- ____ HLA antibody screen
- ____ HLA genotype
- ____ HLA typing
- ____ HLA match
- ____ HLA phenotype
- ____ Hyperacute rejection
- ____ Immunosuppressive agent
- ____ Indirect allorecognition
- ____ Major histocompatibility antigens
- ____ Mixed lymphocyte response
- ____ Syngeneic graft
- ____ Zenograft

# CHAPTER OUTLINE

## INTRODUCTION

Transplantation is a potentially lifesaving treatment for end-stage organ failure, cancers, autoimmune diseases, immune deficiencies, and a variety of other diseases. Over 28,000 solid-organ (kidney, pancreas, liver, heart, lung, small intestine) transplants were performed in the United States,[1] and approximately 50,000 hematopoietic stem cell transplants were performed worldwide in 2006.[2] The number of transplants performed is a testament to the numerous developments over the past few decades in patient management pre- and post-transplant and in the technologies for organ/stem cell acquisition and sharing. Of critical importance has been the continued elucidation of the immunologic mechanisms of graft rejection and graft-versus-host disease, in particular the role of human leukocyte antigens (HLA) and the development of pharmacological agents that interfere with various components of the immune system to promote sustained graft survival.

The HLA system (covered in detail in Chapter 3) is the largest immunologic barrier to successful allogeneic organ transplantation. It consists of cell surface proteins that play a central role in immune recognition and initiation of immune responses. Because of the ubiquitous presence of these proteins on the surface of nucleated cells and their extensive degree of polymorphism, an allogeneic response may result in graft rejection in solid-organ and stem cell transplantation or graft-versus-host disease in stem cell transplantation.

## HISTOCOMPATIBILITY SYSTEMS

The classical (transplant) HLA antigens, also known as **major histocompatibility antigens,** include the class I

(HLA-A, B, and C) and class II (HLA-DR, DQ, and DP) proteins. HLA proteins are encoded by a set of closely linked genes on the short arm of chromosome 6 in the major histocompatibility complex (MHC). The HLA genes are inherited as **haplotypes** from parental chromosomes **(Fig. 17–1)**. Offspring receive one maternal and one paternal HLA haplotype. Based on this Mendelian inheritance, there is a 25 percent chance that any two siblings will inherit the same two haplotypes (i.e., are HLA identical), a 50 percent chance of being HLA haploidentical (i.e., share one of two HLA haplotypes), and a 25 percent chance of being HLA nonidentical (i.e., share neither HLA haplotype).

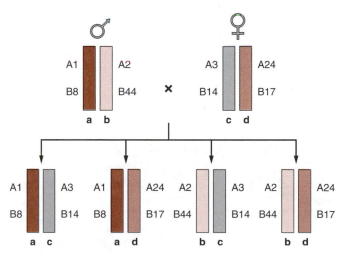

**FIGURE 17–1.** HLA genes are linked and inherited in Mendelian fashion as haplotypes. One paternal (a or b) and one maternal (c or d) haplotype is passed to each offspring. Four different combinations of haplotypes are possible in offspring. Elucidation of haplotype sharing between siblings is an important assessment in the search for a transplant donor.

Recombination can take place, resulting in the inheritance of unexpected haplotypic combinations; however, this occurs in less than 1 percent of families that are HLA typed.

HLA proteins are heterodimeric molecules. Class I proteins are the product of the HLA-A, B, and C genes and are expressed on the cell surface covalently bound to beta-2-microglobulin. Class I heterodimers are codominantly expressed on virtually all nucleated cells. Class II heterodimers are the products of the HLA-DRB1 + DRA1, HLA-DQB1 + DQA1, and DPB1 + DPA1 genes. Class II heterodimers are codominantly expressed primarily on antigen-presenting cells (e.g., dendritic cells, monocytes, macrophages, B lymphocytes).

As discussed in Chapter 3, HLA proteins have critical roles for the development and functioning of the innate and adaptive immune systems. They serve as recognition elements for antigen receptors on T lymphocytes, thus initiating adaptive immune responses. In addition, they serve as ligands for regulatory receptors on natural killer cells in the innate immune response. The CD8 molecule on cytotoxic T lymphocytes interacts with class I HLA proteins in addition to the HLA + peptide complex, while the CD4 molecule on the T helper cell subset interacts with class II HLA proteins in addition to the HLA + peptide complex.

A cardinal feature of the genes encoding the HLA proteins is an extensive degree of allelic polymorphism. The HLA system is the most polymorphic genetic system in humans **(Table 17–1)**. This degree of polymorphism is believed to have resulted from the need to bind peptides from an innumerable array of pathogenic organisms and thus generate protective immune responses. While this has successfully enabled populations to survive infectious challenges, it severely restricts the ability to transplant foreign tissues or cells between any two individuals.

## Minor Histocompatibility Antigens

A second set of transplantation antigens was identified based on studies in mice and humans demonstrating tissue rejection in MCH-identical transplants and based on outcomes of human stem cell transplants between HLA-identical siblings in whom graft-versus-host disease has developed.[3] Early experimental studies documented a "slower" rejection pace mediated by these transplantation antigens, thus their name—minor histocompatibility antigens (mHAs).

mHAs are non-HLA proteins that demonstrate polymorphism in amino acid sequence within a species. Both X-linked and autosomally encoded mHAs have been identified. Introducing a polymorphic variant of one of these proteins from one individual into another individual who possesses a different polymorphic variant (via transplantation of tissue or cells) can induce a recipient immune response to the donor variant. The immune response is mediated by CD4 and/or CD8 T cells recognizing a variant protein in the context of the recipient MHC molecule. This response is analogous to the reaction to a foreign microbial antigen. Several different types of mHAs have been identified, including proteins encoded by the male Y chromosome, proteins for which the recipient has a homozygous gene deletion, proteins that are autosomally encoded, and proteins that are mitochondrial DNA encoded.[3]

## MIC Antigens

The MHC class I–related chain A (MICA) encodes a cell surface protein that is involved in gamma/delta T-cell responses. MICA is polymorphic with over 50 allelic variants. MIC proteins are expressed on endothelial cells, keratinocytes, fibroblasts, epithelial cells, dendritic cells, and monocytes, but they are not expressed on T or B lymphocytes.[4] As such, MICA proteins could serve as targets for allograft immune responses. Antibodies to MICA antigens have been detected in as many as 11 percent of kidney transplant patients.[5] MICA antibodies have been associated with rejection episodes and decreased graft survival.

## ABO Blood Group Antigens

The ABO system is the only blood group system that impacts clinical transplantation. Anti-A or anti-B antibodies develop in individuals lacking the corresponding blood group antigens. ABO blood group incompatibility is a barrier to solid-organ transplantation, because these antibodies can bind the corresponding antigens that are expressed on the vascular endothelium. Binding activates the complement cascade, which can lead to **hyperacute rejection** of the transplanted organ. As such, recipient–donor pairs must be ABO identical or compatible to avoid this adverse outcome. For example, an individual of blood group A will possess anti-B antibodies and can thus receive an organ only from an ABO-A or O donor. Likewise, a B-expressing individual has anti-A antibodies and can receive an organ only from an ABO-B or O donor. Recently, approaches using plasma exchange and intravenous immunoglobulin administration have allowed successful transplantation of kidneys from ABO-incompatible donors by lowering ABO antibody to levels that allow transplantation to proceed without risk of hyperacute rejection.[6]

| Table 17–1. | Approximate Number of HLA Antigens and Alleles Defined at the Six Classical Transplant Loci | |
| --- | --- | --- |
| **HLA LOCUS** | **# ANTIGENS** | **# ALLELES** |
| A | 28 | 506 |
| B | 61 | 851 |
| C | 10 | 276 |
| DRB1 | 24 | 559 |
| DQB1 | 9 | 81 |
| DPB1 | 6 | 126 |

## Killer Immunoglobulin–like Receptors

Another polymorphic genetic system that impacts allogeneic transplantation is the killer immunoglobulin-like receptor (KIR) system.[7] KIRs are one of several types of cell surface molecules that regulate the activity of natural killer (NK) lymphocytes. Within the KIRs are activating and inhibitory receptors that vary in number and type on any individual NK cell. The balance of signals received by the activating and inhibitory receptors governs the activity of the NK cell (see Fig. 2–12). Included among the functions of NK cells are secretion of cytokines and non-MHC restricted cytotoxicity.

The ligands for the inhibitory KIRs have been defined as several of the MHC class I molecules, including specific HLA-A, -B, and -C proteins. Normally, an NK cell encounters self class I MHC proteins as it circulates in the body. This interaction between MHC protein and the inhibitory KIR maintains the NK cells in a quiescent state. If an NK cell encounters a cell lacking or having decreased class I expression, inhibitory receptors are not occupied and an inhibitory signal loss occurs, resulting in NK cell activation.

The regulatory role of KIRs has been exploited in haploidentical stem cell transplantation.[8] Stem cell donors have been selected for recipients who lack a corresponding class I MHC protein for the donor's inhibitory KIR type. This results in alloreactivity by NK cells that repopulate the recipient after transplant. These alloreactive NK cells have been shown to mediate a graft-versus-leukemia reaction and prevent relapse after transplantation.

## ALLORECOGNITION

Transplantation of cells or tissues between two individuals is classified by the genetic relatedness of the donor and the recipient. An **autograft** is the transfer of tissue from one area of the body to another of the same individual. A **syngeneic graft** is the transfer of cells or tissues between identical twins. An **allograft** is the transfer of cells or tissue between two individuals of the same species. Lastly, a **xenograft** is the transfer of tissue between two individuals of a different species. Most transplantation falls into the category of allografting. As stated earlier, HLA disparity between donor and recipient will result in a vigorous immune response to the foreign MHC antigens and is the primary stimulus of graft rejection. The response to foreign MHC antigens is characterized by strong cellular and humoral immune responses.

The recipient immune system recognizes foreign HLA proteins via two distinct mechanisms—direct and indirect allorecognition[9] **(see Fig. 17–2).** In **direct allorecognition,** recipient T cells bind and respond directly to foreign (allo) HLA proteins on graft cells. Although an individual T lymphocyte can recognize self-HLA + peptide, foreign HLA proteins may mimic a self-HLA + peptide complex

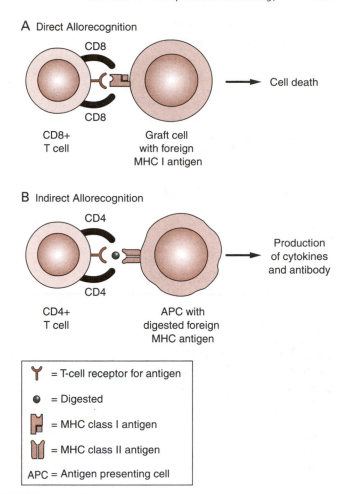

**A**  Direct Allorecognition

CD8

CD8

CD8+
T cell

Graft cell
with foreign
MHC I antigen

→ Cell death

**B**  Indirect Allorecognition

CD4

CD4

CD4+
T cell

APC with
digested foreign
MHC antigen

→ Production
of cytokines
and antibody

Y = T-cell receptor for antigen

● = Digested

⊓ = MHC class I antigen

∐ = MHC class II antigen

APC = Antigen presenting cell

**FIGURE 17–2.** Direct versus indirect allorecognition. *(A)* In direct allorecognition, cytotoxic T cells bind directly to foreign HLA proteins on graft cells. *(B)* In indirect allorecognition, foreign MHC antigens are presented by phagocytic cells, and CD4+ T cells respond.

due to similarities in structure of the allo-HLA protein itself or to structural similarities of allo-HLA protein + peptide. Either way, direct allorecognition is characterized by a high frequency (up to 2 percent) of responding T cells[9] compared to the responder frequency in a typical T-cell response to a foreign antigen.

The high frequency of responding T cells may be due to several factors, including recognition of multiple amino acid disparities by multiple T-cell clones; the presence of multiple different peptides on an allogeneic cell that are each recognized by different T-cell clones; and the presence of many foreign molecules per cells, resulting in activation of T cells with low affinity, which normally would not be stimulated. The **mixed lymphocyte response (MLR)** is an in vitro correlate of direct allorecognition.[5]

**Indirect allorecognition** is the second -pathway by which the immune system recognizes foreign HLA proteins.[10] Indirect allorecognition is analogous to the normal mechanism of recognition of foreign antigens, as it involves the uptake, processing, and presentation of foreign HLA proteins by recipient antigen-presenting cells to recipient

T cells. Indirect allorecognition plays a predominant role in acute and chronic rejection.

The effector responses against transplanted allogeneic tissue include direct cytotoxicity, delayed-type hypersensitivity responses, and antibody-mediated mechanisms. Antibody may mediate antibody-dependent cellular cytotoxicity reactions and may fix complement, resulting in cell death. Rejection episodes vary in the time of occurrence and the effector mechanism that is operative.

## TRANSPLANT REJECTION

### Hyperacute Rejection

Hyperacute rejection occurs within minutes to hours after the vascular supply to the transplanted organ is established. This type of rejection is mediated by preformed antibody that reacts with donor vascular endothelium. ABO, HLA, and certain endothelial antigens may elicit hyperacute rejection. Binding of preformed antibodies to the alloantigens activates the complement cascade and clotting mechanisms and leads to thrombus formation. The result is ischemia and necrosis of the transplanted tissue.[11]

Hyperacute rejection is seldom encountered in clinical transplantation. Donor–recipient pairs are chosen to be ABO identical or compatible, and patients awaiting transplantation are screened for the presence of preformed HLA antibodies. In addition, the absence of donor HLA specific antibodies is confirmed prior to transplant by the performance of a crossmatch test. These approaches have virtually eliminated hyperacute rejection episodes.

Some individuals possess very low levels of donor-specific antibody in the pretransplant period. In these cases, antibody-mediated rejection may take place over several days. This has been termed **accelerated rejection.**[9,12] Like hyperacute rejection, accelerated rejection involves intravascular thrombosis and necrosis of donor tissue.

### Acute Cellular Rejection

Days to weeks after transplant, individuals may develop **acute rejection.** This is a cellular-type rejection but may involve antibody as well.[11] Acute rejection is characterized by parenchymal and vascular injury. Interstitial cellular infiltrates contain a predominance of CD8-positive T cells as well as CD4 T cells and macrophages. CD8 cells likely mediate cytotoxic reactions to foreign MHC-expressing cells, while CD4 cells likely produce cytokines and induce delayed-type hypersensitivity (DTH) reactions. Antibody may also be involved in acute graft rejection by binding to vessel walls, activating complement, and inducing transmural necrosis and inflammation as opposed to the thrombosis typical of hyperacute rejection. The development and application of potent immunosuppressive drugs that target multiple pathways in the immune response to alloantigens has improved early graft survival of solid-organ

transplants by reducing the incidence of acute rejection and by providing approaches for its effective treatment. However, it is chronic rejection that remains the most significant cause of graft loss after the first year post-transplant, because it is not readily amenable to treatment.

### Chronic Rejection

**Chronic rejection** results from a process of graft arteriosclerosis characterized by progressive fibrosis and scarring with narrowing of the vessel lumen due to proliferation of smooth muscle cells.[13] Several predisposing factors impact the development of chronic rejection, including prolonged cold ischemia, reperfusion, acute rejection episodes, and toxicity from immunosuppressive drugs. Chronic rejection is also thought to have an immunologic component, presumably a delayed-type hypersensitivity reaction to foreign HLA proteins.[9] This is indicated in studies employing animal models of graft arteriosclerosis in which mice lacking IFN gamma do not develop graft arteriosclerosis. In addition, similar studies support an important role for CD4 T cells and B cells in this process. Cytokines and growth factors secreted by endothelial cells, smooth muscle cells, and macrophages activated by IFN gamma stimulate smooth muscle cell accumulation in the graft vasculature.

## GRAFT-VERSUS-HOST DISEASE

Stem cell transplants (and less commonly lung and liver transplants) are complicated by a unique allogeneic response—**graft-versus-host disease (GVHD).** Recipients of stem cell transplants for hematologic malignancies typically have depleted bone marrow prior to transplantation as a result of the chemotherapy used to treat the malignancy. Next, donor bone marrow or, more commonly, peripheral blood stem cells are infused. The infused products often contain some mature T cells. These cells have several beneficial effects, including promotion of engraftment, reconstitution of immunity, and mediation of a graft-versus-leukemia effect. However, these mature T cells may also mediate GVHD.

**Acute GVHD** occurs during the first 100 days postinfusion and targets the skin, gastrointestinal tract, and liver.[14] In mismatched allogeneic stem cell transplantation, the targets of GVHD are the mismatched HLA proteins, while in matched stem cell transplantation, minor histocompatibility antigens are targeted. The infused T cells can mediate GVHD in several ways, including a massive release of cytokines due to large-scale activation of the donor cells by MHC mismatched proteins and by infiltration and destruction of tissue.

The incidence and severity of GVHD is related to the match status of the donor and recipient as well as other factors.[15] In efforts to reduce the incidence and severity of GVHD, several approaches are taken, including immunosuppressive therapy in the early post-transplant period and removal of T lymphocytes from the graft. T-cell reduction is very effective in lowering the incidence of GVHD, but it can also reduce the graft-versus-leukemia (GVL) effect of the infused cells and increase the incidence of graft failure.

Beyond 100 days post-transplant, patients may experience chronic GVHD. This condition resembles autoimmune disease, with fibrosis affecting the skin, eyes, mouth, and other mucosal surfaces.

## IMMUNOSUPPRESSIVE AGENTS

There is a growing list of agents that are employed to suppress antigraft immune responses in solid-organ and stem cell transplantation. **Immunosuppressive agents** are used in several ways, including induction and maintenance of immune suppression and treatment of rejection. Combinations of different agents are frequently used to prevent graft rejection. However, the immunosuppressed state (and graft survival) induced by these agents comes at a price of increased susceptibility to infection, malignancies, and other associated toxic side effects. There are several classes of immunosuppressive agents, which are briefly discussed in the following sections.

### Corticosteroids

Corticosteroids are potent anti-inflammatory and immunosuppressive agents used for immunosuppression maintenance. At higher doses, they are used to treat acute rejection episodes. Steroids act by blocking production and secretion of cytokines, inflammatory mediators, chemoattractants, and adhesion molecules. These activities decrease macrophage function and alter leukocyte-trafficking patterns. However, long-term use is associated with several complications, including hypertension and diabetes mellitus.

### Antimetabolic Agents

Anti-metabolic agents interfere with the maturation of lymphocytes and kill proliferating cells.[16] Azathioprine was the first such agent employed. It has been replaced in large part by mycophenolate mofetil, which has a more selective effect on lymphocytes compared to azathioprine and thus fewer side effects.

### Calcineurin Inhibitors

Cyclosporine and FK-506 (tacrolimus) are compounds that block signal transduction in T lymphocytes, resulting in impairment of cytokine syntheses, including IL-2, 3, 4, and interferon-gamma.[16] Inhibition of cytokine synthesis blocks the growth and differentiation of T cells, impairing the antigraft response. Rapamycin (sirolimus)[17] is an agent that inhibits T-cell proliferation by binding to specific intracellular proteins, including mammalian target of rapamycin (mTOR).

### Monoclonal Antibodies

Several monoclonal antibodies that bind to cell surface molecules on lymphocytes are used as induction agents and to treat severe rejection episodes. OKT3 is a mouse monoclonal antibody the binds to the CD3 receptor on human lymphocytes.[16] Binding of OKT3 to the CD3-positive T-cell surface has several outcomes. Binding may modulate CD3 from the cell surface, rendering the affected T cells nonfunctional. Higher doses of antibody deplete T cells from the circulation via complement-mediated lysis or opsonization for removal by phagocytic cells.

Two anti-CD25 monoclonal antibodies are available for use in transplant patients.[18] Basiliximab and dacluzimab both bind the CD25 (IL2 receptor) and thus interfere with IL2-mediated T-cell activation. It may also deplete CD25-expressing cells. An additional monoclonal antibody that targets the CD52 receptor found on T and B lymphocytes is alemtuzumab, which may be used for induction therapy at the time of transplantation.[18] A problem with monoclonal antibody preparations administered to patients is the development of anti-mouse antibody.

### Polyclonal Antibodies

Two polyclonal anti-T-cell antibody preparations are used to treat severe rejection. Thymoglobulin is an antithymocyte antibody prepared in rabbits, and ATGAM is a polyclonal antiserum prepared from immunization of horses. Both are potent immunosuppressive agents that deplete lymphocytes from the circulation. The development of these anti-mouse antibodies can interfere with the activity of the monoclonal antibody. A drawback associated with administration of polyclonal antibody preparations is the development of serum sickness due to antibody responses to the foreign immunoglobulin.

## CLINICAL HISTOCOMPATIBILITY TESTING

Appreciation of the beneficial role of **HLA matching**[9,19] and the detrimental role of antibody to HLA proteins[12] on graft survival provided the impetus for development and application of specialized testing to aid in the selection of the most appropriate donors for patients needing transplantation. Histocompatibility laboratories provide specialized testing for both solid-organ and stem cell transplantation programs. Two main activities are carried out by these laboratories in support of transplantation, HLA typing, and **HLA antibody screening**/identification.

### HLA Typing

**HLA typing** is the phenotypic or genotypic definition of the HLA antigens or genes in a transplant candidate or donor. For clinical HLA testing, phenotypes or genotypes of the classical transplant antigens or genes are determined (HLA-A, B,

Cw, DR, DQ). This information is used to find the most suitable donor–recipient combination from an immunologic standpoint. It must be stressed that other considerations go into the choice of a particular donor for any given patient, be it a solid-organ or stem cell transplant.

## HLA Phenotyping

The classic procedure for determining the **HLA phenotype** is the **complement-dependent cytotoxicity (CDC)** test. Panels of antisera or monoclonal antibodies that define individual or groups of immunologically related HLA antigens are incubated with lymphocytes from the individual to be HLA typed. Purified T lymphocytes are used for HLA class I typing, while purified B lymphocytes are used for HLA class II typing. After incubation with the antisera, complement is added. In the presence of bound antibody, which occurs only if the lymphocyte expresses the HLA antigen targeted by the antisera, complement is activated and cells are killed. A vital dye is then added that distinguishes live cells from dead when they are viewed microscopically. Using this assay, an extensive array of HLA antigens can be defined (Table 17–1).

There are several limitations to the CDC method for HLA typing. Viable lymphocytes must be used, which demands timely performance of the assay. Separation of T and B lymphocytes is required for definition of class I versus class II antigens. The source of antisera for HLA typing is not always consistent or reliable. Thus, reagents can vary in quality or quantity over time. Finally, the level of resolution (i.e., the ability to distinguish two closely related yet distinct HLA antigens) is limited. The limits of resolution don't significantly impact the role of this technology for matching solid-organ donors and recipients. However, for unrelated stem cell transplantation, a higher level of resolution is required. DNA-based (molecular) HLA typing methods are now commonly employed in histocompatibility laboratories, because they address the limitations of CDC-based methods and are amenable to higher throughput formats.

## HLA Genotyping

Molecular-based HLA genotyping methods use polymerase chain reaction (PCR)–based amplification of HLA genes followed by analysis of the amplified DNA to identify the specific HLA allele or group of alleles.[20] The most common approaches for analysis include PCR amplification of HLA genes with panels of primer pairs, each of which amplifies specific alleles or related allele groups. Amplification is detected by agarose gel electrophoresis **(Fig. 17–3).** Only those primer pairs that bind to the target gene result in detection of an amplification product. The HLA type is then identified by determining which primers resulted in amplification. A second common approach for HLA genotyping is to perform a single PCR reaction that will amplify all HLA gene variants at a specific locus (referred to as a *generic*

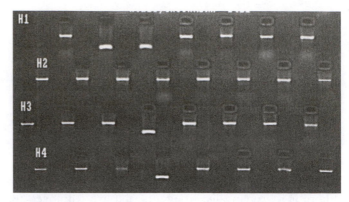

**FIGURE 17–3.** An example of a PCR with sequence-specific primers (PCR-SSP) analysis of the HLA-DQB1 locus. Each lane of this ethidium bromide stained agarose gel contains the amplification product of an individual PCR reaction. Each reaction contains primers to a ubiquitous gene and should demonstrate amplification (the larger band in each lane). This serves as an internal control to document successful amplification in each reaction. Each reaction also contains primers specific for various HLA-DQB1 alleles. An amplification product of small size is seen in several lanes, indicating the presence of the target HLA-DQB1 gene for those specific primers. The particular pattern of amplified primers is assessed to determine the HLA- DQB1 type of the sample. (Color Plate 14).

*amplification*). The amplified gene is then subjected to hybridization with a panel of DNA probes, each specific for a unique HLA allele or allele group. Only those probes that specifically hybridize to the amplified DNA will be detected. The **HLA genotype** is determined by assessing which probes hybridized. A third common method for HLA genotyping is sequencing of PCR-amplified HLA genes.

HLA genotyping overcomes the limitation of CDC-based HLA phenotyping. Cells do not need to be viable in order to obtain DNA for HLA genotyping. Typing reagents are chemically synthesized; thus, there is no reliance on human donors of antisera. HLA genotyping can provide varying levels of resolution that can be tailored to the specific clinical need. DNA-based typing can provide results at a level of resolution comparable to CDC-based typing (antigen equivalent) or can provide allele-level results (required for matching of unrelated stem cell donors and recipients). Allele-level HLA typing has demonstrated the incredible extent of polymorphism within the HLA loci (Table 17–1).

## HLA Antibody Screening and Identification

Antibodies to HLA antigens can be detected in candidates and recipients of solid-organ transplants. These antibodies develop in response to multiple blood transfusions; to prior HLA-mismatched transplants; and, in women, to multiple pregnancies. Because of the potential adverse impact HLA antibodies can have on graft survival, patients awaiting solid-organ transplantation are screened periodically for their presence.[12] If detected, the specificity (which HLA proteins they bind) of the antibodies is then determined so that donors possessing those HLA antigens can be eliminated from consideration for donation to that patient. Patients are tested monthly for the presence of HLA antibodies while they are waiting for an organ offer. Antibody screening and identification is also performed post-transplantation to aid in the diagnosis of antibody-mediated rejection and to assess the effectiveness of therapy for antibody-mediated rejection.

The methods used for antibody detection and identification have changed significantly in recent years. The CDC method used for HLA typing is also used for HLA antibody detection and identification. In this case, panels of lymphocytes with defined HLA phenotypes are incubated with the patient's serum. If the serum contains HLA antibodies, they will bind to those lymphocytes in the panel that express the cognate HLA antigen. Binding is detected by addition of complement and a vital dye to assess cell death microscopically. In some scenarios, the level of antibody in a patient serum may be below a level detectable by the CDC assay. In these cases, antihuman globulin (AHG) may be added to the CDC assay to increase the test's sensitivity. The AHG-CDC assay can detect lower levels of antibody as well as isotypes of bound antibody that don't activate complement and thus wouldn't normally be detected in the standard CDC assay. The proportion of lymphocytes in the panel (usually 30 to 60 unique lymphocyte preparations are included in the panel) that are killed by the patient's serum is referred to as the *percent panel reactive antibody* (%PRA). In addition, the specificity of the antibodies can be determined by evaluating the phenotype of the panel cells.

Enzyme-linked immunosorbent assay (ELISA) has been developed in recent years as a substitute for CDC-based HLA antibody testing.[21] ELISA assays utilize purified HLA antigens bound to the wells of microtiter plates. Patient serum is added to the wells of the plate, and if HLA-specific antibody is present, it will bind. Bound antibody is detected by addition of an enzyme-labeled anti-immunoglobulin reagent. Addition of substrate results in a color change in the wells that have bound antibody. The wells of the ELISA plate may contain a pool of HLA antigens, thus serving as a qualitative screen for the presence of HLA antibody in a serum. Alternatively, each well may contain HLA antigens representing a single donor and thus can be used in a fashion analogous to a CDC-based analysis, allowing %PRA and specificity to be determined.

Another approach for antibody detection and identification is flow cytometry.[22] Antibody in patient serum can be incubated with latex beads that are coated with HLA antigens, either from a single donor or a single purified HLA protein. Patient serum is incubated with the beads, and bound antibody is detected by adding an FITC-labeled anti-IgG reagent **(Fig. 17–4)**. A more recent version of flow cytometry–based antibody detection is the multiplex bead array system that can assess binding of up to 100 different HLA antigens in a single tube using a dedicated flow-based detection system.[23] Flow cytometry–based methods are the most sensitive technology for detecting HLA antibodies. In addition, they can provide the most specific determination of the specificity of HLA antibodies when beads coated with a single HLA antigenic type are used.

Once a donor has been identified for a particular patient, a donor–recipient **crossmatch** test is performed to confirm the absence of donor-specific antibody. Donor lymphocytes are incubated with recipient serum in a CDC assay to verify a lack of binding as detected by microscopic analysis after addition of a vital dye. Alternatively, binding of antibody can be detected by flow cytometry using an FITC-labeled anti-IgG reagent. As for antibody screening and identification, the flow cytometric crossmatch is the most sensitive method for detecting donor-specific antibody.[12]

## SUMMARY

The immune system's ability to recognize and respond to the myriad of infectious agents that humans encounter has obvious benefits. However, the mechanisms that impart this ability make the transplantation of organs and cells between allogeneic individuals difficult. The target of the response to transplanted tissues is HLA proteins. These proteins play critical roles as antigen-presenting molecules for CD4 and CD8 T cells, resulting in the phenomenon of MHC restriction. While an individual's immune system develops to respond to the foreign proteins presented on its own MHC antigens, it responds even more intensely to foreign MHC proteins. Both the humoral and cellular arms of the immune system contribute to this allogeneic immune response and mediate graft rejection. Even in the face of this intense response, transplantation has become an effective treatment for a variety of diseases due to the development of immunosuppressive agents that block the immune system from responding to the allogeneic MHC proteins in the transplanted tissue. Unfortunately, these agents also block immune response to infectious organisms and tumors. In concert with the development of immunosuppressive drugs, defining the MHC antigens of donors and recipients and monitoring the allospecific immune response are critical components of clinical transplantation and contribute to the continually improved outcomes of transplantation.

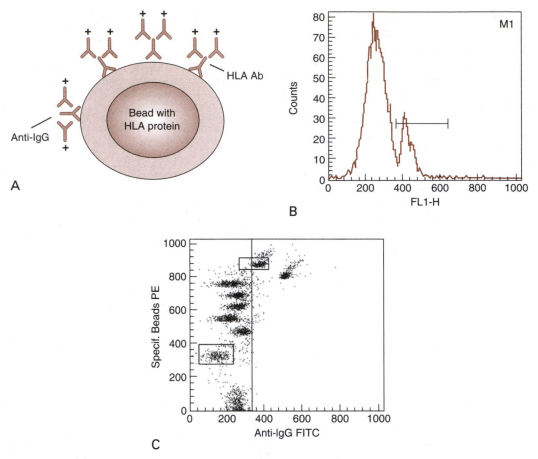

FIGURE 17–4. *(A)* Flow cytometric detection and identification of HLA antibodies employs latex beads that are coated with HLA proteins from individual donors or single HLA molecules. For qualitative determination of the presence of HLA antibodies, multiple beads, each coated with the product of an individual donor, are pooled together so as to represent the majority of common HLA antigens. They are then incubated with patient serum. To determine the specificity of HLA antibodies in a serum sample, beads coated with a single HLA protein species can be incubated with patient serum. Once incubated with serum, both bead types are then incubated with an FITC-labeled anti-IgG reagent that will detect the presence of antibodies bound to the bead. *(B)* Single-parameter histogram display of an HLA class I antibody screen. A pool of HLA-coated beads was incubated with a patient serum, washed, and then incubated with an FITC-labeled anti-IgG reagent. Unbound FITC-labeled reagent was washed away and the beads analyzed for fluorescence on a flow cytometer. The large peak represents beads with no bound antibody, while the smaller peak to the right indicates the presence of HLA antibody bound to approximately 19 percent of the HLA class I coated beads. This represents a positive HLA class I antibody screen. *(C)* Nine individual clusters of latex beads, each coated with a single HLA class I antigen species, are identified in the dual-parameter dot plot of the serum from *(B)*. The HLA antigen coated on each bead is indicated to the right of the bead. The bead coated with HLA-A11 has shifted to the right relative to the other beads, indicating that the HLA antibodies in this patient's serum are specific for the A11 antigen.

# CASE STUDY

A 40-year-old mother of three needs to have a second kidney transplant. Her first transplant was lost due to chronic rejection. The mother's HLA typing, HLA antibody, and ABO blood group status was determined. The patient was found to have antibodies to HLA-B35 by complement-dependent cytotoxicity testing with a panel of lymphocytes. The HLA type and blood group were also determined for two of her siblings and two close friends (who were also siblings) who are interested in donating a kidney to the patient. From the available donors, who would be the most compatible for donation to this patient?

| IDENTIFICATION | BLOOD GROUP | A | B | CW | DR | DQ |
|---|---|---|---|---|---|---|
| Recipient | O | 1,2 | 8,44 | 7,5 | 17,4 | 2,7 |
| Sibling 1 | O | 1,11 | 8,35 | 7,4 | 17,1 | 2,5 |
| Sibling 2 | A | 3,11 | 7,35 | 7,4 | 15,1 | 6,5 |
| Friend 1 | B | 2,24 | 57,7 | 6,7 | 7,15 | 2,6 |
| Friend 2 | O | 2,24 | 57,7 | 6,7 | 7,15 | 2,6 |

# EXERCISE

## HLA HAPLOTYPE SEGREGATION ANALYSIS

### Principle

Serological HLA typing provides information about the HLA protein polymorphisms expressed on the cell surface of an individual. HLA phenotype information is limited to the alloantigens that are recognized by the reagent panel selected for a particular indication. Each reagent panel consists of polyclonal antisera or monoclonal antibodies selected to recognize private or shared HLA specificities and HLA antigens. An HLA class I panel might detect the products of HLA-A, -B, -C loci; a class II panel might recognize the products of the DR and DQ loci. Donor–recipient matching for renal (kidney) transplantation is usually based on the HLA-A, -B, -DR, because these antigens seem to be the most immunogenic. By convention, HLA phenotypes are written as a string of antigens (e.g., HLA-A1, 3; B7, 8; DR7, 17). If only one HLA antigen is identified for a locus, then an X or blank is inserted. To help distinguish these possibilities, retyping with a different panel might be needed, or the entire family might be typed. Family typing is essential if the goal is to find a genotypic HLA-identical donor (i.e., a sibling who shares two haplotypes with a patient). Each parent–child combination will share only one haplotype. Segregation analysis involves inspection of phenotype data from parental and offspring generations of a nuclear family so that the four haplotypes can be inferred from the HLA phenotype data. Haplotype segregation analysis is based on the principle that HLA genes are transmitted en bloc and yields the HLA genotype of the individual.

Sequence-based HLA typing is a method of direct allele typing. Segregation analysis using the HLA allele assignments of family members is still needed to define the segregating haplotypes. Predicted haplotypes of some individuals can be deduced without family studies if the particular HLA alleles at closely linked loci exhibit linkage disequilibrium. By referring to published allele frequency tables for the appropriate ethnic group, the two haplotypes of many individuals can be assigned.

### Procedure

1. Arrange the HLA phenotypes in the order in which the corresponding genes are arranged on chromosome 6, from centromeric (left) to telomeric (right), to recognize and interpret rare intra-HLA recombination events that occur in approximately 1 to 2 percent of families.

2. Identify the antigens at each locus from one parent that could only have come from the father and designate these as haplotypes (a) and (b) or could only have been inherited from the mother (haplotypes [c] and [d], where [a, b, c, d] is a shorthand representation of the inferred haplotypes). For each child, list the two haplotypes that can account for the phenotype of the child (i.e., ac, ad, bc, bd).

3. Write out each of the four haplotypes (i.e., HLA-DQ_, DR_, B_, C_, A_) where the underline would be replaced with the number corresponding to the particular antigen assigned to each locus in the string.

4. If there is no antigen available to assign a given locus, insert X after the locus designation. A blank X may reflect homozygosity at the locus.

5. Each child will inherit one paternal haplotype and one maternal haplotype. If an extra haplotype is required to explain the data, then consider the following possibilities: (a) incomplete typing or missed antigen, (b) incorrect typing, (c) nonpaternity, or (d) interlocus crossover during meiosis in one of the parents.

### Jones Family Genotype Analysis Worksheet

1. Using the following worksheet, deduce the haplotypes that segregate in the Jones family. The HLA phenotypes of the Jones family are listed in the centromeric → telomeric order.

| | | | | |
|---|---|---|---|---|
| Father: | DQ2,X DR13,17 | B8,X | Cw7,X A1,24 | |
| (a) | DQ___ DR___ B___ | Cw___ A___ | | |
| (b) | DQ___ DR___ B___ | Cw___ A___ | | |
| Mother: | DQ1,X DR1,13 | B35,60 | Cw3,w4 A2,3 | |
| (c) | DQ___ DR___ B___ | Cw___ A___ | | |
| (d) | DQ___ DR___ B___ | Cw___ A___ | | |
| Child 1: (patient) | DQ1,2 DR1,17 | B8,35 | Cw4,w7 A3,24 | |
| ( ) | DQ___ DR___ B___ | Cw___ A___ | | |
| ( ) | DQ___ DR___ B___ | Cw___ A___ | | |
| Child 2: | DQ1,2 DR13,17 | B8,60 | Cw3,w7 A2,24 | |
| ( ) | DQ___ DR___ B___ | Cw___ A___ | | |
| ( ) | DQ___ DR___ B___ | Cw___ A___ | | |
| Child 3: | DQ1,2 DR13,17 | B8,60 | Cw3,w7 A1,2 | |
| ( ) | DQ___ DR___ B___ | Cw___ A___ | | |
| ( ) | DQ___ DR___ B___ | Cw___ A___ | | |
| Child 4: | DQ1,2 DR13,X | B8,60 | Cw3,w7 A1,2 | |
| ( ) | DQ___ DR___ B___ | Cw___ A___ | | |
| ( ) | DQ___ DR___ B___ | Cw___ A___ | | |
| Child 5: | DQ1,2 DR1,13 | B8,35 | Cw4,w7 A1,3 | |
| ( ) | DQ___ DR___ B___ | Cw___ A___ | | |
| ( ) | DQ___ DR___ B___ | Cw___ A___ | | |

2. Using the (a, b, c, d) as an abbreviation for the four haplotypes, which paternal and maternal haplotypes were present in each of the five children?

3. Which sibling is the best match for Child 1, who is in need of an organ transplant, and why?

## Interpretation of Results

HLA genotyping is important in histocompatibility testing, especially when serotyping data is incomplete and the possibility of a related donor is under consideration. The chance that two siblings will be HLA identical by sharing a paternal and a maternal haplotype is 1:4, or 25 percent. The chance that two siblings share one haplotype is 1:2, or 50 percent. The chance that two siblings share zero haplotypes is 1:4, or 25 percent, following the Mendelian principle. If a child needing a renal transplant shares two haplotypes with a sibling (e.g., patient: a, c/sibling: a, c), then it follows that they probably share the same HLA antigens at closely linked loci that may not have been typed, such as –DP, or at a locus where the phenotype assignment is problematic.

Allele typing by DNA-based methods yields the genotype directly at the coding level. However, DNA typing results, taken alone, provide no information about whether the allele is expressed. Although HLA expression is codominant, certain virus infections and cancers interfere with HLA gene expression and thus alter the phenotype.

# REVIEW QUESTIONS

1. The type of allograft rejection associated with vascular and parenchymal injury with lymphocyte infiltrates is which of the following?

   a. Hyperacute rejection
   b. Acute cellular rejection
   c. Acute humoral rejection
   d. Chronic rejection

2. Antigen receptors on T lymphocytes bind HLA class II molecules with the help of which accessory molecule?

   a. CD2
   b. CD3
   c. CD4
   d. CD8

3. Patients at risk for graft-versus-host disease (GVHD) include each of the following, except recipients of

   a. bone marrow transplants.
   b. lung transplants.
   c. liver transplants.
   d. irradiated leukocytes.

4. HLA molecules exhibit all of the following properties, except that they

   a. belong to the immunoglobulin superfamily.
   b. are heterodimeric.
   c. are integral cell membrane glycoproteins.
   d. are monomorphic.

5. Kidney allograft loss from intravascular thrombosis without cellular infiltration 5 days post-transplant raises the suspicion level about which primary rejection mechanism?

   a. Hyperacute rejection
   b. Accelerated humoral rejection
   c. Acute humoral rejection
   d. Acute cellular rejection

6. Which reagents would be used in a direct (forward) donor–recipient crossmatch test?

   a. Donor serum and recipient lymphocytes + rabbit serum complement
   b. Recipient serum and donor lymphocytes + rabbit serum complement
   c. Donor stimulator cells + recipient responder cells + complete culture medium
   d. Recipient stimulator cells + donor responder cells + complete culture medium

7. The indirect allorecognition pathway involves which one of the following mechanisms?

   a. Processed peptides from polymorphic donor proteins restricted by recipient HLA class II molecules
   b. Processed peptides from polymorphic recipient proteins restricted by donor HLA class I molecules
   c. Intact polymorphic donor protein molecules recognized by recipient HLA class I molecules
   d. Intact polymorphic donor protein molecules recognized by recipient HLA class II molecules

8. Which immunosuppressive agent selectively inhibits IL-2 receptor-mediated activation of T cells and causes clearance of activated T cells from the circulation?

   a. Mycophenolate mofetil
   b. Cyclosporine mofetil
   c. Corticosteroids
   d. Daclizumab

# References

1. www.unog.org.

2. Appelbaum, FR. Hematopoietic-cell transplantation at 50. N Eng J Med 357:1472–1475, 2007.

3. Simpson, E, Scott, D, James, E, et al. Minor H antigens: Genes and peptides. Transpl Immunol 10:115–123, 2002.

4. Zwirner, NW, Dole, K, and Stastny, P. Differential surface expression of MICA by endothelial cells, fibroblasts, keratinocytes, and monocytes. Hum Immunol 60:323–330, 1999.

5. Zou, Y, Stastny, P, Susal, C, Dohler, B, and Opelz, G. Antibodies against MICA antigens and kidney-transplant rejection. N Eng J Med 357:1293–1300, 2007.

6. Thielke, J, Kaplan, B, and Benedetti, E. The role of ABO-incompatible living donors in kidney transplantation: State of the art. Semin Nephrol 27:408–413, 2007.

7. Rarag, SS, Fehinger, TA, Ruggeri, L, Velardi, A, and Caliguri, MA. Natural killer cell receptors: New biology and insights into the graft-versus-leukemia effect. Blood 100:1935–1947, 2002.

8. Ruggeri, L, Capanni, M, Urbani, E, et al. Effectiveness of donor natural killer cell alloreactivity in mismatched hematopoietic transplants. Science 295:2097–2100, 2002.

9. Abbas, A, Lichtman, AH, and Pillai, S. Cellular and molecular immunology, ed. 6. Saunders, Philadelphia, 2007, pp. 375–396.

10. Afzali, B, Lechler, RI, and Hernandez-Fuentes, MP. Allorecognition and the alloresponse: Clinical implications. Tissue Antigens 69:545–556, 2007.

11. Leichtman, AB. Primer on Transplantation. American Society of Transplant Physicians, Thorofare, 1998, pp. 217–222.

12. Gebel, HM, Bray, RA, and Nickerson, P. Pre-transplant assessment of donor-reactive, HLA-specific antibodies in renal transplantation: Contraindication vs. risk. Am J Transplant 3:1488–1500, 2003.

13. Colvin, RB. Chronic allograft nephropathy. N Eng J Med 349:2288–2290, 2003.

14. Goker, H, Haznedaroglu, IC, and Chao, NJ. Acute graft vs. host disease: pathobiology and management. Experimental Hematology. 29(3):259–277, 2001.

15. Copelan, EA. Hematopoietic stem-cell transplantation. N Eng J Med 354:1813–1826, 2006.

16. Halloran, PF, and Lui, SL. Primer on Transplantation. American Society of Transplant Physicians, Thorofare, 1998, pp. 93–102.

17. Augustine, JJ, Bodziak, KA, and Hricik, DE. Use of sirolimus in solid organ transplantation. Drugs 67:369–391, 2007.

18. Buhaescu, I, Segall, L, Goldsmith, D, and Covic, A. New immunosuppressive therapies in renal transplantation: Monoclonal antibodies. J Nephrol 18:529–536, 2005.

19. Lee, SJ, Klein, J, Haagenson, M, et al. High-resolution HLA matching contributes to the success of unrelated donor marrow transplantation. Blood 110:4576–4583, 2007.

20. Schmitz, JL. Molecular diagnostics for the clinical laboratorian, ed. 2. Humana Press, New York, 2005, pp. 485–493.

21. Lucas, DP, Paparounis, ML, Myers, L, et al. Detection of HLA class I-specific antibodies by the QuikScreen enzyme-linked immunosorbent assay. Clin Diag Lab Immunol. 4:252–257, 1997.

22. Bray, RA, Nickerson, PW, Kerman, RH, and Gebel, HM. Evolution of HLA antibody detection: Technology emulating biology. Immunol Res 29:41–54, 2004.

23. Colombo, MB, Haworth, SE, Poli, F, et al. Luminex technology for anti-HLA antibody screening: Evaluation of performance and of impact on laboratory routine. Cytometry B Clin Cytom 72:465–471, 2007.

# Tumor Immunology

Diane L. Davis, PhD, MT, SC, SLS (ASCP), CLS(NCA)

## LEARNING OBJECTIVES

*After finishing this chapter, the reader will be able to:*

1. Compare and contrast the normal cell and the tumor cell and describe the process by which tumors develop.

2. Discuss evidence to support and to refute the theories of immunosurveillance and immunoediting.

3. Define *tumor-associated antigen* (TAA) and list the categories of common tumor markers, giving examples of each category.

4. Describe the principles of how tumor markers may be appropriately used for screening, diagnosis, and disease classification/monitoring.

5. Discuss the impact of disease prevalence and test sensitivity/specificity on the clinical value of a test.

6. Describe characteristics of an ideal tumor marker.

7. List and describe the laboratory techniques used for tumor marker analysis, including the advantages and disadvantages of each, with particular attention to the effects of antigen excess, antibody cross-reactivity, and heterophile antibodies in immunoassays.

8. For each of the following tumor markers, describe how it is best used clinically: alpha-fetoprotein (AFP), β-2 microglobulin, CA-15.3, CA-19.9, CA-125, calcitonin, carcinoembryonic antigen (CEA), clusters of differentiation (CD) in WBC, estrogen/progesterone receptors, fecal occult blood, HER2/neu, human chorionic gonadotropin (hCG), monoclonal immunoglobulins and light chains, parathyroid hormone (PTH), prostate-specific antigen (PSA), and thyroglobulin (TG).

9. Compare and contrast passive versus active immunotherapy, describing common techniques used in each.

## KEY TERMS

- ___ Anaplastic
- ___ Antibody conjugates
- ___ Benign
- ___ Cytogenetics
- ___ Dissemination
- ___ Dysplasia
- ___ Graft versus leukemia
- ___ High dose hook effect
- ___ Immunoediting
- ___ Immunohistochemistry
- ___ Immunosurveillance
- ___ Immunotherapy
- ___ Immunotoxins
- ___ Induction
- ___ In situ
- ___ Invasion
- ___ Mass spectrometry (MS)
- ___ Metastasis
- ___ Microarray
- ___ Neoplasia
- ___ Oncofetal antigen
- ___ Oncopeptidomics
- ___ Proteomics
- ___ Proto-oncogenes
- ___ Susceptibility genes
- ___ Tumor-associated antigen (TAA)
- ___ Tumor infiltrating lymphocyte (TIL)
- ___ TNM system
- ___ Tumor suppressor genes

## INTRODUCTION AND DESCRIPTION OF TUMORS

Tumor immunology is the study of the antigens associated with tumors, the immune response to tumors, the tumor's effect on the host's immune status, and the use of the immune system to help eradicate the tumor.

Tumor immunology is best understood with a background on differences between tumor cells and normal cells.[1] Normal cell growth and division are regulated processes designed to rapidly produce new cells when necessary, inhibit cell division when sufficient cells are present, and limit cell life span (programmed cell death, or apoptosis). Regulatory genes that promote cell division, the **proto-oncogenes,** can cause uninhibited cell division if their expression is altered or if they are mutated into oncogenes. Similarly, mutations or malfunctions in **tumor suppressor genes** that remove growth-inhibitory signals can cause tumors. Tumors, therefore, are composed of cells that possess many of the attributes of the normal cells from which they arose but have accelerated or dysregulated growth. Similarity to normal tissue is one reason why the immune system does not automatically eradicate all tumors.

If a tumor does not invade surrounding tissue and normal body function is largely preserved, it is said to be **benign.** Malignant tumors can invade surrounding tissues and greatly disrupt normal body function. **Metastasis** is when the malignant cells travel through the body, causing new foci of malignancy until body function is so disrupted that death occurs. Malignant cells typically differ visually from normal cells, are metabolically more active to support their growth, and express different genes or different levels of gene products as compared to normal cells.[1] For example, leukemic cells can have aberrant morphology and express different surface antigens either in type or amount.

The conversion of a normal cell to a malignant cell is typically a process, not an event.[2] During the **induction** phase, cells are exposed to a variety of environmental insults, including chemical carcinogens, oncogenic viruses, and radiation (ionizing and ultraviolet). Cancer may only develop as the result of multiple mutations caused by these insults, and it more readily develops in cells genetically predisposed to these mutations. During the induction phase, which may take months to years, cells exhibit **dysplasia** or abnormal growth that is not yet considered **neoplasia,** or consistent with a tumor.

The **in situ** phase of cancer is when neoplastic cells have formed but are confined to the tissue of origin. If the cells are malignant, the cancer proceeds to the **invasion** phase and then to **dissemination** throughout the body, usually via the blood and lymphatics. Treatment is far more effective the earlier the malignancy is detected, but detection is far more difficult in the early stages, as there are fewer cells to detect and they more closely resemble normal cells if they are dysplastic rather than neoplastic.[2]

The progeny of the cell that undergoes transformation are monoclonal in origin, meaning they are initially identical phenotypically and genotypically. This can be an important feature in diagnosing malignancy. As rapid uncontrolled proliferation continues, mistakes can occur in DNA replication, causing cellular phenotypic and genotypic heterogeneity to develop.[1,2] This ability to mutate may help cancer cells escape from both the immune system and from chemotherapeutic agents, as described below. Further, it complicates identification of reliable tumor markers, as marker expression may change over time.

In pathology, tumors more similar to fetal or embryonic tissue are classified as poorly differentiated, or **anaplastic,** while well-differentiated tumors are more similar to normal tissue. Generally, the poorly differentiated tumors are more aggressive and lead to poorer patient prognosis. Tumors are also classified by the **TNM system** by the size of the primary tumor (T), the involvement of adjacent lymph nodes (N), and the detection of metastasis (M).[1]

## IMMUNOSURVEILLANCE

**Immunosurveillance** by the immune system to eradicate cancer cells as they form has long been postulated. There is increased incidence of tumors in those with deficient immune systems such as the elderly and in immunosuppressed individuals, but this is not proof of the existence of immunosurveillance. Increased life span implies increased exposure to carcinogens, which cause tumors. In immunosuppressed people, many tumors are essentially infections, as they are of viral rather than spontaneous origin. Further, the incidence of nonviral tumors in T-cell-deficient individuals is not increased, although this may be due to adequate NK cell activity.[3–5] These topics are still under study.

There is, however, evidence that supports the hypothesis that the immune system provides tumor surveillance for the body:

- NK cells, T lymphocytes (**tumor infiltrating lymphocytes [TIL]**), and macrophage infiltrates have been demonstrated in some tumors, and they are associated with a better prognosis.[3]
- A common characteristic of many tumors is loss of MHC expression and subsequent poor antigen presentation, allowing tumor cells to escape from T cells.[3]
- Certain therapeutic advances directed toward up-regulating the immune system to fight a particular cancer have shown some success.[3]
- Spontaneous regression of some tumors has been observed.[4]

If immunosurveillance is indeed occurring, mechanisms by which tumors escape is important to determine. Some tumor antigens may be poorly immunogenic, particularly if they are very similar to normal self antigens and induce immune tolerance. The tumor cell may lack MHC class I, class II, or accessory molecule expression. The tumor may be resistant to the immune response, or the tumor's growth rate may exceed the ability of the immune response to destroy it, particularly in people with deficient immune systems. Soluble antigen released by the tumor may bind to the T-cell receptor, thereby preventing interaction with the tumor cell. In addition, the local environment of some tumors has been shown to be immunosuppressive, including detection of immunosuppressive cytokines such as transforming growth factor–β.[3,5–7]

It is also possible that immunosurveillance itself is ultimately responsible for tumors that can escape the immune system because of **immunoediting**.[5] In the "elimination" phase of immunosurveillance, tumors are sufficiently immunogenic to be eliminated by the immune system. During the "equilibrium" stage, as mutations occur over time, cells that are less immunogenic have a growth advantage. Finally, in the "escape" phase, cancer cells have mutated beyond the immune system's ability to control them.

Although research has been unable to immediately determine the extent and precise mechanisms of tumor immunosurveillance, research into the manipulation of the immune system to fight cancers is ongoing and discussed later in this chapter.

## TUMOR–ASSOCIATED ANTIGENS

**Tumor-associated antigens (TAA)** are antigens present in the tumor tissue in higher amounts than in normal tissue.[3] They are often the products of mutated genes and viruses, but they can also arise from aberrant expression of normal genes. For example, **oncofetal tumor antigens** are most highly expressed in both normally developing fetal tissue and in certain kinds of cancers. Tumors also generally express normal antigens and products from their tissue of origin. Virtually no tumor-associated antigens are tumor-specific, because they also have been found in some noncancerous human tissue.[4] The perfect tumor-associated antigen unique to a particular tumor could aid in the screening, diagnosis, histopathologic evaluation, staging, monitoring, localization, and immunotherapy of various malignancies, but such a perfect antigen has not yet been found.

## PRINCIPLES OF LAB TESTS FOR SCREENING, DIAGNOSING, AND MANAGING TUMORS

Screening tests are used in ostensibly normal people to detect occult cancer. Diagnostic tests are those that help determine differential diagnosis, tumor stage, prognosis, and therapy selection. These are two very different functions, and the ability of lab tests to perform all these functions well is still imperfect.

Disease prevalence profoundly impacts the test's usefulness. Bayes' theorem probability calculation shows the following:

- A "good" cancer test with 99 percent sensitivity and 95 percent specificity
  - will be positive in 99 out of 100 people with disease;
  - will be negative in 95 out of 100 people without disease.
- If the cancer rate in the population is 0.1 percent, then 98 percent of positives would be false positives. At a 1 percent cancer rate, the false-positive rate is still 83 percent.
- Assuming that a clinician can identify this cancer by signs and symptoms 75 percent of the time, if this same test is applied, the false-positive rate is 1.7 percent.

Tests for differential diagnosis, then, generally perform relatively well, because the clinical suspicion of cancer translates to a higher cancer prevalence in the population being tested. The presumptions for screening tests are that a relatively low number of people being screened actually have cancer and that it would be worse to miss a cancer than to do further testing on a normal person to exclude cancer. The concept of a normal or reference range doesn't really apply, as it may be difficult to determine with certainty that a reference population does not have cancer, and values from normal and cancerous populations may overlap. Cutoff values for tumor markers are typically selected above the point at which further testing will be done, so cutoff values for screening tests are generally set with the expectation that there will be an extremely high number of false positives due to low disease prevalence. This is not a benign choice, as additional testing can be invasive, costly, or anxiety-provoking.

Therefore, widespread use of a laboratory test to screen for cancer is justified if [8–10]:

- the tumor is an important health problem for the population being screened;
- there is a recognizable early symptom or marker that can be used for screening with reasonably high sensitivity and specificity;
- it is a tumor for which treatment at an early stage is more successful than at a later stage;
- the screening test is acceptable to the population;
- the costs and benefits of the screening test are acceptable to the population.

The benefits include improved survival time, less radical treatment needed for tumors detected earlier, and reassurance for those with negative results. The costs include longer morbidity in patients whose prognosis is not changed, overtreatment of questionable diagnoses, misleading reassurance for those with false-negative results, anxiety and possible morbidity from more invasive testing for those with false-positive results, the actual physical hazards of the screening tests, and the actual dollar costs of the screening test.[8–10] To improve the cost-to-benefit ratio, selected subgroups, such as patients with a family history of a cancer, should be screened when possible instead of the entire population.

Differential diagnosis of tumor type can be done by tissue/cell morphology and detection of tumor markers directly from tumor tissue. **Immunohistochemistry** can detect expressed antigens using labeled antibodies, and molecular techniques such as fluorescent in situ hybridization (FISH) can detect abnormal gene expression using nucleic acid probes[11] (see Chapter 11). The requirements for using a tumor marker to facilitate differential diagnosis by the pathologist are less stringent than the requirements for using tests for widespread screening. To be helpful in pathological diagnosis, the marker must be differentially expressed in the tumor of origin and other tumors, which may have a similar appearance histologically.

These markers must be combined with other clinical results, because the differentiation that occurs with transformation sometimes can result in loss of the marker. This false-negative situation is relatively common. In addition, the DNA changes that occur with malignant transformation sometimes can cause expression of a marker that is not normally associated with the tumor type in question, although this occurrence is relatively uncommon.

Disease management with laboratory tests is typically done with serial determinations of a tumor marker.[12] A baseline level at initial diagnosis is established. As the disease and treatments progress, additional levels are determined to establish prognosis, monitor the results of therapy, and detect recurrence. This is an area in which many tumor markers are best used clinically, because it is not the absolute value of the tumor marker that is important but rather the upward or downward trend when the marker's biological half-life is considered. Serial determinations done to aid the clinician in making important decisions concerning the therapeutic regimen must be done by the same methodology so that changes are due to actual alterations in the patient, not differences in methods.[12] An idealized model of using tumor markers to guide therapy is shown in **Figure 18–1**.

Problems with prostate-specific antigen (PSA) are a good illustration of the dilemmas associated with tumor markers.[2,10,12,13] No other tissue in men is known to produce PSA, so it is very specific for the prostate gland and increases in

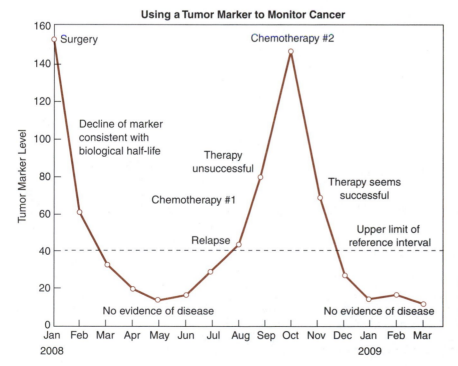

FIGURE 18–1. Tumor marker analysis. A curve showing a sample scenario monitoring a cancer patient for tumor recurrence and for therapy efficacy using levels of a tumor-associated antigen.

almost all prostate cancers. However, in a healthy person, the amount of PSA produced is directly related to the gland's size, and many men develop benign enlarged prostates as they age. Further, as men age, they are more likely to develop prostate cancer, but they are less likely to die from it. In other words, as men age, there are prostate cancers that can and should be left alone. It is recommended that PSA screening cease once a man's remaining life expectancy is less than 10 years. Great effort has been expended to discriminate between benign prostatic hypertrophy, weakly aggressive cancers, and highly aggressive cancers using PSA. If the free-to-bound ratio of PSA is low or the rate of PSA is increasing at a rate that exceeds 0.5 ng/mL per year[13] (PSA velocity), this is more associated with cancer and is justification for a biopsy. Due to the fact that an increased PSA does not always indicate a cancerous state or an aggressive cancer that must be treated, the net benefit to the widespread PSA screening currently done in the United States may be questionable.[10]

## LAB TESTS FOR TUMOR MARKER DETECTION

Clinicians screen for the presence of malignancies by a variety of methods.[2] Commonly used tests include stool occult blood and colonoscopy for colorectal carcinoma, Papanicolaou smear for cervical cancer, self-exams for breast and testicular cancer, x-ray mammography for breast cancer, and digital rectal exam for prostate cancer. Laboratory tests can provide important adjunct information to patient histories and physical exams.

Broadly, the three types of laboratory methods for cancer screening and diagnosis are gross and microscopic morphology of tumors, detection of antigen/protein tumor markers, and DNA/RNA molecular diagnostics. These techniques are complementary in that many of the DNA changes and subsequent mRNA expression result in the altered antigens/proteins detected or morphology visualized, so the choice of method often depends on convenience, cost, sensitivity, and specificity.

Pathologists and histology labs process suspected tumor tissue with gross dissection and preparation of slides for microscopic analysis. A variety of special stains, nucleic acid probes, and tumor marker antibodies can be applied to the slides to enhance the visible features. Even so, evaluation of morphology and staining patterns can be very subjective, and classification categories can be rather broad. Considerable skill is required to accurately diagnose cancer by morphology alone, and final diagnosis is often made with supplemental clinical information and additional testing, which is described below.[14]

Some of the molecular diagnostic techniques that have become increasingly routine include the following:

- **Cytogenetic studies:** Many cancers are associated with particular karyotypes. However, as more precise knowledge of the exact gene defects present in various cancers is gained, testing for the aberrant genes is becoming more prevalent.[14]

- **Nucleic acid amplification techniques:** Polymerase chain reaction (PCR) and its variants increase the inherent level of DNA or RNA, allowing the detection of small populations of cancer cells (including circulating cells in metastasis) and the detection of mutations, deletions, and gene rearrangements/translocations.[14] (See Chapter 11 for a complete discussion of PCR.)

- **Fluorescent in situ hybridization (FISH):** Nucleic acid probes capable of binding to sequences of interest are tagged with fluorophors and applied to cells. Cells containing the sequence of interest can be visualized with fluorescent microscopes. Similar techniques using nonfluorescent labels such as enzymes and silver stains are also becoming available.

Candidate DNA/RNA sequences for genetic screening of cancers abound, but most are still in the research stage. The *BCR-ABL* translocation associated with chronic myelogenous leukemia is a well-respected marker for this disease,[15] and monoclonal expression of B-cell DNA rearrangement is present almost exclusively in multiple myeloma or other lymphoid malignancy.[16] Most other phenotypically related cancers have heterogeneous genetic causes, so universal and reliable genetic abnormalities are not yet described. The future may lie with **microarray** tests that are currently being developed with multiple nucleic acid tests contained on a single chip to allow for simultaneous testing of a sample for multiple genes. One potential use of this technology is detection and semiquantitation of mRNA expression in cells to distinguish patterns (rather than single markers) consistent with cancer.[14]

Some genetic abnormalities are associated with an increased risk of developing a cancer or with a poorer prognosis. Examples of **susceptibility genes** are the BRCA-1 and BRCA-2 mutations linked with an increased risk of breast, ovarian, and prostate cancers.[10] An example of a prognostic marker is overexpression of the Her2/neu oncogene. Breast cancers with this oncogene tend to be more aggressive but will more likely respond to certain therapies (trastuzumab).[10]

Antigen/protein tumor markers are substances expressed by cancer cells or by the body in response to the presence of cancer. The ideal tumor marker has the following characteristics:

- It must be produced by the tumor or as a result of the tumor and must be secreted into some biological fluid that can be analyzed easily and inexpensively for levels.
- Its circulating half-life must be long enough to permit its concentration to rise with increasing tumor load.
- It must increase to clinically significant levels (above background control levels) while the disease is still treatable and with few false negatives (sufficient sensitivity).
- The antigen must be absent from or at background levels in all individuals without the malignant disease in question to minimize false-positive test results (sufficient specificity).[2,10,12]

Non-nucleic acid tumor markers generally fall into seven categories: cell surface markers, proteins, oncofetal antigens, carbohydrate antigens, blood group antigens, enzymes/isoenzymes, and hormones.[12] Examples are shown in **Table 18–1**. Most are detected by immunologic methods with antibodies to distinct epitopes on the molecules. Prostate-specific antigen (PSA), for example, is an enzyme, but it is typically detected as an antigen.

Tumor markers are not always directly associated with the malignant transformation. Often, they are the normal products of the tissue of origin being expressed, and this is more likely if the tumor is well differentiated. For example, endocrine gland tumors often produce generous amounts of hormone that the tissue of origin produces.

Although there are scores of possible tumor markers in the literature, less than a dozen have FDA approval as such.[10,12] However, many non-FDA-approved markers are available to clinicians, with a notation on the lab report stating that results are for research use only. The National Academy of Clinical Biochemistry has developed a set of very useful consensus guidelines regarding the clinical use of tumor markers.[10] They list methods and markers for a variety of purposes that have acceptable evidence of validity. These guidelines recommend very few markers for screening/early detection and still recommend using adjunct tests or screening high-risk populations. These markers are listed in **Table 18–2**. All other recommended markers have various uses in diagnosis and disease monitoring. Some of

the most common and useful markers are listed in **Table 18–3**, along with important noncancerous conditions that cause elevations.

The new field of **proteomics** employs **mass spectrometry (MS)** to identify and quantify an array of proteins simultaneously present in a sample. This has given birth to a new field called **oncopeptidomics**.[17] Protein profiling in cancer patients will aid in the discovery of new tumor markers or patterns of protein expression that are consistent with cancer. Oncopeptidomics may allow more subtle increases of tumor markers to have diagnostic significance, since multiple markers can be measured and the overall pattern assessed, but this is currently only at the research stage.

There are some important aspects to laboratory testing for tumor markers. Most tumor markers are detected using antibodies because of the specificity of antibodies and the general reliability of immunoassays. However, there are some important limitations to using antibodies as reagents. Antibodies are directed at specific epitopes, and the antibodies from different manufacturers may vary greatly in terms of what is measured, particularly if monoclonal antibodies are used. This makes it important to use the same method for monitoring patients over time, and clinicians should be aware of this if patients change clinics or laboratories. It also means that if laboratories switch methods, they must provide a transition period during which specimens are measured by both methods and specimens are archived until new data is established for each patient.[10]

**Table 18-1. Categories of Protein/Antigen Tumor Markers[2,12]**

| TUMOR MARKER CLASS | EXAMPLES | DISEASE ASSOCIATIONS |
|---|---|---|
| Cell surface markers | Estrogen/progesterone receptors | Prognosis for hormone therapy in breast cancer |
| | CD markers on white blood cells | Clonality and lineage of white blood cell neoplasms |
| Proteins | Thyroglobulin (TG) | Well-differentiated papillary or follicular thyroid carcinoma |
| | Immunoglobulins (Ig) and Ig light chains (Bence Jones proteins) | Multiple myeloma and lymphoid malignancies |
| Oncofetal antigens | Alpha-1-fetoprotein (AFP) | Germ cell carcinoma, hepatocellular carcinoma |
| | Carcinoembryonic antigen (CEA) | Colorectal carcinoma and some others |
| Carbohydrate antigens | CA 125 | Ovarian cancer |
| | CA 15-3 | Breast cancer |
| Blood group antigens | CA 19-9 (related to Lewis antigens) | Pancreatic and gastrointestinal cancers |
| Enzymes/isoenzymes | Prostate-specific antigen (PSA) | Prostate cancer |
| | Alkaline phosphatase (ALKP) | Bone and liver cancer |
| | Neuron specific enolase | Neural tissue neoplasms |
| Hormones | Human chorionic gonadotropin (hCG) | Germ cell carcinoma, trophoblastic tumors |
| | Calcitonin | Medullary thyroid cancer |
| | Gastrin | Pancreatic gastrinoma |

**Table 18–2. Tumor Markers Useful for Cancer Screening Professional Consensus Recommendations from the National Academy for Clinical Biochemistry Lab Medicine Practice Guidelines[10]**

| CANCER TYPE | MARKER | ADJUNCT TEST | POPULATION RECOMMENDED |
|---|---|---|---|
| Prostate | Prostate-specific antigen (PSA, total and free) | Digital rectal exam | Men over 50 and with at least 10 years of life expectancy |
| Colorectal | Fecal occult blood | Genetic testing | Subjects over 50 years old for occult blood; genetic testing in high-risk subjects |
| Liver | Alpha-1-fetoprotein (AFP) | Ultrasound | High-risk subjects |
| Ovarian | Carbohydrate antigen 125 (CA 125) | Ultrasound | Subjects with family history of ovarian cancer |

**Table 18–3. Common Tumor Markers[2,10,12,27]**

| MARKER | CANCER(S) | USES* | NORMAL SOURCES | NONCANCEROUS CONDITIONS WITH ELEVATIONS | COMMENTS |
|---|---|---|---|---|---|
| AFP | Nonseminomatous testicular Germ cell Liver | 1, 2, 3, 4 | Fetal liver and yolk sac, adult liver | Pregnancy, non-neoplastic liver disease | Screening for high-risk populations for liver cancer such as those with liver cirrhosis and chronic hepatitis In germ cell tumors, both AFP and hCG are elevated. |
| β–2 microglobulin | Lymphocyte malignancies | 2 | MHC class I | Inflammatory and high cell turnover conditions | Higher levels imply poor prognosis in multiple myeloma. |
| Calcitonin and Ca++ | Familial medullary thyroid carcinoma | N/A | Thyroid | In hypercalcemia, increased calcitonin is expected. Serum Ca++ may be low when calcitonin is elevated in medullary carcinoma. | Can be elevated in other forms of cancer. |
| CD markers | White blood cell (WBC) | N/A | All WBCs | WBC increase such as infection | An array of CD markers are associated with WBC malignancies. |
| CEA | Colorectal Breast | 2, 3, 4 | Tissues of entodermal origin | Renal failure, non-neoplastic liver and intestinal disease, age | Values increased with age and in smokers. |
| CA125 | Ovarian adenocarcinoma | 1, 2, 3, 4 | Various | Endometriosis, pelvic inflammatory disease, uterine fibroids, and pregnancy | Don't collect specimen during menstruation (false increase). |
| CA15-3 | Breast Can be increased in pancreatic, lung, colorectal, ovarian, and liver cancers | 4 | Mammary tissue | Benign breast disease Benign liver disease | Epitope of episialin. 15-3 is monoclonal antibody. Others are 27.29 and 549. |
| CA 19-9 | Pancreatic | 1, 2, 4 | Sialyated Lewis[a] blood group antigen | Benign hepatobiliary and pancreatic conditions | Can be elevated in some nonpancreatic malignancies. Subjects who are Lewis a and b negative cannot synthesize CA 19-9. |

## Table 18-3. Common Tumor Markers[2,10,12,27]—Cont'd

| MARKER | CANCER(S) | USES* | NORMAL SOURCES | NONCANCEROUS CONDITIONS WITH ELEVATIONS | COMMENTS |
|---|---|---|---|---|---|
| ER/PR | Breast adenocarcinoma | 2 | Breast | N/A | ER/PR + breast cancers benefit from estrogen/progesterone reduction therapy. |
| Fecal occult blood | Colorectal cancer | N/A | N/A | Sources of peroxidase in feces other than blood (certain foods) | Heme functions as a peroxidase and can be detected chemically. Better specificity with antibodies against globin chains of hemoglobin. |
| hCG | Nonseminomatous testicular cancer Germ cell trophoblastic (hydatidiform mole, choriocarcinoma) | 1, 2, 3, 4 | Placenta | Pregnancy | hCG high homology with luteinizing hormone (LH). Malignancies can produce free alpha and beta chains as well as intact alpha/beta dimer. Immunoassays that detect only intact hCG should not be used for tumor marker detection. In germ cell tumors, both AFP and hCG are elevated. |
| HER2/neu | Breast | 2 | Growth factor gene in all cells | N/A | Cancer associated with overexpression of HER2/neu and good response to monoclonal antibody therapy (trastuzumab) |
| Monoclonal free Ig light chains | Plasma cell, B lymphocytes | 1, 2, 3, 4 | Normal Igs are polyclonal. Few free light chains exist. | Monoclonal gammopathy of undetermined significance (MGUS), amyloidosis, nonsecretory myeloma | Bence Jones proteins are free Ig light chains in urine detected by heating. This method is largely historic. |
| Monoclonal Igs | Plasma cell, B lymphocytes | 1, 2, 3, 4 | Normal Igs are polyclonal. | Monoclonal gammopathy of undetermined significance | Monoclonal IgG/IgA— multiple myeloma Monoclonal IgM— Waldenström's macroglobulinemia |
| PSA | Prostate | 1, 2, 3, 4 | No tissues other than prostate | UTI/prostatitis, benign prostatic hypertrophy | Levels directly proportional to prostate size. Many elevations are benign or not clinically significant. Decreased percent of free PSA and ≥0.5 mg/mL/year increase (PSA velocity) more associated with malignancy. Collect specimen before ejaculation, digital rectal exam, or prostate manipulation. |

*Continued*

| Table 18-3. | Common Tumor Markers[2,10,12,27]—Cont'd | | | | |
|---|---|---|---|---|---|
| MARKER | CANCER(S) | USES* | NORMAL SOURCES | NONCANCEROUS CONDITIONS WITH ELEVATIONS | COMMENTS |
| PTH and Ca++ | Parathyroid carcinoma | 1, 2, 3, 4 | Parathyroid glands | In hypocalcemia, increased PTH is expected. Serum Ca++ may be high when PTH is elevated in parathyroid carcinoma. | PTH has a short half-life, so levels are done intraoperatively to ensure complete parathyroid tumor removal. |
| TG | Thyroid | 3, 4 | Thyroid | TG reflects thyroid mass, injury, and TSH levels. Thyroid markers (T4, TSH) generally normal in thyroid cancer. | Assays must simultaneously test for thyroglobulin antibodies (false decrease). Often tested after TSH stimulation to see if TG increases. Also can withhold thyroid medication to increase TSH in patients with thyroid gland removed. |

Abbreviations: AFP = alpha-1-fetoprotein ; CA = carbohydrate antigen; Ca++ = serum calcium; CD = clusters of differentiation in WBC; CEA = carcinoembryonic antigen; ER/PR = estrogen/progesterone receptors; hCG = human chorionic gonadotropin; Ig = immunoglobulins; PTH = parathyroid hormone; PSA = prostate-specific antigen; TG = thyroglobulin; UTI = urinary tract infection
* NACB recommendations: 1 = diagnosis/case finding; 2 = staging/prognosis; 3 = detecting recurrence; 4 = monitoring therapy

While antibodies are employed for their specificity, it is not absolute. Antibodies will cross-react with similar structures, and this is particularly problematic when the cross-reacting substances are in excessive amounts, as can occur in cancer. For example, hCG is made of an alpha subunit and a beta subunit. The alpha subunit is virtually identical to the alpha subunit of luteinizing hormone (LH), and the beta subunits are 80 percent homologous, so epitope choice is quite important. Further, assay configuration influences what is measured. Cancers may produce free alpha and beta chains in addition to intact hCG, so an immunochemical method that relies only on beta chain epitopes to minimize LH interference will measure something completely different than a method that sandwiches intact hCG between an antialpha capture antibody and an antibeta labeled antibody.[10]

By virtue of unchecked growth and aggressive metabolism, some tumors may produce massive amounts of tumor marker molecules. The prozone effect is a well-known limitation of antibody-based assays in which antigen saturation of antibodies inhibits the cross-linkage required to visualize the reaction. In immunoassays, a similar phenomenon has been called the **high-dose hook effect**,[18] and the result is a falsely decreased measurement, as shown in **Figure 18–2.** It is critical that criteria be developed to identify situations in which the hook effect may be present so that specimens can be diluted and accurate results obtained. A related problem of antigen excess in automated systems is specimen carryover, so in addition to diluting the specimen with excessive antigen, the specimen being tested immediately after it may need to be repeated.

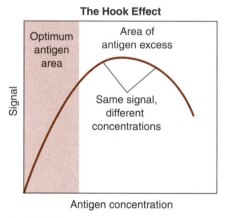

FIGURE 18–2. The high-dose hook effect. Antigen excess can saturate antibodies, and the intended "sandwich" configurations cannot form, leading to a false decrease in signal.

Finally, because many of the antibodies used in immunoassays are animal in origin, heterophile antibodies in specimens can interfere profoundly with results.[18] In a tragic case involving false-positive hCG results from an automated analyzer, several women had unnecessary chemotherapy or hysterectomies for presumed undetected cancer.[19] Although heterophile antibodies are mostly associated with false increases by mechanisms similar to that shown in **Figure 18–3,** false decreases are also possible. Antibody-blocking reagents are commercially available (e.g., Scantibodies) to block heterophile antibodies in suspicious specimens, and many manufacturers are employing blocking agents within the routine reagents. Specimens with

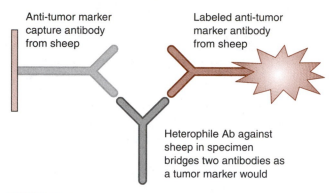

**Mechanism of false-positives
due to heterophile antibodies**

Anti-tumor marker
capture antibody
from sheep

Labeled anti-tumor
marker antibody
from sheep

Heterophile Ab against
sheep in specimen
bridges two antibodies as
a tumor marker would

**FIGURE 18–3.** Heterophile antibody interference. Heterophile antibodies can cause both false decreases and false increases, depending on their reactivity against the antibody species used in an assay. However, as shown, false increases are most likely.

nonlinear behavior on dilution or with discrepant results using different methods or after applying antibody-blocking reagents may have heterophile antibodies and should not be reported until the issue is resolved.

## IMMUNOTHERAPY

**Immunotherapy** is the final aspect of tumor immunology to be discussed. The possibility of stimulating the patient's own immune system to respond to tumor-associated antigens has long intrigued scientists. This chapter cannot cover all the different protocols, but increasing knowledge concerning tumors and the immune system has led to new research and recent optimism in this area.

Immunotherapeutic methods used can be separated into two types: passive or active immunotherapy. Passive immunotherapy involves transfer of antibody, cytokines, or cells to patients who may not be able to mount an immune response. With active immunotherapy, patients are treated in a manner that stimulates them to mount immune responses to their tumors.

### Passive Immunotherapy

Passive transfer of allogeneic cellular immunity from one person to another to fight cancer has many barriers because of possible recipient rejection of foreign cells, graft-versus-host disease (GVHD), and the fragility of live cells, although research models are being studied. Inducing a patient's own cellular immunity is far more likely to be successful, as discussed in the next section. However, a form of GVHD called **graft versus leukemia** has been demonstrated with transfer of allogeneic T cells and is associated with improved patient prognosis.[20] Therefore, successful passive transfer of anticancer T cells is theoretically possible.

Adoptive T-cell therapy has been attempted using several models.[21] For example, T cells from allogeneic donors can be immunized against tumors. After recipients are immunosuppressed to prevent rejection and to eliminate T suppressor mechanisms, they receive the T cells. One strategy in this model to treat GVHD is to genetically engineer the allogeneic T cells with a "suicide switch." This gene makes the cells vulnerable to a drug that will immediately eliminate them in the event of GVHD.

Other strategies for adoptive T-cell therapy use autologous T cells.[21] Tumor-infiltrating lymphocytes (TILs) can be harvested and expanded in vitro using IL-2. The patient is then lymphodepleted to remove T suppressor cells, and high concentrations of TILs are transfused. Similarly, autologous T cells can be harvested, exposed to cancer antigens, expanded with IL-2, and then returned to the patient. Attempts have also been made to insert genetically engineered T-cell receptors into autologous T cells.[20]

Passive transfer of antibody to treat cancer almost always employs monoclonal antibodies. "Naked" monoclonal antibodies against cancer could induce antibody-dependent cell-mediated cytolysis (ADCC), complement-mediated lysis, or opsonization. If the antibodies are directed toward particular receptors, they could trigger a desirable action in the cell such as inducing apoptosis or inhibiting growth signals. **Antibody conjugates,** or **immunotoxins,** are antibodies conjugated to toxins or radioisotopes on the premise that they can kill cancer cells while leaving adjacent cells intact. In order for these techniques to work, the following are required:[22]

- Antibodies must be directed at a cell surface antigen with high density.
- The antigen must be present on the primary tumor and on all metastatic foci.
- Normal tissues must be free from the antigen or not susceptible to the toxin.
- The antibodies must have sufficient access to the tumor tissue (i.e., the tumor burden is not such that certain portions escape exposure to the antibodies).

The obstacles involved in immunotherapy with antibodies are:

- tumor heterogeneity with regard to antigenic expression;
- antigenic modulation or the loss of antigen from the tumor cells.
- failure of antibodies to penetrate tumor tissue.
- failure of antibody–toxin conjugates to internalize into the cell after binding and release toxin.
- toxic effects on other tissues, particularly the hematopoietic organs.
- the limited amount of toxin that can be linked to the antibody without destruction of binding activity.
- host immune response to the injected antibody.
- circulating antigen forming immune complexes with the antibodies, removing them from circulation.

**Table 18–4** shows the cancer immunotherapy antibodies currently available in the United States.[22] Most antibodies are artificially engineered, as the development of heterophile

## Table 18-4.   Currently Available FDA-Approved Antibodies for Cancer Therapy[22]

| ANTIBODY BRAND NAME | GENERIC NAME | COMPOSITION | ANTIGEN TARGET | THERAPEUTIC USE |
|---|---|---|---|---|
| Avastin | Bevacizumab | Humanized IgG1 monoclonal with murine binding region for VEGF | Vascular endothelial growth factor (VEGF) | Prevent blood vessel formation in tumors. Eradicate tumors through lack of blood supply, especially colorectal cancers and nonsmall cell lung cancers |
| Bexxar | Tositumomab | Iodine-131 ($^{131}$I) murine IgG2a lambda monoclonal plus unlabeled tositumomab | CD 20– on B cells | Radioactive immunotherapy non-Hodgkins lymphoma |
| Campath | Alemtuzumab | Humanized IgG1 monoclonal with murine binding region for CD 52 | CD52– on almost T and B cells as well as some other WBC | Antibody-dependent lysis of lymphocytes in chronic lymphocytic leukemia |
| Erbitux | Cetuximab | Chimeric monoclonal-murine Fab variable portion and human IgG1 kappa Fc portion | Epidermal growth factor receptor (EGFR) | Reduced proliferation of cancers expressing EGFR, especially colorectal cancers and their metastases, head and neck cancers |
| Herceptin | Trastuzumab | Humanized IgG1 kappa monoclonal with murine binding region for HER2 | HER2/neu | Reduced proliferation of breast cancers overexpressing HER2/neu through ADCC, anti-angiogenesis, reduced cell signaling for growth |
| Mylotarg | Gemtuzumab ozogamicin | Humanized IgG4 kappa monoclonal with murine binding region for CD33 linked to calicheamicin | CD33 on leukemic blasts and immature myelomonocytic cells | Toxin immunoconjugate therapy—antibody is internalized and toxic calicheamicin kills cells in acute myelogenous leukemia |
| ProstaScint | Capromab pendetide | Indium-111 ($^{111}$In) murine IgG1 kappa monoclonal | Prostate-specific membrane antigen | Radioactive immunotherapy of prostate cancer |
| Rituxan | Rituximab | Chimeric monoclonal-murine Fab variable portion and human IgG1 kappa Fc portion | CD 20– on B cells | ADCC, complement lysis, and induced apoptosis when two CD20 molecules bind in non-Hodgkins lymphoma |
| Zevalin | Ibritumomab | Yttrium-90 ($^{90}$Y) labeled chimeric monoclonal-murine Fab variable portion and human IgG1 kappa Fc portion plus unlabeled rituximab | CD 20– on B cells | Radioactive immunotherapy of non-Hodgkins lymphoma |

antibodies in patients receiving therapy is a significant interference. The chimeric antibodies splice animal (usually murine) variable Fab onto human Fc for a final composition of about 25 percent animal and 75 percent human. "Humanized" antibodies splice the portion of animal antibody required for epitope binding to human antibody for a final composition of about 5 percent animal and 95 percent human. This improves antibody half-life, which is naturally long in the absence of heterophile antibodies. Long antibody half-life is desirable for therapeutic effects, but it also prolongs negative effects. This is particularly a problem for antibodies conjugated to radioisotopes, which cause bone marrow toxicity and myelosuppression.[22,23]

Currently, immunotherapeutic antibodies are most effective against hematologic malignancies, small tumors, and micro metastases, not bulky tumors.[22,23] Antibodies poorly penetrate tumor mass, because they are large molecules, and they bind to the first available antigen encountered on the outside of the tumor. Surgical removal or debulking of a tumor may ideally precede the use of antibodies. Further, since there is usually more than one path for cell growth, antibodies are rarely, if ever, used alone. Combination therapy with chemotherapeutic agents or other treatments is usually recommended.[22]

Radiolabeled antibodies are particularly effective because of the "bystander" or "crossfire" effect seen with high-energy isotopes that can kill up to several hundred cells. This is particularly advantageous for tumors with heterogeneous antigen expression and could allow antibodies to kill cells that are not expressing antigen at all. An additional use for radiolabeled antibodies is imaging studies to locate foci of cancer. However, their use must be managed to minimize bone marrow toxicity, although this toxicity is generally reversible.[22,23]

Currently, there are no FDA-approved antibody–toxin conjugates, although denileukin diftitox, a recombinant IL-2 coupled with modified diphtheria toxin, has been approved for T-cell lymphoma. Only one antibody–drug conjugate (gemtuzumab ozogamicin) has been approved.[22] Conjugation can theoretically allow the use of "ultratoxic" drugs and some extreme cytotoxins, because the agent's delivery is limited and focused by the antibody. Several cytotoxins are under study, including diphtheria toxin, *Pseudomonas* exotoxin, abrin, ricin, and saporin. Since toxins have their own binding mechanisms, antibodies must bypass the normal mechanism or the toxin must be modified. Further, some cytotoxins must be internalized to be effective, so the antibody must target an epitope that would be internalized.[22]

## Active Immunotherapy

The goal of active immunotherapy is to have the patient develop an immune response that will help eliminate the tumor. Nonspecific stimulation by adjuvants such as Bacillus Calmette Guerin (BCG) was first attempted, and superficial bladder cancer is still treated with BCG.[24] Improved technology has allowed the production of novel adjuvants and selective use of stimulatory cytokines (TNF-α, IFN-γ, IL-1, IL-2, and so on) in immunocompetent patients to enhance the natural antitumor response and the artificial vaccine-induced response.[6]

Other attempts at stimulating host immune systems have involved transfection of normal cells or isolated tumor cells with genes for cytokine production and injection of the modified cells into or around the tumor.[25] This has been done with many cytokines, including TNF-α, interferons, IL-2, and granulocyte monocyte–colony stimulating factor (GM-CSF). Of the cytokines transfected, GM-CSF has shown the most promise.[25]

Cancer vaccines have been of great interest to researchers. When specific viruses are associated with a cancer, vaccine construction is relatively straightforward, since viral antigens are obviously foreign. The vaccine for human papillomavirus (HPV) to prevent cervical cancer is an excellent example. It is important to note that many viruses have several serotypes, not all of which may be associated with cancer, so vaccines must be protective against the appropriate epitopes. HPV

vaccines, for example, are directed epitopes that prevent initial infection with carcinogenic serotypes but do not help treat established cervical cancer, as these epitopes are down-regulated in cancer cells.[7] Therefore, a distinction exists between prophylactic vaccines and therapeutic ones.

In the absence of a viral cause of a cancer, prophylactic vaccination is more difficult, since many of the antigens expressed on tumors, as stated previously, appear to some degree on normal tissue. High-affinity cytotoxic T lymphocytes against tumor-associated antigens (TAA) are often deleted by tolerance pathways.[20] Further, just the expression of an antigen on a tumor does not automatically make it a suitable vaccine target, since coexpression with MHC I and obligatory accessory molecules is required for adequate T-cell response. Vaccination with tumor lysates and peptide antigen vaccines have had limited success. This is at least partly due to the heterogeneity of antigens presented on tumors and the few "public antigens" common to all tumors and the many "private antigens" unique to an individual's tumor. Designing custom vaccines for each individual is obviously more difficult than designing more universal vaccines.

Various strategies have been attempted to identify sufficiently immunogenic antigens and how to present them to T cells. They are too numerous to outline here. However, an example is the strategy to prime dendritic cells (DCs), which are particularly potent antigen-presenting cells that can stimulate both humoral and cellular immunity and immune tolerance reactions. The general principle of this technique is that a DC line is cultured from the patient and then exposed to tumor antigen. Antigen exposure may be done using coculture with purified tumor antigens or tumor lysate, fusion of DCs with tumor cells, DC phagocytosis of dead tumor cells, or transfection of RNA.[26] The DCs are reintroduced in the patient by various measures (intravenously, subcutaneously, and so on) as a vaccine. Preliminary research has demonstrated some success with these vaccines, but the details of optimal antigens, DC priming, and modes of DC delivery are still being evaluated.

It remains to be seen which, if any, of the numerous immunization protocols currently under study will work. These protocols will be important adjuncts to traditional therapies in which tumors will first be debulked and then the immune system will eradicate residual tumor and micrometastases.[25] The increased understanding of tumor immunology in recent years has made this a field of active study and increased optimism.

## SUMMARY

Tumor immunology is the study of the antigens associated with tumors, the immune response to tumors, the tumor's effect on the host's immune status, and the use of the immune system to help eradicate the tumor. Cancer begins with changes in one normal cell, and these changes allow the cell to grow and proliferate without regard to normal growth signals or controls. As these abnormal cells grow and continue to mutate, they may show differences in gene expression both in type and amount. Antigens expressed in greater amounts in tumor tissue are called tumor-associated antigens.

There is evidence that immunosurveillance may protect against growth of some tumors. T cells and NK cells can recognize tumor cells as foreign and destroy them. Ultimate development of cancer may be due to immunoediting by cellular immunity. Very immunogenic tumor cells are eliminated, creating an environment that allows tumor cells to evade the immune system.

The clinical laboratory's role in detecting and monitoring cancer is based on the presence of various tumor markers. These include altered antigen/receptor expression, abnormal genes, overproduced cellular products, and substances produced in response to the tumor. Assessment of tumor markers has been applied for tumor screening, diagnosis, histopathologic evaluation, staging, disease monitoring, localization of metastasis, and therapy selection.

Disease prevalence in a population profoundly affects the clinical utility of tumor marker testing. Existence of disease in asymptomatic populations will be low, so the majority of positive tumor marker tests will be false positives. Few tumor markers are recommended for screening, and most should be used in conjunction with other tests or in high-risk populations. Disease prevalence is higher in populations being differentially diagnosed or monitored for known cancer, so the utility of tumor marker assays for these purposes is far superior. Tumor marker tests are generally best utilized to follow the course of a known cancer, since the marker's trend up or down is more important than its absolute value.

Both passive and active immunotherapy directed at appropriate tumor markers have begun to show some signs of success. While most immunotherapy is still at the research stage, several monoclonal antibodies have gained FDA approval for cancer treatment. The human papillomavirus vaccine is FDA approved for cancer prevention, so the continued identification of tumor markers and elucidation of the immune system's response against cancer is worthwhile.

# CASE STUDIES

1. A 45-year-old woman went to her physician's office after noticing a lump during her breast self-exam. She had a strong family history of breast cancer. The lump was detected on mammography and was found to be a 0.5 cm mass that was adherent to her skin. Analysis found her CA-15.3 levels to be 60 IU/mL, which is double the upper limit of the reference interval. After surgery, the levels of CA-15.3 dropped, but at a rate that was slower than the biological half-life. They remained above 30 IU/mL. The tumor morphology indicated malignancy, so it was tested for Her2/neu expression, which was elevated, and estrogen/progesterone receptors, which were negative.

## Questions

a. Do you think that there is residual tumor, and why?

b. In addition to chemotherapy, what other therapy would you recommend, and why?

c. What type of therapy is unlikely to be successful, and why?

2. Several weeks ago, a 25-year-old woman had a thyroidectomy to remove a well-differentiated follicular carcinoma. After surgery, her thyroglobulin (TG) level decreased to undetectable. She remains asymptomatic but was asked to discontinue her thyroid hormone replacement therapy for 2 weeks and return for the laboratory determinations indicated in the table below:

| | PATIENT RESULTS | REFERENCE RANGE |
|---|---|---|
| TG | 7 ug/L | <5 ug/L in athyroidic patients |
| Anti-TG antibodies | None detected | <1:10 |
| Thyroid-stimulating hormone (TSH) | 10.7 mU/L | 0.4–4.2 mU/L |

## Questions

a. What test above is done to ensure accuracy of the TG test? Is this TG measurement likely to be accurate or not?

b. What test above is done to verify that residual thyroid cancer is likely to be producing TG? Is remaining cancer being stimulated or not?

c. What does this TG level indicate in the patient?

3. A 66-year-old black male went to a urologist complaining of frequent urination with only small volumes of urine, creating great urgency. During the digital rectal exam, the urologist felt an enlarged prostate with no distinct nodules or abnormal areas. The patient's serum level of prostate-specific antigen (PSA) was determined and compared to the level from the previous year. The physician also asked that the bound-to-total PSA ratio be determined. The test results are shown below.

| Laboratory Results | | |
|---|---|---|
| TEST | PATIENT RESULTS | REFERENCE INTERVAL |
| PSA October 2008 | 3.9 ng/mL | 0–3.5 ng/mL |
| PSA October 2007 | 3.5 ng/mL | 0–3.5 ng/mL |
| Bound/free PSA | 25.8% | ≥23.4% |

## Questions

a. Do any tissues other than the prostate produce PSA? Could there be another source of the PSA in this case?

b. What is PSA velocity?

c. Should this man have a biopsy? Do you think this man has cancer? Why?

d. At what point is it unethical to test for PSA?

# EXERCISE

## SEMIQUANTITATIVE PSA MEMBRANE TEST FOR THE DETECTION OF ELEVATED SERUM LEVELS OF PSA

### Principle*

This is a solid-phase chromatographic capture membrane enzyme immunoassay for the detection of PSA in patient serum. Elevated PSA is found in men with prostate cancer and in men with benign prostatic hypertrophy. Often, age-adjusted cutoffs are used or compared to previous measurements (PSA increase velocity). This assay uses an internal standard of 4 ng/mL to allow a visual comparison of the specimen reaction to determine if it exceeds 4. Patients without tumors rarely have levels above 10 ng/mL, but many patients with tumors and those with benign prostatic hypertrophy will be in the 4 to 10 ng/mL range. A positive above 4 will warrant further investigation with a quantitative test and a digital rectal examination.

This rapid test for PSA performs according to the following principle: The membrane of the test cassette is impregnated with murine monoclonal antihuman PSA as the immobilized antibody in the test region and with immobilized antimurine antibody in the internal standard and control regions. Antibodies in the internal standard region are adjusted to reflect a positive reaction consistent with 4 ng/mL of PSA. Antihuman PSA monoclonal conjugate labeled with red-colored gold is impregnated in the cassette but not immobilized. When serum is applied, PSA in the patient's serum reacts with the red-colored monoclonal mouse anti-PSA. Through the capillary effect in the membrane of the test cassette, the reaction mixture is carried to each of the areas with immobilized antibodies. If PSA is present, it will be captured by anti-PSA in the test region, and the red-labeled antibody can be visualized. Mobilized red-gold antimurine antibodies are bound in the internal standard and control regions by the murine antiglobulin, independent of the existence of PSA. After the device is incubated at room temperature for 10 minutes, a visual interpretation is performed. No line in the test region or one lighter in color than the 4 ng/mL line is a negative result, and a line as dark or darker than the 4 ng/mL standard is a positive result (Fig. 18–4).

In this test system, the high-dose hook effect (prozone) has been observed at concentrations exceeding 500 ug/mL. Further, free PSA reacts slightly better than complexed PSA, reducing the test's specificity for cancer as compared to other quantitative methods.

**SERATEC PSA Test Cassette**

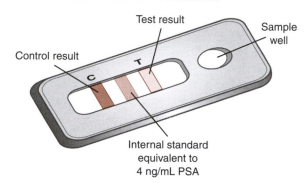

**FIGURE 18–4.** A schematic showing the Seratec PSA test cassette. In this example, the patient line T has more PSA than internal standard, representing 4 ng/mL control, and the control line C indicates a valid reaction. *(This test is available as seratec PSA semi-quant [ref psm400t] from Serological Research Institute, Joan Matthew, 3053 Research Drive, Richmond, CA 94806, USA [Telephone: 1-510-223-737; Fax: 1-510-222-8887; e-mail: contact@seratec.com or jmatthew@serological.com]. Above information taken from seratec PSA semi-quant [ref psm400t] literature rev. May 2005.)*

---

* This test is available from Seratec (Telephone: + 49 551 50480-0; Fax: + 49 551 50480-80; e-mail: seratec@t-online.de).

# REVIEW QUESTIONS

1. How can normal cells become malignant?

   a. Overexpression of oncogenes
   b. Underexpression of tumor-suppressing genes
   c. Viral infection
   d. All of the above

2. Which of the following best summarizes the concept of tumor development via immunoediting?

   a. Cytokines produced by tumor cells are toxic to T cells expressing receptors for tumor-associated antigens.
   b. Cells that can escape the immune system have a growth advantage over more immunogenic tumor cells that are destroyed by T cells during immunosurveillance.
   c. T-cell activity causes an up-regulation of MHC expression on tumor cells that allows them to escape the immune system.
   d. Expression of secreted tumor-associated antigen saturates T-cell receptors and renders them incapable of binding to the actual tumor cells.

3. A woman goes 3 days per week to a tanning bed for 20 minutes of UV exposure per visit. Which stage of cancer is this?

   a. Induction
   b. In situ
   c. Invasion
   d. Dissemination

4. If a disease is present in 1 in every 10,000 individuals, and a marker can detect this disease with 100 percent sensitivity and 95 percent specificity, what would be the number of false positives for each cancer found?

   a. 5
   b. 50
   c. 500
   d. 5000

5. Each of these markers may be elevated in multiple myeloma *except*

   a. CA-125.
   b. β-2 microglobulin.
   c. monoclonal intact immunoglobulin molecules.
   d. free monoclonal light chains from the immunoglobulin molecule.

6. Both AFP and hCG exhibit serum elevations in

   a. pregnancy.
   b. ovarian germ cell carcinoma.
   c. nonseminomatous testicular cancer.
   d. all of the above.

7. Calcitonin and parathyroid hormone levels should not be evaluated as indicating possible tumors without also measuring serum

   a. CEA.
   b. calcium.
   c. thyroglobulin antibodies.
   d. thyroid hormones (TSH, T4).

8. Consensus guidelines indicate enough evidence to use all of the following for cancer screening in the groups indicated *except*

   a. CA-125/women of reproductive age.
   b. AFP/subjects at high risk for liver cancer.
   c. fecal occult blood/people over 50 years of age.
   d. PSA/men over 50 with at least 10 years of life expectancy.

9. A 57-year-old man had a massive tumor removed from his colon. His serum specimen had the following results using an automated ELISA antibody sandwich assay for CEA. The stated linearity of the test is 100 ug/L. What should be done?

| | ABSORBANCE | TEST RESULT | FINAL RESULT USING DILUTION FACTOR |
|---|---|---|---|
| Undiluted specimen | 1.026 | 107.1 ug/L | 107.1 ug/L |
| Specimen × 10 | 1.269 | 125.7 ug/L | 1257.0 ug/L |
| Specimen × 100 | 0.995 | 95.8 ug/L | 9580.0 ug/L |
| Specimen × 1000 | 0.101 | 9.6 ug/L | 9600.0 ug/L |

   a. Retest all specimens using a different kit lot.
   b. Retest the specimen at 1:10,000 and 1:100,000 dilutions.
   c. Retest the specimen using heterophile antibody blocking reagent.
   d. Retest any specimen pipetted after the undiluted specimen and report 9580.0 ug/L for this specimen.

10. A tumor found in the prostate does not stain with antibody to PSA. Is this proof that the tumor came from a different organ?

    a. Yes
    b. No

11. In order to use a tumor marker to monitor the course of the disease, which of the following must be true?

    a. The laboratory measures the marker with the same method over the entire course of the patient's treatment.
    b. The marker must be released from the tumor or because of the tumor into a body fluid that can be obtained and tested.
    c. The marker's half-life is such that the marker persists long enough to reflect tumor burden but clears fast enough to identify successful therapy.
    d. All of the above.

12. Which of the following markers could be elevated in benign liver disease?

    a. AFP
    b. CEA
    c. CA 15-3
    d. CA 19-9
    e. All of the above

13. Choose the *incorrect* statement.

    a. Serum CA 19-9 levels should not be collected from smokers.
    b. Serum CA-125 specimen should not be collected from women who are menstruating.
    c. Feces for occult blood should not be collected from subjects who recently ate peroxidase-containing foods.
    d. Serum PSA specimens should be collected before any manipulation of the prostate, including digital rectal exam.

14. Immunotoxin antibodies used for cancer therapy are "humanized" to prevent subjects from developing

    a. graft-versus-host disease.
    b. heterophile antibodies.
    c. myelosuppression.
    d. serum sickness.

15. Each marker below is correctly paired with a disease in which it can be used for conditional monitoring *except*

    a. CEA/choriocarcinoma.
    b. CA-15.3/breast adenocarcinoma.
    c. CA 125/ovarian adenocarcinoma.
    d. CA-19.9/pancreatic adenocarcinoma.

# References

1. Caudell, K. Alterations in cell growth and neoplasia. In Porth, C (ed): Essentials of Pathophysiology. Lippincott Williams & Wilkins, Philadelphia, PA, 2004.
2. Elkins, B. Neoplasia. In Kaplan, L, Pesce, A, Kazmierczak, S (eds): Clinical Chemistry: Theory, Analysis and Correlation. Mosby, St. Louis, MO, 2003.
3. Abbas, A, and Lichtman, A. Cellular and Molecular Immunology, ed. 5. WB Saunders, Philadelphia, PA, 2003.
4. Roitt, I, Brostoff, J, and Male, D. Immunology, ed. 6. Mosby, London, England, 2001.
5. Kim, R, Emi, M, and Tanabe, K. Cancer immunoediting from immune surveillance to immune escape. Immunology 121: 1–14, 2007.
6. Rao, V, Dyer, C, Jameel, J, Drew, P, and Greeman, J. Potential prognostic and therapeutic roles for cytokines in breast cancer. Oncol Rep 15(1):179–185, 2006.
7. Leggatt, G, and Frazer, I. HPV vaccines: The beginning of the end for cervical cancer. Curr Op Immunology 19:232–238, 2007.
8. Sturgeon, C. Practice guidelines for tumor marker use in the clinic. Clin Chem 48(8):1151–1159, 2002.
9. Pritzker, K. Cancer biomarkers: Easier said than done. Clin Chem 48(8):1147–1150, 2002.
10. National Academy of Clinical Biochemistry. Laboratory Medicine Practice Guidelines: Tumor Markers. Draft Guidelines 2005. www.nacb.org. Accessed September 2007.
11. Tuma, R. Inconsistency of HER2 raises questions. J Natl Cancer Inst 99(14):1064–1065, 2007.
12. Sokoll, L, and Chan, D. Tumor markers. In Clarke, W, and Dufour, D (eds): Contemporary Practice in Clinical Chemistry. AACC Press, Washington, DC, 2006.
13. Loeb, S, and Catalona, W. Prostate-specific antigen in clinical practice. Cancer Letters 249:30–39, 2007.
14. Cross, D, and Burmester, J. The promise of molecular profiling for cancer identification and treatment. Clin Med & Res, 2(3):147–150, 2004.
15. Melo, J, and Barnes, D. Chronic myeloid leukaemia as a model of disease evolution in human cancer. Nat Rev Cancer 7(6):441–453. 2007.
16. Rose, N, Hamilton, R, and Detrick, B. Manual of Clinical Laboratory Immunology. ASM Press, Washington, DC, 2002.
17. Tammen, H, Zucht, H, and Budde, P. Oncopeptidomics—a commentary on opportunities and limitations. Cancer Letters 249:80–86, 2007.
18. Clarke, W. Immunoassays. In Clarke, W, and Dufour, D (eds): Contemporary Practice in Clinical Chemistry. AACC Press, Washington, DC, 2006.
19. Cole, LA, Rinne, KM, Shahabi, S, and Omrani, A. False positive hCG levels leading to unnecessary surgery and chemotherapy, and needless occurrences of diabetes and coma. Clin Chem 45:313–314, 1999.
20. Xue, S, and Stauss, H. Enhancing immune responses for cancer therapy. Cell Mol Immunol 4(3):173–184, 2007.
21. June, C. Adoptive T cell therapy for cancer in the clinic. J Clin Invest. 117(6):1466–1476, 2007.
22. Sharkey, R, and Goldenberg, D. Targeted therapy of cancer: New prospects for antibodies and immunoconjugates. CA Cancer J Clin 56(4):226–243, 2006.
23. Goldenberg, D, and Sharkey, R. Advances in cancer therapy with radiolabeled monoclonal antibodies. Q J Nucl Med Mol Imaging 50(4):248–264, 2006.
24. Oosterlinck, W. Guidelines on diagnosis and treatment of superficial bladder cancer. Minerva Urol Nefrol 56(1):65–72, 2004.
25. Li, C, Huang, Q, and Kung, H. Cytokine and immuno-gene therapy for solid tumors. Cell Mol Immunol 2(2):81–91, 2005.
26. Schott, M. Immune surveillance by dendritic cells: Potential implication for immunotherapy of endocrine cancers. Endocr Relat Cancer 13(3):779–795, 2006.
27. Wu, A. Tietz Clinical Guide to Laboratory Tests, ed. 4. Saunders, Philadelphia, PA, 2006.

# Serological Diagnosis of Infectious Disease

# 19 Serological and Molecular Detection of Bacterial Infections

*Dorothy Fike MS, MT(ASCP) SBB and Christine Stevens*

## LEARNING OBJECTIVES

*After finishing this chapter, the reader will be able to:*

1. Discuss mechanisms of host defense against bacteria.
2. Discuss how certain bacteria evade the immune system.
3. Describe how the M protein contributes to the virulence of *Streptococcus pyogenes*.
4. Describe symptoms of acute rheumatic fever.
5. Discuss how pathogenesis occurs in glomerulonephritis.
6. List and describe five exoantigens produced by group A streptococci.
7. Discuss reasons for performing antibody rather than antigen testing for sequelae of streptococcal infections.
8. State the principle of the antistreptolysin O (ASO) titer test.
9. Explain how the presence of anti-deoxyribonuclease B (anti-DNase B) is detected.
10. Compare the sensitivity of the streptozyme test to other tests for streptococcal antibodies.
11. Interpret laboratory data to diagnose sequelae of streptococcal infections.
12. Discuss how *Helicobacter pylori* may cause ulcers.
13. Discuss the various types of testing that may be done to detect *H. pylori* infection.
14. Explain the testing that may be done to detect antibodies to *H. pylori*.
15. Discuss how *Mycoplasma pneumoniae* may cause infections.
16. Explain the antibody testing that is performed to detect infections to *Mycoplasma pneumoniae*.
17. Identify serological and molecular techniques to detect rickettsial infections.

## KEY TERMS

____ Acute rheumatic fever
____ Anti-DNase B
____ ASO titer
____ Exoantigen
____ Group A Streptococci
____ *Helicobacter pylori*
____ Lancefield group
____ *Mycoplasma pneumoniae*
____ Poststreptococcal glomerulonephritis
____ Rickettsiae
____ Streptolysin O
____ Streptozyme
____ Spotted Fever
____ Typhus
____ Urease

# CHAPTER OUTLINE

## IMMUNE DEFENSES AGAINST BACTERIAL INFECTIONS AND MECHANISMS OF EVASION

Previous chapters in this text have discussed both innate and specific immune responses that serve as protection from foreign antigens, including bacteria. The first line of defense against pathogens is intact skin and mucosal surfaces that serve as structural barriers. Lysozyme, an enzyme found in many secretions such as tears and saliva, is capable of destroying many bacteria. Other soluble innate components that protect us from pathogenic bacteria are interleukins, prostaglandins, and leukotrienes, which cause fever, and acute phase reactants such as C-reactive protein, haptoglobin, and ceruloplasmin, which either coat bacteria or remove substances that might promote bacterial growth. Phagocytosis by neutrophils, monocytes, and macrophages is another mechanism of innate immunity that will protect us against bacteria. The phagocytic process is enhanced by the activation of the alternative complement cascade, which is triggered by microbial cell walls or other products of microbial metabolism.

The specific immune response includes formation of antibodies that are produced to exotoxins or other secreted bacterial products. Antibody formation is the main defense against extracellular bacteria. Anti-exotoxin antibodies bind to the exotoxin and form immune complexes that are eliminated. Through this process, bacterial toxins are neutralized and effectively prevented from causing pathology. In addition, after antibody formation, the classical pathway of complement is activated, leading to lysis of bacterial cells and enhancement of inflammatory effects. Opsonization and phagocytosis can also occur when the Fc receptor on the phagocytic cell binds to the Fc region of the IgG antibody molecule. Cell-mediated immunity, the other branch of the specific immune response, is helpful in attacking intracellular bacteria, such as *Mycobacterium tuberculosis*, *Legionella pneumophila*, *Listeria monocytogenes*, and *Rickettsia sp.*

Bacteria have developed several ways to inhibit the immune response or make it more difficult for the immune response to occur. Three main mechanisms are avoiding antibody, blocking phagocytosis, and inactivating the complement cascade (Fig. 19–1). One mechanism of evading the effects of antibody occurs through altering bacterial antigens

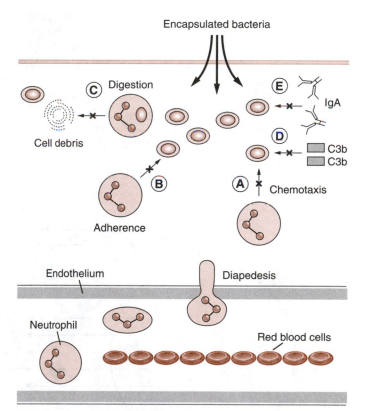

FIGURE 19–1. Ways bacteria are able to evade host defenses. (A) Inhibiting chemotaxis. (B) Blocking adherence of phagocytes to the bacterial cells. (C) Blocking digestion by toxin production, which kills the phagocyte. (D) Inhibiting binding of complement component C3b. (E) Cleavage of IgA.

(epitopes) as a result of genetic mutations. Some streptococci have this capability. In this situation, the specific antibodies developed by the host become ineffective, and responses to the new antigens must develop. Bacteria can also evade the specific immune response through down-regulation of MHC molecules and production of proteases that degrade IgA.[1] *Neisseria gonorrhoeae*, *Haemophilus influenzae*, and *Streptococcus sanguis* are all examples of bacteria that can cleave IgA.[2,3]

However, most of the evasion mechanisms target the process of phagocytosis. Bacteria can mount a defense at several stages in the process, including chemotaxis, adhesion, and digestion.[2,3] Some pathogens such as *Neisseria gonorrhoeae*, for example, inhibit the release of chemotactic factors that would bring phagocytic cells to the area. The cell walls of *S. pyogenes* produce an M protein that interferes with adhesion to the phagocytic cell. Additionally, the presence of a polysaccharide capsule found in such organisms as *Neisseria meningitidis*, *Streptococcus pneumoniae*, *Yersinia pestis*, and *Haemophilus influenzae* inhibits the ability of neutrophils and macrophages to bind to initiate phagocytosis.[3]

Microorganisms use several different mechanisms to resist digestion. Some bacteria can block fusion of lysosomal granules with phagosomes after being engulfed by the phagocyte. *Salmonella* species are able to do this, as can *Mycobacterium tuberculosis* and *Mycobacterium leprae*. In *M. tuberculosis* and *M. leprae* infection, each bacillus is contained in a membrane-enclosed fluid compartment called a *pristiophorus vacuole (PV)*, which does not fuse with the lysosomes. This is due to the complexity of the acid-fast cell walls.

An additional mechanism of resisting digestion involves organisms producing toxins that trigger the release of lysosomal contents into the cytoplasm of the phagocytic cells, subsequently killing these cells. Examples of these toxins are leukocidin, produced by *Staphylococcus*; listeriolysin O, produced by *Listeria monocytogenes*; and streptolysin, produced by *Streptococcus*.[2]

The last major defense some bacteria use is to block the action of complement. Organisms mentioned previously that produce a capsule do not bind the complement component C3b, which is important in enhancing phagocytosis.[3] Such organisms cannot be phagocytized unless coated by opsonins (see Chapter 1). Additionally, some organisms express molecules that disrupt one or more of the complement pathways. Protein H, produced by *S. pyogenes*, binds to C1 but does not allow the complement cascade to proceed further.[3] Another example is group B streptococci, which have sialic acid in their cell walls. This inhibits the complement pathway by degrading C3b.

The rest of this chapter addresses the immunologic response to several important bacteria that cause invasive disease and for which serological testing plays a major role. Molecular methods of detection are also discussed and compared to serological testing.

## GROUP A STREPTOCOCCI

Streptococci are gram-positive spherical, ovoid, or lancet-shaped organisms that are catalase negative and are often seen in pairs or chains.[4] They are divided into groups or serotypes on the basis of certain cell wall components. The outermost cell wall component contains two major proteins known as M and T, and these determine the serogroup or serotype (Fig 19-2). The serotype is based on minor variations in the proteins that can be identified serologically. Interior to the protein layer is the group-specific carbohydrate that divides streptococci into 20 defined groups, designated A through H and K through V. These are known as the **Lancefield groups,** based on the pioneering work of Dr. Rebecca Lancefield. Some strains possess a hyaluronic acid capsule outside the cell wall that contributes to the bacterium's antiphagocytic properties.

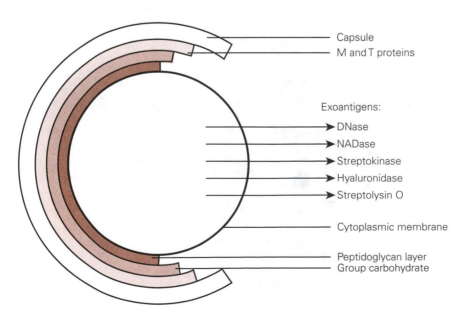

Capsule
M and T proteins

Exoantigens:
DNase
NADase
Streptokinase
Hyaluronidase
Streptolysin O

Cytoplasmic membrane

Peptidoglycan layer
Group carbohydrate

**FIGURE 19–2.** Diagram of antigenic components of *Streptococcus pyogenes*.

*Streptococcus pyogenes*, which belongs to Lancefield group A, is one of the most common and ubiquitous pathogenic bacteria and causes a variety of infections. The M protein is the major virulence factor of the group. It is a filamentous molecule consisting of two alpha-helical chains twisted into a ropelike structure that extends out from the cell surface. There is a net-negative charge at the amino-terminal end that helps to inhibit phagocytosis. In addition, presence of the M protein limits deposition of C3 on the bacterial surface, thereby diminishing complement activation.[5,6] Immunity to **group A streptococci** appears to be associated with antibodies to the M protein. There are more than 100 serotypes of this protein, and immunity is serotype-specific.[6,7] Therefore, infections with one strain will not provide protection against another strain.

Additional virulence factors include **exoantigens** or exotoxins, proteins excreted by the bacterial cells as they metabolize during the course of streptococcal infections. Pyrogenic exotoxins A, B, and C are responsible for the rash seen in scarlet fever and also appear to contribute to pathogenicity.[7,8] Antibodies are produced to the following exoantigens: enzymes **streptolysin O,** deoxyribonuclease B (DNase B), hyaluronidase, nicotinamide adenine dinucleotidase (NADase), and streptokinase.

Culture and rapid screening methods are routinely used for diagnostic testing early in the infection. However, diagnosis of the sequelae such as glomerulonephritis and acute rheumatic fever is best achieved by detection of antibodies. For this reason, laboratory methods for detecting antibodies to these streptococcal products are presented in this chapter.

## Clinical Manifestations of Group A Streptococcal Infection

*Streptococcus pyogenes* cause infections ranging from pharyngitis to life-threatening illnesses such as necrotizing fasciitis and streptococcal toxic shock syndrome. The two major sites of infections in humans are the upper respiratory tract and the skin, with pharyngitis and impetigo being the most common clinical manifestations.[9] Symptoms of pharyngitis include fever, chills, severe sore throat, headache, tonsillar exudates, petechiae on the soft palate, and anterior cervical lymphadenopathy.[9] The most common skin infection is streptococcal pyoderma, or impetigo, characterized by vesicular lesions on the extremities that become pustular and crusted. Such infections tend to occur in young children.[7]

Other acute or suppurative complications include otitis media, scarlet fever, erysipelas, cellulites, puerperal sepsis, and sinusitis. Septic arthritis, acute bacterial endocarditis, and meningitis also can result from a pharyngeal infection.[5,7]

Severe invasive infections with group A streptococci have also been associated with toxic shock syndrome and necrotizing fasciitis.[9,10] Toxic shock syndrome is a life-threatening multisystem disease that initiates as a skin or soft tissue infection and may proceed to shock and renal failure due to overproduction of cytokines.[4,9]

Necrotizing fasciitis results from a skin infection that invades the muscles of the extremities or the trunk. The onset is quite acute and is a medical emergency. Exotoxins produced by *S. pyogenes* cause a rapidly spreading infection deep in the fascia, resulting in ischemia, tissue necrosis, and septicemia if not treated promptly. The disease may be associated with predisposing conditions, such as chronic illness in the elderly or varicella in children, but healthy persons can be affected as well.[10,11] Reporting of necrotizing fasciitis and toxic shock syndrome is part of a surveillance program conducted by the Centers for Disease Control and Prevention. While the incidence of this syndrome has declined in the United States, a significant number of cases are still reported each year.[12]

The two main damaging sequelae to group A streptococcal infections are acute rheumatic fever and **poststreptococcal glomerulonephritis.**[4] These conditions result from the host response to infection. Serological testing plays a major role in the diagnosis of these two diseases, because the organism itself may no longer be present.

**Acute rheumatic fever** develops as a sequela to pharyngitis or tonsillitis in 2 to 3 percent of infected individuals. It does not occur as a result of skin infection. The latency period is typically 1 to 3 weeks after onset of the sore throat. Characteristic features of acute rheumatic fever include fever, pain caused by inflammation in the joints, and inflammation of the heart.

The disease is most likely due to antibodies or cell-mediated immunity originally produced against streptococcal antigens but that cross-react with human heart tissue.[4,13] Chief among the antibodies are those directed toward the M proteins, which have at least three epitopes that resemble antigens in heart tissue, permitting cross-reactivity to occur. Titers of some antibodies may remain high for several years following infection.

The second main complication following a streptococcal infection is glomerulonephritis, a condition characterized by damage to the glomeruli in the kidney. This condition may follow infection of either the skin or the pharynx, while rheumatic fever follows only upper respiratory infections.[9] It is most common in children between the ages of 2 and 12 and is especially prevalent in the winter months.[14]

Symptoms of glomerulonephritis may include hematuria, proteinuria, edema, and hypertension. Patients may also experience malaise, backache, and abdominal discomfort.[15] Renal function is usually impaired because the glomerular filtration rate is reduced, but renal failure is not typical. The most widely accepted theory for the pathogenesis of poststreptococcal glomerulonephritis is that it results from deposition of antibody-streptococcal antigen immune complexes in the glomeruli. These immune complexes stimulate an inflammatory response that damages the kidney and impairs function due to release of the lysosomal contents of leukocytes and activation of complement.[4,14]

## Detection of Group A Streptococcal Antigens

Diagnosis of acute streptococcal infections typically is made by culture of the organism from the infected site. The specimen is plated on sheep blood agar and incubated. If group A streptococcus is present, small translucent colonies with a clear zone of beta hemolysis around them will be visible. Presumptive identification is made on the basis of susceptibility to bacitracin, testing for L-pyrrolidonyl-β-naphthylamide (PYR) activity, or growth in the presence of trimethoprim-sulfamethoxazole.[9]

As an alternative to culture, commercial kits have been developed to detect group A streptococcal antigen using throat swabs. Antigen is extracted by either enzymatic or chemical means, and the process takes anywhere from 2 to 30 minutes, depending on the particular technique. Either enzyme immunoassay (EIA) or latex agglutination is then used to identify the antigen. Many of these tests require no more than 2 to 5 minutes of hands-on time, providing a distinct advantage over culture. However, while the specificity is high, the sensitivity of the test varies with the type of procedure done. Recent developments using enzyme immunoassays have improved the test's sensitivity, but cultures should be performed when rapid test results are negative.[7,16] Molecular methods, including hybridization of specific rRNA sequences and real-time PCR (polymerase chain reaction), have also been developed as a means to rapidly detect group A streptococcal infections.[17]

Serotyping and molecular techniques can be used to identify a particular strain of group A streptococcus associated with an epidemic. Serotyping involves identification of M-protein antigens by precipitation with type-specific antisera. More than 80 different serotypes have been identified by this method. However, serotyping has limitations, including limited availability of typing sera, new M types that do not react with the antisera, and difficulty in interpreting the results.[16] Genotyping techniques involving PCR amplification of a portion of the *emm* gene, which codes for the M protein, followed by sequence analysis, circumvents these problems.[17] Pulsed field gel electrophoresis (PFGE) has also been used for epidemiological studies. DNA from group A streptococcus is separated by using an alternating current to obtain a unique pattern, or "fingerprint." The patterns from multiple sources may be compared when there is a group A streptococcal outbreak.[16]

## Detection of Streptococcal Antibodies

Culture or rapid screening methods are extremely useful for diagnosis of acute pharyngitis. However, serological diagnosis must be used to identify rheumatic fever and glomerulonephritis, because the organism is unlikely to be present in the pharynx or on the skin at the time symptoms appear.[13] Group A streptococci elaborate more than 20 exotoxins, and it is the antibody response to one or more of these that is used as documentation of nonsuppurative disease. Some of the exotoxin products include streptolysins O and S; deoxyribonucleases A, B, C, and D; streptokinase; NADase; hyaluronidase; diphosphopyridine nucleotidase; and pyrogenic exotoxins[4] (see Fig. 19–2).

The antibody response to these streptococcal products is variable due to several factors, such as age of onset, site of infection, and timeliness of antibiotic treatment. The most diagnostically important antibodies are the following: anti-streptolysin O (ASO), anti-DNase B, anti-NADase, and anti-hyaluronidase. Assays for detection of these antibodies can be performed individually or through use of the **Streptozyme** kit which detects antibodies to all these products (see the exercise at the end of the chapter). During group A streptococcal infections, other antibodies are made to cellular antigens, such as the group A carbohydrate and the M protein.[16] Generally, detection of these antibodies is done in research or reference laboratories, since commercial reagents are not available.

Serological evidence of disease is based on an elevated or rising titer of streptococcal antibodies. The onset of clinical symptoms of rheumatic fever or glomerulonephritis typically coincides with the peak of antibody response, so a serum specimen tested at the time should demonstrate an elevation of the concentration of these antibodies. If acute and convalescent phase sera are tested in parallel, a fourfold rise in titer (a two-tube difference in the doubling serial dilutions) is considered significant. The use of at least two tests for antibodies to different exotoxins is recommended, because production of detectable ASO does not occur in all patients. The most commonly used tests are those for ASO and anti-DNase B.[9] Anti-hyaluronidase tests are not available commercially, and testing for these antibodies is performed only in research or reference laboratories.

### Antistreptolysin O (ASO) Testing

ASO tests detect antibodies to the streptolysin O enzyme produced by group A streptococcus, which is able to lyse red blood cells. Presence of antibodies to streptolysin O indicates recent streptococcal infection in patients suspected of having acute rheumatic fever or poststreptococcal glomerulonephritis following a throat infection.

The classic hemolytic method for determining the **ASO titer** was the first test developed to measure streptococcal antibodies. This test was based on the ability of antibodies in the patient's serum to neutralize the hemolytic activity of streptolysin O.

The traditional ASO titer involves dilution of patient serum, to which a measured amount of streptolysin O reagent is added. These are allowed to combine during an incubation period after which reagent red blood cells are added as an indicator. If enough antibody is present, the streptolysin O is neutralized and no hemolysis occurs. The titer is reported as the reciprocal of the highest dilution demonstrating no hemolysis. This titer may be expressed in either Todd units (when the streptolysin reagent standard is used) or in international units (when the World Health Organization international standard is used).[16]

The range of expected normal values is variable and depends on the patient's age, the geographic location, and the season of the year. ASO titers tend to be highest in school-age children and young adults. Thus, the upper limits of normal must be established for specific populations.[16] Typically, however, a single ASO titer is considered to be moderately elevated if the titer is at least 240 Todd units in an adult and 320 Todd units in a child.[16]

Because of the labor-intensive nature of the traditional ASO titer test, and because the streptolysin O reagent and the red cells used are not stable, ASO testing is currently performed by nephelometric methods in the routine clinical laboratory. Nephelometry has the advantage of being an automated procedure that provides rapid, quantitative measurement of ASO titers.[16] The antigen used in this technique is purified recombinant streptolysin. When antibody-positive patient serum combines with the antigen reagent, immune complexes are formed, resulting in an increased light scatter that the instrument converts to a peak rate signal. All results are reported in international units, which are extrapolated from the classic hemolytic method described previously. When using the nephelometric method, the upper limits of normal for different populations have not been established, so each laboratory must determine its own upper limit of normal.

ASO titers typically increase within 1 to 2 weeks after infection and peak between 3 to 6 weeks following the initial symptoms (e.g., sore throat).[13] However, an antibody response occurs in only about 85 percent of acute rheumatic fever patients within this period. Additionally, ASO titers usually do not increase in individuals with skin infections.[5]

## Anti-DNase B Testing

Testing for the presence of **anti-DNase B** is clinically useful in patients suspected of having glomerulonephritis preceded by streptococcal skin infections, as ASO antibodies often are not stimulated by this type of disease.[4] In addition, antibodies to DNase B may be detected in patients with acute rheumatic fever who have a negative ASO test result.

DNase B is mainly produced by group A streptococci, so testing for anti-DNase B is highly specific for group A streptococcal sequelae.[6] Macrotiter, microtiter, EIA, and nepelometric methods have been developed for anti-DNase testing. The classic test for the measurement of anti-DNase B activity is based on a neutralization methodology. If anti-DNase B antibodies are present, they will neutralize reagent DNase B, preventing it from depolymerizing DNA. Presence of DNase is measured by its effect on a DNA-methyl-green conjugate. This complex is green in its intact form, but when hydrolyzed by DNase, the methyl green is reduced and becomes colorless. An overnight incubation at 37°C is required in some testing methodologies to permit antibodies to inactivate the enzyme. Tubes are graded for color, with a 4+ indicating that the intensity of color is unchanged, and a 0 indicating a total loss of color. The result is reported as the reciprocal of the highest dilution demonstrating a color intensity of between 2+ and 4+.

Normal titers for children between the ages of 2 and 12 years range from 240 to 640 units.[13]

Nephelometry provides an automated means of testing that can be used for rapid quantitation of anti-DNase B. In this method, immune complexes formed between antibodies in patient serum and DNase B reagent generate an increase in light scatter. Results are extrapolated from values from the classic method and are reported in international units per mL.[16]

## Streptozyme Testing

The Streptozyme test is a slide agglutination screening test for the detection of antibodies to several streptococcal antigens. Sheep red blood cells are coated with streptolysin, streptokinase, hyaluronidase, DNase, and NADase so that antibodies to any of the streptococcal antigens can be detected. Reagent red blood cells are mixed with a 1:100 dilution of patient serum. Hemagglutination represents a positive test, indicating that antibodies to one or more of these antigens are present.

The test is rapid and simple to perform, but it appears to be less reproducible than other antibody tests. In addition, more false positives and false negatives have been reported for this test than for the ASO and anti-DNase B assays.[9] Because a larger variety of antibodies are included in this test, the potential is higher for detection of streptococcal antibodies. However, single-titer determinations are not as significant as several titrations performed at weekly or biweekly intervals following the onset of symptoms.[16] The Streptozyme test is an excellent screening tool, but it should be used in conjunction with the ASO or DNase when sequelae of group A streptococcal infection are suspected.

## HELICOBACTER PYLORI

### Characteristics of *Helicobacter Pylori* Infections

*Helicobacter pylori* has become an important organism within the past 20 years. This gram-negative, microaerophilic spiral bacterium is the major cause of both gastric and duodenal ulcers.[18,19] *H. pylori* is found worldwide, affecting 30 percent of the populations in developed countries and more than 90 percent of the populations in developing countries.[18] Since 1994, the National Institutes of Health has recommended that individuals with gastric or duodenal ulcers caused by *H. pylori* be given antibiotic treatment along with the anti-ulcer medications. If untreated, *H. pylori* infection will last for the patient's life and may lead to gastric carcinoma.[18] A variety of techniques have been developed to diagnose *H. pylori* infection due to the prevalence of the organism and the significance of the infection.

The genomic sequences of two strains of the organism have been determined using molecular techniques. There is a large amount of genetic heterogeneity due to the frequent exchange of genetic material between strains. One of the proteins of *H. pylori*, CagA, is highly immunogenic and is one of the virulence factors of the bacterium. The severity of the disease is related to injection of the CagA protein into the gastric epithelial cells. Once the CagA protein is in the epithelial cells, changes occur in the function of the cell's signal transduction pathways and in the structure of the cytoskeleton.[20,21]

A second virulence factor is vacuolating cytotoxin, or VacA. The VacA gene codes for a toxin precursor. Epidemiological studies have shown that if the CagA and VacA genes are present in the strain of bacteria infecting the individual, there is a higher risk of developing gastric or peptic ulcers or gastric carcinoma.[21,22]

## Antigen–Detection Procedures

Since *H. pylori* is found in the stomach, some of the methods to determine if the organism is present require an endoscopy. This includes culturing for *H. pylori*, histologically examining gastric biopsy tissue, and performing a urease biopsy test. The most specific test to detect *H. pylori* infection is culture, but the sensitivity is usually lower than other methods, since the organism is not evenly distributed throughout the tissue.[23] *H. pylori* produces a large amount of urease, so a biopsy urease test may be done to detect the presence of bacteria. The organism is present if there is a color change due to the increase of pH from the breakdown of urea to ammonia and bicarbonate. The biopsy urease test is easy to use, and results can be detected within 2 hours in some test procedures, making it ideal for rapid diagnosis of *H. pylori* infections.[24]

Procedures for detecting *H. pylori* that do not require the use of endoscopy include urea breath testing, enzyme immunoassays for bacterial antigens in the feces, molecular tests for *H. pylori* DNA, and antibody tests. In the urea breath test, the patient ingests urea labeled with radioactive carbon ($^{14}C$) or a nonradioactive $^{13}C$. Urea is metabolized to ammonia and bicarbonate. The bicarbonate is excreted in the breath, and the labeled carbon dioxide is measured by detection of radioactivity for ($^{14}C$) or mass spectrometry analysis for $^{13}C$. This breath technique has excellent sensitivity and specificity, and it is helpful in determining if the bacteria have been eradicated due to antimicrobial therapy; however, it involves the use of radioactivity.[4,23]

Analysis of stool samples before and after antimicrobial therapy for *H. pylori* antigens is mainly done to determine if the bacteria have been eliminated.[23] The test currently uses an enzyme-labeled monoclonal antibody. The sensitivity and specificity of this monoclonal antibody test are 84 to 95 percent and 97 percent, respectively, as compared to the urea breath test. Continued improvement needs to be made in this test procedure to achieve the level of accuracy of the urea breath test.

Noninvasive molecular tests have also been developed to detect *H. pylori* DNA.[23,24] However, PCR-based methods, which detect the presence of the organism in fecal samples, cannot distinguish between living and dead *H. pylori*. Care must be taken when purifying the sample and performing the procedure so that contamination or amplification of exogenous DNA does not occur.[23] There may be residual DNA left after the bacteria have been eradicated. Real-time PCR using TaqMan technology has been developed to determine the patient's bacterial load and has shown good correlation with the urea breath test. Molecular methods are quick and precise and can determine antibiotic resistance as well.[23,24]

## Detection of *Helicobacter Pylori* Antibodies

Serological testing is a primary screening method of determining infection with *H. pylori*. Infections from this organism result in antibody production of IgG, IgA, and IgM. The presence of antibody in the blood of an untreated patient indicates an active infection, since the bacterium does not spontaneously clear. Antibody levels in untreated individuals remain elevated for years. In treated individuals, the antibody concentrations decrease after about 6 months to about 50 percent of the level the patient had during the active infection. This means that if an antibody test is used to detect eradication of *H. pylori*, the pretreatment sample should be stored for a year so that parallel testing can be performed.[25] A decrease in antibody concentration of more than 25 percent must occur for treatment to be considered successful.[25]

Most serological tests in clinical use detect *H. pylori*–specific antibodies of the IgG class. Although IgM antibody is produced in *H. pylori* infections, testing for its presence lacks clinical value, since most infections have become chronic before diagnosis. Thus, IgG is the primary antibody found. IgA testing has a lower sensitivity and specificity than IgG testing, but it may increase sensitivity of detection when used in conjunction with IgG testing.[23]

Measurement of the antibodies may be done by several techniques, including enzyme-linked immunosorbent assays (ELISA), immunoblot, and rapid tests using latex agglutination or flow-through membrane-based enzyme immunoassay. The test methodology of choice for the detection of *H. pylori* antibodies is the ELISA technique, which is reliable and accurate.[25] Tests employing antigens from a pooled extract from multiple and genetically diverse strains yield the best sensitivity, since *H. pylori* is so heterogeneous. Very few, if any, patients produce antibodies to all of the *H. pylori* antigens; most patients produce antibodies against the CagA and VacA proteins. Antibodies to these two proteins indicate a more severe case of gastritis or gastric carcinoma.[23]

There are also a number of rapid tests on the market. It is recommended that samples with positive rapid test results be tested by an ELISA test for correlation. When compared to other techniques for antibody detection of *H. pylori*, ELISA tests are sensitive, specific, and cost-effective for determining the organism's presence in untreated individuals.[23] However, since antibodies are not rapidly cleared after treatment, antibody testing is not as well suited for determining eradication of infection as are other methods. Additionally, individuals who are immunocompromised (the elderly or immunosuppressed individuals) may have a false-negative result with antibody testing.

# MYCOPLASMA PNEUMONIAE

## Characteristics of *Mycoplasma* Infection

*Mycoplasma* is a member of a unique group of organisms that belong to the class *Mollicutes.* These organisms lack cell walls and have a small genome, sterols in their cell membrane, and complex growth requirements. This makes culture of these organisms difficult and time-consuming. The best-known organism of this class is **Mycoplasma pneumoniae,** which is a leading cause of upper respiratory infections worldwide.[26]

*Mycoplasma pneumoniae* infections are found in all age groups. The incubation period is 1 to 3 weeks, and the infection can often spread through households. Symptoms of infection include sore throat, chills, hoarseness, tracheo-bronchitis, and headache. Twenty percent of all community-acquired pneumonias and 20 percent of all hospitalizations for pneumonia in the United States are thought to be due to *Mycoplasma* infections.[26,27] *M. pneumoniae* may remain in the respiratory tract for several months. It can attach to cells in the respiratory tract and cause chronic inflammation.[26] Other complications may be extra-pulmonary, including hemolytic anemia, skin rashes, arthritis, meningoencephalitis, pericarditis, and peripheral neuropathy.[27] An autoimmune response may play a role in these extrapulmonary complications.

## Detection of *Mycoplasma Pneumoniae* by Culture

Because *M. pneumoniae* does not have a cell wall, the organism is sensitive to drying, so transport is extremely important to obtaining a culture.[28] The transport media used can be trypticase soy broth with 0.5 percent albumin, SP4 medium, or a viral transport medium. If the sample cannot be plated immediately, it should be frozen at –70°C.

Culturing of *M. pneumoniae* is not routinely performed from respiratory samples, because the cultures are difficult to grow and require specialized agars. Growth may take several weeks, and serological testing may indicate the presence of *M. pneumoniae* infection before the culture.

## Detection of Antibodies to *Mycoplasma pneumoniae*

For many years, prior to the development of antigen-specific serological tests, laboratory diagnosis of *Mycoplasma pneumoniae* involved testing for cold agglutinins, because these are present in about 50 percent of patients with the infection. Cold agglutinins are autoantibodies that react with the I/i antigens on red blood cells and cause their agglutination at temperatures below 37°C. Development of these antibodies is thought to result from cross-reaction of the I antigen on human red blood cells or from alteration of the red blood cells by the organism.[29]

Testing for cold agglutinins is no longer recommended for the detection of *M. pneumoniae* infections, since some viral infections and collagen vascular diseases also cause production of cold agglutinins.[29] More recently, *M. pneumoniae*–specific serological tests have been developed. These include enzyme immunoassay, particle agglutination, indirect immuno-fluorescence, and complement fixation. Depending on the technique used, IgM, IgG, and IgA classes of antibody to *M. pneumoniae* may be detected.[29] Enzyme immunoassays (EIA) are the most widely used method of detection, because they require a small sample volume and can test large numbers of specimens in an automated format.[26] The EIA procedure may be as sensitive as PCR if enough time has elapsed for antibodies to be formed. It is better to test for the presence of both the IgG and IgM classes of antibody for greater accuracy, but each class of antibody must be tested for separately.[29]

The indirect fluorescent assay (IFA) can also detect IgM or IgG classes of antibody to *M. pneumoniae*. In this test, *Mycoplasma* antigen is attached to a glass slide. Patient serum is placed on the slide and incubated. The slide is then washed, and fluorescent-labeled anti-IgM or anti-IgG is added to the slide and allowed to incubate. After incubation, the slide is washed and observed under a fluorescent microscope. If the screening test is positive, then a serial dilution may be done to determine the concentration of antibody present.[29]

## Molecular Techniques

Molecular techniques provide a more rapid means of detecting *Mycoplasma* infection than culture or serological testing. PCR testing for *Mycoplasma* may be performed using throat swabs, nasophayngeal swabs, sputum, fixed tissue, and cultures. In addition to obtaining rapid results, PCR tests are also advantageous in that only one specimen is required, tissues that have already been processed for histology can be used, and live organisms are not required. However, inhibitors present, especially in nasopharyngeal aspirates, may cause a false-negative reaction.[29] Therefore, a negative PCR test may indicate the need for additional testing by other means.

RNA amplification techniques have also been used. RNA-based amplification methods are highly sensitive due to the large number of rRNA (ribosomal RNA) copies in the *M. pneumoniae* cell, which also indicates that the organism is alive. Nucleic acid amplification methods have been developed that detect several different gene targets, including the ATPase operon gene, the PI adhesion gene, the 16S RNA gene, and the tuf gene. Molecular testing will likely replace serological testing in the future.

# RICKETTSIAL INFECTIONS

## Characteristics of Rickettsial Infections

The **rickettsiae** are short rods, or coccobacilli, that are obligate, intracellular, gram-negative bacteria. The genus

*Rickettsia* is made up of two distinct groups: the **spotted fever** group (SFG) and the **typhus** group (TG). Each is responsible for a different set of diseases. **Table 19–1** contains a partial list of species found in each group. Rickettsial diseases are associated with arthropods, as they spend at least part of their life cycle in an arthropod host before being transmitted to humans.[30] Arthropod hosts include ticks, mites, lice, or fleas. Humans are accidental hosts for rickettsiae except for *Rickettsia prowazekii*, which causes epidemic typhus.[31] Some of the rickettsia are found only in certain areas of the world and are genetically different enough to be considered different species. *R. japonica* is found only in Japan, while *R. rickettsii* is found in the Western Hemisphere. Some species, like *R. typhi*, are found everywhere in the world.[32] In the United States, the main rickettsial diseases are two types of typhus—endemic and epidemic—caused by *R. typhi* and *R. felis*, respectively, and Rocky Mountain spotted fever, caused by *R. rickettsii* (see Table 19–1). These diseases are most prevalent between May and September.[31]

In Rocky Mountain spotted fever, symptoms occur approximately 7 days after a tick bite. These include fever, severe headache, malaise, and myalgia, accompanied by nausea, vomiting, abdominal pain, and sometimes a cough. A rash, which starts on the hands and feet and proceeds to the trunk, appears in 3 to 5 days after the beginning of other symptoms.[30] The organism infects endothelial cells, causing an increase in vascular permeability and focal hemorrhages.

Murine typhus, caused by *R. typhi* (which is carried by fleas), is characterized by a cough and chest infiltrate suggestive of pneumonia. A rash appears in only about one-half of patients.[30] This disease can cause severe manifestations such as seizures, coma, and respiratory failure. Symptoms of disease caused by *R. felis* are not as well defined.

## Serological Diagnosis

Serodiagnosis is currently the method of choice for detecting rickettsial infections. Methods that may be used are probe-based immunoassays and agglutination assays.[32] For many years, antibodies produced in patients with rickettsial infections were detected by an agglutination test known as the Weil-Felix test, which was based on cross-reactivity of the patient's antibodies with polysaccharide antigens present on the OX-19 and OX-2 strains of *Proteus vulgaris* and the OX-K strain of *Proteus mirabilis*.

Current serological assays for rickettsial antibodies are organism-specific and include indirect fluorescent assays (IFA), microimmunofluorescent assays (micro-IF), immunoperoxidase assays (IPA), ELISA, and immunoblot assays (IBA). IFA and IPA require the whole bacterium as the reagent, while ELISA and IBA use rickettsial antigens adsorbed onto a solid phase or nitrocellulose membrane. The IFA test and the micro-IF are currently considered the gold standard for detecting rickettsial antibodies.[32] The IPA, which uses a light microscope instead of a fluorescent microscope to read the slides, has a sensitivity and specificity similar to that of IFA.[32] Testing by both of these methods can detect significant titers of antibodies in Rocky Mountain spotted fever by the second week of infection.[30] However, antirickettsial treatment needs to be started by the fifth day of illness in order to be successful. Thus, serological diagnosis tends to be more retrospective, after treatment has begun.

## Molecular Techniques

Molecular detection of rickettsial infections can be accomplished by performing a PCR using primers that target genes of the TG and SFG groups of organisms. To detect both SFG and TG rickettsiae, the citrate synthase gene and the

| Table 19–1. | Etiology and Ecology of Rickettsial Diseases | | |
| --- | --- | --- | --- |
| **ORGANISM** | **GEOGRAPHICAL LOCATION** | **DISEASE ASSOCIATION** | **MODE OF TRANSMISSION** |
| **Spotted Fever Group (SFG)** | | | |
| *R. rickettsii* | Western Hemisphere | Rocky Mountain spotted fever | Tick bite |
| *R. japonica* | Japan | Japanese spotted fever | Tick bite |
| *R. felis* | North and South America, Europe, Africa | Flea-borne spotted fever | Unknown |
| *R. akari* | United States, Ukraine, Croatia, Korea | Rickettsialpox | Mite bite |
| **Typhus Group (TG)** | | | |
| *R. typhi* | Worldwide | Endemic typhus | Flea feces |
| *R. prowazekii* | Worldwide | Epidemic typhus | Louse feces |
| | Worldwide | Recrudescent typhus | Years after epidemic typhus |

17 kDa antigen gene are used, while the 190 kDa antigen (Omp A) gene and the 120 kDa antigen (OmpB) gene are used only to detect the SFG group.[32] PCR can then be followed by restriction digest or nucleotide sequence analysis of the amplicon, or real-time PCR can be used to definitively identify the rickettsial species. The continued development of real-time PCR holds much promise for the future.

**Table 19–2** summarizes and compares the major types of testing available for all organisms listed in the chapter.

## Table 19–2.   Comparison of Testing Methods for Bacterial Identification

| ORGANISM | TEST METHOD | TESTING PRINCIPLE | COMMENTS |
|---|---|---|---|
| *Group A Streptococcus* | Culture | Plate on blood agar | Takes 24–48 hours |
| | Rapid EIA | Extract antigen from throat swab | Rapid but not as sensitive as culture |
| | PCR | Amplify portions of the emm gene | Need for specialized equipment |
| | Antibody testing | Neutralization of exotoxins (ASO, anti-DNase, etc.) | Used to diagnose strep sequelae |
| | Slide agglutination | Agglutination of red cells coated with exotoxins | Rapid but results not as reliable as other testing; good initial screening tool |
| *Helicobacter pylori* | Urease test | Place biopsy material on urea agar. Color change as urea is broken down | Results in 2 hours. Invasive procedure, and organism may be missed due to uneven distribution in tissue |
| | Urea breath test | Patient ingests radioactive urea; bicarbonate produced, which is breathed out as $CO_2$ | Rapid and sensitive but involves radioactivity |
| | Rapid EIA | To identify antigen in stool specimens | Rapid but not as sensitive as urea breath test. Used to determine success of therapy |
| | Antibody testing | EIA test to determine presence of IgG or IgM | Best for initial screening method. Not as reliable as antigen testing to evaluate therapy |
| | PCR | Amplify specific DNA | Rapid and sensitive but subject to contamination |
| *Mycoplasma pneumoniae* | Culture | Look for growth on specialized agars | Difficult to grow and takes several weeks |
| | Cold agglutinin testing | Antibodies cross-react with I antigen on group O red cells; look for agglutination | Easy to do but not specific for *Mycoplasma* |
| | EIA | Test for presence of IgG and IgM with purified antigens | Sensitive and automated |
| | IFA | Antigen attached to slide and then reacted with antibody. An anti-immunoglobulin with a fluorescent tag is added | Need to have a fluorescent microscope, and slide must be interpreted carefully |
| | DNA or RNA amplification | Amplify either DNA or RNA specific to the organism | Very specific but requires special equipment |
| *Rickettsia sp.* | Weil-Felix reaction | Agglutination of *Proteus* antigens due to cross-reactivity | Easy and inexpensive, but not specific |
| | IFA | Antigen attached to slide and then reacted with antibody. An anti-immunoglobulin with a fluorescent tag is added. | Need to have a fluorescent microscope, and slide must be interpreted carefully. Takes time for antibody to be produced. |

*Continued*

| Table 19–2. | Comparison of Testing Methods for Bacterial Identification—Cont'd | | |
|---|---|---|---|
| ORGANISM | TEST METHOD | TESTING PRINCIPLE | COMMENTS |
| | IPA | Antigen attached to slide and then reacted with antibody. An anti-immunoglobulin with an enzyme tag is added. | Can be read with an ordinary light microscope but takes time for antibody to be produced |
| | PCR | Amplification of specific genes for each group—TG and SFG | Fast and sensitive but requires specialized equipment |

## SUMMARY

While many bacteria are destroyed or inactivated by the immune system, some are able to evade the host's defense mechanisms and cause disease. Some of the mechanisms used to evade the immune system include avoiding antibody by developing new antigens, blocking phagocytosis by means of structural components such as capsules, and inactivating the complement cascade by producing certain proteins. When bacteria are able to overcome host defenses and infection occurs, procedures have been developed that use cultures or molecular techniques to detect the organism itself or that use serological techniques to detect the presence of antibodies produced during infection. The bacteria discussed in this chapter (group A streptococcus, *H. pylori*, *M. pneumoniae*, and *rickettsiae*) can all be detected using these types of procedures.

Although group A streptococcus can be cultured, and rapid detection of the organism is possible, complications such as acute rheumatic fever and poststreptococcal glomerulonephritis can occur, and the organism is no longer present in the body. Testing for streptococcal antibodies is important to detect these sequelae. In group A streptococcal infections, several antibodies are formed to the exoantigens (toxins) that are produced by the bacteria. Anti-streptolysin O and anti-DNase B are the two most common antibodies that are detected in the clinical laboratory. Other antibodies that are produced are anti-hyaluronidase and anti-NADase. Some of the test procedures such as the Streptozyme test detect the presence of more than one antibody. Methods for detecting these antibodies include nephelometry, latex agglutination, and enzyme neutralization.

*H. pylori* causes gastric ulcers, and if the bacteria are not eliminated using antibiotics, patients are at increased risk of developing gastric carcinoma. *H. pylori* infection may be detected by invasive or noninvasive tests. The urease enzyme produced by the organism can be detected from gastric biopsy tissue obtained by endoscopy, or the breath of patients can be analyzed after they ingest urea labeled with a carbon isotope. Serological procedures, such as ELISA, immunoblotting, and rapid latex agglutination or EIA tests, may be used to detect *H. pylori* antibodies in patient serum. PCR methods can be used to detect the presence of *H. pylori* DNA in fecal specimens.

Antibody testing for *Mycoplasma pneumoniae* and *rickettsiae* has been performed for many years. At one time, serological diagnosis of these infections used the principle of cross-reactivity of antibodies produced by patients to nonorganism-specific antigens. Testing for cold agglutinins was commonly included in the testing protocol for *M. pneumoniae*, because a large percentage of these patients produced antibodies to the I/i antigens on red blood cells. Testing for rickettsial infections incorporated the Weil-Felix test, an agglutination method that used strains of *Proteus* bacteria known to cross-react with rickettsial antibodies. Current serological methods used to detect the antibodies in these diseases are more sensitive and organism-specific. Molecular techniques such as PCR have been developed to detect nucleic acid from *M. pneumoniae* and *rickettsiae*. These tests hold much promise for the future.

# CASE STUDIES

1. A 6-year-old boy was brought to the pediatric clinic. His mother indicated he had been ill for several days with fever and general lethargy. The morning of the visit, the boy told his mother that his back hurt, and she had observed what appeared to be blood in his urine. History and physical examination indicated a well-nourished child with an unremarkable health history other than a severe sore throat with fever 3 weeks prior that was medicated with aspirin and throat lozenges. This child's temperature was 101.5°F, and the physician noted edema in the child's hands and feet. Blood and urine specimens were collected for a Streptozyme test, complete blood cell count, and urinalysis. Laboratory test results were as follows:

**Complete Blood Count**

| | |
|---|---|
| Red cell count | Normal |
| Platelet count | Normal |
| White blood cell count | $12.7 \times 10^9$/L (Normal = $4.8$–$10.8 \times 10^9$/L) |

**Urinalysis**

| | |
|---|---|
| Color | red (Normal = straw) |
| Clarity | Cloudy (Normal = clear) |
| Protein | 2+ (Normal = negative/trace) |
| Blood | Large (Normal = none) |

**Streptozyme**
Positive 1:600

## Questions

a. What disorder is indicated by the child's history, physical exam, and laboratory test results?

b. What was the most likely causative agent of the sore throat preceding the current symptoms?

c. Discuss the most widely accepted theory explaining the physiological basis for this disease.

d. Why didn't the physician order throat and/or urine cultures?

2. A 36-year-old female was seen by her physician for pneumonia-like symptoms along with a sore throat and chills. She was also having difficulty breathing. The patient had a temperature of 100.2°F and was producing a moderate amount of sputum. Her physician decided that the probable diagnosis was some type of pneumonia and ordered the following laboratory tests to be performed: complete blood count, sputum culture, tests for influenza virus, and tests for *Mycoplasma pneumoniae*. The results of the tests were as follows:

**Complete Blood Count**

| | |
|---|---|
| Red cell count | Normal |
| White cell count | Somewhat elevated |

**Sputum Culture**
Negative

**Mycoplasma Titer**
Positive 1:64

**Cold Agglutinin Titer**
Positive 1:128

## Questions

a. What is the most probable cause of the pneumonia?

b. Why was the sputum culture negative?

c. Why was the cold agglutinin titer higher than the *Mycoplasma* titer?

# EXERCISE

## STREPTOZYME TEST

### Principle

The Streptozyme rapid slide test is an agglutination test that detects antibodies to five Group A streptococcal exoantigens, including streptolysin O, streptokinase, hyaluronidase, DNase B, and NADase. These antigens are attached to aldehyde-fixed sheep red blood cells. When patient serum is added to these reagent red blood cells, agglutination of the red blood cells occurs if the patient has antibodies to one or more of these antigens.

### Sample Preparation

Blood is collected aseptically. Either serum or plasma may be used, as well as peripheral blood from a fingertip or earlobe. If blood is collected from a finger or ear puncture, a heparinized capillary tube or the tube supplied with the Streptozyme kit may be used. If serum or plasma cannot be tested within 24 hours of collection, it should be stored frozen.

### Reagents, Materials, and Equipment

Streptozyme rapid slide test kit (Wampole Laboratories, Cranbury, NJ), which contains the following:

Streptozyme reagent

Positive control serum

Negative control serum

Calibrated capillary tubes and bulbs

Mirrored glass slide

Additional materials needed:

Stirrers

Test tubes

Isotonic saline (0.85 percent)

Pipettes

> **WARNING:** Because no test method can offer complete assurance that human immunodeficiency virus, hepatitis B virus, or other infectious agents are absent, controls should be handled as though capable of transmitting an infectious disease. The Food and Drug Administration recommends that such material be handled at a biosafety level 2.

> **CAUTION:** The reagents in this kit contain sodium azide, which may react with lead and copper plumbing to form highly explosive metal azides. Upon disposal, flush with a large volume of water to prevent azide buildup.

### Procedure*

1. Dilute serum or plasma sample 1:100 with isotonic saline. If the sample is peripheral blood from the earlobe or fingertip, fill the capillary tube (supplied with the kit) to the line. Without allowing the blood to clot and using the bulb supplied, expel the sample into a tube containing 2.4 mL of isotonic saline. This technique yields an approximate 1:100 dilution.

2. Fill the capillary tube to the mark (0.05 mL) with the diluted specimen. Using the bulb supplied, expel the specimen onto a section of the glass slide provided with the kit.

3. Repeat step 2 for the positive and negative controls, placing each on a section of the slide that borders the patient specimen.

4. Add 1 drop of reagent to each section. Be sure the reagent is mixed well before it is used.

5. Thoroughly mix all samples using a disposable stirrer. Use a clean stirrer for each sample.

6. Rock the mirrored slide back and forth gently for 2 minutes at the rate of 8 to 10 times per minute.

7. At the end of 2 minutes, place the slide on a flat surface and observe for agglutination.

8. Agglutination must be read within 10 seconds. Reading is facilitated by a direct light source above the slide.

> **NOTE:** If the test is positive, a titer can be obtained by preparing a 1:100 primary dilution of patient serum, making further dilutions (as indicated below) and testing each dilution by the above method.

| PREPARATION OF SAMPLE | RESULTING | DILUTION |
|---|---|---|
| 1.0 mL of primary dilution (1:100) | + 1.0 mL saline1:200 | |
| 0.5 mL of primary dilution | + 1.5 mL saline | 1:400 |
| 0.5 mL of primary dilution | + 2.5 mL saline | 1:600 |
| 0.5 mL of primary dilution | + 3.5 mL saline | 1:800 |

*Adapted from the package insert for the Streptozyme rapid slide test by Wampole Laboratories, Division of Inverness Medical Professional Diagnostics, Princeton, NJ.

## INTREPRETATION

A single Streptozyme determination is not significant, and serial titrations should be performed on a weekly or biweekly basis for up to 6 weeks following a streptococcal infection. Any positive serum should be further diluted to determine the titer. Positive results with Streptozyme are often obtained when the ASO titer is negative, because multiple antibodies can be detected. Titers considered to be within normal limits may vary with the season of the year, the geographic location, and the age group of the patients.

# REVIEW QUESTIONS

1. All of the following are protective mechanisms against bacteria *except*

   a. production of fever.
   b. phagocytosis.
   c. activation of complement.
   d. alteration of surface antigens.

2. All of the following are characteristics of streptococcal M proteins *except*

   a. it is the chief virulence factor of group A streptococci.
   b. it provokes an immune response.
   c. antibodies to one serotype protect against other serotypes.
   d. it limits phagocytosis of the organism.

3. An ASO titer and a Streptozyme test are performed on a patient's serum. The ASO titer was negative, showing hemolysis in all patient tubes. The Streptozyme test is positive, and both the positive and negative controls react appropriately. What can you conclude from these test results?

   a. The patient has a high titer of ASO.
   b. The patient has an antibody to a streptococcal exoenzyme other than streptolysin O.
   c. The patient has not had a previous streptococcal infection.
   d. The patient has scarlet fever.

4. Which of the following applies to acute rheumatic fever?

   a. Symptoms begin after either a throat or a skin infection.
   b. Antibodies to group A streptococci cross-react with heart tissue.
   c. Diagnosis is usually made by culture of the organism.
   d. All patients suffer permanent disability.

5. Which of the following indicates the presence of anti-DNase B activity in serum?

   a. Reduction of methyl green from green to colorless
   b. Clot formation when acetic acid is added
   c. Inhibition of red blood cell hemolysis
   d. Lack of change in the color indicator

6. Which of the following is considered to be a nonsuppurative complication of streptococcal infection?

   a. Acute rheumatic fever
   b. Scarlet fever
   c. Impetigo
   d. Pharyngitis

7. All of the following are ways that bacteria can evade host defenses *except*

   a. presence of a capsule.
   b. stimulation of chemotaxis.
   c. production of toxins.
   d. lack of adhesion to phagocytic cells.

8. Antibody testing for Rocky Mountain spotted fever may not be helpful for which reason?

   a. It is not specific.
   b. It is too complicated to perform.
   c. It is difficult to obtain a blood specimen.
   d. Antibody production takes at least a week before detection.

9. Which of the following enzymes is used to detect the presence of *H. pylori* infections?

   a. DNase
   b. Hyaluronidase
   c. Urease
   d. Peptidase

10. Which of the following reasons make serological identification of a current infection with *Helicobacter pylori* difficult?

    a. No antibodies appear in the blood.
    b. Only IgM is produced.
    c. Antibodies remain after initial treatment.
    d. No ELISA tests have been developed.

11. *M. pneumoniae* infections are associated with which antibodies?

    a. Cold agglutinins
    b. Antibodies to ATPase
    c. Antibodies to DNase
    d. Antibodies to *Proteus* bacteria

12. Which of the following best describes the principle of the IFA test for detection of antibodies produced in Rocky Mountain spotted fever?

    a. Proteus antigens are used to determine cross-reactivity.
    b. A light microscope is used to detect antigen–antibody combination.
    c. Whole bacteria are used to detect antibodies.
    d. Antibodies are detected by direct fluorescence.

# References

1. Findley, BB, and McFadden, G. Anti-immunology: Evasion of the host immune system by bacterial and viral pathogens. Cell 124:767–782, 2006.
2. Black, JG. Microbiology Principles and Explorations, ed. 6. Wiley, Hoboken, NJ, 2005, pp. 446–469.
3. Mak, TW, and Saunders, M. The Immune Response: Basic and Clinical Principles. Elsevier Academic Press, Burlington, MA, 2006, pp. 641–694.
4. Forbes, BA, Sahm, DF, and Weissfeld, A. Bailey and Scott's Diagnostic Microbiology, ed. 12. Mosby Elsevier, St. Louis, 2007, pp. 265–280.
5. Fischetti, VA. Streptococcal M protein. Sci Am 264:58, 1991.
6. Larson, HS. Streptococcaccae. In Mahan, CR, and Manuselis, G (eds): Textbook of Diagnostic Microbiology, ed. 2. WB Saunders, Philadelphia, 2000, pp. 345–371.
7. Wessels, MR. Streptococcal and enterococcal infections. In Braunwald, E, Fauci, AS, Kasper, EL, et al. (eds): Harrison's Principles of Internal Medicine, ed. 15. McGraw-Hill, New York, 2001, pp. 901–909.
8. Sauda, M, Wu, W, Conran, P, et al. Streptococcal pyrogenic exotoxin B enhances tissue damage initiated by other Streptococcus pyogenes products. J Infect Dis 184:723–731, 2001.
9. Spellerberg, B, and Brandt, C. Streptococcus. In Murray, PR, Baron, EJ, Jorgensen, JH, et al. (eds): Manual of Clinical Microbiology, ed. 9. ASM Press, Washington, DC, 2007, pp. 412–429.
10. Moses, AE, Goldberg, S, Korenman, Z, et al. Invasive group A streptococcal infections. Israel Emerg Infect Dis 8:421–426, 2002.
11. Davies, HD, McGeer, A, Schwartz, B, et al. Invasive group A streptococcal infections in Ontario, Canada, Ontario Group A Streptococcal Study Group. N Eng J Med 335:547–554, 2001.
12. Centers for Disease Control and Prevention. Summary of notifiable diseases—March 21, 2008. MMWR 55(53):1–94, 2008.
13. Active Bacterial Core Surveillance. Active Bacterial Core Surveillance (ABCs) Report, Emerging Infections Program Network: Group A streptococcus 2006. Available at http://www.cdc.gov/ncidod/dbmd/abcs/survreports/gas06.pdf. Accessed March 2008.
14. Brady, HR, and Brenner, BM. Pathogenesis of glomerular injury. In Braunwald, E, Fauci, AS, Kasper, DL, et al. (eds): Harrison's Principles of Internal Medicine, ed. 15. McGraw-Hill, New York, 2001, pp. 1572–1580.
15. Lang, MM, and Towers, C. Identifying poststreptococcal glomerulonephritis. Nurse Pract 26:34, 2001.
16. Shet, A, and Kaplan, E. Diagnostic methods for group A streptococcal infections. In Detrick, B, Hamilton, RG, and Folds, JD, (eds): Manual of Molecular and Clinical Laboratory Immunology, ed. 7. American Society for Microbiology, Washington, DC, 2006, pp. 428–433.
17. CDC, Biotechnology Core Branch Facility. Introduction to emm typing: M protein gene (emm) typing Streptococcus pyogenes. Available at: http://www.cdc.gov/ncidod/biotech/strep/M-ProteinGene_typing.htm. Accessed March 2008.
18. National Institutes of Health Consensus Conference. Helicobacter pylori in peptic ulcers. JAMA 272:65–69, 1994.
19. Malfertheiner, P, Megraud, F, O'Moran, C, and the European Helicobacter pylori Study Group (EHPSG). Current concepts in the management of Helicobacter pylori infection—the Maastricht 2-2000 Consensus Report. Alim Pharmacol Ther 16:167–180, 200, 2002.
20. Segal, ED, Cha, J, Lo, J, Falkow, S, and Tompkins, LS. Altered states: Involvement of phosphorylated CagA in the induction of host cellular growth changes by Helicobacter pylori. Proc Natl Acad Sci USA 96:14559–14564, 1999.
21. Megraud, F. Impact of Helicobacter pylori virulence in the outcome of gastroduodenal disease: Lessons from the microbiologist. Digest Dis 19:99–103, 2001.
22. Sokic-Milutinovic, T, Wex, T, Todorovic, V, Milosavljevic, T, and Malfertheiner, P. Anti-CagA and anti-VacA antibodies in Helicobacter pylori–infected patients with and without peptic ulcer disease in Serbia and Montenegro. Scand J Gastroenterol 3:222–226, 2004.
23. Dunn, BE, and Phadnis, SH. Serologic and molecular diagnosis of Helicobacter pylori infection and eradication. In Detrick, B, Hamilton, RG, and Folds, JE (eds): Manual of Molecular and Clinical Laboratory Immunology, ed. 7. American Society for Microbiology, Washington, DC, 2006, pp. 462–467.
24. Megraud, F, and Lehours, P. Helicobacter pylori detection and antimicrobial susceptibility testing. Clin Microbiol Rev 20(2):280–322, 2007.
25. Megraud, F, and Fox, JG. Helicobacter. In Murray, PR, Baron, EJ, Jorgensen, JH, et al. (eds): Manual of Clinical Microbiology, ed. 9. ASM Press, Washington, DC, 2007, pp. 947–962.
26. Waites, KB, and Taylor-Robinson, DT. Mycoplasma and ureoplasma. In Murray, PR, Baron, EJ, Jorgensen, JH, et al. (eds): Manual of Clinical Microbiology, ed. 9. ASM Press, Washington, DC, 2007, pp. 1004–1020.
27. Foy, HM. Infections caused by Mycoplasma pneumoniae and possible carrier state in different populations of patients. Clin Infect Dis 17(suppl. 1):S37–S46, 1993.
28. Forbes, BA, Sahm, DF, and Weissfeld, A. Bailey and Scott's Diagnostic Microbiology, ed. 12. Mosby Elsevier, St. Louis, 2007, pp. 525–532.
29. Waites, KB, Brown, MB, and Simecka, JW. Mycoplasma: Immunologic and molecular diagnostic methods. In Detrick, B, Hamilton, RG, and Folds, JE (eds): Manual of Molecular and Clinical Laboratory Immunology, ed. 7. American Society for Microbiology, Washington, DC, 2006, pp. 510–517.
30. Walker, DH, and Bouyer, DH. Rickettsia and orientia. In Murray, PR, Baron, EJ, Jorgensen, JH, et al. (eds): Manual of Clinical Microbiology, ed. 9. ASM Press, Washington, DC, 2007, pp. 1036–1045.
31. Anderson, B, Friedman, H, and Bendinelli, M. Rickettsial Infection and Immunity. Plenum Press, New York, 1997.
32. Hechemy, KE, Rikihisa, Y, Macaluso, K, Burgess, AWO, Angerson, BE, and Thompson, HA. The Rickettsiaceae, Anaplasmataceae, Bartonellaceae, and Coxiellaceae. In Detrick, B, Hamilton, RG, and Folds, JE (eds): Manual of Molecular and Clinical Laboratory Immunology ed. 7. American Society for Microbiology, Washington, DC, 2006, pp. 527–539.

# 20 Serological Response to Parasitic and Fungal Infections

*Patsy C. Jarreau, MHS, CLS(NCA), MT(ASCP)*

## LEARNING OBJECTIVES

*After finishing this chapter, the reader will be able to:*

1. Explain why a host has more difficulty overcoming parasitic diseases than those caused by bacteria or viruses.

2. Discuss outcomes that may follow invasion by a parasite, including a reason for each outcome.

3. List ways parasites evade host defenses.

4. State examples that illustrate how host responses to parasites cause other pathology for the host.

5. Discuss the role of IgE in parasitic infections.

6. State important diagnostic information provided by serological testing for *Toxoplasma gondii*.

7. Explain how serological tests for *Entamoeba histolytica, E. histolytica/dispar, Giardia lamblia, Trichomonas vaginalis,* and *Cryptosporidium parvum* differ from serological tests for other parasites.

8. List possible limitations associated with parasitic serology.

9. List factors that have led to a notable increase in fungal infections in the last 25 years.

10. Describe the etiological and physiological factors to be examined when a mycosis is suspected.

11. Describe the types of immune defenses mounted by the host in response to fungal infections.

12. Discuss the importance of serodiagnosis in making a rapid and presumptive diagnosis of fungal infections.

13. List three areas of testing in which immunologic procedures have major application for mycotic diagnosis.

14. Recognize the clinical disease and epidemiology of aspergillosis, candidiasis, cryptococcosis, and coccidioidomycosis.

15. List at least three serological tests currently used for the serodiagnosis of aspergillosis, candidiasis, cryptococcosis, and coccidioidomycosis.

## KEY TERMS

____ Antigen switching
____ Antigenic variation
____ Aspergillosis
____ Candidiasis
____ Coccidioidomycosis
____ Conida
____ Cryptococcosis
____ Cyst
____ Eosinophil chemotactic factor
____ Fungi
____ Hyphae
____ Mold
____ Mycelium
____ Mycoses
____ Spherule
____ Thermal dimorphism
____ Toxoplasmosis
____ Yeast

# CHAPTER OUTLINE

Conventional laboratory diagnosis of parasitic and fungal diseases is determined by observing morphological features of parasites and culture (in the case of fungi). Though serological testing for parasitic and fungal infections has increased, it is still not widely used. Serological testing for parasites and fungi is limited, and the antigens for both are often cruder than their counterparts for viral and bacterial diagnosis. This results in decreased specificity in many diagnostic procedures. A further similarity between the two groups of organisms is that both parasitic and fungal diseases have received more attention in recent years because of their role as opportunistic infections in immunocompromised patients. These individuals' reduced ability to produce antibodies limits the utility of serological tests. Therefore, it seems appropriate to discuss immunologic factors for these two types of infections in one chapter. This chapter provides information on the immunologic aspects of these infections along with a discussion of available serological testing.

## PARASITIC IMMUNOLOGY

Until the emergence of HIV, parasitic infections were uncommon in the United States. With the spread of AIDS, several infections such as toxoplasmosis, giardiasis, and cryptosporidiosis have become more important problems. Other parasitic diseases such as malaria, schistosomiasis, and leishmaniasis are among the most harmful infective diseases afflicting humans worldwide.[1] A further understanding of parasitic immunology will lead to better diagnosis and control of these diseases and will add to the fundamental knowledge of the immune response. This section covers the various immunologic strategies used by a host as it combats parasitic infections. Specific details about various parasites are considered later in the chapter, as is the diagnostic role of serological testing methods as they relate to each parasite.

When a parasite enters a host, there are several possible results. First, there may be no infection at all, because the host's innate immunity prevents the parasite from establishing an infection. In this case, the host fails to provide either the necessary physical environment or some important nutritional factor(s) needed for the parasite's survival. The host may even produce products that are toxic to the parasite.

In the second possible outcome, the parasite may invade the host, become established, and then be killed and eliminated by host defense mechanisms. These events indicate that an effective immune response has occurred. Typically, the host remains immune to reinfection for some time. This response requires antibody formation and cell-mediated immunity.

The third possible outcome is the reverse of the second—the parasite may overwhelm and kill the host. Reasons for this include an organism that multiplies so rapidly that the host does not have time to mobilize its defenses, the parasite invades a vital organ(s), or the host has an inadequate immune system.

A fourth possible outcome is a long-lasting infection in which the host begins to eliminate the parasite but cannot remove it completely. In the best case, the host controls the disease for an extended period and eventually overcomes and eliminates the parasite. In the worst case, the host ultimately succumbs to the infection and dies.

And, finally, a fifth possible outcome is the host mounts a response that attacks not only the parasite but also host tissues. The effects of this inappropriate response (hypersensitivity or immune disease) may be mild or severe; often the consequences for the parasite are minimal. In fact, most of the pathology associated with a parasitic infection results from the immunologic responses to the offending organism and may be more dangerous for the host than the invader.

### Evasion of Host Defenses

Any parasite's survival depends on its ability to live in a peaceable manner with its host. If the host dies, then so does the parasite. However, when the host recognizes a parasite as a foreign entity, the relationship becomes combative. As a host defends itself, the parasite attempts to evade these defense mechanisms. Parasites are large organisms that are very antigenically complex and have complex life cycles. Different stages of the organism may be found in various body locations. The net result leads to a situation in which the host may partially control the infection but not eliminate the parasite. The host continues to fight with increasingly complex responses until either the host or the parasite prevails. Frequently, there is only an uneasy compromise that can be tipped in favor of either side. Many factors, some known and many others not yet known, work together to preserve the parasite's existence.

If a parasite becomes sequestered within host cells, the parasite is protected. For example, when parasites such as the tissue protozoans invade macrophages or liver cells, they are temporarily hidden from the immune system. The host cannot recognize the parasites while they reside inside these cells.[2] However, eventually they must exit these cells and invade new ones. When they move between cells, they are vulnerable to the host's defenses.

Some parasites disguise themselves by acquiring host antigens. Schistosomes survive in unprotected blood vessels, because the invading form (schistosomula) acquires red blood cell antigens that later help protect the adult from attack by the immune system.[3]

Another process of evasion some parasites employ is called **antigenic variation.** African trypanosomes evade the immune response by periodically changing their surface antigens. A variant surface glycoprotein produces an unlimited group of variable antigen types.[4,5] The host builds antibody, mainly IgM, to the one antigen, thereby reducing the infection. The parasite responds by changing its antigen, making the current antibody ineffective. This switching may occur very rapidly, within 5 to 6 days. The host must then produce a new antibody. This process of **antigen switching** can continue for long periods of time.

Another mechanism of escape involves antigen shed from the parasite. For example, *Entamoeba histolytica* can shed antigens.[2] Antibody is formed and attaches to the antigen. Since the antigen is not attached to the parasite, the immune response is unable to harm the offending organism.

Molecular mimicry may result from parasitic antigens that are similar to antigens normally found on host tissue. This may lead to autoimmune problems such as the cardiac and intestinal consequences that occur in the late stages of Chagas disease.[2]

Along with these specific mechanisms parasites use to evade the host's immune system, there are numerous non-specific factors that interfere with the normal operation of the system as a whole. When a host eliminates a bacterial or viral infection, the immune system rests until a new encounter occurs. Parasitic infections, however, are chronic, because the host is rarely able to totally eliminate the source of infection. The immune system is forced to remain active. Often the result is immunosuppression, disruption of normal B-cell and T-cell functions, and hypersensitivity reactions. For example, schistosomes have mechanisms that

can down-regulate the host's immune system. This immune modulation promotes the parasite's survival but also limits severe damage to the host. As a result, adult schistomes can live in the human host for up to 40 years before finally being eliminated.[6,7] All of these complicated mechanisms along with a multitude of other evasive mechanisms either contribute to or directly cause the pathology seen in parasitic diseases.

## Immunologic Response to Parasites

Innate and adaptive immune responses are important in protecting the host from parasitic infection. Working in concert, several cell types—including B and T lymphocytes, natural killer cells, macrophages, other antigen-presenting cells, granulocytes, and mast cells—actively participate in the recognition and elimination of parasites from the host. Soluble substances, including immunoglobulins, complement, and cytokines, also participate in the host's ability to overcome parasitic infections.

Innate immune responses are critical in the early recognition of an infection. As part of the innate immune defense, neutrophils act as phagocytes to destroy both intracellular and extracellular parasites. Hydrogen peroxide kills extracellular organisms while neutrophilic granules destroy ingested organisms. Because natural killer (NK) cells can be activated without prior exposure to the pathogen, they are important in the early defense against parasitic infection. NK cells produce gamma interferon (IFN-$\gamma$), which inhibits the replication of intracellular parasites.[8] Complement activation provides protection through the production of chemotactic components, opsonization for enhanced phagocytosis, and lysis of extracellular parasites.

Cellular immunity is responsible for the production of cytokines and chemokines, which enhance the cytotoxic function of effector cells, increase the numbers of immune cells, and attract immune cells to the site of infection. Many protozoan parasites are effectively reduced or eliminated by macrophages that are activated by sensitized T cell–generated cytokines such as interferon-$\gamma$ and the migration inhibitory factor. Other cytokines such as interleukin-3 and granulocyte-monocyte colony-stimulating factor act on cells of the myeloid line to cause an increase in neutrophils, eosinophils, and macrophages; thus, additional effector cells are recruited to combat the infection.

The immunoglobulin response to parasites includes formation of IgM, IgG, IgA, and IgE antibodies. Specific antibody can damage protozoa, neutralize parasites by blocking attachment to the host cell, prevent the spread of the parasite, promote complement lysis, and enhance phagocytosis and destruction through antibody-dependent cellular cytotoxy. Helminth infections in particular are characterized by eosinophilia and high levels of IgE. IgE binds to mast cells and basophils. When specific antigen–antibody combinations occur, mast cells degranulate and release chemotactic factors, histamine, prostaglandins, and other mediators. One of the most important mediators released is **eosinophil chemotactic factor,** which attracts eosinophils to the infected area. Eosinophils can destroy helminths by degranulation or through antibody-dependent cellular cytotoxicity. It is believed that the ability to produce IgE evolved mainly for the purpose of dealing with parasitic infections.[3]

Although antibodies are detectable in serum and may be useful guides when diagnosing diseases caused by parasites, they have little or no correlation with the course or prognosis of the disease. Later protection from reinfection by the parasite cannot be predicted on the basis of circulating antibody levels, nor can any other useful information be gained by measuring cellular responses.

However, serology can be used to identify parasites that are present in organs or other deep tissues such as the brain or muscle and that are not recoverable in blood, urine, or feces. If a person travels to an endemic area, becomes infected with a parasite, and then returns to a nonendemic area, a positive serology test can indicate a recent infection. Conversely, a positive test result in a person who lives in an endemic area may only reflect a previous parasitic infection. Because antibody levels may remain elevated for years, the positive result may not relate to the patient's current condition.

## Serology in Protozoan Diseases

Falciparum malaria and African trypanosomiasis continue to produce high mortality rates despite intense efforts to control the parasites responsible for these diseases. Relatively mild diseases such as amebiasis, giardiasis, and toxoplasmosis are found worldwide but have become significant problems for patients who have suppressed immune systems. Immunosuppressive drugs used to treat cancer, prevent rejection of transplanted organs, and, more importantly, treat diseases such as AIDS have caused increased susceptibility to these infections. Infections with *Cryptosporidium parvum, Cyclospora cayetanensis,* and several *Microsporidium* species have become more prevalent, especially in immunocompromised hosts. Because protozoa can live in the blood, the gastrointestinal tract, organ tissues, and macrophages, clinical manifestations and host responses are quite varied. Toxoplasmosis and other representative protozoan diseases for which serological testing is useful are presented here.

### Toxoplasmosis

**Toxoplasmosis** results from infection with *Toxoplasma gondii,* a ubiquitous protozoan parasite that infects humans by ingestion of infective **cysts** (oocysts). It is thought that cysts are transferred by hand-to-mouth contact from contaminated soil or cat litter or by ingesting oocysts in raw or partially cooked pork, mutton, or beef. Transmission may also occur through blood transfusions or organ transplantation. Cats are known to be definitive hosts for this parasite, but other definitive hosts must also exist, since nearly 24 percent of the U.S. population over age 12 is infected with this parasite.[9]

This disease is nearly always asymptomatic or may present with a mild lymphadenopathy. Rarely, the parasite reaches the central nervous system (CNS) or the eye. Invasion of the CNS can be fatal but typically occurs only in immunosuppressed patients.[10] This is one of the more common opportunistic infections seen in individuals with AIDS.

Encysted organisms can be found in any tissue **(Fig. 20–1).** These cysts may remain viable for years, which explains why immunosuppressed patients can exhibit symptoms long after initial infection. The greatest concern, however, is that *Toxoplasma* species can cross the placenta. If the fetus is exposed during the first trimester, death nearly always occurs as a result of CNS damage. Infection during the second trimester may result in hydrocephaly, blindness, or other nervous system damage. Later infection may result in blindness or mild CNS defects. However, women who are exposed to this parasite before pregnancy do not transmit the infection to the fetus.

*T. gondii* is capable of replicating inside human macrophages. The parasite can survive indefinitely here, because the organism can prevent the fusion of lysosomes with phagosomes. Normally a phagocytic cell digests the material within the phagolysosome, but in this case, digestion does not occur. The macrophages' ability to kill the parasite is greatly increased if the parasite is first opsonized by antibody. Antibody-coated *Toxoplasma* organisms trigger phagocytosis, which ultimately destroys the organism. Immunocompromised patients often have severe problems with this infection, a fact that further confirms the role played by antibody in controlling this disease.

Serological testing plays an important role in diagnosing toxoplasmosis, because isolation of the organism requires tissue biopsy. Generally, seroconversion to an antibody-positive state, a fourfold increase in the titer of IgG, or high levels of IgM and IgG antibodies are considered diagnostic. However, detectable elevations of IgM may persist for months to years,

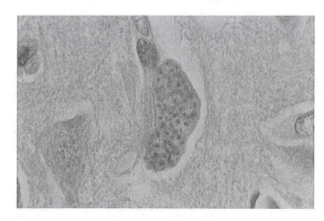

└────────────┘ 50 μm

**FIGURE 20–1.** Pseudocyst of *Toxoplasma gondii* seen in a brain section. *(From Leventhal, R and Cheadle, RF. Medical Parasitology:A Self-Instructional Text. Ed 5. FA Davis, Philadelphia, color plate 127, 2002, with permission.) See Color Plate 15.*

making determination of acute infection difficult. IgA levels can also be detected in early infection and can persist for 3 to 9 months. Concurrent elevations of IgM and IgA indicate early infection and are used to screen pregnant women.[2]

Enzyme immunoassays (EIA) for IgM, IgG, or IgA and indirect fluorescent antibody (IFA) assays for IgG are available and should be performed when congenital toxoplasmosis is suspected. IFA testing has been widely used, but EIA is the method of choice,[11] as it is more sensitive, less difficult to perform, and easier to interpret. Elevated titers of IgG, IgM, or IgA antibody classes suggest that infection has occurred within the previous 3 to 9 months. Elevated IgG titers without IgM antibody suggest an older infection. Paired samples whose collection is separated by 3 weeks are tested to confirm the presence of recent infection. In a recent infection, titers of both of these antibody classes will rise. Newborns with congenital toxoplasmosis usually have detectable IgM antibody. Presence of elevated IgM titers in the mother's serum further supports the diagnosis **(Table 20–1).** Specific IgA antibody assays provide even more sensitive methods for early detection and confirmation of congenital toxoplasmosis and should be performed on newborns suspected of harboring the parasite. Early diagnosis and maternofetal treatment can reduce fetal infection to mild or subclinical. Prenatal congenital toxoplasmosis can be diagnosed by performing polymerase chain reaction (PCR) technology on amniotic fluid to detect *T. gondii* DNA.[12]

Currently, there are no useful serological procedures for diagnosing CNS infection in immunocompromised patients.[9,11] These individuals often do not produce detectable levels of specific antibody against the parasite, and procedures to detect circulating antigen appear to lack sensitivity. PCR is, therefore, the method of choice to detect *T. gondii* DNA in CSF.

## Other Protozoa

Serum antibody studies are not used to identify several protozoa, because conventional methods of identification are easier to perform and provide more definitive results. *Entamoeba histolytica, Entamoeba histolytica/dispar, Cryptosporidium parvum, Giardia lamblia,* and *Trichomonas vaginalis* are all parasites that are usually identified by microscopic examination of specimen materials. Feces are tested for *E. histolytica, E. histolytica/dispar, C. parvum,* and *G. lamblia;* urine or vaginal discharge is tested for *T. vaginalis.* However, immunologic procedures directed toward identifying the organism or a soluble antigen found in the specimen are extremely helpful. The identification rates for each test compare favorably with conventional identification techniques, but immunologic procedures offer an important advantage, because a technologist who is not experienced in parasitology can successfully perform them. Direct fluorescent antibody (DFA) and enzyme-linked immunosorbent assay (ELISA) kits are available for these organisms. The DFA methods use monoclonal antibody labeled with fluorescein isothiocyanate against the parasite's cell wall to visualize the initial antibody-parasite complex (see Fig. 10–5, color plate 10) Autofluorescence of *Cyclospora cayetanensis* is a characteristic of the organism that is used as an additional diagnostic technique for identifying this parasite in feces, but it can lead to confusion and incorrect interpretation of DFA reactions performed to detect other parasites, such as *C. parvum.*[13]

EIA methods employ enzyme conjugated to either antigen or antibody, depending on the assay being performed. The ELISA methods capture organisms or soluble antigen by adding patient samples to antibody-coated wells. The enzyme conjugate is then added. The appropriate substrate for the enzyme employed is then added. The wells are washed between each step of the procedure to remove antibodies or antigens that are not attached. A change in chromogen color indicates the presence of bound antigen. The more color produced, the greater the concentration of the patient antibody or antigen. (More details about this procedure are given in this chapter's laboratory exercise.)

PCR techniques have been developed to identify species of *Plasmodium, Toxoplasma, Giardia, Trypanosoma, Leishmania, Cryptosporidium, Entamoeba, Microsporidia, Babesia,* and *Cyclospora.* Many of these procedures are available in reference laboratories but are not yet used in the routine laboratory. PCR testing has been compared to microscopy in the identification of many parasites. Though specificity is equal, most studies indicate that PCR is more sensitive. It is easier to interpret but more difficult and time-consuming to perform. It also provides the ability to genotype.[12–14]

The FDA has recently approved a rapid EIA diagnostic test for malaria. The procedure derives results in approximately 15 minutes. It allows the differentiation of *Plasmodium falciparum* from less virulent malaria parasites. Though malaria is rare in the United States, cases are diagnosed in individuals who travel to endemic countries. Since the disease is uncommon, diagnosis may be delayed. Death can be prevented if the disease is diagnosed and treated early. Rapid testing allows faster diagnosis and leads to earlier treatment.[15] Other rapid tests are available for the diagnosis of *Cryptosporidium, Giardia, Cyclospora,* and other parasitic

| TABLE 20–1. | Interpretation of Toxoplasma Serological Test Results | |
|---|---|---|
| TITER IIF–IgG | EIA–IgM | INTERPRETATION |
| <1:16 | Negative | No evidence of exposure |
| 1:16 | Negative | Infection probably acquired more than 1 year ago |
| 1:1024 | 1:4–1:256 | Infection probably acquired within the past 18 months |
| >1:1024 | 1:1024 | Recent infection, probably acquired within the past 4 months |

IIF = indirect immunofluorscence; EIA = enzyme immunoassay

infections. These tests are useful in diagnosing foodborne and waterborne illnesses.

## Helminth Infections

Phagocytosis by macrophages and neutrophils can destroy larval stages of helminths. It has been long recognized that eosinophils and mast cells play an important role in the defense against tissue parasites. IgE-coated mast cells recruit eosinophils to the site of infection. Eosinophils degranulate and kill the organisms through oxygen-dependent and oxygen-independent mechanisms.[3]

Intestinal helminth infections are relatively simple to diagnose, because eggs, adult round worms, and segments of tapeworms are easily recovered from stool specimens. However, larvae or embryos of some tapeworm species can exit the host's intestine and migrate to other tissues. The pathology produced by these wandering parasites depends on the damage caused to the invaded organ or tissue. Because symptoms are often vague or mimic other disease processes, it is difficult to identify the parasite as the causative agent. Serodiagnostic tests can provide helpful information when investigating these problems, especially in cysticercosis and echinococcosis. Current methods include IFA tests; slide, tube, and precipitin tests; complement fixation; particle agglutination tests; and enzyme-linked immunoassays, among others. Most commercial kit systems are based on an ELISA system. DNA probes are used in immunoblot methods at the Centers for Disease Control and Prevention (CDC) to diagnose cysticercosis, echinococcosis, paragonimiasis, and schistosomiasis. **Table 20–2** lists tests performed at the CDC. Samples for CDC processing must be submitted via state health laboratories. The CDC does not accept specimens sent directly by private laboratories or physicians.

| TABLE 20–2. | Antibody Detection Tests for Parasites Offered at the Centers for Disease Control and Prevention | |
|---|---|---|
| **DISEASE** | **ORGANISM** | **TEST** |
| Amebiasis | Entamoeba histolytica | Enzyme immunoassay (EIA) |
| Babesiosis | Babesia microti / Babesia sp. WA1 | Immunofluorescence (IFA) |
| Chagas disease | Trypanosoma cruzi | IFA |
| Cysticercosis | Larval Taenia solium | Immunoblot (Blot) |
| Echinococcosis | Echinococcus granulosus | EIA, Blot |
| Leishmaniasis | Leishmania braziliensis / L. donovani / L. tropica | IFA |
| Malaria | Plasmodium falciparum / P. malariae / P. ovale / P. vivax | IFA |
| Paragonimiasis | Paragonimus westermani | Blot |
| Schistosomiasis | Schistosoma sp. / S. mansoni | FAST-ELISA |
| | S. haematobium / S. japonicum | Blot |
| Strongyloidiasis | Strongyloides stercoralis | EIA |
| Toxocariasis | Toxocara canis | EIA |
| Toxoplasmosis | Toxoplasma gondii | IFA-IgG, EIA-IgM |
| Trichinellosis (Trichinosis) | Trichinella spiralis | EIA |

Courtesy of the Centers for Disease Control and Prevention, Division of Parasitic Diseases. Send an e-mail to dpdx@cdc.gov or call the Division of Parasitic Diseases at (770) 488-4431 for information on the following diseases or organisms for which serology tests are not available at CDC but may be available elsewhere within the United States or abroad: African trypanosomiasis; Angiostrongylus; Anisakis; Baylisascaris procyonis; Echinococcus multilocularis; Fasciola hepatica; Filariasis; Gnathostoma.

## Limitations of Parasitic Serology

As in all clinical laboratory areas, it is important in clinical immunology to find the most straightforward and economic procedure for each test method. However, it is also important to consider the specificity and sensitivity of the method when choosing a procedure. Because no external proficiency testing program is currently offered in the area of parasitic serology except for diagnosis of *Toxoplasma* and *Babesia microti*,[11] it is very difficult to evaluate the quality of commercial products. In the United States, commercial kit manufacturers must obtain FDA approval before selling their products. The FDA requires only that a new method be equivalent to a method that has already been approved. Researchers at the CDC have expressed concern that, over time, the quality of new test kits may drift in a negative direction, because a new kit may not be quite as good as the one used for comparison but may still receive approval.[16] Because commercial kits for the diagnosis of some parasitic diseases are not available, individual laboratories develop their own methods using antigen purchased from various sources. This fact and the lack of proficiency testing places the burden of quality assurance on the individual laboratory. Due to the difficulty in procuring and preparing antigens that are highly specific for these parasites, a large variation occurs in the results reported by various laboratories. According to the CDC, unexpected results should be confirmed by another laboratory.

Another problem affecting the choice of a procedure is timing. A procedure may detect only a certain class of antibody such as IgM; thus, the test must be performed when the patient is producing IgM, or the diagnosis may be missed. A particular antibody produced against a certain stage in a parasite's life cycle may not be recovered by a given procedure, so again timing is important. It must not be forgotten that related organisms produce similar antigens, which, in turn, induce the formation of cross-reacting antibodies. This problem reduces the specificity of a procedure. Although all of these problems must be considered, it should be emphasized that with a clear understanding of parasitology and the principles of immunology, useful diagnostic information can be provided for the physician.

## FUNGAL IMMUNOLOGY

Fungal infections are usually well controlled in humans as long as the immune system functions properly. **Fungi** that are normally considered nonpathogenic may cause mild to very severe pathology in immunocompromised individuals. A rapidly growing population of immunocompromised individuals exists as a result of several factors, the most important being the prevalence of immunodeficiency diseases such as AIDS. Other factors are the increased use of medications such as broad-spectrum antibiotics for bacterial infections and immunosuppressive agents for treatment of cancer and transplantation patients. Because of the immunocompromised

status of these individuals, a substantial increase in the prevalence of fungal infections has occurred, and mycoses have become a serious health issue around the world. According to the U.S. National Center for Statistics, fungal infections were the seventh most common cause of infectious-disease-related death in 1992, and the number of deaths due to fungal disease had increased threefold since 1980.[17] This time period parallels the introduction of HIV in the United States. Fungal diseases are often the first opportunistic diseases detected in patients with AIDS. One of the most common opportunistic diseases in patients with AIDS is pneumonia caused by *Pneumocystis carinii*, also known as *Pneumocystis jiroveci*. This organism was first characterized as a parasite but now is designated a fungus, because it has a greater gene sequence homology with fungi than with parasites.[18] Many saprophytic fungi formerly dismissed as cultural contaminants are now reported as opportunistic pathogens.[19]

## Characteristics of Fungi

Fungi are eukaryotic cells with nuclei and rigid cell walls. Fungi have two fundamental structural forms, appearing either as filamentous **molds** or **yeasts;** sometimes they appear in both forms. Molds are composed of **hyphae** and **conidia.** Hyphae are filamentous tubular branching structures that intertwine to form a dense mat called a **mycelium.** Conidia are asexual reproductive structures produced at the tip or along the sides of fertile hyphae. Yeasts are unicellular and reproduce asexually by budding.

Although most fungi are monomorphic, some exhibit **thermal dimorphism.** These dimorphs reproduce both as molds, at 25°C to 30°C, and as yeasts, at 35°C to 37°C. The mycelial mold form is the saprophytic state found in nature; the yeast form is the parasitic or pathogenic state found in tissue in disease, with the exception of *Coccidioides immitis*, which grows as a **spherule** at 35°C to 37°C. The thermal dimorphs are the etiologic agents of serious systemic **mycoses** that can be life-threatening.

## Mycotic Infections (Mycoses)

Of the greater than 80,000 species of fungi that have been identified, less than 400 are considered pathogens. Ninety percent of the fungal infections affecting humans and animals are caused by less than 50 species.[20] Though most pathogenic fungi are found in water, soil, or decaying organic matter, some exist in humans as normal flora. Fungal diseases are generally not spread from person to person. Those fungi that are etiologic agents of human infection are normally soil saprophytes that have been traumatically introduced into body tissues or accidentally inhaled into the lungs. These exogenous pathogens can grow at the relatively elevated temperature of the human body and can survive cellular defenses. A few endogenous organisms—for example, the yeast *Candida albicans*—also can cause infection when the host defense is deficient for only a brief period.[19]

Mycoses are clinically classified as superficial, cutaneous, subcutaneous, and systemic. The most common human pathogens are *Coccidioides*, *Blastomyces*, *Histoplasma*, and *Paracoccidioides*. These organisms usually cause lung disease but may also become systemic and damage any organ of the body.[21] Due to the increased incidence of mycoses in immunocompromised patients, a new classification called *opportunistic* has been added.[20] Many fungi that cause opportunistic infections are normally considered nonpathogenic. The most common opportunistic organisms are *Candida*, *Aspergillus*, *Cryptococcus*, and *Zygomycetes*. Identifying the etiologic agent is critical for treating and managing the patient when a fungal infection has been established. Because culture does not always reveal the infectious agent, immunologic procedures can provide the first presumptive evidence of the infection.[22]

## Immune Response to Fungi

Host immunity, including the innate and adaptive responses to bacteria and viruses, has been widely studied. Much less has been done to investigate the role of these responses in combating fungal infections. The development of a fungal infection depends on the virulence of the fungus, the number of infecting fungi inhaled or injected into the tissue, and the host's immune status.[19] The ability of the organism to survive at 37°C at a neutral pH and the production of toxins are factors that affect the virulence of the fungus.[21] Natural or innate resistance to fungal infection is very high. Physical barriers such as skin and mucous membranes provide primary defense against fungal invasion. Effector cells such as neutrophils, macrophages, and dendritic cells play an early role in the defense against organisms that breach the physical barriers. These cells possess germline-encoded receptors that allow recognition of fungi and subsequent killing of the organisms through phagocytosis.[23] Although the body produces antibodies to fungi, humoral immunity and complement play only minor roles in the immune response to fungi. Opsonization is not necessary for phagocytosis of most fungi, but it is required for phagocytosis of *Cryptococcus neoformans*.[23] Cellular immunity is the most important defense against fungal infection. In the majority of cases, the cellular defenses of normal persons are sufficient, and infections resolve spontaneously.

## Serology in Mycotic Diseases

Diagnosis of fungal infections depends on the patient's history, clinical symptoms, and the identification of the organism. Fungi are identified by culture, recognizing the organism's growth rate and the presence of distinctive colonial and microscopic morphological characteristics. Although the humoral response to fungi is not the major defense against fungal infection, antibodies are produced against the invading organisms. Antibody detection, antigen detection, and the identification of fungi in patient specimens or culture are the three areas in which immunologic procedures have found major application. Because fungi grow so slowly, isolation and morphological identification of fungi usually cannot be accomplished in less than 5 days. Therefore, the rapid availability of results in serological testing makes them an important tool in diagnosing fungal infections. Culture often fails to detect or identify the infectious agent. In many cases, positive serological test results stimulate continued efforts to isolate and identify the etiologic agent in culture.[22] Serological tests also can yield information used to monitor the effects of treatment with therapeutic agents.

Selecting the tests to be performed depends on the etiologic agent of the mycosis. The clinician must provide the laboratory with all the pertinent information available, including the patient's symptoms, history of other past or present infections, and medical treatments that have left the patient immunocompromised or debilitated. The patient's occupation, place of residence, and record of travel are also important, because some occupations expose an individual to opportunistic or pathogenic fungi that might not otherwise have been considered, and many fungi are endemic to specific geographic areas. Because serological tests are effective at different stages of mycotic disease and because the stage of the disease may not be known, the best procedure is to use a combination of serological tests and a variety of related antigens to identify the antibodies of the etiologic agent. Serial dilutions of serum should be made after an initial 2- to 3-week interval (of the acute phase), midway through an infection, and after recovery (the convalescent phase) to determine if and how the titer is changing. Titers of 1:32 or a fourfold or greater rise in titer are significant in making a diagnosis as long as the patient is immunocompetent. In immunocompromised individuals, testing for antigens rather than antibodies must be performed.

Serodiagnostic tests are commercially available with different degrees of sensitivity and specificity for aspergillosis, blastomycosis, candidiasis, coccidioidomycosis, cryptococcosis, histoplasmosis, paracoccidioidomycosis, and sporotrichosis. Some of these tests are available in routine laboratories (see **Table 20–3**).

The following discussion provides information on four of the fungal infections for which serological testing is used.

## Aspergillosis

*Aspergillus* species are found worldwide in soil and air, in decaying vegetation, and on stored grains **(Fig. 20–2)**. Aspergillosis is an opportunistic infection predominantly caused by *Aspergillus fumigatus*, *A. flavus*, *A. niger*, and *A. terreus*. Other pathogenic species of *Aspergillus* are involved with less frequency. Typical clinical infections may be colonizing, allergic, or disseminating, depending on the pathological findings in the host. Disseminated aspergillosis usually occurs in severely immunocompromised hosts.[24]

Pulmonary colonization is usually a primary condition induced by inhalation of large numbers of conidia. Allergic bronchopulmonary aspergillosis is characterized by allergic

| Table 20–3. Serological and Molecular Testing Used for Fungal Infections | | |
| --- | --- | --- |
| ORGANISM | SEROLOGICAL TESTING | MOLECULAR DIAGNOSTIC TESTING |
| Aspergillus sp. | Immunodiffusion | Not routinely available |
|  | Counterimmunoelectrophoresis |  |
|  | Enzyme immunoassay |  |
| Blastomyces dermatitidis | Immunodiffusion | Not routinely available |
|  | Enzyme immunoassay |  |
|  | Complement fixation |  |
| Candida albicans | Immunodiffusion | PNA-FISH |
|  | Counterimmunoelectrophoresis |  |
|  | Latex agglutination |  |
|  | Enzyme immunoassay |  |
| Coccidioides immitis | Complement fixation | Performed on isolates of the organism (used for confirmation) |
|  | Immunodiffusion (exoantigens test) |  |
|  | Latex agglutination |  |
|  | Tube precipitin test |  |
|  | Precipitation |  |
|  | Enzyme immunoassay |  |
| Cryptococcus neoformans | Latex agglutination antigen test | Not routinely available (research labs only) |
|  | Tube agglutination |  |
|  | Enzyme immunoassay |  |
|  | Indirect immunofluorescence |  |
| Dematiaceous organisms | Not useful | Not routinely available (research labs only) |
|  | Only useful in screening for allergy to organisms |  |
| Dermatophytes | Not useful | Not routinely available |
| Histoplasma capsulatum | Immunodiffusion (exoantigens test) | Performed on isolates of the organism |
|  | Complement fixation |  |
|  | Skin test for delayed or immediate hypersensitivity |  |
|  | Latex agglutination |  |
|  | Counterimmunoelectrophoresis |  |
|  | Radioimmunoassay for antibody |  |
|  | Direct fluorescent antibody assay for antigen in tissue |  |
| Paracoccidiodes brasiliensis | Immunodiffusion | Available in reference labs |
|  | Complement fixation |  |
| Penicillium marneffei | Immunodiffusion | Not routinely available |
| Sporothrix schenckii | Immunodiffusion (exoantigens test) | Not routinely available |
| Zygomycetes | Not useful | Not routinely available |

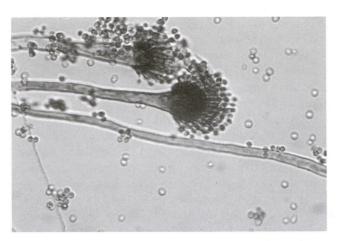

FIGURE 20–2. Aspergillus fumigatus; LPCB stain × 450.

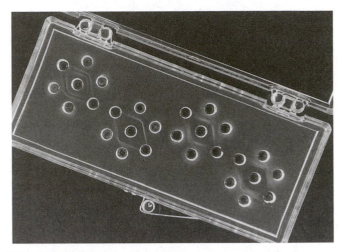

FIGURE 20–3. Immunodiffusion patterns of selected fungal antibodies. *(Courtesy of Immunomycologies, Norman, OK.)*

reactions to the toxins and the endotoxins of *Aspergillus* species. Allergy, asthma, or transient pulmonary infiltrates may develop when hypersensitive individuals are exposed repeatedly to large numbers of conidia.[19] Disseminating or invasive aspergillosis is usually found in immunocompromised individuals with chronic granulomatous disease.[25] The following sections provide information regarding serological testing for aspergillosis.

## Immunodiffusion and Counterimmunoelectrophoresis Tests

Ouchterlony immunodiffusion (ID) or counterimmunoelectrophoresis (CIE) for antibodies are methods available for aspergillosis testing. In the ID or CIE methods, the presence of one or more lines of serum precipitins is suggestive but not conclusive evidence of an active infection. Three or more lines are associated with aspergilloma (fungus ball) or with invasive aspergillosis if the patient is not anergic. For test results to be valid, the *Aspergillus* reference antiserum must demonstrate three or more bands with *Aspergillus* reference antigen. Nonspecific banding can be caused by C-reactive protein. The immunodiffusion tests are positive only in immunocompetent patients **(Fig. 20–3).**

## Enzyme Immunoassay

An EIA method has been developed to detect the serum galactomannan antigen of *Aspergillus*. This test is more sensitive than immunodiffusion tests and is therefore more valuable for diagnosis of aspergillosis in immunocompromised patients. Results are available in about 3 hours rather than the usual 4 weeks required for culture. Invasive aspergillosis has a mortality rate of 50 to 100 percent. Earlier identification of the organism expedites the administration of antifungal drugs and reduces mortality.[26]

## Candidiasis

Infections with *Candida albicans* and several other *Candida* species are collectively called **candidiasis.** *Candida albicans* is considered the most common cause of all serious fungal diseases. Although it is a normal endogenous inhabitant of the alimentary tract and the mucocutaneous regions of the body, it can become an opportunistic pathogen in debilitated and immunocompromised hosts. Systemic involvement is rare except when the yeasts are seeded into the body in large numbers through indwelling catheters, organ transplantation, or needles of drug abusers. Prolonged therapy with antibiotics or treatment with steroids and corticosteroids may also lead to systemic involvement.[19]

Intact skin and mucous membranes are barriers to invasion of this fungus. Cellular defenses protect against mucocutaneous infection. Most individuals also have some antibodies to *C. albicans*. Opsonic serum factors and the ability of polymorphonuclear cells to phagocytize the yeast cells are also believed to play a part in immunity.[19] Hematogenous dissemination occurs in patients with neutropenia. A number of serological tests for candidiasis have been developed, but their clinical utility has been hampered by the occurrence of false-positive results in patients who are colonized with *Candida* or who have superficial infections, and the frequency of false-negative results in immunocompromised patients who fail to produce sufficient antibody.[22] Some of the serological tests for candidiasis are discussed next.

## Immunodiffusion and Counterimmunoelectrophoresis Tests

ID and CIE methods for antibodies give comparable results, and both reliably detect antibodies in systemic candidiasis in immunocompetent hosts. A heat-stable cytoplasmic antigen is used with positive-control sera containing at least three of the seven known precipitins. Formation of one or more bands between the reagent antigen and patient's serum is considered a positive reaction. Systemic candidiasis is presumptively identified when serial dilutions of specimens show an increasing number of precipitin bands or convert from negative to positive. The patient's symptoms, direct smears, and cultures should be considered to validate positive ID and CIE tests.[22]

## Latex Agglutination (LA)

The LA test for antibodies is quantitative and can be of diagnostic and prognostic value. Latex particles sensitized with a homogenate antigen of *C. albicans* are reacted with patient sera and control sera. When this screening test is positive, a serial dilution is performed and reported as the highest dilution giving a 2+ reaction. A titer of 1:4 suggests an early infection, colonization, or a nonspecific reaction. A titer of 1:8 or greater, conversion from a negative to a positive test, or a fourfold increase in titer is presumptive evidence of invasive infection. A fourfold decrease in titer may indicate successful therapy.[22]

## Enzyme Immunoassay for Candida Antigen

Antibody detection tests have little or no value in immunocompromised patients; therefore, tests for antigenemia must be performed for these patients. Antigen tests include EIA and the reverse passive agglutination test. A double-antibody sandwich EIA method can be used to detect antigenemia.

## Reverse Passive Agglutination Test

A reverse passive LA test is also available for detecting antigenemia.[22] A study found that when a titer of 1:8 was used to indicate a positive test result, the sensitivity was 50 percent and the specificity was 73 percent.[27]

## Coccidioidomycosis

*Coccidioides immitis* is the etiologic agent of **coccidioidomycosis.** The fungus is endemic in the southwestern United States, especially in California's San Joaquin Valley (where it is called "valley fever") and in northern Mexico. *C. immitis* is a mold found primarily in alkaline desert soil in hot, semiarid regions. Animals, especially desert rodents, are vectors. The infectious conidia become airborne in dust storms or when disrupted by earthquakes or construction projects. Primary pulmonary coccidioidomycosis results from inhalation of dust containing the fungus. Sixty percent of infections are asymptomatic and self-limiting in immunocompetent individuals.[28] Hosts who are symptomatic may develop an acute primary pulmonary disease resembling the flu that resolves without treatment, a chronic progressive pulmonary disease, or secondary infections. Dissemination to the skin (erythema nodosum), bones, subcutaneous tissues, lymph nodes, and meninges is rare.

The antigen developed for serological identification of circulating antibodies of *C. immitis* is coccidioidin, which is an antigen filtrate of broth cultures of mycelial growth. Serological tests are important in the diagnosis and management of coccidiomycosis. Serological methods available for coccidioidomycosis are discussed below.

## Complement Fixation

Complement fixation (CF) is the most widely used quantitative serodiagnostic method for identifying *C. immitis* infections.[22] Complement-fixing antibodies of the IgG class develop in 3 to 6 months after the onset of symptoms. Titers of 1:2 to 1:4 are presumptive evidence of an early infection and should be repeated in 3 to 4 weeks. A titer of 1:16 is indicative of an active infection, particularly when accompanied by a positive ID test. Titers greater than 1:16 occur in 90 to 95 percent of patients with disseminated coccidioidomycosis. Titers parallel the severity of the mycoses.[25] Serum, cerebrospinal fluid (CSF), pleura, peritoneum, and joint fluids can be assayed by CF. A titer of 1:2 or higher in CSF is indicative of coccidioidal meningitis 95 percent of the time. False-negative results occur in patients with solitary pulmonary lesions. Cross-reactions in patients with acute histoplasmosis will occur as false-positive reactions.[22]

## Tube Precipitation (TP) Test

Precipitating IgM antibodies appear in 1 to 3 weeks after infection in 90 percent of symptomatic patients; therefore, a positive TP test can be an early indication of a primary infection. If precipitins are formed in any dilution of this test, it is considered diagnostic. The precipitins disappear within 4 to 6 months in 80 to 90 percent of patients with coccidioidomycosis, even in cases with dissemination. This makes the test of little prognostic value. The TP test is, however, highly specific with very few cross-reactions.[19,22,28,29]

## Immunodiffusion

Agar gel double ID tests are as sensitive as complement fixation tests and are not subject to anticomplementary reactions. The ID method is the most commonly used screening test for the diagnosis of coccidioidomycosis. When diffusion bands form lines of identity with the reference antisera, the bands represent the reaction of coccidioidin antigen and patient antibody. Single bands typically indicate chronic infection. Two or more bands usually indicate active disease or dissemination. Serum dilutions can be performed for quantification of coccidioidin antibodies. This test is highly specific when reference antisera are used.[19,29]

## Latex Agglutination

Latex particles sensitized with coccidioidin are reacted with inactivated patient serum to detect antibodies to the organism. This procedure is not recommended for testing CSF or diluted sera, because many false reactions occur. The LA test is positive early in the course of the disease, but as many as 10 percent of the cases of coccidioidomycosis confirmed by culture or serology give false-negative results with an LA test. Because false-positive results are common, a CF test or an ID test should be performed for confirmation when LA screening tests are positive.[19,22,29]

## Enzyme Immunoassay

EIA tests for IgG and IgM antibodies are available for use with serum or CSF. Positive EIA tests should be confirmed with CF or TP tests, because the EIA test is not absolutely specific.[22]

## Cryptococcosis

*Cryptococcus neoformans* is the etiologic agent of **cryptococcosis**. Pigeons are the chief vector, and *C. neoformans* is found where pigeons roost and defecate. After an individual inhales the yeast, cryptococcosis may be asymptomatic and unapparent, or it may develop as a symptomatic pulmonary infection. Encapsulation and the ability to synthesize melanin are the significant virulence factors. Untreated infections with *C. neoformans* have a predilection for disseminating to the CNS and the brain. In disseminated disease, the yeast spread is hematogenous. Any organ or tissue of the body may be infected, but localization outside the lungs or brain is relatively uncommon. There is little humoral response elicited by infections with *C. neoformans*, whether the patient is immunosuppressed or not. In normal patients, subclinical infection usually is resolved rapidly by growth-inhibiting substances present in body fluids.[19] Serious clinical disease is found in patients with debilitating illnesses and immunosuppression; AIDS patients especially are predisposed to disseminated infections. Primary and secondary cutaneous cryptococcosis are regularly encountered clinical manifestations in immunosuppressed patients.[19,22]

Meningitis occurs in approximately two-thirds of the infections that disseminate. The predilection of the fungus for the CNS is postulated to be due to the absence of inhibitory factors in spinal fluid and the minimal phagocytic response found there.[19]

### The Latex Particle Agglutination (LPA) Antigen Test

When cryptococcosis is first suspected, the capsular polysaccharide antigen of *C. neoformans* can be detected. An india-ink stain can be performed to demonstrate the polysaccharide capsule of *Cryptococcus* **(Fig. 20-4)**, but because of its higher sensitivity and specificity, latex agglutination for cryptococcal antigen is now recommended.[21,30] Inactivated serum or spinal fluid and positive and negative human reference sera are each mixed with latex particles

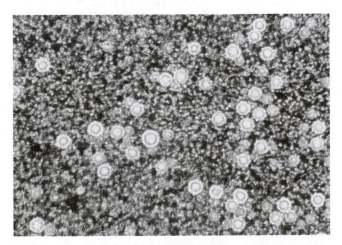

**FIGURE 20-4.** India ink preparation; *Cryptococcus neoformans* × 1000. *(From Kern, ME. Medical Mycology: A Self-Instructional Text. FA Davis, Philadelphia, 1985, p. 53, with permission.)*

sensitized with rabbit anticryptococcus globulin in rings on a test slide. The test is read macroscopically for agglutination. To be valid, the negative control must be negative, and the positive control must show 2+ agglutination. The presence of any agglutination when assaying a patient specimen is considered a positive test if controls are acceptable. Results may be quantitated by performing a serial dilution. The titer is reported as the highest dilution showing 2+ agglutination. A titer of 1:2 suggests infection, but a titer of 1:4 or greater is evidence of an active infection. Higher titers correlate with the severity of infection. Positive titers are found in CSF in 95 percent of cases involving the CNS.

Cross-reactions may occasionally occur due to rheumatoid factor (RF) or circulating antibodies that bind with nonreactive polysaccharide in immune complexes. Treating the serum or CSF specimens with a protease that destroys RF and cleaves antibodies in the immune complexes eliminates these reactions. Extraction of RF and circulating antibodies in serum can also be accomplished by treatment with ethylenediaminetetraacetic acid (EDTA) and boiling for 5 minutes. False-positive results in spinal fluid can be eliminated simply by heating the specimen in a boiling water bath.[22,29]

### Enzyme-Linked Immunoassay

An EIA test is available to detect antigens of *C. neoformans* in both serum and CSF. The EIA method for antigen detection is more sensitive than the latex agglutination procedure but takes more time to perform.[22,29]

While tests for antibodies to *C. neoformans* are not as widely used as antigen tests, they may be helpful in determining patient prognosis. Two methods available for antibody detection are the tube agglutination (TA) test and the indirect fluorescent antibody test.

### Tube Agglutination (TA) Test

The TA test can be used as both a qualitative screening test and a semiquantitative test to detect antibodies to *C. neoformans*. Serum or CSF from patients with suspected *C. neoformans* infection is heat inactivated to destroy complement. The serum or spinal fluid, an anticryptococcus positive control, and a negative control of rabbit serum are each mixed in test tubes with a *Cryptococcus* antigen suspension of weakly encapsulated yeast cells. The tubes are incubated and then refrigerated overnight. Reactions are read for agglutination. The positive control must read 3+ to 4+ in order for the test to be valid. Tests with reactions greater than the negative control are considered positive. The test can be made semiquantitative by performing a serial dilution and following the same procedure as that for the screening test. The titer is reported as the highest dilution showing any degree of agglutination. A titer of 1:2 or greater suggests a current or recent infection with *C. neoformans*. Approximately 90 percent of patients with pulmonary cryptococcosis will demonstrate antibody titers in the TA test. As the mycosis progresses, antigens begin to appear with a decrease in antibody production. Following treatment, a decrease in antigen titers and a reappearance of antibodies indicate a good prognosis. The TA test has a specificity of 89 percent with extrameningeal infections.[22,29,30]

### Indirect Fluorescent Antibody Test

Indirect immunofluorescence tests are also available for the detection of antibodies to *C. neoformans*. They are most valuable when antigen tests are negative; moreover, they can be combined with antigen tests to determine the patient's prognosis. A positive test suggests a recent or current infection with *C. neoformans* or a cross-reaction with another fungus. IFA tests have a specificity of 77 percent and a sensitivity of 50 percent. Both false-negative and false-positive results may occur.

## Molecular Testing

Screening clinical samples for fungi using molecular testing is not commonly performed. The development of cost-effective screening methods for fungal infections is impaired by the large number of pathogens that exist. A panel of PCR primers for fungal infections common in immunocompromised patients would be extremely useful for screening.[25] Though not commonly performed in routine laboratories, PCR assays are available for many fungi in reference laboratories.

Another molecular technique used for detecting fungal antigens is peptide nuclear acid fluorescent in situ hybridization (PNA-FISH). This technique utilizes small PNA polymer probes that are labeled with a fluorescent dye to identify PNA sequences on chromosomes. This procedure is currently used to differentiate *Candida albicans* from other *Candida* species.[31] See Table 20–3 for molecular tests used for specific mycoses.

## SUMMARY

Serological testing for parasitic and fungal diseases is less routine than for other infectious diseases, because test availability is limited and diagnosis is usually made from culture and morphological features of the organisms. However, some serological tests are available and can be useful for detecting these diseases.

Clearly the nature of the immune response as related to parasitic infections is complex. Most parasitic diseases are diagnosed by more direct methods such as fecal, blood, or urine examination. Therefore, serological procedures are not frequently needed. However, clinical manifestations of several parasitic diseases such as toxoplasmosis are not always clear-cut. In these cases, it may be possible to confirm the diagnosis serologically. In the United States, serum for such studies is often sent to a state public health reference laboratory for serological testing. Occasionally, a state laboratory may send specimens to the CDC in Atlanta, Georgia. Many private laboratories also offer testing for the more common parasites such as *Entamoeba histolytica*, *Entamoeba histolytica/dispar*, *Trichinella spiralis*, *Giardia lamblia*, and *Toxoplasma gondii*. *T. gondii* is also included as part of the ToRCH (Toxoplasma, rubella, cytomegalovirus, and herpes) panel, which is used to evaluate congenital and neonatal infections of newborn infants.

Tests used in parasitic serology cover the full range of methods available in immunology. Table 20–2 illustrates that everything from latex agglutination to countercurrent electrophoresis has been used or is currently being used to identify and quantify antibodies against parasites. New diagnostic procedures can be expected in the future, especially as molecular technology to detect parasitic nucleic acids develops, but these tests will remain expensive for some time. In underdeveloped countries in which parasitic infections are common, high cost will limit the benefits from these procedures.

Identification of fungal agents in culture, direct mounts, or histopathologic preparations of clinical specimens is not always possible. Serological tests are therefore useful for both the diagnosis and prognosis of patients with fungal infections. Positive serological tests are often the first suggestive evidence of mycotic infection. Tests for fungal antibodies and fungal antigens are available. Assays with different degrees of sensitivity and specificity for aspergillosis, candidiasis, coccidioidomycosis, and cryptococcosis were presented in this chapter. Serodiagnostic test findings should be used in conjunction with the patient's symptoms, history, and other clinical findings. Because cross-reactions are sometimes encountered, it is recommended that a battery of tests be utilized to more accurately interpret test results. While molecular tests have been developed for fungal infections, they are mainly performed in reference laboratories at the time of this writing. Table 20–3 provides a summary of the mycoses presented in this chapter and the serological and molecular tests that may be useful for their diagnosis.

# CASE STUDY

An otherwise healthy newborn develops a fever and a respiratory infection a few days after birth. He also has a slightly enlarged liver. The family has a cat that spends a great deal of time outdoors. The mother cleans the cat's litter box and did so throughout her pregnancy. It is suspected that the child may have congenital toxoplasmosis. The following serological test was performed on the mother and the baby. The results are listed below:

| TEST | MOTHER | BABY |
|------|--------|------|
| T. gondii IgG | 1:256 | 1:512 |

Questions:

a. Evaluate the baby's status related to *T. gondii* infection.

b. What additional testing should be performed to confirm the baby's status?

# EXERCISE

## GIARDIA LAMBLIA ANTIGEN TESTING BY A SANDWICH ELISA METHOD

### Principle

The qualitative determination of *Giardia lamblia* trophozoite and cyst antigens in feces is an enzyme immunoassay that employs rabbit and mouse antisera. *Giardia*-specific antigen (GSA 65) is a 65K MW glycoprotein produced in abundance by *Giardia* protozoa as they multiply in the intestinal tract. The test sample is added to a microtiter sample well. During the first incubation, GSA 65 antigens present in the stool supernate are captured by antibody (anti-GSA 65) bound to the well. After washing to remove unbound substances, enzyme conjugate comprised of the second anti-*Giardia* antibody and the enzyme (horseradish peroxidase) is added. During the second incubation, this antibody "sandwiches" the antigen. After washings to remove unbound enzyme conjugate, substrate is added that develops color in the presence of the bound enzyme complex. Presence of color indicates a positive reaction.

### Reagents, Materials, and Equipment

Test kit such as ProSpect Giardia, which contains the following:

Test strips: microplate containing anti-*Giardia* antibody (eight wells per strip)

Test strip holder

Enzyme conjugate—mouse monoclonal anti-*Giardia* antibody with thimerosal

Positive control

Negative control

Substrate—tetramethylbenzidine (TMB) in buffer

Wash buffer 10X concentration

Stop solution—1.0 N hydrochloric acid

Specimen dilution buffer

Other materials required but not provided in the kit include the following:

Stool specimen collection containers

Wash bottle or dispenser for wash buffer

Timer that measures minutes

Distilled or deionized water

Optional materials include the following:

Microplate reader

Micropipettes

Plastic or glass disposable test tubes

### Sample Collection, Storage, and Preparation

Specimen is collected in the same manner as that used for examination of stool for ova and parasites. The specimen should be stored at 2°C to 8°C and tested within 48 hours. If the sample cannot be assayed with 48 hours, the specimen should be frozen at –20°C to –70°C. Specimens preserved with 10 percent formalin, MF, or SAF fixatives should be tested within 2 months. Specimens that have been concentrated or fixed with PVA are not suitable for testing with this assay.

### Dilution in Wells

Label one tube for each specimen. Add 0.4 mL specimen dilution buffer to each tube. Coat one swab with specimen, and vigorously mix into specimen dilution buffer. Express as much fluid as possible before removing the swab from the tube, and discard the swab. Put a transfer pipette into the tube. If specimen is watery or preserved, mix by shaking. No further preparation is necessary.

### Procedure*

Run positive and negative controls with each run.

1. Break off the required number of wells (number of samples plus two for controls) and place in a strip holder. Return the remainder of the strips to the foil pouch, and reseal tightly.

2. Add four drops of the negative control to well 1 and four drops of positive control to well 2. (Do not dilute the controls.)

3. Add 100 µL of sample dilution buffer to each of the remaining wells.

4. Add one drop of the stool specimen to each test well. Samples can be added directly or prediluted in tubes before adding to wells.

5. Incubate the microtiter plate at room temperature (20°C to 25°C) for 60 minutes.

6. Shake out or aspirate the contents of the wells. Wash by filling each well with diluted wash buffer. Avoid generating bubbles in the wells. Decant by shaking out or aspirating contents of the wells. Repeat wash procedure for a total of three washes. After the last wash, decant contents. Invert strip and vigorously tap it on a clean paper towel.

---

*Adapted from the ProSpect Giardia Microplate Assay (revised January 7, 2005), Remel Inc., Thermo Fisher Scientific.

7. Add four drops (200 μL) of enzyme conjugate to each well.

8. Incubate for 30 minutes at room temperature.

9. Decant and wash each well five times, as described in step 6.

10. Add four drops (200 μL) of color substrate to each well.

11. Incubate the microplate for 10 minutes.

12. Add one drop of stop solution to each well. Mix wells by tapping the strip holder on the counter.

13. Read reactions within 10 minutes after adding stop solution. Read visually or at 450 nm if a microtiter reader is used.

## Interpretation of Results

### Visual

The color of each well should be compared to the color chart included in the test kit.

Positive control: At least 1+ yellow color intensity

Negative control: Colorless

Positive test: Any sample well that has yellow color of at least 1+ intensity

Negative test: Colorless

### Microtiter Reader

Zero the reader on air. Read all wells at 450 nm. Subtract the absorbance reading of the negative control from the absorbance readings of all other wells.

Positive control: $\geq 0.300$

Negative control: $\leq 0.100$

Positive test: $\geq 0.050$

Negative test: $\leq 0.050$ (tests with faint yellow color should be repeated)

## Comments

*Giardia lamblia* is a protozoan parasite that lives in the intestinal tract. Giardiasis is the most common parasitic disease diagnosed in the United States and, according to the CDC, causes an estimated 20,000 infections each year. Transmission of the infection occurs through ingestion of fecally contaminated food or water. This disease is common in day-care centers and in institutions where people are confined for extended periods. Giardiasis is also commonly diagnosed in homosexual men. Symptoms of the acute disease include diarrhea, nausea, weight loss, malabsorption, abdominal cramps, flatulence, and anemia. Because acute, chronic, and asymptomatic infections occur and because symptoms are similar to those of many other intestinal diseases, it is important to accurately diagnose the disease so that appropriate treatment can be administered.

Diagnosis of giardiasis is frequently made by observation of the parasite in fecal preparations. This method relies on an experienced technologist to correctly identify the organism. When an insufficient number of samples are examined, the diagnosis is often missed because the excretion of organisms is frequently intermittent. Other more invasive methods such as sigmoidoscopy or biopsy have also been used. The alternate approach, an ELISA method, such as the one presented in this exercise, offers a rapid noninvasive technique that does not require the observation and identification of an intact organism. These results suggest that immunologic procedures can play a significant role in the diagnosis of some parasitic diseases.

# REVIEW QUESTIONS

1. Compared to a host's response to the mumps virus, overcoming a parasitic infection is more difficult for the host because of which of the following characteristics of parasites?
   a. Large size
   b. Complex antigenic structures
   c. Elaborate life cycle
   d. All of the above

2. Most of the pathology associated with parasitic infections results from which of the following?
   a. Symbiotic relationships with the host
   b. Elaborate parasitic life cycles
   c. Immune response to the offending organism
   d. Innate defense mechanisms of the host

3. Parasites are able to evade host defenses by which of the following means?
   a. Acquisition of host antigens
   b. Changing surface antigens
   c. Sequestering themselves within host cells
   d. All of the above

4. The chronic nature of parasitic infections is due to the host's
   a. inability to eliminate the infective agent.
   b. type I hypersensitivity response to the infection.
   c. ability to form a granuloma around the parasite.
   d. tendency to form circulating immune complexes.

5. Clinical information provided by studying the immune response to parasitic diseases
   a. aids in correctly diagnosing the disease.
   b. predicts the prognosis of the disease.
   c. determines the possibility of reinfection by the parasite.
   d. All of the above

6. The presence of both IgM and IgG antibody in toxoplasmosis infections suggests that the infection
   a. occurred more than 2 years ago.
   b. occurred less than 18 months ago.
   c. is chronic.
   d. has resolved itself.

7. IgE is an important component of the immune response to infections caused by
   a. *Toxoplasma gondii.*
   b. *Giardia lamblia.*
   c. *Cryptosporidium parvum.*
   d. *Schistosoma mansoni.*

8. Which of the following are factors that have enabled saprophytic fungi to cause infections in humans?
   a. Their ability to survive the body's cellular defenses
   b. Their traumatic introduction into body tissues
   c. Use of antibiotics and immunosuppressive agents
   d. All of the above

9. In congenital toxoplasmosis, the newborn has elevated levels of what class of immunoglobulin?
   a. IgA
   b. IgG
   c. IgM
   d. IgE

10. When a mycosis is suspected, patient information must be acquired for all of the following *except*
    a. symptoms and physical examination.
    b. occupation, residence, and travel.
    c. medical treatment and medications.
    d. an exercise program.

11. The most significant defense against fungal infections is
    a. cellular immunity.
    b. humoral immunity.
    c. phagocytosis.
    d. complement activation.

12. Serodiagnosis is most important in making a rapid and presumptive diagnosis of fungal infections when
    a. the patient is under 12 or over 50 years of age.
    b. the patient has an undiagnosed acute or chronic respiratory infection.
    c. cultures of specimens are positive.
    d. histological tissue slide preparations are positive.

13. Because the stage of the mycosis is often not known, what is the best way to proceed when initiating serodiagnosis?
    a. Use a skin test in an endemic area, because a positive skin test is diagnostic.
    b. Use a combination of serological tests.
    c. Serial testing is excessive; a single test is always diagnostic.
    d. Use a single, specific antibody test.

14. After infection has been established, serodiagnostic tests are most likely to be positive in which of the following cases?
    a. The patient has developed a state of anergy.
    b. The patient is immunocompromised.
    c. The patient is immunocompetent.
    d. The tests were taken before antibodies had time to develop.

15. Which best describes nonspecific cross-reactions that occur in fungal serological tests?

    a. Occur as a result of crude unpurified antigens
    b. Occur with only one genus of fungi
    c. Do not interfere with fungal identification
    d. Tend to remain at high titer as a mycosis develops

16. Two serological tests currently used for the diagnosis of aspergillosis and candidiasis are

    a. complement fixation (CF) and enzyme immunoassay (EIA).
    b. immunodiffusion (ID) and counterimmunoelectrophoresis (CIE).
    c. counterimmunoelectrophoresis (CIE) and complement fixation (CF).
    d. enzyme immunoassay (EIA) and immunodiffusion (ID).

17. A 27-year-old man from Ohio, diagnosed with AIDS, developed chest pains and after a short period of time also developed severe headaches with dizziness. His hobby was raising messenger pigeons. His physician ordered a sputum culture and spinal tap, and both were positive for a yeastlike fungus. These findings are most consistent with infection by

    a. *Candida albicans.*
    b. *Coccidioides immitis.*
    c. *Cryptococcus neoformans.*
    d. *Histoplasma capsulatum.*

18. Which of the following serological tests detects the polysaccharide capsule antigen in serum and CSF of patients with suspected infection with *Cryptococcus neoformans*?

    a. Complement fixation (CF)
    b. Hypersensitivity skin test
    c. Latex agglutination (LA)
    d. Hemagglutination test

19. What is the most widely used quantitative serological test for identification of antibodies in infection with *Coccidioides immitis*?

    a. Complement fixation (CF)
    b. Latex agglutination (LA)
    c. Exoantigen test
    d. Fluorescent antibody test

## ACKNOWLEDGEMENT

The author would like to thank Russell F. Cheadle, MS, MT(ASCP), and Norma B. Cook, MA, MT(ASCP), for their contributions to this chapter in previous editions.

## References

1. World Health Organization. Revised Global Burden of Disease (GBD) 2002 Estimates: Mortality, incidence, prevalence, YLL, YLD and DALYs by sex, cause and region, estimates for 2002 as reported in the World Health Report 2004.
2. Garcia, LS. Diagnostic Medical Parasitology, ed. 5. American Society for Microbiology Press, Washington, DC, 2007, pp. 567–591.
3. Male, D, Brostoff, J, and Roitt, I. Immunology, ed. 7. Mosby Elsevier, Philadelphia 2006, pp. 277–298.
4. John, DT, and Petri, WA. Markell and Voge's Medical Parasitology, ed. 9. Saunders/Elsevier, Philadelphia, 2006, p. 112.
5. Barry, JD. The relative significance of mechanisms of antigenic variation in African Trypanosomes. Parasitol Today 13:212–218, 1997.
6. Jenkins, SJ, Hewitson, JP, Jenkins, GR, et al. Modulation of the host's immune response by schistosome larvae. Parasite Immunol 27:385–393, 2005.
7. Collier, L, Balows, A, and Sussman, M (eds). Topley and Wilson's Microbiology and Microbial Infections, ed. 9, vol. 5. Oxford University Press, New York, 1998, pp. 69–70.
8. Papazarharia, M, Athanasiadis, GI, Papadoupoulos, E, et al. Involvement of NK cells against tumors and parasites. Int J Biol Markers 22(2):144–153, 2007.
9. Jones, JL, Kruszon-Moran, D, Wilson, M, et al. Toxoplasma gondii infection in the Unites States: Seroprevalence and risk factors. Am J Epidemiol 154:357–365, 2001.
10. Wilson, M, Jones, JL, and McAuley, JB. Toxoplasma. In Murray, PR, Baron, EJ, Jorgensen, JH, et al. Manual of Clinical Microbiology, ed. 9, vol. 1. American Society for Microbiology Press, Washington, DC, 2007, pp. 2070–2081.
11. Wilson, W, Schantz, PM, and Nutman, T. Molecular and immunologic approaches to the diagnosis of parasitic infections. In Detrick, B, Hamilton, RG, and Folds, JD (eds): Manual of Clinical Laboratory Immunology, ed. 7. American Society for Microbiology, Washington, DC, 2006, pp. 557–568.

12. Christoph, J, Kattnew, E, Seitz, HM, and Reiter-Owana I. Strategies for the diagnosis and treatment of prenatal toxoplasmosis—a survey (abstract). Z Geburtshilfe Und Neonatologie 208(1):10–16, 2004.

13. Morgan, UM, Pallant, L, Dwyer, BW, et al. Comparison of PCR and microscopy for detection of *Cryptosporidium parvum* in human fecal specimens: Clinical trial. J Clin Microbiol 36:995–998, 1998.

14. Aviles, H, Belli, A, Armijos, R, et al. PCR detection and identification of *Leismania* parasite in clinical specimens in Ecuador: A comparison with classical diagnostic methods. J Parasitol 85(2):181–187, 1999.

15. FDA clears for marketing first quick test for malaria. http://www.fda.gov/bbs/topics/NEWS/2007/New01659.html. Released June 26, 2007. Accessed July 27, 2007.

16. Wilson, M, and Schantz, P. Nonmorphologic diagnosis of parasitic infections. In Balows, A, Hausler, WJ, et al. (eds): Manual of Clinical Microbiology, ed. 6. American Society for Microbiology, Washington, DC, 1991, pp. 717–726.

17. The Fifth NIAID Workshop in Medical Mycology: Epidemiology. http://www3.niaid.nih.gov/research/topics/fungal/meetings.htm. Accessed August 10, 2007.

18. Stringer, JR, Beard, CB, Miller, RF, and Wakefield, AE. A new name (*Pneumocystis jerovici*) for Pneumocystis from humans. Emerging infectious diseases [serial online] September 8, 2002. http://www.cdc.gov/ncidod/EID/vol8no9/02-0096.htm.

19. Rippon, JW. Medical Mycology: The Pathogenic Fungi and Pathogenic Actinomycetes, ed. 3. WB Saunders, Philadelphia, 1988.

20. Brooks, GF. Jawetz, Melnick & Adelberg's Medical Mycology, ed. 24. McGraw-Hill Medical, London, 2007.

21. Forbes, BA, Sahm, DF, Weissfeld, AS. Bailey and Scott's Diagnostic Microbiology, ed. 12. Mosby Elsevier, Philadelphia, 2007, pp. 542–627.

22. Reiss, E, Kaufman, L, Kovacs, A, et al. Clinical immunomycology. In Rose, NR, et al.: Manual of Clinical Immunology, ed. 6. American Society for Microbiology, Washington, DC, 2002, pp. 559–583.

23. Hohl, TM, Rivera, A, and Pamer, E. Immunity to fungi. Curr Opin Immunol 18(4):465–472, Aug. 2006.

24. Washington, WC, Koneman, EW, Allen, SD, et al. Koneman's Color Atlas and Textbook of Diagnostic Microbiology, ed. 6. Lippincott Williams and Wilkins, Philadelphia, 2006, pp. 1151–1243.

25. Forbes, BA, Sahm, DF, and Weissfeld, AS. Laboratory methods in basic mycology. In Bailey and Scott's Diagnostic Microbiology, ed. 12. Mosby Elsevier, Philadelphia, 2007, pp. 628–716.

26. FDA News. U.S. Food and Drug Association. May 16, 2003.

27. Petri, MG, Konig, J, Moecke, HP, Gramm, HJ, et al. Epidemiology of invasive mycoses in ICU patients: A prospective multicenter study in 435 non-neutropenic patients. Paul-Ehrlich Society for Chemotherapy, Divisions of Mycology and Pneumonia Research. Intensive Care Med 23:317–325, 1997.

28. Centers for Disease Control. Coccidiomycosis. http://www.cdc.gov/ncidod/dbmd/diseaseinfo/coccidiomycosis. Accessed November 29, 2007.

29. McGinnis, MR, and Tilton, RC. Immunologic diagnosis of fungal infection. In Howard, DA, et al. (eds): Clinical and Pathogenic Microbiology, ed. 2. Mosby, St. Louis, MO, 1994, pp. 641–648.

30. Package insert. Cryptococcal Latex Agglutination System (CALAS), Meridian Bioscience, Inc. Rev. March 2002.

31. Wilson, DA, Joyce, MJ, Hall, LS, et al. Multicenter evaluation of Candida albicans peptide nucleic acid fluorescent in situ hybridization probe for characterization isolates from blood cultures. J Clin Microbiol 43(6):2909–2912, 2005.

# Spirochete Diseases

21

*Marc Golightly, PhD, Candace Golightly, MS, MLT(ASCP), and Christine Stevens*

## LEARNING OBJECTIVES

*After finishing this chapter, the reader will be able to:*

1. Describe identifying characteristics of *Treponema pallidum* and *Borrelia burgdorferi*.
2. Explain how syphilis and Lyme disease are transmitted.
3. Discuss the different stages of syphilis.
4. Discuss the advantages of direct fluorescent staining for *T. pallidum* over darkfield examination without staining.
5. Define *reagin*.
6. Distinguish treponemal from nontreponemal tests for syphilis.
7. Describe the principle of the following tests for syphilis: Venereal Disease Research Laboratory (VDRL), rapid plasma reagin (RPR), fluorescent treponemal antibody absorption (FTA-ABS), and agglutination assays.
8. Give reasons for false-positive reagin test results.
9. Compare and contrast sensitivity and specificity of treponemal and nontreponemal testing for the various stages of syphilis.
10. Discuss the advantages and disadvantages of polymerase chain reaction (PCR) and enzyme immunoassay (EIA) testing for syphilis.
11. Discuss limitations of cerebrospinal fluid (CSF) testing for neurosyphilis and testing for congenital syphilis.
12. Describe early and late manifestations of Lyme disease.
13. Relate various aspects of the immune response to Lyme disease to disease stages.
14. Compare immunofluorescence assay (IFA), EIA, and immunoblot testing for Lyme disease as to sensitivity and ease of performance.
15. Discuss causes of false positives and false negatives in serological testing for Lyme disease.

## KEY TERMS

- *Borrelia burgdorferi*
- Chancre
- Congenital syphilis
- Erythema migrans
- Flocculation
- FTA-ABS test
- Gummas
- Immunoblotting
- Nontreponemal tests
- Polymerase chain reaction (PCR)
- Prozone
- Reagin
- RPR test
- Tertiary syphilis
- *Treponema pallidum*
- Treponemal tests
- VDRL test

347

## CHAPTER OUTLINE

Spirochetes are long, slender, helically coiled bacteria containing *axial filaments*, or *periplasmic flagella*, which wind around the bacterial cell wall and are enclosed by an outer sheath.[1] These gram-negative, microaerophilic bacteria exhibit a characteristic corkscrew flexion or motility. Diseases caused by these organisms have many similarities, including a localized skin infection that disseminates to numerous organs as the disease progresses, a latent stage, and cardiac and neurological involvement if the disease remains untreated. This chapter discusses disease manifestations and testing for the two major spirochete diseases, syphilis and Lyme disease. Serological testing plays a key role in diagnosis of these diseases, because isolation of the organism itself is difficult to accomplish in the laboratory, and clinical symptoms are not always apparent.

## SYPHILIS

Syphilis remains the most commonly acquired spirochete disease in the United States today.[2,3] It is typically spread through sexual transmission. Although the incidence of cases in the United States reached an all-time low of 2.2 cases per 100,000 individuals in 2000,[4] it has been increasing from 2000 to 2005 (latest data available at time of writing).[3] In this period, there has been a dramatic increase in primary and secondary syphilis. Homosexual transmission between men is responsible for much of this increase.[3,5,6] In fact, in 2000, this group accounted for 6 percent of the syphilis cases in this country; in 2005, over 60 percent of syphilis occurred in this group. Neurosyphilis (usually rare) is also appearing in the homosexual HIV-positive male population.[7] Also troubling has been the first reported increases of syphilis in the female population in over 10 years.[3]

In countries such as the United Kingdom in western Europe, the incidence also appears to be on the rise again.[8–10] Likewise, primary and secondary syphilis rates in China are rapidly increasing; in 2005, they were substantially higher than most developed countries, including the United States.[11] Thus, despite the current emphasis on safe sexual practices, syphilis remains a major health problem in many areas of the world. Early detection of the disease is of major importance. This chapter presents characteristics of the organism and the disease and discusses the most frequently used methods of identification.

## Characteristics of the Organism

The causative agent of syphilis is *Treponema pallidum,* subspecies *pallidum*, a member of the family Spirochaetaceae. Organisms in this family have no natural reservoir in the environment and must multiply within a living host. Three other pathogens in this group are so morphologically and antigenically similar to *T. pallidum* that all but one are classified as subspecies.[12] These other organisms are *T. pallidum* subspecies *pertenue*, the agent of yaws; *T. pallidum* subspecies *endemicum*, the cause of nonvenereal endemic syphilis; and *T. carateum*, the agent of pinta. Yaws is found in the tropics, pinta is found in Central and South America, and endemic syphilis is found in desert regions.

*T. pallidum* (which will hereafter be used to refer to subspecies *pallidum*) varies in length from 6 to 20 mm and in width from 0.1 to 0.2 mm, with 6 to 14 coils (**Fig. 21–1**).[1,13] The outer membrane of *T. pallidum* is a phospholipid bilayer with very few exposed proteins. Several identified membrane proteins, called *treponemal rare outer membrane proteins (TROMPs)*, have been characterized.[14] It appears that the scarcity of such proteins delays the host immune response.

## Mode of Transmission

Pathogenic treponemes are rapidly destroyed by heat, cold, and drying out, so they are almost always spread by direct contact. Sexual transmission is the primary mode of dissemination, and this occurs through abraded skin or mucous membranes coming in contact with an open lesion. Approximately 30 to 50 percent of the individuals who are exposed to a sexual partner with active lesions will acquire the disease.[13] Congenital infections can also occur during

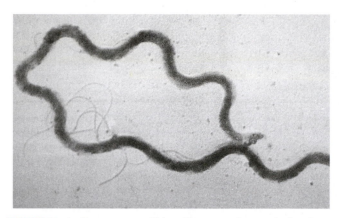

FIGURE 21-1. *Treponema pallidum.* Electron micrograph showing the coils and periplasmic flagella. *(Courtesy of CDC Archives, Atlanta, GA)*

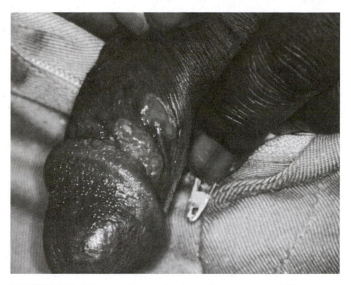

FIGURE 21-2. Primary chancre in the early stage of syphilis. *(Courtesy of CDC/M. Rein, VD)*

pregnancy. Transmission to the fetus is possible in mothers with clinically latent disease.

Other potential means of transmission include parenteral exposure through contaminated needles or blood, but this is extremely rare. For the past 30 years, the lack of transfusion-transmitted syphilis in the United States has actually called into question the necessity of testing potential donors for presence of the disease.[15] However, current guidelines (2007) by the American Red Cross for blood donation requires waiting 12 months after treatment for syphilis before donating.[16] Because syphilis can only be transmitted by means of fresh blood products, the use of stored blood components has virtually eliminated the possibility of transfusion-associated syphilis.[13]

## Stages of the Disease

Once contact has been made with a susceptible skin site, endothelial cell thickening occurs with aggregation of lymphocytes, plasma cells, and macrophages.[17] The initial lesion, called a **chancre,** develops between 10 and 90 days after infection, with about 21 days being the average.[8] A chancre is a painless, solitary lesion characterized by raised and well-defined borders **(Fig. 21-2).** In men these usually occur on the outside of the penis, but in women they may appear in the vagina or on the cervix and thus may go undetected. This primary stage lasts from 1 to 6 weeks, during which time the lesion heals spontaneously.

If the initial chancre is untreated, about 25 percent of such cases progress to the *secondary stage,* in which systemic dissemination of the organism occurs. This stage is usually observed about 1 to 2 months after the primary chancre disappears, but in up to 15 percent of reported cases, the primary lesion may still be present.[18] Symptoms of the secondary stage include generalized lymphadenopathy, or enlargement of the lymph nodes; malaise; fever; pharyngitis; and a rash on the skin and mucous membranes.[9,13,18] The rash may appear on the palms of the hands and the soles of the feet.[13] Involvement of the central nervous system may occur earlier than previously suspected, because viable organisms have been found in the cerebrospinal fluid (CSF) of several patients with primary or secondary syphilis.[12] Approximately 40 percent of patients with secondary syphilis may exhibit neurological signs such as visual disturbances, hearing loss, tinnitus, and facial weakness.[8] Lesions persist from a few days up to 8 weeks. After this time, spontaneous healing occurs, as in the primary stage.

The *latent stage* follows the disappearance of secondary syphilis. This stage is characterized by a lack of clinical symptoms. It is arbitrarily divided into early latent (less than 1 year's duration) and late latent, in which the primary infection has occurred more than 1 year previously. Patients are noninfectious at this time, with the exception of pregnant women, who can pass the disease on to the fetus even if they exhibit no symptoms.

About one-third of the individuals who remain untreated develop **tertiary syphilis.**[8,13] This stage appears anywhere from months to years after secondary infection. Typically, this occurs most often between 10 and 30 years following the secondary stage.[8,13] Tertiary syphilis has three major manifestations: gummatous syphilis, cardiovascular disease, and neurosyphilis.

**Gummas** are localized areas of granulomatous inflammation that are most often found on bones, skin, or subcutaneous tissue. Such lesions can reach up to several centimeters in diameter, and they contain lymphocytes, epithelioid cells, and fibroblastic cells.[18] They may heal spontaneously with scarring, or they may remain destructive areas of chronic inflammation. It is likely that they represent the host response to infection.

Cardiovascular complications usually involve the ascending aorta, and symptoms are due to destruction of elastic tissue, especially in the ascending and transverse segments of the aortic arch.[18] This may result in aortic aneurysm, thickening of the valve leaflets causing aortic regurgitation, or narrowing of the ostia, producing angina pectoris.[13]

*Neurosyphilis* is the complication most often associated with the tertiary stage, but it actually can occur anytime after the primary stage and can span all stages of the disease. In immunodeficient individuals such as HIV patients, there has been a large rise in the incidence of early neurosyphilis.[7] During the first 2 years following infection, however, central nervous system involvement often takes the form of acute meningitis.

Late manifestations of neurosyphilis include *tabes dorsalis*, a degeneration of the lower spinal cord, and general paresis, or chronic progressive dementia. It usually takes more than 10 years for these to occur, but both are the result of structural central nervous system damage and cannot be reversed. Fortunately, these symptoms are now very rare because of early detection and treatment with penicillin.[8,13]

## Congenital Syphilis

Congenital syphilis occurs when a woman who has early syphilis or early latent syphilis transmits treponemes to the fetus. Due in large measure to a national plan launched by the Centers for Disease Control and Prevention, the occurrence of congenital syphilis dropped to 529 cases in the year 2000 and continued to drop through 2004,[19,20] despite increases in primary and secondary syphilis. Although the disease can be transmitted at any stage of pregnancy, typically the fetus is most affected during the second or third trimester, and fetal or perinatal death occurs in approximately 10 percent of the cases.[18]

Infants who are liveborn often have no clinical signs of disease during the first few weeks of life. Some may remain asymptomatic, but between 60 and 90 percent of such infants develop later symptoms if not treated at birth.[21] Inflammation of the umbilical cord, called *necrotizing funisitis*, may be the first indication of the disease.[13,22] The infant may exhibit clear or hemorrhagic rhinitis, or runny nose. Skin eruptions, in the form of a macropapular rash that is especially prominent around the mouth, the palms of the hands, and soles of the feet, are also common.[9] Other symptoms include generalized lymphadenopathy, hepatosplenomegaly, jaundice, anemia, painful limbs, and bone abnormalities such as saddle nose or saber shins.[12,13,19] Neurosyphilis may occur in up to 60 percent of infants with congenital disease.[23]

## Nature of the Immune Response

The primary body defenses against treponemal invasion are intact skin and mucous membranes. Once the skin is penetrated, T cells and macrophages play a key role in the immune response. Primary lesions show the presence of both CD4+ and CD8+ T cells. Cytokines produced by these cells activate macrophages, and it is ultimately phagocytosis by macrophages that heals the primary chancre.[18] The protective role of antibody is uncertain, however, as coating of treponemes with antibody does not necessarily bring about their destruction.[14] In fact, circulating immune complexes may actually prevent the host from synthesizing further specific treponemal antibody.[24] *T. pallidum* is also capable of coating itself with host proteins, which delays the immune system's recognition of the pathogen.[13] The rare treponemal proteins, or TROMPS, are important in bringing about complement activation that ultimately kills the organism.[14] However, the chronic nature of the disease is an indicator that the organisms are able to evade the immune response. Treponemes may persist in the host for years if antibiotic therapy is not obtained.

## Laboratory Diagnosis

Traditional laboratory tests for syphilis can be classified into three main types: direct detection of spirochetes, nontreponemal serological tests, and treponemal serological tests. These vary in sensitivity and ease of performance. Principles and procedures of each type of testing are discussed below and are compared and summarized in **Table 21–1**.

### Direct Detection of Spirochetes

Direct detection of spirochetes can be accomplished by dark-field microscopy or fluorescent antibody testing. The performance of either test requires that the patient have active lesions.

#### Dark-Field Microscopy

Primary and secondary syphilis can be diagnosed by demonstrating the presence of *T. pallidum* in exudates from skin lesions.[2,12] In dark-field microscopy, a dark-field condenser is used to keep all incident light out of the field except for that captured by the organisms themselves. It is essential to have a good specimen in the form of serous fluid from a lesion. This is usually obtained by cleaning the lesion with sterile saline and rubbing it with clean gauze. Pathogenic treponemes are identified on the basis of characteristic corkscrew morphology and flexing motility.[13]

Because observation of motility is the key to identification, specimens must be examined as quickly as possible, before they become dried out. False-negative results can occur due to delay in evaluating the slides, an insufficient specimen, or pretreatment of the patient with antibiotics.[13] Thus, a negative test does not exclude a diagnosis of syphilis. In addition, an experienced microscopist should perform testing. If a specimen is obtained from the mouth or the rectal area, morphologically identical nonpathogens can be found, so these must be differentiated from the true pathogens.

#### Fluorescent Antibody Testing of a Specimen

The use of a fluorescent-labeled antibody is a sensitive and highly specific alternative to dark-field microscopy. This can be performed by either a direct method, which uses a fluorescent-labeled antibody conjugate to *T. pallidum*, or an indirect method using antibody specific for *T. pallidum* and

## Table 21–1. Comparison of Tests Used for the Diagnosis of Syphilis

| TEST | ANTIGEN | ANTIBODY | COMMENTS |
|---|---|---|---|
| **Direct Microscopic** | | | |
| Darkfield | *T. pallidum* from patient | None | Requires active lesion. Must have good specimen, experienced technologist; inexpensive |
| Fluorescent antibody | *T. pallidum* from patient | Antitreponemal antibody with fluorescent tag | Requires active lesion. More specific than darkfield; specimen does not have to be live |
| **Nontreponemal** | | | |
| VDRL | Cardiolipin | Reagin | Flocculation; good for screening tests, treatment monitoring, spinal fluid testing; false positives |
| RPR | Cardiolipin | Reagin | Modified VDRL with charcoal particles. More sensitive than VDRL in primary syphilis |
| TRUST | Cardiolipin | Reagin | Uses red particles to visualize the reaction; similar to RPR |
| **Treponemal** | | | |
| FTA-ABS | Nichols strain of *T. pallidum* | Antitreponemal | Confirmatory; specific, sensitive; may be negative in primary stage |
| EIA | Treponemal or recombinant | Antitreponemal | Simple to perform; can be automated; not as sensitive as FTA-ABS |
| | Enzyme-labeled treponemal antigen | Anti-IgG or anti-IgM, antitreponemal antibody from patient | Simple to perform; sensitive in primary syphilis, but sensitivity decreases in later stages |
| MHA-TP or Serodia TP-PA | Sheep RBCs or gel particles sensitized with *T pallidum* sonicate | Antitreponemal | Not as sensitive as FTA-ABS |
| DNA probe | Patient DNA matched to treponemal DNA | None | Technically demanding; very specific; lacks sensitivity |

VDRL = venereal disease research laboratory; RPR = rapid plasma reagin; TRUST = toluidine red unheated serum test; FTA-ABS = fluorescent treponemal antibody absorption; EIA = enzyme immunoassay; MHA-TP = microhemagglutination assay for antibodies to *Treponema pallidum*; TP-PA = *T. pallidum* particle agglutination; DNA = deoxyribonucleic acid.

a second labeled anti-immunoglobulin antibody.[12] An advantage of this method is that live specimens are not required. A specimen can be brought to the laboratory in a capillary tube, and fixed slides can be prepared for later viewing. Even after fixing, treponemes can be washed off the slide, so each slide must be handled individually, and rinsing must be carefully done.[12] The use of monoclonal antibodies has made this method very sensitive and specific.[12] However, monoclonal antibodies can still cross-react with other subspecies of *T. pallidum*, and this must be taken into account when making a diagnosis.

## Serological Tests

If a patient does not have active lesions, as may be the case in secondary or tertiary syphilis, then serological testing for antibodies is the key to diagnosis. Serological tests can be classified as nontreponemal or treponemal, depending on the reactivity of the antibody that is detected.

**Nontreponemal tests,** which detect antibody to cardiolipin, have traditionally been used to screen for syphilis because of their high sensitivity and ease of performance. However, false-positive results are common because of the nonspecific nature of the antigen. Therefore, any positive results must be confirmed by a more specific **treponemal test,** which detects antibodies to *T. pallidum*.

### Nontreponemal Tests

Nontreponemal tests determine the presence of **reagin,** an antibody that forms against cardiolipin, a lipid material from damaged cells. This is found in the sera of patients with syphilis and several other disease states. An antigen that is a combination of cholesterol, lecithin, and cardiolipin is used in the reaction to detect the nontreponemal reaginic antibodies, which are either of the IgG or IgM class. The term *reagin* should not be confused with the same word that was originally used to describe IgE. They are not the same. Fortunately, the term *reagin* in reference to IgE is rarely used today.

The traditional nontreponemal tests are based on flocculation reactions in which patient antibody complexes with the cardiolipin antigen. **Flocculation** is a specific type of precipitation that occurs over a narrow range of antigen concentrations. The antigen consists of very fine particles.

In general, nontreponemal tests are positive within 1 to 4 weeks after the appearance of the primary chancre.[2,12] Titers usually peak during the secondary or early latent stages. In primary disease, between 13 and 41 percent of individuals appear nonreactive, but by the secondary stage, almost all patients have reactive test results.[2,12] However, testing of sera from patients in the secondary stage is subject to false negatives because of the **prozone** phenomenon (antibody excess). Typically this creates a nonreactive pattern that is granular or rough in appearance.[12] If a prozone is suspected, serial twofold dilutions of the patient's sera should be made to obtain a titer.

Reagin titers tend to decline in later stages of the disease, even if the patient remains untreated. After several years, about 25 percent of untreated syphilis cases were shown to become nonreactive for reagin.[13] This decline occurs more rapidly in individuals who have received treatment. A first-time infection, if in the primary or secondary stage, should show a fourfold decrease in titer by the third month following treatment and an eightfold decrease by 6 to 8 months.[18] Following successful treatment, tests typically become completely nonreactive within 1 to 2 years.

Examples of nontreponemal tests include Venereal Disease Research Laboratory (VDRL), rapid plasma reagin (RPR), toluidine red unheated serum test (TRUST), unheated serum reagin (USR), and reagin screen test (RST). The RPR and the VDRL are the most widely used of these tests.

## Venereal Disease Research Laboratory Test

The **VDRL test,** which was designed by the Venereal Disease Research Laboratories, is both a qualitative and quantitative slide flocculation test for serum, and there is a modification for use on spinal fluid.[25] Antigen for all tests must be prepared fresh daily and is done so in a highly regulated fashion. The antigen is an alcoholic solution of 0.03 percent cardiolipin, 0.9 percent cholesterol, and 0.21 percent lecithin. Basically, the antigen suspension is prepared by adding the VDRL antigen via a dropper to a buffered saline solution while continuously rotating on a flat surface; attention must be paid to required rotation speed and timing. A daily calibrated Hamilton syringe is used to deliver one drop of antigen for the slide test. If the delivery is off by more than 2 drops out of 60, the syringe must be cleaned with alcohol and recalibrated.

The serum specimens to be tested are heated at 56°C for 30 minutes to inactivate complement, and 0.05 mL is pipetted into a ceramic ring of a glass slide. Three control sera—nonreactive, minimally reactive, and reactive—are pipetted into rings on the glass slide in the same manner. Sera and patient samples are spread out to fill the entire ring. One drop (1/60 mL) of the VDRL antigen is then added to each ring. The slide is rotated for 4 minutes on a rotator at 180 rpm. It is read microscopically to determine the presence of flocculation, or small clumps. The results are recorded as reactive (medium to large clumps), weakly reactive (small clumps), or nonreactive (no clumps or slight roughness).[25] Tests must be performed at room temperature within the range of 23°C to 29°C (73°F to 85°F), because results may be affected by temperature changes. All sera with reactive or weakly reactive results must be tested using the quantitative slide test, in which twofold dilutions of serum ranging from 1:2 to 1:32 are initially used. Sera yielding positive results at the 1:32 dilution are titered further.

The VDRL test and some of the newer ELISA tests are the only ones routinely used for the testing of spinal fluid.[12,13] For VDRL spinal fluid testing, the antigen volume used is less than the serum test and is at a different concentration. In addition, different slides are used (Boerner agglutination slides). The test is read microscopically, as in the VDRL serum test. If a test is reactive, twofold dilutions are made and retested following the same protocol. A positive VDRL test on spinal fluid is diagnostic of neurosyphilis, because false positives are extremely rare.[13]

## Rapid Plasma Reagin (RPR) Test

The RPR is a modified VDRL test involving macroscopic agglutination. The cardiolipin-containing antigen suspension is bound to charcoal particles, which make the test easier to read. The suspension is contained in small glass vials, which are stable for up to 3 months after opening. The antigen is similar to the VDRL antigen with the addition of ethylenediaminetetraacetic acid (EDTA), thimerosal, and choline chloride, which stabilize the antigen and inactivate complement so that serum does not have to be heat-inactivated before use. Patient serum (approximately 0.05 mL) is placed in an 18 mm circle on a plastic-coated disposable card using a capillary tube or Dispenstir device. Antigen is dispensed from a small plastic dispensing bottle with a calibrated 20-gauge needle. One free-falling drop is placed onto each test area, and the card is mechanically rotated under humid conditions.[2] Cards are read under a high-intensity light source, and if flocculation is evident, the test is positive. All reactive tests should be confirmed by retesting using doubling dilutions in a quantitative procedure. The RPR test appears to be more sensitive than the VDRL in primary syphilis.[13]

## Standard Treponemal Serological Tests

Treponemal tests detect antibody directed against the *T. pallidum* organism or against specific treponemal antigens. The two main types of treponemal tests include the fluorescent treponemal antibody absorbed (FTA-ABS) test and agglutination tests. Typically, these tests are more difficult to perform and are more time-consuming than non-treponemal tests, so they have been traditionally used for confirmation rather than screening.

## Fluorescent Treponemal Antibody Absorption Test

One of the most used confirmatory tests is the **FTA-ABS test,** an indirect fluorescent antibody test. A dilution of heat-inactivated patient serum is incubated with a sorbent consisting of an extract of nonpathogenic treponemes (Reiter strain). This removes cross-reactivity with treponemes other than *T. pallidum.* Slides used for this test have the Nichols strain of *T. pallidum* fixed to them. They are kept frozen until use and then are equilibrated at room temperature for 30 minutes.

Diluted patient samples and controls are measured and applied to individual wells on the test slide. Slides are then incubated in a covered moist chamber at 37°C for 30 minutes. They are rinsed with deionized water and placed in a Coplin jar with phosphate-buffered saline for 5 minutes. After a second rinsing, the slides are air-dried, and antibody conjugate (antihuman immunoglobulin conjugated with fluorescein) is added to each well. Slides are reincubated as before, and a similar washing procedure is followed. Mounting medium is applied, and coverslips are placed on the slides. They are examined under a fluorescence microscope as soon as possible.

If specific patient antibody is present, it will bind to the *T. pallidum* antigens. The antibody conjugate will, in turn, only bind where patient immunoglobulin is present and bound to the spirochetes. When slides are read under a fluorescence microscope, the intensity of the green color is reported on a scale of 0 to 4+. No fluorescence indicates a negative test, and a result of 2+ or above is considered reactive.[12] A result of 1+ means that the specimen was minimally reactive, and the test must be repeated with a second specimen drawn in 1 to 2 weeks.[12] Experienced personnel are required to read and interpret fluorescent test results.

The FTA-ABS is highly sensitive and specific, but it is time-consuming to perform. This test is usually positive before reagin tests, although 20 percent of primary syphilis cases are nonreactive.[24] In secondary and latent syphilis, tests are usually 100 percent reactive. Once a patient is reactive, that individual remains so for life. Although there are fewer false positives compared to reagin tests, reactivity is seen with other treponemal diseases, notably yaws and pinta.[13]

## Agglutination Tests

Several varieties of passive hemagglutination tests have been used to detect specific treponemal antibody. These are no longer available in the United States, and particle agglutination tests such as the Serodia TP-PA test have largely replaced microhemagglutination tests.[22] Particle agglutination tests use colored gelatin particles coated with treponemal antigens and are more sensitive in detecting primary syphilis.[18] In the Serodia TP-PA test, patient serum or plasma is diluted in microtiter plates and incubated with either *T. pallidum*–sensitized gel particles or unsensitized gel particles as a control. Presence of *T. pallidum* antibodies is indicated by agglutination of the sensitized gel particles, which form a latticelike structure that spreads to produce a smooth mat that covers the well's surface. In wells containing a sample that is negative for the antibody, the gel particles settle to the well's bottom and form a compact button.

## Comparison and Testing Strategy of Traditional Nontreponemal and Treponemal Serological Tests

Nontreponemal tests are inexpensive, simple to perform, and can yield quantitative results. Thus, they are extremely useful as a screening tool, in monitoring the progress of the disease, and in determining the outcome of treatment. The main disadvantage is that they are subject to false positives. Transient false positives occur in diseases such as hepatitis, infectious mononucleosis, varicella, herpes, measles, malaria, and tuberculosis, and during pregnancy.[12] Chronic conditions causing sustained false-positive results include systemic lupus erythematosus, leprosy, intravenous drug use, autoimmune arthritis, advanced age, and advanced malignancy.[2,18]

A reactive nontreponemal test should be confirmed by a more specific treponemal test. In pregnancy, this is especially important, because nontreponemal titers from a previous syphilis infection may increase nonspecifically.[2,14] Under the following conditions, titers can be considered to be a nonspecific increase: lesions are absent, the increase in titer is less than fourfold, and documentation of previous treatment is available.[2]

Although treponemal tests are usually reactive before reagin tests in primary syphilis, they suffer from a lack of sensitivity in congenital syphilis and neurosyphilis. Nontreponemal tests should be used for these purposes.[2,13] Treponemal tests, while more difficult to perform, have been traditionally used as confirmatory tests to distinguish false-positive from true-positive reagin results. They also help establish a diagnosis in late latent syphilis or late syphilis, because they are more sensitive than nontreponemal tests in these stages.[2] **Table 21–2** compares sensitivities of some of the most widely used serological tests.

## Newer Technologies in Syphilis Testing

### Enzyme Immunoassay

Several enzyme immunoassay (EIA) tests have been developed for serodiagnosis of syphilis. One of these, Reagin II, uses a cardiolipin antigen similar to that used in the VDRL test. This method can easily screen large number of samples, and it is reported to have a sensitivity of 93 percent in primary syphilis.[26] However, it also has a slightly higher rate of false positives than RPR tests.

Other EIA tests have been developed to capture a specific class of antibody, either IgM or IgG. Microtiter wells are coated with antibody to IgM or IgG and are reacted with patient serum. Treponemal antigens that are labeled with an enzyme are then added **(Fig. 21–3)**. These have a fairly

| Table 21–2. | Sensitivity of Commonly Used Serological Tests for Syphilis | | | |
|---|---|---|---|---|
| STAGE TEST | PRIMARY (%) | SECONDARY (%) | LATENT (%) | LATE (%) |
| **Nontreponemal (Reagin) Tests** | | | | |
| Venereal Disease Research Laboratory Test (VDRL) | 78 | 100 | 95 | 71(37–94) |
| Rapid plasma reagin card test (RPR) | 86 | 100 | 98 | 73 |
| **Specific Treponemal Tests** | | | | |
| Fluorescent treponemal antibody absorption (FTA-ABS) test | 84 | 100 | 100 | 96 |
| *T. pallidum* microhemagglutination assay (MHA-TP) | 76 | 100 | 97 | 94 |

Adapted from LaSalsa, et al. Spirochete infections. In Henry, JB (ed): Clinical Diagnosis and Management by Laboratory Methods, ed. 21. WB Saunders, Philadelphia, 2007, Table 58-1.

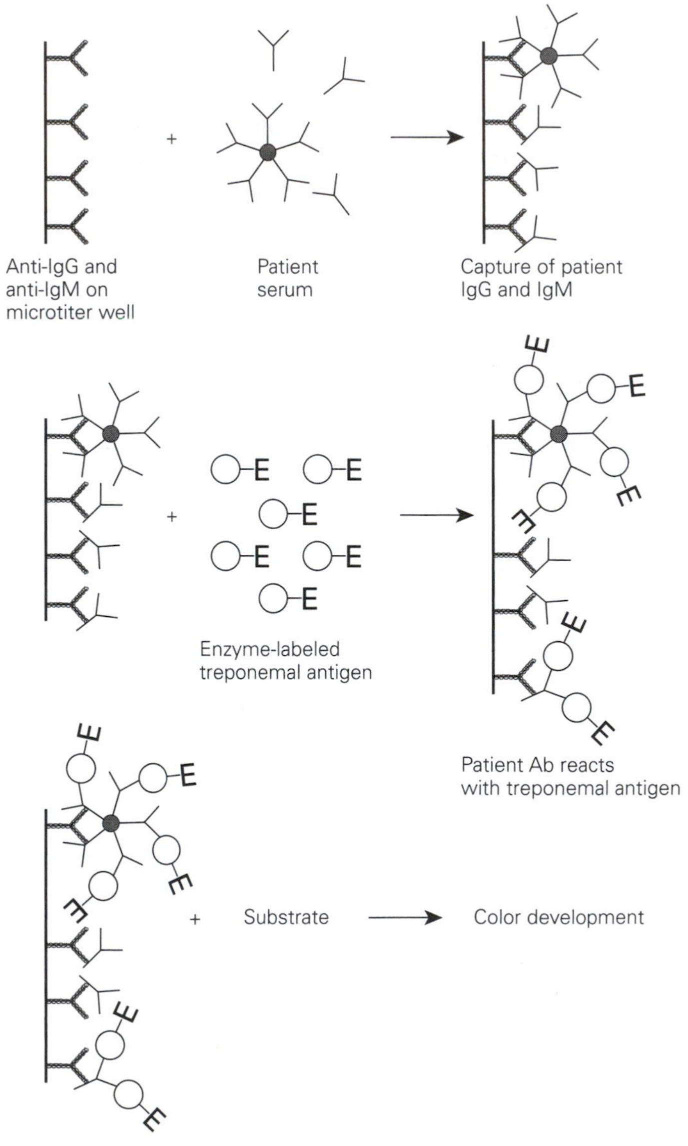

FIGURE 21–3. Antibody capture enzyme-linked immunosorbent assay (ELISA) test. Only specific antitreponemal antibody will react with enzyme-labeled antigen.

Anti-IgG and anti-IgM on microtiter well

Patient serum

Capture of patient IgG and IgM

Enzyme-labeled treponemal antigen

Patient Ab reacts with treponemal antigen

+ Substrate → Color development

high sensitivity in primary syphilis, but the sensitivity decreases as the disease progresses.[27] Specificity is similar to other treponemal tests. EIA tests are especially useful in diagnosing congenital syphilis in infants, as they look for presence of IgM, which cannot cross the placenta.

The EIA tests have continued to improve, with the driving force being the rising incidence of syphilis worldwide. Sensitivities and specificities are being reported as high as 99 percent and 98 percent, respectively, in large trials. The positive and negative predictive values likewise are high (99.3 percent and 97.2 percent, respectively).[28,29] With the ease of performance of EIAs, improved sensitivity and specificity, and because false positives may exceed the true positives in low-risk populations, a change in the testing strategy has been proposed and adapted in high-volume testing centers.[30] Under this scheme, the testing order is reversed from the traditional nontreponemal screening followed by confirmatory treponemal testing strategy. Patients would be screened by the EIA test followed by an RPR or equivalent test. If the initial EIA was negative, no further testing would be done unless early syphilis is suspected (i.e., prior to seroconversion). If the EIA was positive and the subsequent RPR was positive, then it would be considered positive for syphilis. If the initial EIA was positive followed by a negative RPR, then an FTA-ABS or equivalent would be performed. If that testing was positive, then late or latent syphilis or previous history of syphilis would be considered. If negative, then it would be considered negative for syphilis at this time, and careful evaluation of patient history should be considered regarding possible reevaluation at a later date.

### Polymerase Chain Reaction Technique

**Polymerase chain reaction (PCR)** technology, which involves isolating and amplifying a sequence of DNA that is unique to a particular antigen, has been applied to testing of various tissues, including kidney, lymph nodes, eye, and skin, as well as to spinal fluid and swab samples for the presence of treponemes. While there are many variations of this procedure, basically DNA is extracted from the sample and then amplified or increased using a DNA polymerase enzyme and a primer pair that starts the reaction. The newly made DNA is then subjected to agarose gel electrophoresis using a technique known as *Southern blotting*. Nitrocellulose paper is used to make a copy or blot of the gel. A labeled probe, which is a nucleotide sequence specific to the DNA sequence being tested for, is added to the nitrocellulose paper. The probe will adhere only to a complementary strand of DNA. Presence of the radiolabel on the nitrocellulose paper confirms the presence of treponemal antigen **(Fig. 21–4).**

Early studies demonstrated that PCR is an extremely sensitive technique, capable of detecting as little as one treponeme in a CSF sample.[31] For other fluids, especially serum, although the specificity appears to be 100 percent, sensitivity is closer to 70 percent.[32] More recently, in the United Kingdom, it has been offered as a diagnostic test for early syphilis in conjunction with the traditional testing in a clinical trial. This study found the sensitivity and specificity for swab specimens in early syphilis was also high (94.7 percent and 98.6 percent, respectively).[33] PCR has been used in conjunction with fine-needle aspiration of material from the inguinal lymph nodes. Preliminary results indicate that this could be a useful new tool for diagnosis when serological testing is not conclusive.[34]

Other specimens such as whole blood, CSF, and amniotic fluid can be tested by PCR; however, further research is required before these specimens are used in clinical practice.[35] Newer advances in this technology include real-time PCR, which is semiautomated and extremely fast. Most importantly, real-time PCR can discriminate between azithromycin-resistant and azithromycin-susceptible strains of *T. pallidum* in clinical samples. The implications for early proper treatment are obvious.[36] Unfortunately, at this time, the lack of commercial kits and nonstandardization has largely hampered the large-scale use of this technology for syphilis.[13]

## Special Diagnostic Areas

### Congenital Syphilis

Nontreponemal tests for congenital syphilis performed on cord blood or neonatal serum detect the IgG class of antibody.[37] It is difficult to differentiate passively transferred IgG maternal antibodies from those produced by the neonate, so there are problems in establishing a definitive diagnosis. Late maternal infection may result in a nonreactive test because of low levels of fetal antibody. Additionally, testing the infant's spinal fluid for presence of treponemes often lacks sensitivity.[38] Nontreponemal titers in the infant that are higher than the mother may be a good indicator of congenital disease, but this does not always occur.[12]

Several approaches have focused on detecting IgM in the infant. An FTA-ABS test for IgM alone lacks sensitivity, and the test is subject to interference because of the presence of rheumatoid factor.[38] However, an IgM capture assay is more sensitive, and a Western blot assay (see Chapter 8 for details) using four major treponemal antigens has demonstrated a high sensitivity and specificity.[12]

Currently, it is recommended that in high-risk populations, nontreponemal tests be performed on both mother and infant at birth, regardless of previously negative maternal tests. Since symptoms are not always present at birth, if congenital syphilis is suspected because of maternal history, tests should be repeated on infant serum within a few weeks.[21] If infection is present in the infant, the titer will remain the same or will increase. The Western blot test is recommended to confirm congenital syphilis.[13]

### Cerebrospinal Fluid Test

CSF is typically tested to determine whether treponemes have invaded the central nervous system. Such testing is usually more reliable if central nervous system symptoms are present. The traditional test performed on spinal fluid is the VDRL, which is a highly specific indicator of neurosyphilis.[13] If blood contamination of the specimen is not present, a positive VDRL confirms neurosyphilis.[17] However, sensitivity is lacking, because samples from fewer than 70 percent of patients with active neurosyphilis have given positive tests.[13,18] If a negative test is obtained, other indicators such as increased lymphocyte and elevated total protein (>45 mg/dL) count, are used as signs of active disease.[17] PCR has been advocated in diagnosing neurosyphilis and may play an important role in the future; however, the clinical availability of the test is limited, as discussed above.[13,35]

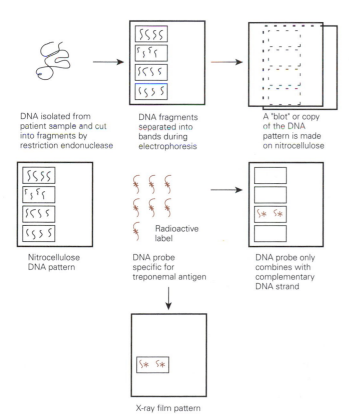

| DNA isolated from patient sample and cut into fragments by restriction endonuclease | DNA fragments separated into bands during electrophoresis | A "blot" or copy of the DNA pattern is made on nitrocellulose |

| Nitrocellulose DNA pattern | DNA probe specific for treponemal antigen | DNA probe only combines with complementary DNA strand |

Radioactive label

X-ray film pattern

**FIGURE 21–4.** Southern blotting technique for determining the presence of treponemal DNA.

## Treatment

Penicillin is still the drug of choice for treating primary or secondary syphilis. A single intramuscular injection is usually effective.[39] Doxycycline can be used as an alternative if the patient is allergic to penicillin. In addition, azithromycin has been also commonly used; however, resistant strains are arising.[36] Neurosyphilis is treated with crystalline penicillin or procaine penicillin to achieve a high enough concentration in the central nervous system. Probenecid is recommended for use along with penicillin in neurosyphilis patients.[39] For congenital syphilis, crystalline penicillin is administered for 10 days.

## LYME DISEASE

Lyme disease was first described in the United States in 1975 when an unusually large number of cases of juvenile arthritis appeared in a geographically clustered rural area around Old Lyme, Connecticut (hence the disease name), in the summer and fall. Two mothers recognized this and brought it to the attention of health officials. Due to the epidemiological features of this newly described "Lyme arthritis," transmission by an arthropod vector was suggested.[40] In 1982, the agent was isolated and identified as a new spirochete. It was given the name **Borrelia burgdorferi** after Willy Burgdorfer (first author in the original description).[41] The clinical features of Lyme disease were soon recognized to go beyond the arthritis, and it is now known to be a multisystem illness involving the skin, the nervous system, the heart, and the joints. Lyme disease is the most common vector-borne disease in the United States with approximately 20,000 cases being reported each year (2003 to 2005). The number of cases being reported per year has doubled since 1991. According to the CDC, this reflects both a true increase in the frequency of disease as well as better recognition and reporting.[42]

## Characteristics of the Organism

Several species of *Borrelia* are known to be the causative agents of Lyme disease. In North America, it is exclusively *B. burgdorferi sensu stricto*, while in Europe several species are known to cause Lyme disease (*B. afzelii*, *B. garinii*, *B. sensu stricto*, and occasionally other *Borrelia* species).[43,44] All share similar characteristics and for simplicity will be referred to as *B. burgdorferi*. The organism is a loosely coiled spirochete, 5 to 25 mm long and 0.2 to 0.5 mm in diameter.[1,43] The outer membrane, which consists of glycolipid and protein, is extremely fluid and only loosely associated with the organism. Several important lipoprotein antigens, labeled OSP-A through OSP-F, are located within this structure and are actually encoded by plasmids.[44] There are also surface proteins that allow the spirochetes to attach to mammalian cells.

Just underneath the outer envelope are 7 to 11 *endoflagella* or *periplasmic flagella*. These run parallel to the long axis of the organism and are made up of 41 kDa subunits that elicit a strong antibody response. This immunodominant characteristic is of diagnostic importance, since the response is not only strong but is also very early. Unfortunately, the flagellin subunit has homology to that of other nonpathogenic and pathogenic spirochetes, notably *B. recurrentis* and *T. pallidum*, causing cross-reactivity issues in serological testing.[1,45] Due to this, a large number of uninfected people have low levels of antibodies to the 41 kDa protein.[46] While this is usually not a problem in the current diagnostic scheme of testing, it can become an issue when these individuals become ill with certain viruses that are known polyclonal B-cell activators (such as Epstein-Barr virus). In this case, this normally low-level antibody becomes high enough to cause biological false positivity. The organism divides by binary fission approximately every 12 hours. It can be cultured in the laboratory in a complex liquid medium (Barbour-Stoenner-Kelly) at 33°C, but it is difficult to isolate from patients, and the spirochetemia is short-lived and generally found only early on in illness.[43] Cultures often must be incubated for 6 weeks or longer to detect growth and are therefore of little diagnostic utility.[1]

The main reservoir host is the white-footed mouse (*Peromyscus leucopus*), although in California and Oregon the spirochete is also harbored by the dusky-footed woodrat.[44] The tick infectivity rate on the West Coast is very low, thought, in part, to be due to a large number of ticks feeding on the western fence lizard whose blood is bactericidal for the spirochete.[47] Vectors are several types of *Ixodes* ticks: *I. scapularis* in the Northeast and Midwest United States, *I. pacificus* in the West, *I. ricinus* in Europe, and *I. persulcatus* in Asia. The lone star tick (*A. americanum*) is also known to carry the organism but is not thought to transmit the disease. White-tailed deer are the main host for the tick's adult stage **(Fig. 21–5)**. Nymphs and adult stages of the tick can transmit the disease. The peak feeding is in the late spring/early summer and the fall, which corresponds to the peak biphasic occurrence of Lyme disease.[1] Larvae forms of the ticks generally cannot transmit the disease, because they have not yet had a blood meal from which to pick up the organisms, and ova infection is extremely rare. The tick must feed for a period of time before the spirochete can be transmitted. Most agree that the risk for transmission is very low when ticks have fed for less than 36 hours, and one study finds transmission is still low at 72 hours.[48]

## Stages of the Disease

Lyme disease resembles syphilis in that manifestations occur in several stages. These have been characterized as (1) localized rash, (2) early dissemination to multiple organ systems, and (3) a late disseminated stage often including arthritic symptoms.[49] Because these stages are not always sharply delineated, however, it may be easier to view Lyme disease as a progressive infectious disease that involves diverse organ systems.

The clinical hallmark of early infection is the rash known as **erythema migrans (EM),** which appears between 2 days

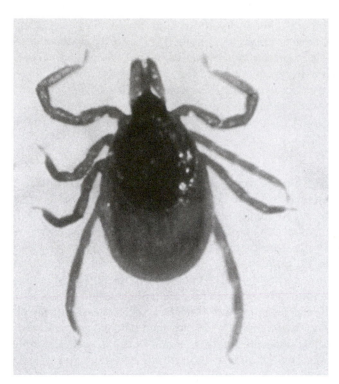

**FIGURE 21–5.** Adult tick *I. scapularis*, which transmits Lyme disease. *(Courtesy of Steven M. Opal, MD, Assistant Professor of Medicine, Brown University, Providence, RI)*

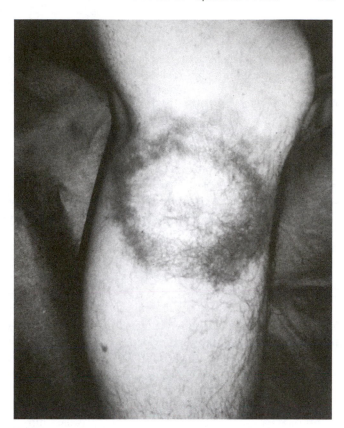

**FIGURE 21–6.** Erythema chronicum migrans rash, which appears after a tick bite in Lyme disease. *(Courtesy of Steven M. Opal, MD, Associate Professor of Medicine, Brown University, Providence, RI)*

and 2 weeks after a tick bite.[50] EM is a small red papule where the bite occurred, which rapidly expands to form a large ringlike erythema and often a central area that exhibits partial clearing **(Fig. 21–6)**. The clinical diagnosis of early Lyme disease relies on the recognition of this characteristic rash, which should be at least 5 cm in diameter. At this stage, the patient may be asymptomatic or have nonspecific flulike symptoms such as malaise, headache, fever, arthralgias, and fatigue.[13,51,52] The EM usually continues to expand for over a week, and even if untreated, gradually fades within 3 to 4 weeks. Unfortunately, approximately 20 percent of patients do not develop the rash.[49,51,52] At this early stage, the antibody response is minimal and most serologies are negative.

Early dissemination occurs via the bloodstream and occurs in days to weeks following the EM rash. The skin, nervous system, heart, or joints may be affected. Approximately 10 to 15 percent of patients will display multiple skin lesions.[44] There is often migratory pain in the joints, tendons, muscles, and bones. If treatment is not obtained, neurological or cardiac involvement is seen in about 15 percent of patients within 4 to 6 weeks after the onset of infection.[44,53] Cardiac involvement typically manifests itself as varying degrees of atrioventricular block. Occasionally, acute myopericarditis or mild left ventricular dysfunction are also seen.[49] The most prevalent neurological sign is facial palsy.[44,54] This is a peripheral neuritis that usually involves one side of the face. Other peripheral nerve manifestations include pain and weakness in the limb that

was bitten. The central nervous system may be involved as well, and this is termed *neuroborreliosis*. Some patients develop sleep disturbances, mild chronic confusional states, or difficulty with memory and intellectual functioning.[49] An aseptic meningitis, characterized by severe headache, photophobia, and mild elevation of spinal fluid protein, can also be seen.[13]

Late Lyme disease may develop in some untreated patients months to years after acquiring the infection.[55] The major manifestations of late Lyme disease are arthritis and late neuroborreliosis (peripheral neuropathy and encephalomyelitis). Between 50 and 60 percent of these individuals will develop brief attacks of arthritis.[44,54] This usually affects the large joints, especially the knee, and is episodic in nature. Many of these patients had earlier signs of dissemination of the organism, including secondary skin lesions and neurological signs such as stiffness of the neck. All of these usually respond well to conventional antibiotic treatment.[48] Treatment-resistant arthritis has been reported to be associated with particular human leukocyte antigen (HLA–DRB) alleles.[44] Despite resolution of objective manifestations of *Borrelia* infection after antibiotic treatment, a small percentage of patients continue to have fatigue, concentration and short-term memory problems, and musculoskeletal pain. Some of these symptoms are self-limiting and last less than 6 months, while others may last greater than 6 months.[56] There is a large body of evidence that suggests these symptoms are not due to continuing persistence of infection. The interested reader is referred to a recent article in which "post–Lyme disease syndromes" and "chronic Lyme disease" are reviewed in detail.[56]

## Nature of the Immune Response

The immune response in Lyme disease is highly variable and complex. A well-documented humoral and cellular response is known to exist. Spirochete lipoproteins also trigger production of macrophage-derived cytokines, which further enhance the immune response.[44] However, the clinical effectiveness of these responses is certainly questionable and not necessarily protective, because late Lyme disease occurs despite high levels of circulating antibody and cellular responses.

## Laboratory Diagnosis

Diagnosis of Lyme disease is a clinical one with the laboratory testing used as supporting evidence. Unfortunately, the clinical diagnosis is often difficult for reasons discussed above. If the characteristic rash is present, this can be used as a presumptive finding, but as many as 20 percent of patients do not get or do not recognize the rash. Direct isolation of the organism from skin scrapings, spinal fluid, or blood is possible, but the yield of positive cultures is extremely low. Therefore, culture is not used as a routine diagnostic tool.

The antibody response is variable and may not be detectable until 3 to 6 weeks after the tick bite. The IgM response occurs first followed by the IgG response. The IgG response does not peak until the third and fourth weeks of infection.[50,51] These antibody responses are also not mutually exclusive and can be variable (e.g., an IgM response can occur in late Lyme disease). In most cases of acute early Lyme disease (first 2 weeks), serological testing is too insensitive to be diagnostically helpful.[55] If patients with symptoms are tested in less than 7 days after infection, seropositivity is only about 30 percent.[51,57] Therefore, the decision to start treatment for early Lyme disease must be made before seroconversion, like many acute infectious diseases. However, untreated seronegative patients having symptoms for 6 to 8 weeks are unlikely to have Lyme disease, and other possible diagnoses should be pursued.[48] Antibiotic therapy begun shortly after the appearance of EM may delay or abrogate the antibody response. In chronic Lyme disease, negative serologies have been attributed to previous antibiotic therapy; however, the scientific support of this theory is not strong.[56]

The CDC currently recommends a two-tiered approach to providing laboratory support for the diagnosis of Lyme disease.[57,58] It is recommended that patients with clinical evidence of Lyme disease be screened with an IFA or EIA test. If this serology is positive or borderline, a Western blot should be performed on that specimen as supplemental testing. Under no circumstances should Lyme testing be performed in the absence of supporting clinical evidence. A positive test performed under these circumstances has only a 6 percent positive predictive value (even when done in an endemic area), while it rises to >97 percent when clinical symptoms and history are present and consistent with Lyme disease.[59] Some of the current testing procedures are discussed and compared in **Table 21–3**.

### Immunofluorescence Assay (IFA)

The IFA was the first test used to evaluate the antibody response in Lyme disease, followed by various forms of enzyme immunoassays shortly thereafter. The IFA assay is fairly easy to put together, which is why it is usually the first assay on the market in many infectious disease arenas. Basically, microscope slides are coated with antigen from whole or processed spirochetes (supplied by the manufacturer already coated), and then patient serum (in doubling dilutions) is added and allowed to react. An antihuman globulin with a fluorescent tag attached is added next and reacts with any specific antibody bound to the spirochetes on the slide. Typically, a test result is only considered positive if a titer of 1:256 is obtained,[57] although this varies between manufacturers. As mentioned above, specimens obtained in the first few weeks are usually negative, as the level of antibody present is below the detection limit of this (and other) assays.[57] As might be expected, other closely related organisms such as *B. recurrentis* (relapsing fever), *T. denticola* and others (associated with periodontal disease), and *T. pallidum* (syphilis) may cross-react and cause biological false-positive results.[45] Autoimmune connective tissue diseases such as rheumatoid arthritis and systemic lupus erythematosus can also produce false positives in the IFA assay for Lyme disease and the FTA assay for syphilis.[60] An astute technologist can recognize a false positive by the beaded fluorescent pattern it produces. Reading of fluorescent patterns tends to be very subjective and requires highly trained individuals. However, if performed correctly by experienced personnel, the test can provide sensitive and accurate results. This test is ideal for low-volume testing.

### Enzyme Immunoassay (EIA)

EIA testing is quick, reproducible (not subjective), relatively inexpensive, and lends itself well to automation and high-volume testing.[57] There are many forms of this assay based on different diagnostic philosophies that revolve around the antigen used for the assay. Antigen preparations that have been used are crude sonicates of the organism, purified proteins, synthetic proteins, and recombinant proteins. The manufacturer's selected antigen is then coated onto 96-well microtiter plates or strips by various proprietary methods. Patient sera is added and allowed to incubate with the antigen. After a washing step, antihuman globulin conjugated with an enzyme tag such as alkaline phosphatase is added to each well. Adding specific substrate produces a color change. Plates are read in a spectrophotometer, and the antibody is

| **Table 21–3.** | **Comparison of Tests for the Diagnosis of Lyme Disease** | | |
|---|---|---|---|
| **TEST** | **ANTIGEN** | **ANTIBODY** | **COMMENTS** |
| IFA | Whole or processed *B. burgdorferi* | Anti-*Borrelia* antibody from patient, antihuman globulin with fluorescent tag | Difficult to perform; false positives; subjective |
| EIA | Sonicated *B. burgdorferi* | Anti-*Borrelia* antibody from patient, antihuman globulin with enzyme tag | Easy to perform; false positives; more sensitive than IFA |
| | Purified flagellin protein | Antiflagellin antibody from patient, antihuman globulin with enzyme tag | Easy to perform; highly specific; sensitive in early Lyme disease |
| | C6 peptide | Conserved region of surface lipoprotein (VlsE) | Easy to perform; highly specific; initial studies promising; sensitive in early and late Lyme disease |
| DNA probe | Patient DNA matched to *Borrelia* DNA | None | Technically demanding, very specific; lacks sensitivity |

IFA = immunofluorescence assay; EIA = enzyme immunoassay; DNA = deoxyribonucleic acid

quantitated based on color intensity. EIAs are not subjective, and the titer is based on a continuum range rather than twofold doubling of patient's sera in the IFA. Therefore, a more accurate measurement of the specific antibody is possible.[57]

Like the IFA, drawbacks of EIA include a lack of sensitivity during the early stages of Lyme disease and specificity problems. The sensitivity for early serum specimens has been reported to be anywhere from 58 to 92 percent.[61] The differences in using various antigens is usually manifested in trade-offs between increasing sensitivity at the expense of specificity versus increasing specificity at the expense of sensitivity. Unfortunately, the technical adaptations of the EIA have not resulted in high enough sensitivity and specificity to replace the two-tier method of testing.[55] The specificity issues are generally similar to the IFA assay; however, there are no clues (beaded pattern) that a particular sample may be a false positive. Again, false positives occur with syphilis and other treponemal diseases such as yaws and periodontal disease, as well as relapsing fever and leptospirosis.[1,61] If serum is absorbed to decrease cross-reactivity, this also decreases specific Lyme antibody titers. Additionally, patients with infectious mononucleosis, Rocky Mountain spotted fever, and other autoimmune diseases have been also known to be positive with EIA.[57] Lyme disease patients do not test positive with RPR, so this may be helpful if syphilis is in the differential diagnosis.[57]

## Western Blot

**Immunoblotting,** or Western blotting, is a method that, in many systems, is a confirmatory test (e.g., HIV testing). Likewise, in Lyme disease testing, it is the second test in the CDC-recommended two-tier testing scheme.[58,62] However, the Lyme disease immunoblot is very complex **(Fig. 21–7)**

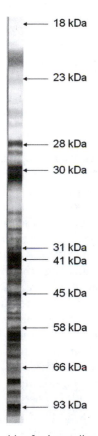

FIGURE 21–7. Immunoblot for Lyme disease.

and does not provide the same level of confidence as simpler systems such as with HIV.[63] In Lyme disease, the immunoblot is generally referred to as supplemental testing. The technique consists of electrophoresis of *Borrelia* antigens in an acrylamide gel and then transfer of the resulting pattern to nitrocellulose paper. This step is performed by the manufacturer, and nitrocellulose antigen strips are provided in the test kit. These strips are reacted with patient serum and developed with an antihuman globulin (either anti-IgG or anti-IgM) to which an enzyme label is attached. The further incubation with the enzyme's substrate allows for visualization of any antibody that has bound to a particular antigen. The reactivity is then scored and interpreted.

Ten proteins are used in the CDC-recommended interpretation of this test. They are designated by their molecular weights: 18, 23, 28, 30, 39, 41, 45, 58, 66, and 93 kDa.[58] For a result to be considered positive for presence of specific IgM antibody, two of the following bands must be present: 23(Osp C), 39, and 41 (flagellin) kDa.[64,65] An IgG immunoblot is considered positive if any 5 of the 10 bands listed above are positive.[64,65] Due to the complexity of the Lyme immunoblots, testing and interpretation of blots should be done only in qualified laboratories that follow CDC-recommended evidence-based guidelines on immunoblot interpretations.[66] As previously stated, the currently accepted testing protocol calls for a two-step approach with the use of EIA or IFA as initial screening tools. Then, if a test is equivocal or positive, it should be further tested by Western blot.[58] Current CDC recommendations do not advise testing seropositive/borderline patients for IgM antibodies if they have had symptoms for more than 4 weeks for the reasons outlined above. Serological evidence of Lyme disease in these patients is indicated by a positive result in the IgG immunoblot.[58]

### Polymerase Chain Reaction

In testing for Lyme disease, the PCR has found a niche in certain scenarios. While only a few organisms need to be present for detection under optimal conditions, the number of spirochetes in infected tissues and body fluids is low, making specimen collection, transport, and preparation of DNA critical to these clinical specimens and sensitivity an issue.[55]

Several probes for target DNA that is present only in strains of *B. burgdorferi* have been made and used in PCR testing.[55,67] The procedure involves extracting DNA from the patient sample followed by amplification using specific primers, DNA polymerase, and nucleotides. Once a sufficient amount of the unknown DNA is made, this is combined with a known DNA probe to see if hybridization takes place. The single-stranded *Borrelia* DNA probe will bind only to an exact complementary strand, thus positively identifying the presence of the organism's DNA in the patient sample. This is much more specific than testing for antibody, because there is little cross-reactivity. Specificity of recent PCR studies has ranged from 93 percent to 100. However, sensitivity remains an issue. In a series of studies, the median sensitivity of PCR on skin biopsies was 69 percent; of blood components, 14 percent; of CSF, 38 percent; and of synovial fluid, 78 percent. However, the range of sensitivities in any one type of specimen is quite large, suggesting the testing remains to be standardized.[13,55] Furthermore, it would be hard to clinically justify a skin biopsy for PCR as a diagnostic method for an EM rash in most cases.

However, in difficult diagnostic neurological and arthritic cases, PCR on CSF and synovial fluid is often employed. PCR for *Borrelia* still has limited availability.

### Treatment

*Borrelia* is sensitive to several orally administered antibiotics, including penicillins, tetracyclines, and macrolides. For adult early Lyme disease and early disseminated Lyme disease, doxycycline, cefuroxime axetil, or amoxicillin are the recommended drugs of choice.[48,49] For young children, amoxicillin and cefuroxime axetil are used, and if the child is over 8 years of age, doxycycline. Prophylaxis, full-course treatment, or serological testing of all patients with tick bites is not recommended. A single dose of doxycycline may be offered to adults and children over 8 years of age. Macrolides are not recommended as a first-line therapy for early Lyme disease, as they are less effective.[48] Under rare circumstances, an individual with a tick bite may be fully treated: (1) if the tick was identified as a nymph or adult *I. scapularis*; (2) if the tick was attached for more than 36 hours; (3) if treatment can be started within 72 hours of tick removal; (4) if the local infection rate of ticks is over 20 percent; or (5) if doxycycline is not contraindicated.[48] Neuroborreliosis requires the use of intravenous therapy. Ceftriaxone, cefotaxime, or penicillin G are the antibiotics used for this purpose.[51] Currently there are no effective vaccines for humans. A human vaccine made with the Osp-A surface antigen has had limited usefulness, has been associated with side effects, and has been recalled from the market.[68]

### SUMMARY

Syphilis and Lyme disease are the two major diseases caused by spirochetes. Spirochetes are distinguished by the presence of axial filaments that wrap around the cell wall inside a sheath and give the organisms their characteristic motility.

Syphilis is caused by the organism *Treponema pallidum*, subspecies *pallidum*. The disease is acquired by direct contact, usually through sexual transmission. The disease can be separated into four main clinical stages. An untreated patient may progress from the primary stage to the secondary stage, in which systemic dissemination of the organism occurs. The latent stage follows the disappearance of the secondary stage. Patients are usually free of clinical symptoms, but serological tests are still positive, and transmission to the fetus can occur at this stage. About one-third of the individuals who remain untreated develop tertiary syphilis. Early diagnosis and treatment help to prevent later complications.

Direct laboratory diagnosis involves detecting the organism from a lesion, using either dark-field microscopy, fluorescence microscopy, or PCR. If an active lesion is not present, diagnosis must be made on the basis of serological tests. These can be classified as either nontreponemal or treponemal. Nontreponemal tests determine the presence of reagin. The VDRL, RPR, and RST tests are examples of such tests. These are good screening tests for low-volume testing laboratories, because they are fairly sensitive and simple to perform. However, they lack specificity, and specimens with positive results must be confirmed with a more specific treponemal antibody test.

Traditional treponemal antibody tests include the FTA-ABS and particle agglutination. These detect antibody formed against the organism itself. Treponemal tests are more specific and sensitive in early stages of the disease. Titers of these antibodies remain detectable for life, while nontreponemal titers drop after successful treatment. New developments in testing include EIA technology and PCR. EIAs test for antibody to specific treponemal antigens, and class separation of antibodies is possible. For large-volume testing, the EIA is now the recommended screening test followed by confirmation with the RPR or equivalent test.

Lyme disease represents the most common vector-borne infection in the United States today. The organism responsible is a spirochete named *Borrelia burgdorferi*, which is transmitted by the deer tick. Although an expanding red rash is often the first symptom noted, the disease can be characterized as a progressive infectious syndrome involving diverse organ systems. Despite resolution of objective manifestations of *Borrelia* infection after antibiotic treatment, a small percentage of patients continue to have fatigue; concentration and short-term memory problems; and musculoskeletal pain, which, in some are self-limiting and last less than 6 months, and in others last greater than 6 months. There is a large body of evidence against these symptoms being due to continuing persistence of infection.

The presence of IgM and IgG cannot usually be detected until 3 to 6 weeks after symptoms initially appear. Current testing protocol involves screening with IFA or EIA and follow-up of equivocal or positive tests with immunoblotting. All serological findings must be interpreted carefully and in conjunction with clinical diagnosis.

# CASE STUDIES

1. A 30-year-old woman saw her physician, complaining of repeated episodes of arthritis-like pain in the knees and hip joints. She recalled having seen a very small tick on her arm about 6 months prior to the development of symptoms. No rash was ever seen, however. A blood specimen was obtained with the following results: rheumatoid arthritis—negative; lupus—negative; RPR—negative; EIA test for Lyme disease—indeterminate.

### Questions

a. Does the absence of a rash rule out the possibility of Lyme disease?

b. What might cause an indeterminate EIA test ?

c. What confirmatory testing would help in determining the cause of the patient's condition?

2. A mother who had no prenatal care appeared at the emergency room in labor. A baby boy was safely delivered, and he appeared to be normal. A blood sample was obtained from the mother for routine screening. An RPR test performed on the mother's serum was positive. The mother had no obvious signs of syphilis and denied any past history of the disease. She indicated that she had never received any treatment for a possible syphilis infection. Cord blood from the baby also exhibited a positive RPR result.

### Questions

a. Is the baby at risk for congenital syphilis?

b. What is the significance of a positive RPR on a cord blood?

c. How should these results be handled?

# EXERCISE

## RPR CARD TEST FOR SEROLOGICAL DETECTION OF SYPHILIS

### Principle

The RPR (rapid plasma reagin) 18 mm circle card test is a nontreponemal serological test for syphilis that detects reagin, an antibody formed against cardiolipin during the progress of the disease. The antigen consists of cardiolipin mixed with carbon particles, cholesterol, and lecithin. If antibody is present in the patient specimen, flocculation occurs with coagglutination of the carbon particles, resulting in black clumps against the white background of the plastic-coated card. Nonreactive specimens appear to have an even, light-gray color.

### Sample Preparation

Either plasma or serum can be used for this procedure. Collect blood by venipuncture using aseptic technique. Centrifuge the specimen at a force sufficient to sediment cellular elements. Keep the plasma or serum in the original collecting tube. Heat inactivation is not necessary for this procedure.

### Reagents, Materials, and Equipment

1. Macro-Vue 18 mm Circle Card Test Kit, which contains the following:

Antigen suspension: 0.003 percent cardiolipin, 0.020 to 0.022 percent lecithin, 0.09 percent cholesterol, EDTA (0.0125 mol/L), Na2HPO4 (0.01 mol/L), 0.1 percent thimerosal (preservative), 0.02 percent charcoal, 10 percent choline chloride (w/v), and distilled water. Refrigerate to store. Unopened ampules have a shelf life of 12 months from date of manufacture. Once opened, antigen in the dispensing bottle may be used for approximately 3 months or until the expiration date.

Brewer diagnostic cards: specially prepared plastic-coated cards designed for use with the RPR card antigen.

Dispenstirs

Needles, 20 gauge

Stirrers

Dispensing bottle

Serological pipette, 1 mL

Controls: known reactive and weakly reactive sera prepared from pooled rabbit sera and nonreactive pooled human sera. These need to be stored at 4°C and may be used until the expiration date on the label.

A rotator, 100 rpm, circumscribing a circle 2 cm in diameter with an automated timer and a cover containing a moistened sponge or blotter.

> WARNING: Because no test method can offer complete assurance that human immunodeficiency virus, hepatitis B virus, or other infectious agents are absent, specimens and these reagents should be handled as though capable of transmitting an infectious disease. The Food and Drug Administration recommends such material be handled at a Biosafety Level 2.

### Procedure*

1. Controls, RPR card antigen suspension, and test specimens should be at room temperature for use. The antigen suspension should be checked with controls using the regular test procedure. Only those suspensions that give the prescribed reactions should be used.

2. Attach the needle to the tapered fitting on the dispensing bottle.

3. To prepare the antigen suspension, vigorously shake the ampule for 10 to 15 seconds to resuspend the antigen and disperse any carbon particles lodged in the neck of the ampule. Overagitating will produce a coarse antigen, so disregard any particles left in the neck of the ampule after this time.

4. Snap the ampule neck, making sure that all the antigen is below the break line. Withdraw all the antigen into the dispensing bottle by collapsing the bottle and using it as a suction device.

5. To check the delivery of the needle, place it firmly on a 1 mL pipette. Fill the pipette with antigen suspension. Holding the pipette in a vertical position, count the number of drops delivered in 0.5 mL. This should be 30±1 drops for a yellow 20-gauge needle.

6. Hold a Dispenstir device between the thumb and forefinger near the sealed end. Squeeze and do not release until open end is below the surface of the specimen. Hold the specimen tube vertically to minimize stirring up the cellular elements when using original blood tube. Release finger pressure to draw up the sample.

7. Hold Dispenstir in a vertical position over the card test area. Do not touch the surface of the card. Squeeze, allowing one drop to fall onto card.

8. Measure out controls in the same manner.

9. Gently shake antigen-dispensing bottle before use. Hold in a vertical position, and dispense several drops into

---

* Adapted from the package insert for the Macro-Vue RPR 18 mm Circle Card Test (Brewer Diagnostic Kit), manufactured by Becton Dickinson and Company, Cockneysville, MD.

bottle cap to make sure the needle passage is clear. Place one free-falling drop onto each test or control area. Return test droplets from the bottle cap to the dispensing bottle. Do not mix antigen and specimen. Mixing is accomplished during rotation.

10. Rotate for 8 minutes, under humidifying cover, on a mechanical rotator at 100 rpm.

11. Immediately following mechanical rotation, briefly rotate by hand with tilting of the card (three to four to-and-fro motions). Read macroscopically in the "wet" state under a high-intensity incandescent lamp or strong daylight.

12. Report as reactive any specimen showing characteristic clumping, ranging from slight but definite to marked and intense. Report as nonreactive any specimen showing slight roughness or no clumping.

13. Upon completion of tests, remove the needle from the dispensing bottle and rinse with distilled or deionized water. Do not wipe the needle, because this may remove the silicon coating and affect accuracy of delivery.

> NOTE: There are only two possible reports with the card test: reactive or nonreactive, regardless of degree of activity. Any specimen demonstrating slight but definite clumping is always reported as reactive.

## Interpretation

The diagnosis of syphilis should not be made on a single reactive result without the support of a positive history or clinical evidence. As with all cardiolipin antigen tests, biological false positives are possible with a number of diseases and conditions. Therefore, reactive specimens should be subjected to further serological study, including confirmatory testing.

RPR card tests should not be used for spinal fluids. Additionally, the Public Health Service has indicated that little reliance may be placed on cord blood serological tests for syphilis.

Lipemia will not interfere with the card tests. However, if the degree of lipemia is so great that antigen particles are obscured, the specimen should be considered unsatisfactory. Hemolyzed specimens are acceptable unless they are so hemolyzed that printed material cannot be read through them.

# REVIEW QUESTIONS

1. *Treponema pallidum* and *Borrelia burgdorferi* can be distinguished from each other on the basis of which of the following?
   a. Only *T. pallidum* has axial filaments.
   b. Only *B. burgdorferi* has an outer sheath.
   c. Only *B. burgdorferi* can be grown in the laboratory on artificial media.
   d. Only *T. pallidum* stimulates IgM production to the membrane proteins.

2. False-positive nontreponemal tests for syphilis may be due to which of the following?
   a. Infectious mononucleosis
   b. Systemic lupus
   c. Pregnancy
   d. All of the above

3. In the fluorescent treponemal antibody absorption (FTA-ABS) test, what is the purpose of absorption with Reiter treponemes?
   a. It removes reactivity with lupus antibody.
   b. It prevents cross-reactivity with antibody to other *T. pallidum* subspecies.
   c. It prevents cross-reactivity with antibody to nonpathogenic treponemes.
   d. All of the above.

4. Which test is recommended for testing cerebrospinal fluid for detection of neurosyphilis?
   a. RPR
   b. VDRL
   c. FTA-ABS
   d. Enzyme immunoassay

5. Advantages of direct fluorescent antibody testing to *T. pallidum* include all of the following *except*
   a. reading is less subjective than with dark-field testing.
   b. monoclonal antibody makes the reaction very specific.
   c. slides can be prepared for later reading.
   d. careful specimen collection is less important than in dark-field testing.

6. Which of the following is true of reagin?
   a. It can be detected in all patients with primary syphilis.
   b. It is antibody directed against cardiolipin.
   c. Reagin tests remain positive after successful treatment.
   d. It is only found in patients with syphilis.

7. Which syphilis test detects specific treponemal antibodies?
   a. RPR
   b. VDRL
   c. FTA-ABS
   d. Agglutination

8. Which of the following is true of treponemal tests for syphilis?
   a. They are usually negative in the primary stage.
   b. Titers decrease with successful treatment.
   c. In large-volume testing, they should be used as screening tests.
   d. They are subject to a greater number of false positives than reagin tests.

9. An RPR test done on a 19-year-old woman as part of a prenatal workup was negative but exhibited a rough appearance. What should the technologist do next?
   a. Report the result out as negative.
   b. Do a VDRL test.
   c. Send the sample for confirmatory testing.
   d. Make serial dilutions and do a titer.

10. Treponemal EIA tests for syphilis are characterized by all of the following *except*
    a. they are adaptable to automation.
    b. they are useful in diagnosing secondary or tertiary syphilis.
    c. subjectivity in reading is eliminated.
    d. they can be used to distinguish between IgG and IgM antibodies.

11. Which of the following tests is the most specific during the early phase of Lyme disease?
    a. IFA
    b. EIA
    c. Immunoblotting
    d. Isolation of the spirochete

12. False-positive serological tests for Lyme disease may be due to all of the following *except*
    a. shared antigens between *Borrelia* groups.
    b. cross-reactivity of antibodies.
    c. resemblance of flagellar antigen to that of *Treponema* organisms.
    d. a patient in the early stage of the disease.

13. Advantages of PCR testing for syphilis include all of the following *except*

    a. it is extremely specific.
    b. many false positives are eliminated.
    c. testing of serum is extremely sensitive.
    d. it can be used on CSF.

14. A 24-year-old man who had just recovered from infectious mononucleosis had evidence of a genital lesion. His RPR test was positive. What should the technologist do next?

    a. Report out as false positive.
    b. Do a confirmatory treponemal test.
    c. Do a VDRL.
    d. Have the patient return in 2 weeks for a repeat test.

15. A 15-year-old girl returned from a camping trip. Approximately a week after her return, she discovered a small red area on her leg that had a larger red ring around it. Her physician had her tested for Lyme disease, but the serological test was negative. What is the best explanation for these results?

    a. She definitely does not have Lyme disease.
    b. The test was not performed correctly.
    c. Antibody response is often below the level of detection in early stages.
    d. Too much antibody was present, causing a false negative.

16. Which of the following is a true statement about late manifestations of Lyme disease?

    a. Treatment cannot reverse complications.
    b. Both central and peripheral nervous systems may be affected.
    c. Cardiac or neurological damage occurs in all cases.
    d. Arthritis appears only in elderly patients.

17. Problems encountered in IFA testing for Lyme disease include all of the following *except*

    a. cross-reactivity with antibodies to syphilis.
    b. false negatives in the later stages of disease.
    c. false positives with rheumatoid factor.
    d. subjectivity in the reading of fluorescent patterns.

## References

1. The spirochetes. In Forbes, BA, Sahm, DF, and Weissfeld, AS: Bailey and Scott's Diagnostic Microbiology, ed. 11. Mosby, St. Louis, MO, 2002, pp. 595–602.
2. Pope, V, Larsen, SA, and Schriefer, M. Immunological methods for the diagnosis of spirochetal diseases. In Rose, NR, et al: Manual of Clinical Laboratory Immunology, ed. 5. American Society for Microbiology, Washington, DC, 1997, pp. 510–525.
3. 2005 Syphilis surveillance project annual report (August 1, 2008) CDC. http://www.cdc.gov/STD/Syphilis2005/default.htm.
4. Centers for Disease Control and Prevention. Primary and secondary syphilis—United States, 2000–2001. MMWR 51(43): 971–973, 2002.
5. Centers for Disease Control and Prevention. Primary and secondary syphilis among men who have sex with men—New York City, 2001. MMWR 51(38):853–856, 2002.
6. Centers for Disease Control and Prevention. Outbreak of syphilis among men who have sex with men—Southern California, 2000. MMWR 50(38):117–120, 2001.
7. Symptomatic early neurosyphilis among HIV-positive men who have sex with men—four cities, United States, January 2002–June 2004. MMWR 56(25):625–628, 2007.
8. Schiff, E, and Lindberg, M. Neurosyphilis. South Med J 95:1083–1087, 2002.
9. Doherty, L, et al: Syphilis: Old problem, new strategy. BMJ 325:153–165, 2002.
10. Nicholl, A, and Hamers, FF. Are trends in HIV, gonorrhoea, and syphilis worsening in western Europe? BMJ 324:1324–1327, 2002.
11. Chen, ZQ, Zhang, GC, Gong, ZD. Syphilis in China: Results of a national surveillance program. *Lancet*:369:132–138, 2007.
12. Pope, V, Norris, SJ, and Johnson, R. Treponema and other host-associated spirochetes. In Murray, PR, et al. (eds): Manual of Clinical Microbiology, ed. 9. American Society for Microbiology, Washington, DC, 2007, pp. 987–1003.
13. LaSala, PR, and Smith, MB. Spirochete infections. In McPherson, RA and Pincus, MR (eds): Henry's Clinical Diagnosis and Management by Laboratory Methods, ed. 21. WB Saunders, Philadelphia, 2007, pp. 1059–1073.
14. Blanco, DR, Miller, JN, and Lovett, MA. Surface antigens of the syphilis spirochete and their potential as virulence determinants. Emerg Infect Dis 3:11–20, 1997.
15. Orton, S, Liu, H, Dodd, R, and Williams, A. Prevalence of circulating Treponema pallidum DNA and RNA in blood donors with confirmed-positive Syphilis tests. Transfusion 42:94–99, 2002.
16. American Red Cross. Blood donation eligibility guidelines. http://www.redcross.org/services/biomed/0,1082,0_557_,00.html. Accessed August 1, 2008.

17. Goldmeier, D, and Hay, P. A review and update on adult syphilis, with particular reference to its treatment. Int J STD AIDS 4:70–82, 1993.

18. Lukehart, SA. Syphilis. In Kasper, D, et al. (eds): Harrison's Principles of Internal Medicine, ed. 16. McGraw-Hill, New York, 2005, pp. 977–984.

19. Congenital syphilis—United States, 2000. MMWR 50:573–577, 2001.

20. CDC's Updated Plan to Eliminate Syphilis in the United States, 2006 national STD prevention conference, May 8, 2006.

21. Chhabra, RS, et al. Comparison of maternal sera, cord blood, and neonatal sera for detecting presumptive congenital syphilis: Relationship with maternal treatment. Pediatrics 91:88–91, 1993.

22. Guarner, J, et al. Testing umbilical cords for funisitis due to Treponema pallidum infection, Bolivia. Emerg Infect Dis 6:487–492, 2000.

23. Michelow, IC, et al. Central nervous system infection in congenital syphilis. N Engl J Med 346:1792–1798, 2002.

24. Pavia, CS, and Drutz, DJ. Spirochetal diseases. In Stites, DP, Terr, AI, and Parslow, TG (eds): Medical Immunology, ed. 9. 1997, pp. 739–747.

25. Larsen, SA, et al (eds): A Manual of Tests for Syphilis. American Public Health Association, Washington, DC, 1998.

26. Pope, V, et al. Comparison of the Serodia Treponema pallidum Particle Agglutination, Captia Syphilis-G, and SpiroTek Reagin II tests with standard test techniques for diagnosis of syphilis. J Clin Microbiol 38:2543–2545, 2000.

27. Van der Sluis, JJ. Laboratory techniques in the diagnosis of syphilis: A review. Genitourin Med 68:413–419, 1992.

28. Woznicova, V, and Valisova, Z. Performance of CAPTIA SelectSyph-G Enzyme-linked immunosorbent assay in syphilis testing of a high risk population: Analysis of discordant results. J Clin Microbiol 45(6):1794–1797, 2007.

29. Knight, C, Crum, M, and Hardy, R. Evaluation of the LIAI-SON chemiluminescence immunoassay for diagnosis of syphilis. Clin Vac Immunol 14:710–713, 2007.

30. Pope, V. Use of treponemal test to screen for syphilis. Infect Med 21:399–404, 2004.

31. Noordhoek, G, et al. Detection by polymerase chain reaction of Treponema pallidum DNA in cerebrospinal fluid from neurosyphilis patients before and after antibiotic treatment. J Clin Microbiol 29:1976–1984, 1991.

32. Grimprel, E, et al. Use of polymerase chain reaction and rabbit infectivity testing to detect Treponema pallidum in amniotic fluid, fetal and neonatal sera, and cerebrospinal fluid. J Clin Microbiol 29:1711–1718, 1991.

33. Palmer, H, Higgins, S, Herring, A, and Kingston, M. Use of PCR in the diagnosis of early syphilis in the United Kingdom. Sex Transm Infect 79:479–483, 2003.

34. Kouznetsov, AV, and Prinz, JC. Molecular diagnosis of syphilis: The Schaudinn-Hoffmann lymph-node biopsy. Lancet 360:388–389, 2002.

35. Woznicova, V, Votava, M, and Flasarova, M. Clinical specimens for PCR detection of syphilis. Epidemiol Mikrobiol Immunol 56:66–71, 2007.

36. Pandori, M, et al. Detection of Azithromycin resistance in Treponema pallidum by real-time PCR. Antimicrob Agents Chemother 51:3425–3430, 2007.

37. Patel, JA, and Chonmaitree, T. Syphilis screen at delivery: A need for uniform guidelines. Am J Dis Child 147:256–258, 1993.

38. Sanchez, PJ, et al. Evaluation of molecular methodologies and rabbit infectivity testing for the diagnosis of congenital syphilis and neonatal central nervous system invasion by Treponema pallidum. J Infect Dis 167:148–157, 1993.

39. Workowski, KA, and Levine, WC. Sexually transmitted diseases treatment guidelines—2002. MMWR 51(RR06):1–80, 2002.

40. Steere, A, et al. Lyme arthritis: An epidemic of oligoarticular arthritis in children and adults in three Connecticut communities. Arthritis Rheum 20:7–17, 1977.

41. Burgdorfer, W, et al. Lyme disease—A tick-borne spirochetosis? Science 216:1317, 1982.

42. Centers for Disease Control and Prevention. Lyme disease—United States, 2003–2005. MMWR 56(23):573–576, 2007.

43. Wilske, B, Johnson, B, and Schriefer, R. Borrelia. In Murray, PR, et al. (eds): Manual of Clinical Microbiology, ed. 9. American Society for Microbiology, Washington, DC, 2007, pp. 971–986.

44. Steere, AC. Lyme disease. N Engl J Med 345:115–124, 2001.

45. Magnarelli, LA, Miller, JN, Anderson, JF, and Riviere, GR. Cross-reactivity of nonspecific Treponemal antibodies in serologic tests for Lyme disease. J Clin Micro 28:1276–1279, 1990.

46. Grodzicki, RL, and Steere, AC. Comparison of immunoblotting and indirect enzyme-linked immunosorbent assay using different antigen preparations for diagnosing early Lyme disease. J Infect Dis 1988; 157(4):790–797.

47. Lane, RS, and Quistad, GB. Borreliacidal factor in the blood of the western fence lizard (Sceloporus occidentalis). J Parasitol 84:29–34, 1998.

48. Wormser, GP, Dattwyler, RJ, Shapiro, ED, et al. The clinical assessment, treatment, and prevention of Lyme disease, human granulocytic anaplasmosis, and Babesiosis: Clinical practice guidelines by the Infectious Diseases Society of America. Clin Inf Dis 43:1089–1134, 2006.

49. Steere, AC. Lyme borreliosis. In Kasper, D, et al. (eds): Harrison's Principles of Internal Medicine, ed. 16. McGraw-Hill, New York, 2005, pp. 995–998.

50. Centers for Disease Control Division of Vector-Borne Infectious Diseases. Lyme disease: Diagnosis. http://www.cdc.gov/ncidod/dvbid/lyme/ld_humandisease_diagnosis.htm. Accessed August 1, 2008.

51. Smith, RP, et al. Clinical characteristics and treatment outcome of early Lyme disease in patients with microbiologically confirmed erythema migrans. Ann Intern Med 136:421–428, 2002.

52. Hercogova, J. Review: Lyme borreliosis. Int J Dermatol 40:547–550, 2001.

53. Nadelman, RB, et al. Prophylaxis with single-dose doxycycline for the prevention of Lyme disease after an Ixodes scapularis tick bite. N Engl J Med 345:79–84, 2001.

54. Kalish, RA, et al. Evaluation of study patients with Lyme disease, 10–20 year follow-up. J Infect Dis 183:453–460, 2001.

55. Aguero-Rosenfeld, ME, Wang, G, Schwartz I, and Wormser, GP. Diagnosis of Lyme borreliosis. Clin Micro Rev 18:484–509, 2005.

56. Feder, HM, Johnson, BJ, O'Connell, S, et al. A critical appraisal of "Chronic Lyme Disease." N Engl J Med 357:1422–1430, 2007.

57. Johnson, B. Lyme disease: Serodiagnosis of Borrelia burgdorferi sensu lato infection. In Rose, NR, et al. (eds): Manual of Molecular and Clinical Laboratory Immunology, ed. 7.

American Society for Microbiology, Washington, DC, 2006, pp. 493–500.

58. Centers for Disease Control and Prevention. Recommendations for test performance and interpretation from the Second National Conference on Serological Diagnosis of Lyme Disease. MMWR 44:590, 1995.

59. Golightly, MG. Laboratory considerations in the diagnosis and management of Lyme borreliosis. Am J Clin Path 99:168–174, 1993.

60. McKenna, C, Schroeter, A, Kierland, R, et al. The fluorescent treponemal antibody absorbed (FTA-ABS) test beading phenomenon in connective tissue diseases. Mayo Clin Proc 48:545–548 1973.

61. Brown, SL, Hansen, SL, and Langone, JJ. Role of serology in diagnosis of Lyme disease. JAMA 282:62–66, 1999.

62. Pfister, HW, Wilske, B, and Weber, K. Lyme borreliosis: Basic science and clinical aspects. Lancet 343:1013–1016, 1994.

63. Golightly, MG, and Benach, J. Tick-Borne diseases. Rev Clin Micro 10(1):1–10, 1999.

64. Engstrom, SM, Shoop, E, and Johnson, RC. Immunoblot interpretation criteria for serodiagnosis of early Lyme disease. J Clin Microbiol 33:419–427, 1995.

65. Dressler, F, et al. Western blotting in the serodiagnosis of Lyme disease. J Infect Dis 167:392–400, 1993.

66. Centers for Disease Control and Prevention. Notice to readers: Caution regarding testing for Lyme disease. MMWR 54:125–126, 2005.

67. Rosa, PA, and Schwan, TG. A specific and sensitive assay for the Lyme disease spirochete Borrelia burgdorferi using the polymerase chain reaction. J Infect Dis 160:1018–1029, 1989.

68. Lyme Info. Lyme disease vaccine. http://www.lymeinfo.net/vaccine.html. Accessed August 1, 2008.

# Serology and Molecular Detection of Viral Infections

## 22

*Linda E. Miller, PhD, I,MP(ASCP)SI*

## LEARNING OBJECTIVES

*After finishing this chapter, the reader will be able to:*

1. Differentiate between the different hepatitis viruses and their modes of transmission.
2. Correlate the various serological markers of hepatitis with their diagnostic significance.
3. Indicate the laboratory methods that are most commonly used to screen for, confirm, or monitor hepatitis virus infections.
4. Associate the Epstein-Barr virus (EBV) with the specific diseases it causes.
5. Correlate the heterophile antibody and antibodies to the EBV with their clinical significance.
6. Indicate the laboratory methods used to test for heterophile antibodies and EBV antibodies.
7. List the diseases associated with varicella-zoster virus, rubella virus, rubeola virus, and mumps virus.
8. State the most common serology method used to detect antibodies to these viruses.
9. Explain how serology is used to detect current infection with or immunity to each of the preceding viruses.
10. Discuss the clinical significance of cytomegalovirus, human T lymphotropic virus type I, and human T lymphotropic virus type I.
11. Discuss the laboratory methods used to detect exposure to the preceding viruses.
12. Correlate viral IgM and IgG antibodies with their clinical significance in terms of detecting current infections, congenital infections, or immunity to infections.
13. Discuss the role of molecular tests in diagnosing and monitoring patients with viral infections.

## KEY TERMS

- Anti–HBe
- Anti–HBs
- Cytomegalovirus (CMV)
- Epstein-Barr virus (EBV)
- HBeAg
- HBsAg
- Hepatitis
- Herpes simplex virus
- Human T-cell lymphotropic virus (HTLV)
- IgM anti–HBc
- Mumps virus
- Rubella virus
- Rubeola virus
- Varicella-zoster virus (VZV)

# CHAPTER OUTLINE

## IMMUNE DEFENSES AGAINST VIRAL INFECTIONS AND VIRAL ESCAPE MECHANISMS

Viruses are submicroscopic particles, whose size is measured in nanometers. Their basic structure consists of a core of DNA or RNA packaged into a protein coat, or capsid. In some viruses, the capsid is surrounded by an outer envelope of glycolipids and proteins derived from the host cell membrane. It is remarkable that these tiny particles are capable of causing severe, and sometimes lethal, disease in humans, ranging from childhood infections, inflammatory diseases with predilection for a specific organ, disseminated disease in immunocompromised patients, cancer, and congenital abnormalities.

Viruses are obligate intracellular pathogens that rely on the host cell for their replication and survival. They infect their host cells by attaching to specific receptors on the cell surface; penetrating the host cell membrane; and releasing their nucleic acid, which then directs the host cell's machinery to produce more viral nucleic acid and proteins. These components assemble to form intact viruses that are released by lysis of the cell or by budding off the cell's surface. The free virions can then infect neighboring host cells and begin new replication cycles that promote dissemination of the infection. Viruses can thus be present in the host as both freely circulating particles and intracellular particles during the viral replication cycle. A number of immunologic mechanisms are required to attack the virus in its different states, and successful defense against viral infections requires a coordinated effort among innate immunity, humoral immunity, and cell-mediated immunity.

Innate immunity provides the first line of protection against viral pathogens. Two important nonspecific defenses against viruses involve type I interferons and NK cells.[1,2] Virus-infected cells are stimulated to produce IFN-α and IFN-β following recognition of viral RNA by Toll-like receptors (TLR). These interferons inhibit viral replication by inducing the transcription of several genes that code for proteins with antiviral activity—for example, a ribonuclease enzyme that degrades viral RNA. IFN-α and IFN-β also enhance the activity of NK cells, which bind to virus-infected cells and release cytotoxic proteins like perforin and granzymes, which cause the cells to die and release their virus particles. These cell-free virions are now accessible to antibody molecules.

When innate defenses are insufficient in preventing viral infection, specific humoral and cell-mediated defenses are activated.[1,2] Virus-specific antibodies are produced by B cells and plasma cells and can attack free virus particles in several ways. Antibodies play a key role in preventing the spread of a viral infection through neutralization. In this process, antibodies specific for a component of the virus that binds to a receptor on the host cell membrane will bind to the virus and prevent it from attaching to and penetrating the cell. Secretory IgA antibodies play an especially important role in this process, because they neutralize viruses in the mucosal surfaces (e.g., respiratory and digestive tracts), which often serve as entryways for the pathogens; meanwhile, IgM and IgG antibodies can bind to viruses in the bloodstream and inhibit dissemination of the infection. In addition, IgG antibodies promote phagocytosis of viruses through their opsonizing activity and promote destruction of viruses through antibody-dependent cell-mediated cytotoxicity (ADCC). IgG and IgM antibodies also activate complement, which can participate in opsonization via C3b or lysis of enveloped viruses by the membrane attack complex. IgM antibodies can also inactivate viral particles by agglutinating them.

While antibodies can attack viruses in many different ways, they cannot reach viruses that have already penetrated host cells. Elimination of intracellular viruses requires the action of cell-mediated immunity. Cytotoxic T cells (CTL) play a key role in this mechanism of defense. Upon activation of CD4+ T helper cells and cytokines, CD8+ CTL become programmed to expand in number and attack the virus-infected cells.[3] To recognize the virus-infected host cell, the T-cell receptor on the CTL must bind to a viral antigen complexed with MHC class I on the surface of the virus-infected host cell **(Fig. 22-1)**. CD8 is a co-receptor in this interaction. Interaction of co-stimulatory molecules, such as B7 and CD28, provides secondary signals necessary for the CTL response. These molecular interactions stimulate the granules in the CTL to release a pore-forming protein called perforin, which produces pores in the membrane of the infected host cell, and proteases called granzymes, which enter the pores. These enzymes activate apoptosis of the host cell, resulting in interruption of the viral-replication cycle and release of assembled infectious virions. The free virions can then be bound by antibodies. The CTL response is powerful and involves a series of cell divisions to produce up to 50,000 times the original number of cells in a period of 1 to 3 weeks.[3]

Despite the variety of defenses that are stimulated against viruses, the immune response is not always successful in totally eliminating these pathogens. That is because viruses have developed several strategies by which they can escape the host's defenses.[1,2] First, viruses are rapidly dividing agents that undergo frequent genetic mutations. These mutations result in the production of new viral antigens, which are not recognized by the initial immune response to the virus. This strategy is used commonly by the influenza virus, with continual antigenic variation, resulting in the emergence of new infectious strains that require annual development of new vaccines to protect the population. Antigenic variation is also employed commonly by other viruses, such as rhinoviruses, which cause the common cold, and human immunodeficiency virus (HIV), which causes AIDS.

Second, some viruses can evade the action of components of the immune system such as interferons, complement proteins, or the lysosomal enzymes in phagocytic cells. For example, the hepatitis C virus can block the degradation of viral RNA induced by the interferons.

Third, viruses can evade the host's defense by suppressing the immune system. Some viruses, like the cytomegalovirus (CMV), rubeola, and HIV, accomplish this by reducing the expression of MHC molecules on the surface of virus-infected cells, making them less likely to be recognized by T lymphocytes. Other viruses can alter the function of certain cells of the immune system after directly infecting them. For example, the **Epstein-Barr virus (EBV)** causes polyclonal activation of the B lymphocytes it infects, and HIV suppresses the function of the CD4+ T helper cells. EBV can also suppress the immune system by causing a cytokine imbalance.

Finally, some viruses, such as CMV, varicella-zoster virus, and HIV, can remain in a latent state by integrating their nucleic acid into the genome of the host cells they infect. In this way, the virus can remain silent within the host cell and is protected from the immune system, sometimes for years, before it is stimulated to replicate again by exposure to other infectious agents or by decline of the host's immune defenses.

By utilizing these mechanisms, viruses have remained successful pathogens to humans for many years, causing a range of mild to life-threatening diseases. Rapid, reliable laboratory detection of these pathogens is essential for early patient diagnosis and treatment and for prompt implementation of measures to prevent further spread of the virus to other members of the population.

## LABORATORY TESTING FOR VIRAL INFECTIONS

As our knowledge of viruses has increased, so has the development of laboratory assays to detect viral infections. While serological assays have been used for this purpose for many years, molecular assays have been developed more recently and have added much to the area of viral detection as they have been integrated into the clinical laboratory. Both serology and molecular assays have become some of the most important and frequently performed tests in clinical immunology and microbiology. Serological and molecular tests for viral infections can be easily and rapidly performed by the clinical laboratory; therefore, they play an essential role in helping physicians establish a presumptive diagnosis so that treatment may be initiated promptly. Serological tests are also important in monitoring the course of infection, detecting past infections, and assessing immune status, while molecular tests have enhanced our ability to detect active infection and are essential in guiding antiviral therapy.

In general, presence of virus-specific IgM antibodies in patient serum indicates a current or recent viral infection, while IgG antibodies to the virus signify either a current or past infection and, in most cases, immunity. Specific IgM antibody in the newborn's serum indicates a congenital infection with a virus; on the other hand, IgG antibodies in the infant's serum are mainly maternal antibodies that have crossed the placenta. Current infections in the adult or newborn may also be indicated by immunoassays for viral antigens in serum or other clinical samples from the patient

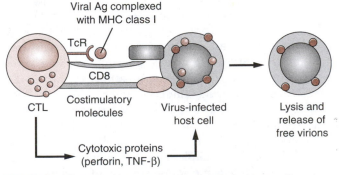

**FIGURE 22-1.** Binding of a CTL to a virus-infected host cell.

or by the presence of viral nucleic acids that molecular methods can detect.

This chapter discusses some of the most important viral infections detected by serology and molecular methods. These include the hepatitis viruses, herpes viruses, measles, mumps, rubella, and human T-cell lymphotropic viruses. Laboratory tests for the human immunodeficiency virus are discussed separately in Chapter 23.

## HEPATITIS

**Hepatitis** is a general term that means inflammation of the liver. It can be caused by several viruses and by noninfectious agents, including ionizing radiation, chemicals, and autoimmune processes. The primary hepatitis viruses, which are listed in **Table 22–1,** affect mainly the liver. Other viruses, such as cytomegalovirus, Epstein-Barr virus, and herpes simplex virus, can also produce liver inflammation, but it is secondary to other disease processes. This section will focus on the primary hepatitis viruses. The hepatitis A virus (HAV) and the hepatitis E virus (HEV) are transmitted primarily by the fecal-oral route, while the hepatitis B virus (HBV), the hepatitis D virus (HDV), and the hepatitis C virus (HCV) are transmitted mainly by the parenteral route (i.e., through contact with blood and other body fluids). All may produce similar clinical manifestations. The early, or acute, stages of hepatitis are characterized by general flulike symptoms such as fatigue, fever, myalgia, loss of appetite, nausea, vomiting, diarrhea or constipation, and mild to moderate pain in the right upper quadrant of the abdomen.[4,5]

Progression of the disease leads to liver enlargement (hepatomegaly) and tenderness, jaundice, dark urine, and light feces. Initial laboratory findings typically include elevations in bilirubin and in the liver enzymes, most notably alanine aminotransferase (ALT).[4,5] These findings are nonspecific indicators of liver inflammation and must be followed by specific serological or molecular tests to identify the cause of hepatitis more definitively. The specific laboratory tests used to detect each type of hepatitis are listed in Table 22–1.

## Hepatitis A

HAV is a nonenveloped, single-stranded ribonucleic acid (RNA) virus that belongs to the *Hepatovirus* genus of the *Picornaviridae* family.[4–6] It is responsible for an estimated 1.5 million clinical cases of hepatitis and tens of millions of HAV infections worldwide.[7] HAV is transmitted primarily by the fecal-oral route, by close person-to-person contact, or by ingestion of contaminated food or water.[4–8] Conditions of poor personal hygiene, poor sanitation, and overcrowding facilitate transmission. Rarely, transmission through transfusion of contaminated blood has been reported and may occur during a short period within the acute stage of infection when a high number of viral particles can be found in the source blood.[8]

Following an average incubation period of 28 days, the virus produces symptoms of acute hepatitis in the majority of infected adults; however, most infections in children are asymptomatic.[6,7] The infection does not progress to a chronic state and is usually self-limiting, with symptoms typically resolving within 2 months. Massive hepatic necrosis resulting in fulminant hepatitis and death are rare and occur mainly in those patients with underlying liver disease or advanced age.[6]

HAV antigens are shed in the feces of infected individuals during the incubation period and the early acute stage of infection, but they usually decline to low levels shortly after symptoms appear and are not a clinically useful indicator of disease.[7] Serological tests for antibody are therefore critical in establishing diagnosis of the infection. Acute hepatitis A is routinely diagnosed in symptomatic patients by demonstrating the presence of IgM antibodies to HAV.[4,5,7] These antibodies are most commonly detected by a solid-phase antibody-capture enzyme immunoassay (EIA) in which IgM in the patient serum is bound to anti-μ antibodies on a solid phase and detected after the addition of HAV antigen, followed by an enzyme-conjugated anti-HAV IgG.[4] IgM anti-HAV is usually detectable at the onset of clinical symptoms and declines to undetectable levels within 6 to 12 months.[4,6,7] Tests for total HAV antibodies detect predominantly IgG and are available in a competitive inhibition EIA format.[4,7] IgG antibodies persist for life, and a positive total anti-HAV in the context of a negative IgM anti-HAV indicates that the patient has developed immunity to the virus, either through natural infection or vaccination.[6] Several molecular methods have also been developed to detect HAV RNA, the most common format being reverse transcriptase polymerase chain reaction (RT-PCR).[4,9] These methods may be used for early detection of HAV in clinical samples during outbreaks of the illness but are used more commonly to detect the virus in samples of food or water suspected of transmitting the virus.[4,9]

A vaccine consisting of formalin-killed HAV was licensed in the mid-1990s to prevent hepatitis A. This vaccine has resulted in a significant decrease in the number of HAV infections in the United States, to the lowest number of cases ever recorded.[7,8] While the vaccine was originally recommended for only high-risk individuals, it is now recommended for routine immunization of children aged 12 to 23 months. It is also recommended for persons traveling to geographical areas where hepatitis A is endemic, for homosexual men, for users of illicit drugs, for persons working with HAV-infected primates or with HAV in a research laboratory, for persons who need clotting factor concentrates, and for persons with chronic liver disease.[8] Routine vaccination is not likely to be implemented by the developing world, where asymptomatic HAV infection is usually acquired during childhood and results in life-long immunity.[7] Infection with HAV may be prevented in nonimmunized individuals who have been exposed to the virus by intramuscular injection of immune globulin, a sterile preparation of pooled human plasma that contains antibodies to HAV, or by prophylactic administration of the hepatitis A vaccine.[7,8]

## Table 22–1. Summary of the Hepatitis Viruses and Their Associated Serological and Molecular Markers

| HEPATITIS VIRUS | TYPE/ FAMILY | TRANSMISSION | PROGRESSION TO CHRONIC STATE | COMPLICATIONS | SEROLOGICAL/ MOLECULAR MARKERS | CLINICAL SIGNIFICANCE |
|---|---|---|---|---|---|---|
| Hepatitis A (HAV) | RNA *Picornaviridae* | Fecal, oral | No | Low risk of fulminant liver disease | • IgM anti-HAV<br>• Total anti-HAV<br><br>• HAV RNA | • Acute hepatitis A<br>• Immunity to hepatitis A<br>• Detection of HAV in clinical, food, or water samples |
| Hepatitis B (HBV) | DNA *Hepadnaviridae* | Parenteral, sexual, perinatal | Yes | 10 to 90 percent of cases may develop chronic hepatitis (depending on age), with increased risk for liver cirrhosis and hepatocellular carcinoma | • HBsAg<br>• HBeAg<br><br>• IgM anti-HBc<br>• Total anti-HBc<br>• anti-HBe<br>• anti-HBs<br>• HBV DNA | • Active hepatitis B infection<br>• Active hepatitis B with high degree of infectivity<br>• Current or recent acute hepatitis B<br>• Current or past hepatitis B<br>• Recovery from hepatitis B<br>• Immunity to hepatitis B<br>• Acute, atypical, or occult hepatitis B; viral load may be used to monitor effectiveness of therapy |
| Hepatitis C (HCV) | RNA *Flaviviridae* | Parenteral, sexual, perinatal | Yes | Eighty-five percent develop chronic infection, with increased risk of cirrhosis, hepatocellular carcinoma, or autoimmune manifestations | • Anti-HCV<br><br>• HCV RNA | • Current or past hepatitis C infection<br>• Current hepatitis C infection; viral load may be used to monitor effectiveness of therapy; also used to determine HCV genotype |
| Hepatitis D (HDV) | RNA Genus *Deltavirus* | Mostly parenteral, but also sexual, perinatal; HBV infection required | Yes | Increased risk of developing fulminant hepatitis, cirrhosis, or hepatocellular carcinoma | • IgM-anti-HDV<br>• IgG-anti-HDV<br><br>• HDV RNA | • Acute or chronic hepatitis D<br>• Recovery from hepatitis D or chronic hepatitis D<br>• Active HDV infection; viral load may be used to monitor effectiveness of therapy |
| Hepatitis E (HEV) | RNA Hepeviridae | Fecal, oral | No | Fulminant liver failure in pregnant women | • IgM anti-HEV<br>• IgG anti-HEV<br><br>• HEV RNA | • Current hepatitis E infection<br>• Current or past hepatitis E infection<br>• Current hepatitis E infection |

## Hepatitis E

HEV is a nonenveloped, single-stranded ribonucleic acid (RNA) virus that belongs to the genus *Hepevirus*, in the family *Hepeviridae*.[4,10,11] Like HAV, it is transmitted by the fecal-oral route. Most HEV infections are related to consumption of fecally contaminated drinking water in developing regions of Africa, the Middle East, Southeast Asia, and Central Asia, all of which have poor sanitation conditions.[10,11] Infections in the United States and other industrialized countries are rare but have been reported.[12]

Following an incubation period of 3 to 8 weeks, HEV causes an acute, self-limiting hepatitis that lasts 1 to 4 weeks in most people who become infected.[4,11] Fulminant hepatitis, associated with rapidly progressing disease and a high mortality rate, occurs more commonly in pregnant women.[11,13] The reason is not totally clear, but is presumably due to changes in the immune response that occur during pregnancy. Like HAV, the infection does not progress to a chronic carrier state. There is no treatment for hepatitis E, but a recombinant vaccine to prevent the infection is currently undergoing clinical trials.[11,13]

Because HEV is not easily cultured, diagnosis of it relies on serology. Acute infection is indicated by the presence of IgM anti-HEV, which is detectable at clinical onset but declines rapidly in the early recovery period.[4,14] These antibodies are typically identified by highly sensitive enzyme immunoassays that use recombinant and synthetic HEV antigens. Specificity of the assays may be increased by testing for IgA anti-HEV along with the IgM assays.[10] In patients who are suspected of having hepatitis E but who yield a negative IgM test, molecular testing for HEV RNA can be performed, typically by RT-PCR.[4] These assays should be performed on stool samples collected within 3 weeks of clinical onset. Immunoassays for IgG anti-HEV, which persists longer, may be performed to determine previous exposure and seroprevalence of the infection.[4,14] Serological and molecular tests are available to diagnose hepatitis E in some parts of the world but are not licensed in the United States at the time of this writing.

## Hepatitis B

Hepatitis B is a major cause of morbidity and mortality throughout the world. The World Health Organization estimates that HBV has infected 2 billion people worldwide, causing 360 million chronic infections and between 500,000 and 1.2 million deaths each year due to liver disease.[15,16] The virus is highly endemic in the Far East, parts of the Middle East, sub-Saharan Africa, and the Amazon areas. In the United States, which is considered a low-prevalence area, HBV is responsible for 1.25 million chronic infections and over 5,000 deaths annually.[17]

HBV is transmitted through the parenteral route by intimate contact with HBV-contaminated blood or other body fluids, most notably semen, vaginal secretions, and saliva.[5,15,16]

Transmission has thus been associated with sexual contact, blood transfusions, sharing of needles and syringes by intravenous drug users, tattooing, and occupational needle-stick injury. Inapparent transmission of HBV may occur through close personal contact of broken skin or mucous membranes with the virus. Transmission of HBV may also occur via the perinatal route, from infected mother to infant, most likely during delivery.

Several measures have been introduced to prevent HBV infection, including screening of blood donors, treating plasma-derived products to inactivate HBV, implementing infection-control measures, and, most importantly, immunizing with a hepatitis B vaccine.[15] The first vaccine, licensed in 1982, was composed of an antigen called HBsAg (see below) that was purified from inactivated virus particles in plasma from HBV-infected donors. The current vaccines, consisting of recombinant HBsAg produced from genetically engineered yeast, are some of the most widely used vaccines throughout the world. In the United States, hepatitis B vaccine is administered to healthy infants and children as part of their routine immunization schedule and is recommended for high-risk individuals such as health-care workers, homosexual men, hemodialysis patients, persons with multiple sex partners, and infants born to HBV-infected mothers.[15,18] This immunization strategy has been highly successful, resulting in a 75 percent decline in the incidence of acute hepatitis B in the United States from 1990 to 2004.[18] The vaccine can also be administered to individuals thought to be exposed to the virus, along with HBIG (hepatitis B immune globulin), a preparation derived from donor plasma with high concentrations of antibodies to HBV, administered as a means of passive immunization to provide temporary protection.[18]

Despite the preventative measures that have been implemented, a substantial number of HBV infections continue to occur, as discussed above. Infection with HBV results in an average incubation period of 45 to 90 days, followed by a clinical course that varies in different age groups.[4,15,19] Over 90 percent of newborns with perinatal HBV infection remain asymptomatic, while typical symptoms of acute hepatitis are observed in 5 to 15 percent of children aged 1 to 5 years and in 33 to 50 percent of older children, adolescents, and adults. Symptoms may last several weeks to several months. Most HBV-infected adults recover within 6 months and develop immunity to the virus, but about 1 percent develop fulminant liver disease with hepatic necrosis, which has a high rate of fatality.

Development of chronic HBV infection, in which the virus persists in the body for 6 months or more, is independently related to age: chronic hepatitis B develops in about 10 percent of infected adults, 25 to 50 percent of young children, and 80 to 90 percent of infected infants. Chronic infection is also more likely to develop in persons who are immunosuppressed and those who have HIV.[15] Chronic infection with the virus results in inflammation and damage to the liver, and places the patient at increased risk of developing cirrhosis (seen in 20 percent of patients with chronic infection) or hepatocellular carcinoma (100 times the risk of non-HBV carriers).[20]

The virus responsible for hepatitis B, HBV, is a DNA virus belonging to the *Hepadnaviridae* family.[4,5,20,21] Eight genotypes, designated A through H, have been identified; genotype A is the predominant one in the United States and throughout the world. The intact virion is a 42 nm sphere consisting of a nucleocapsid core surrounded by an outer envelope of lipoprotein. The core of the virus contains circular partially double-stranded DNA; a DNA-dependent DNA polymerase enzyme; and two proteins, the hepatitis B core antigen and the hepatitis Be antigen (HBeAg). A protein called the *hepatitis B surface antigen (HBsAg)* is found in the outer envelope of the virus. HBsAg is produced in excess and is found in noninfectious spherical and tubular particles that lack viral DNA and circulate freely in the blood.

These antigens, or antibodies to them, serve as serological markers for hepatitis B and have been used in differential diagnosis of HBV infection, in monitoring the course of infection in patients, in assessing immunity to the virus, and in screening blood products for infectivity. The levels of these markers vary with the amount of viral replication and the host's immune response, and they are useful in establishing the initial diagnosis of hepatitis B and in monitoring the course of infection. Typical patterns of these markers during acute and chronic hepatitis B are shown in **Figures 22–2 and 22-3** and are described below.[4,5,19–21]

The hepatitis B surface antigen, or **HBsAg**, is the first marker to appear, becoming detectable 2 to 10 weeks after exposure to HBV. Its levels peak during the acute stages of infection, then gradually decline as the patient develops antibodies to the antigen and recovers. Serum HBsAg usually becomes undetectable by 4 to 6 months after the onset of symptoms in patients with acute hepatitis B. In patients with chronic HBV infection, HBsAg remains elevated for 6 months or more. HBsAg is thus an indicator of active infection and is an important marker in detecting initial infection, monitoring the course of infection and progression to chronic disease, and screening of donor blood.

The hepatitis Be antigen, or **HBeAg**, appears shortly after HBsAg and disappears shortly before HBsAg in recovering patients. It may be elevated during chronic infection.

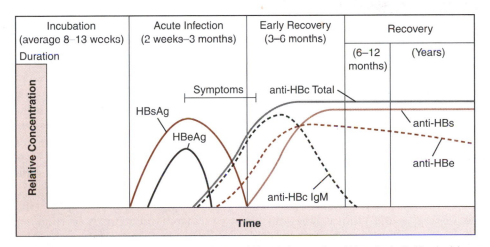

**FIGURE 22–2.** Typical serological markers in acute hepatitis B. © 2008 Abbot Laboratories, Abbot Park, IL. Used with permission.

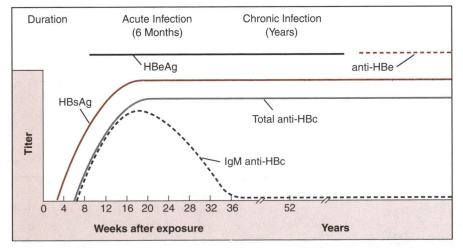

**FIGURE 22–3.** Typical serological markers in chronic hepatitis B. © 2008 Abbot Laboratories, Abbot Park, IL. Used with permission.

This marker is present during periods of active replication of the virus and indicates a high degree of infectivity. The HBcAg is not detectable in serum, because the viral envelope masks it.

As the host develops an immune response to the virus, antibodies appear. First to appear is IgM antibody to the core antigen, or **IgM anti-HBc.** This antibody indicates current or recent acute infection. It typically appears 1 to 2 weeks after HBsAg during acute infection and persists in high titers for 4 to 6 months and then gradually declines. This marker is useful in detecting infection in cases in which HBsAg is undetectable—for example, just prior to the appearance of antibodies to the antigen, in neonatal infections, and in cases of fulminant hepatitis. It is therefore used in addition to HBsAg for the screening of donor blood. IgG antibodies to the core antigen are produced before IgM anti-HBc disappears and then persist for the individual's lifetime. They are the predominant antibodies detected in the test for total anti-HBc, and they can be used to indicate a past HBV infection.

The appearance of antibodies to the HBe antigen, or **anti-HBe,** occurs shortly after the disappearance of HBeAg and indicates that the patient is recovering from HBV infection. Antibodies to HBsAg, or **anti-HBs,** also appear during the recovery period of acute hepatitis B, a few weeks after HBsAg disappears. These antibodies persist for years and provide protective immunity. Anti-HBs are also produced after immunization with the hepatitis B vaccine. Protective titers of the antibody are considered to be 10 mIU/mL of serum or higher.[15,18] Anti-HBs are not produced during chronic HBV infection, in which immunity fails to develop.

Serological markers for hepatitis B are most commonly detected by commercial immunoassays. These are available in a variety of formats, such as enzyme immunoassay and chemiluminescent immunoassay. They are typically automated to ease batch testing in the clinical laboratory, and have excellent sensitivity and specificity.[4,22] An example of an immunoassay for detecting HBsAg is shown in **Figure 22–4.** Because false-positive results can occur, any initial positive results should be verified by repeated testing of the same specimen in duplicate, followed by confirmation with an additional assay, such as an HBsAg neutralization test or by a molecular test that detects HBV DNA.

Several molecular methods have been developed to detect HBV DNA in serum or plasma and are based on target amplification, branched DNA signal amplification, hybridization, or real-time PCR.[21–25] The most sensitive of these is real-time PCR, which can detect as few as 10 copies of HBV DNA per ml.[21] HBV DNA can be detected in the serum about 21 days before HBsAg and may be a useful adjunct in detecting acute HBV infection in certain situations, such as when HBsAg test results are equivocal or in cases of occupational exposures.[21] There has been much debate about the value of testing for HBV DNA in blood donors; however, because of the marginal gain that this

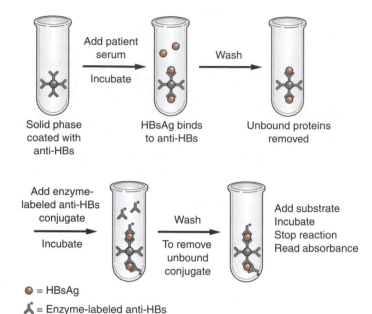

**FIGURE 22–4.** Detection of Hbs antigen by chemiluminescent microparticle immunoassay.

testing would provide over the highly sensitive HBsAg assays in place, nucleic acid testing is currently not used to screen blood donors.[26] Other uses of HBV DNA testing are to evaluate the effectiveness of antiviral therapy in patients with chronic hepatitis B, to diagnose atypical cases of hepatitis B originating from mutations in the HBV genome that cause HBsAg tests to be negative, to diagnose cases of occult hepatitis B infection in which patients are positive for HBV DNA but negative for serological markers for hepatitis B, and to determine the state of virus replication in patients with chronic infection.[20,21,27] HBV genotyping assays have also been developed. They are currently used as a research tool but may be employed in clinical settings in the future to help determine patient responsiveness to specific therapies.[4]

## Hepatitis D

Hepatitis D, also known as *delta hepatitis*, is a parenterally transmitted infection that can occur only in the presence of hepatitis B. This is because HDV is a defective virus that requires the help of HBV for its replication and expression. The only member within the *Deltavirus* genus, HDV consists of a circular RNA genome and a single structural protein called *hepatitis delta antigen* within its core, surrounded by a viral envelope that is of HBV origin and contains the HBsAg.[4,5,28,29] In low-prevalence areas, such as the United States and northern Europe, HDV is largely confined to intravenous drug users, whereas in endemic areas of the world, such as the Mediterranean basin and parts of South America and Asia, most cases appear to result from inapparent parenteral routes.[4,30]

Although about 20 million people worldwide are believed to be infected with HDV, the number of new infections appears to be declining, most likely due to the implementation of the hepatitis B vaccine.[4,5]

Hepatitis D can either occur as a co-infection with hepatitis B, in which infection of HDV and HBV occurs simultaneously, or as a superinfection, in which HDV infects individuals who are already chronic HBV carriers. Clinically, co-infections usually resemble infection with HBV alone, with most patients experiencing an acute self-limited hepatitis in which both viruses are cleared within a few months.[4,30] Only 1 to 3 percent of cases progress to a chronic state. In contrast, superinfections result in a greater risk of developing fulminant hepatitis or chronic liver disease with an accelerated progression toward cirrhosis, liver decompensation, and hepatocellular carcinoma.[4,30]

Detection of hepatitis D has been aided tremendously by the development of molecular methods to detect HDV RNA, a marker of active viral replication that is present in all types of active hepatitis D infections.[4] HDV RNA is detected by reverse-transcriptase PCR assays, which are highly sensitive, specific, and quantitative.[4,31] These assays can be used not only to detect HDV infection, but also to monitor patients during antiviral therapy.

Hepatitis D infection is also indicated by the presence of anti-HDV in the patient's serum, which can be detected by immunoassays employing hepatitis D antigen.[4,30,31] While IgM anti-HDV may be used to detect acute hepatitis D infections, its appearance may be delayed, it may persist for only a short period of time, and it may be missed.[4,5] In contrast, high titers of IgM and IgG antibodies are associated with chronic infection.[4,30]

## Hepatitis C

Hepatitis C is a major public health problem, having infected over 4 million people in the United States and over 170 million people worldwide.[5,32] It is the cause of the majority of infections previously classified as "nonA-nonB" before the discovery of HCV in 1989.[5]

Hepatitis C is transmitted mainly by exposure to contaminated blood, with intravenous drug use being the main source of infection.[5,33] Blood transfusion was also a major source of infection before 1992, when routine screening of blood donors for HCV antibody was implemented, but testing has reduced this risk to about 0.001 to 0.01 percent per unit of blood transfused.[33] Other risk factors for acquiring hepatitis C include organ transplantation before 1992, occupational exposures to contaminated blood; chronic hemodialysis; and possibly intranasal cocaine use, body piercing, and tattooing. Sexual transmission of HCV is thought to be less common but is higher in those who have had multiple sex partners or a history of sexually transmitted diseases.[5,33–35] Perinatal transmission has been estimated to occur at a rate of about 6 percent.[33,35]

HCV has an average incubation period of 7 weeks (range is 2 to 30 weeks) and produces symptoms of acute hepatitis

in only about 20 percent of cases.[5,33,35] Although the majority of infections are asymptomatic, the infection is problematic, because about 85 percent of persons develop chronic infection, which leads to cirrhosis in about 20 percent of these individuals.[33,35] Cirrhosis develops slowly, over 20 to 25 years, causing damage to the liver and posing an increased risk of developing hepatocellular carcinoma. End-stage liver disease related to HCV is now the leading cause for liver transplantation.[34–37] Patients with chronic HCV infection may also develop extra-hepatic manifestations, including mixed essential cryoglobulinemia with immune complexes containing HCV particles; glomerulonephritis, vasculitis, or other autoimmune manifestations; neuropathy; ophthalmological symptoms; and dermatologic manifestations.[33] Early detection of HCV would help in preventing these complications but occurs infrequently, due to the asymptomatic nature of the infection in most individuals. Clearance of the infection may occur spontaneously or may require treatment with antiviral drugs, the standard treatment involving a combination of pegylated interferon-α and ribavirin.[4,38,39]

HCV is an enveloped, single-stranded, positive-sense RNA virus belonging to the family *Flaviviridae* and the genus *Hepacivirus*.[4,5,33] Its genome contains an open reading frame whose 3′ end codes for the nucleocapsid core protein (C) and the envelope proteins (E1 and E2/NS1) and whose 5′ end encodes nonstructural proteins (NS2, NS3, NS4A, NS4B, NS5A, and NS5B).[4,5] Scientists have discovered six different genotypes of the virus, designated 1 through 6, and numerous subtypes for each, indicated by lowercase letters.[4,5,33] Genotype 1 is predominant in the United States. HCV has a high mutation rate, which allows it to escape the immune response and persist in the host. This has also created difficulty in developing an effective vaccine.

Because HCV is a difficult virus to culture, demonstration of the infection has relied on other laboratory methods. Both serological tests and molecular tests have been developed to identify persons with HCV infection. Serological tests are used in the screening of blood and organ donors for HCV infection and in the initial diagnosis of symptomatic patients.[4,39,40] This testing involves detection of HCV IgG antibody by third-generation enzyme immunoassays or chemiluminescent immunoassay methods, which use recombinant and synthetic antigens developed from the conserved domains of the C, NS3, NS4, and NS5 proteins.[4,41] Improvements in the serological assays for anti-HCV over the years have enabled antibodies to be detected earlier than previous methods—about 4 to 6 weeks after infection.[4,5]

While the specificity of these methods is excellent, false-positive results may occur due to cross-reactivity present in persons with other viral infections or autoimmune disorders; therefore, any positive results from an anti-HCV screening test should be confirmed.[4,39] The traditional confirmatory method was the recombinant immunoblot assay (RIBA), which detects antibodies to different HCV antigens that have been immobilized onto a nitrocellulose strip by a colorimetric reaction.[35] However, RIBA has been replaced in many laboratories by molecular methods, which are more sensitive and less labor-intensive.[5,33,36]

In recent years, detecting and monitoring HCV infection have been significantly improved by the implementation of molecular tests. Molecular assays that detect HCV RNA have been developed as qualitative and quantitative tests. Qualitative tests distinguish between the presence or absence of HCV RNA in a clinical sample and are used to confirm infection in HCV-antibody-positive patients, to detect infection in antibody-negative patients who are suspected of having HCV, to screen blood and organ donors for HCV, and to detect perinatal infections in babies born to HCV-positive mothers.[36] The most commonly used qualitative method is reverse transcriptase polymerase chain reaction (RT-PCR), but a highly sensitive transcription mediated amplification (TMA) test has recently been developed as well.[36] These tests can detect HCV infection within 1 to 3 weeks after exposure—much earlier than serological methods.[36,37]

Quantitative tests are performed by RT-PCR, real-time PCR, or branched DNA amplification (bDNA).[36,42] They are used to monitor the amount of HCV RNA, or "viral load," carried by patients before, during, and after antiviral therapy in chronically infected individuals. The ultimate goal of such therapy is to achieve a sustained virological response (SVR), in which the patient continuously tests negative for HCV RNA 6 months after therapy is completed.[36,38] The initial viral load level has also been used as a prognostic tool, since those with a low initial viral load are most likely to achieve an SVR.[36,43]

Another type of molecular assay for HCV is the genotyping test, which determines the exact genotype and subtype of the virus responsible for the patient's infection. Genotyping tests are ideally performed by sequence analysis, although other methods, including a subtype-specific RT-PCR and a line-probe assay have also been developed for this purpose.[4,36] It is important to determine the patient's HCV genotype in order to determine optimal treatment in terms of the dose of antiviral drugs administered and the duration of therapy. Studies have shown that patients with genotypes 1 and 4 require more aggressive treatment, with higher doses of antiviral drugs administered for a longer period of time, in contrast to patients with genotypes 2 and 3, who are more likely to reach an SVR with a shorter course of treatment using lower drug doses.[36–38] In the future, molecular tests will most likely play an important role in evaluating the effectiveness of new antiviral drugs in eradicating this devastating virus.

## Viruses with Uncertain Association with Hepatitis

During the 1990s, researchers discovered two additional viruses in the sera of patients with hepatitis who were not infected with any of the well-characterized hepatitis viruses described above.[4,44–46] These viruses, termed *hepatitis G virus*

(*HGV*, also known as *GB virus type C* or *GBV-C*) and *torquetenovirus* (*TTV*, also known as *transfusion-transmitted virus*), are prevalent throughout the world in persons with or without clinical hepatitis, but their role as etiologic agents of hepatitis remains under debate.[4,47–49]

HGV is an enveloped, single-stranded RNA virus in the *Flaviviridae* family.[4,48] It is transmitted by the bloodborne route, perinatal route, and possibly through sexual contact. Detection of the virus has been based primarily on RT-PCR methods, which amplify HGV RNA.[4,50] Serology tests based on EIA have also been developed and, like RT-PCR, are used largely as a research tool.[4,50] Studies indicate that antibodies to the HGV envelope protein E2 may be associated with recovery from hepatitis G infection.

TTV is a single-stranded non-enveloped DNA virus belonging to the genus *Annellovirus*.[4,49] Parenteral transmission of the virus through contaminated blood has been clearly evidenced, and presence of the virus in stool, bile, and saliva, suggest transmission by the fecal-oral and respiratory routes as well. Detection of TTV is performed by PCR, primarily for research purposes.[4,51] The selection of primers for the PCR is especially important in influencing the test results, since the virus has a tremendous amount of genetic diversity, with over 30 different genotypes discovered. To date, there are no validated serological tests to detect antibody to TTV.[4,49]

## HERPES VIRUS INFECTIONS

The herpes viruses are large, complex DNA viruses that are surrounded by a protein capsid, an amorphous tegument, and an outer envelope.[52,53] These viruses are all capable of establishing a latent infection with lifelong persistence in the host. The *Herpesviridae* family includes eight viruses that can cause disease in humans: the herpes simplex viruses (HSV-1 and HSV-2); varicella-zoster (also known as *human herpes virus-3* or *HHV-3*); the Epstein-Barr virus (HHV-4); cytomegalovirus (HHV-5); and the human herpes viruses 6, 7, and 8 (HHV-6, HHV-7, and HHV-8), the latter of which has been associated with Kaposi's sarcoma. This chapter covers clinical manifestations and laboratory diagnosis of some of these viruses.

### Epstein–Barr Virus

The Epstein-Barr virus (EBV) causes a wide spectrum of diseases, including infectious mononucleosis, lymphoproliferative disease, and several malignancies.[54–56] EBV infections most commonly result from intimate contact with salivary secretions from an infected individual. While transmission of the virus can occur through other mechanisms, such as blood transfusions, bone marrow and solid organ transplants, sexual contact, and perinatal transmission, these routes appear to be much less frequent.[54–57]

In developing nations of the world and lower socioeconomic groups living under poor hygiene conditions, EBV infections usually occur during early childhood, whereas in industrialized nations with higher standards of hygiene, infections are typically delayed until adolescence or adulthood. However, by adulthood, more than 90 percent of individuals have been infected, as evidenced by the presence of EBV antibodies in their serum.

EBV selectively infects host cells that are positive for the CD21 molecule, which serves as a receptor for both the virus and the C3d protein of complement.[53,55] The virus initially infects epithelial cells in the oropharynx, where it enters a lytic cycle, characterized by viral replication, lysis of host cells, and release of infectious virions until the acute infection is resolved.[54] The virions also infect B lymphocytes, which spread the virus throughout the lymphoreticular system. The virus-infected B cells become polyclonally activated, proliferating and secreting a number of antibodies, including EBV-specific antibodies; heterophile antibodies; and autoantibodies such as cold agglutinins, rheumatoid factor, and antinuclear antibodies.[54-56] In healthy individuals, this process is kept in check by the immune response of natural killer cells and specific cytotoxic T cells. However, EBV can persist in the body indefinitely in a small percentage of B cells, in which it establishes a latent infection. Periodic reactivation of the virus results in viral shedding into the saliva and genital secretions, even in healthy, asymptomatic individuals.[54-56]

Several antigens have been identified in EBV-infected cells that are associated with different phases of the viral infection, and antibodies to these antigens have become an important diagnostic tool.[54-56] Antigens produced during the initial stages of viral replication in the lytic cycle are known as the *early antigens (EA)*. These antigens can be further classified into two groups based on their location within the cells: EA-D, which has a diffuse distribution in the nucleus and cytoplasm, and EA-R, which is restricted to the cytoplasm only. The late antigens of EBV are those that appear during the period of the lytic cycle following viral DNA synthesis. They include the viral capsid antigens (VCAs) in the protein capsid and the membrane antigens in the viral envelope. Antigens appearing during the latent phase include the EBV nuclear antigen (EBNA) proteins, EBNA-1, EBNA-2, EBNA-3A, EBNA-3B, EBNA-3C, and EBNA-LP, and the latent membrane proteins (LMPs), LMP-1, LMP-2A, and LMP-2B (Table 22-2).

The clinical manifestations of EBV vary with the host's age and immune status. Infections in infants and young children are generally asymptomatic or mild, while primary infections in healthy adolescents or adults commonly result in infectious mononucleosis (IM).[55-59] More than half of patients with IM present with three classic symptoms: fever, lymphadenopathy, and sore throat. Other symptoms, including splenomegaly, hepatomegaly, and periorbital edema, may also be seen. Symptoms usually last for 2 to 4 weeks, but fatigue, myalgias, and need for sleep can persist for months. Although these symptoms are essential in diagnosing IM,

| Table 22-2. | Epstein-Barr Virus Antigens | |
|---|---|---|
| **EARLY ACUTE PHASE** | **LATE PHASE** | **LATENT PHASE** |
| EA-R (early antigen restricted) | VCA (viral capsid antigen) | EBNA (EBV nuclear antigens) |
| EA-D (early antigen diffuse) | MA (membrane antigen) | EBNA-1, -2, -3A, -3B, -3C, -LP |
| | | Latent membrane proteins (LMP-1, -2A, -2B) |

they can also be caused by many other infectious agents, so laboratory testing plays an important role in differentiating IM from other infections.

Characteristic laboratory findings in patients with IM include an absolute lymphocytosis of greater than 50 percent of the total leukocytes and at least 10 percent atypical lymphocytes (which are predominately activated cytotoxic T cells).[55,58,59,60] Serological findings include presence of a heterophile antibody and antibodies to certain EBV antigens.

By definition, heterophile antibodies are antibodies that are capable of reacting with similar antigens from two or more unrelated species. The heterophile antibodies associated with IM are IgM antibodies produced as a result of polyclonal B-cell activation and are capable of reacting with horse red blood cells, sheep red blood cells, and bovine red blood cells. These antibodies are produced by 40 percent of patients with IM during the first week of clinical illness and by up to 90 percent of patients by the fourth week.[55] They disappear in most patients by 3 months after the onset of symptoms but can be detected in some patients for up to 1 year.[55] Because the heterophile antibody is present in most patients during the acute phase of illness, testing for this antibody is typically performed as a screening test for IM in patients who present with symptoms of the disease.

For many years, the heterophile antibody of IM was detected by a rapid slide agglutination method called the "Monospot," which tested the ability of serum absorbed with guinea pig kidney or beef erythrocyte antigens to agglutinate horse red blood cells. The antibody could then be titered by incubating serial dilutions of the patient's serum with sheep red blood cells in the Paul-Bunnell test. These methods have been replaced today by rapid latex agglutination tests or solid phase immunoassays using purified bovine red blood cell extract as the antigen. Studies have shown that the sensitivity of these kits varies from 71 to 95 percent in adults but is significantly lower in children under 12 years (25 to 50 percent).[59] The specificity of the kits ranges from 82 to 99 percent, depending on the assay.[59] False-positive results, although uncommon, can occur in patients with lymphoma, viral hepatitis, malaria, and autoimmune disease.[55]

Negative heterophile antibody results occur in about 10 percent of adult patients with IM and up to 50 percent of children less than 12 years old.[59] In these patients, who demonstrate symptoms of IM but are negative for the heterophile antibody, further testing for EBV-specific antibodies is indicated.[54,55,59] These antibodies are most often detected by indirect immunofluorescence assays (IFA) using EBV-infected cells or ELISA techniques using recombinant or synthetic EBV proteins.[54,59] While both methods have a high level of sensitivity (95 to 99 percent), IFA tests have a higher level of specificity and are considered the "gold standard" of EBV serology methods. However, many laboratories prefer ELISA tests, because they are less time-consuming and easier to interpret.[54] More recently, methods employing chemiluminescence-based detection of the antibodies have also become available.[58,61] IgM antibody to the VCA is the most useful marker for acute IM, because it usually appears at the onset of clinical symptoms and disappears by 3 months.[54,55] IgG anti-VCA is also present at the onset of IM but persists for life and can thus indicate a past infection. Antibodies to EA-D are also seen during acute IM, and anti-EBNA appears during convalescence.[54,55] A summary of serological responses during acute, convalescent, and post-IM is shown in **Table 22–3.**

Some individuals develop chronic active EBV infection, with severe, often life-threatening IM-associated symptoms that persist or recur for months after the acute illness.[60,62] In addition, EBV has been associated with several malignancies, both hematologic (e.g., Burkitt's lymphoma and Hodgkin's disease) and nonhematologic (e.g., nasopharyngeal carcinoma and gastric carcinoma).[55,58,60] EBV can also cause lymphoproliferative disorders in immunocompromised patients, including central nervous system lymphomas in patients with AIDS, X-linked lymphoproliferative disease in males with a rare genetic mutation, and post-transplant lymphoproliferative disorders (PTLD) in patients who have received hematopoietic stem cell or solid organ transplants.[55,60,63] These disorders result from the inability of immunosuppressed patients to control primary EBV infection, leading to massive polyclonal expansion of the EBV-infected B cells and life-threatening illness with a high rate of mortality. EBV-associated malignancies can be diagnosed with the help of serology tests for EBV antibodies, immunohistochemical tests to detect EBV antigens in tissue biopsies, and molecular methods to detect EBV DNA in blood and tissue samples.[54,55,60,63,64] Typical patterns of EBV antibodies seen in some of these disorders are shown in Table 22–3. Molecular tests may be more reliable than serology in immunocompromised patients who may not demonstrate a good humoral response, and they are also useful in monitoring viral load in patients with EBV-related malignancies who are undergoing therapy.

## Cytomegalovirus

**Cytomegalovirus (CMV)** is a ubiquitous virus with worldwide distribution. Nearly all persons have been exposed by their elderly years, but communal living and poor personal hygiene facilitate spread earlier in life.[65,66] CMV is spread through close, prolonged contact with infectious body secretions; intimate sexual contact; blood transfusions; solid organ transplants; and perinatally, from infected mother to infant. The virus has been isolated in saliva, urine, stool, vaginal and cervical secretions, semen, breast milk, and blood.[65–67]

Primary, or initial, infections in healthy individuals are usually asymptomatic but result in a self-limiting, heterophile antibody-negative IM-like illness with fever, myalgias, and fatigue in a small percentage of cases.[66,67] An immune response against the virus is stimulated, but the virus persists in a latent state in monocytes, dendritic cells, myeloid progenitor cells, and peripheral blood leukocytes and may be reactivated at a later time in the individual's life.[68]

| Table 22–3. | Serological Responses of Patients with Epstein-Barr Virus–Associated Diseases | | | | | | |
|---|---|---|---|---|---|---|---|
| | **ANTI-VCA** | | | **ANTI-EA** | | | |
| **CONDITION** | **IgM** | **IgG** | **IgA** | **EA–D** | **EA–R** | **ANTI–EBNA** | **HETEROPHILE ANTIBODY (IgM)** |
| Uninfected | – | – | – | – | – | – | – |
| IM | + | ++ | ± | + | – | – | + |
| Convalescent IM | – | + | – | – | ± | + | ± |
| Past infection IM | – | + | – | – | – | + | – |
| Chronic active infection IM | – | +++ | ± | + | ++ | ± | – |
| Post-transplant lymphoproliferative disease | – | ++ | ± | + | + | ± | – |
| Burkitt's lymphoma | – | +++ | – | ± | ++ | + | – |
| Nasopharyngeal carcinoma | – | +++ | + | ++ | ± | + | – |

Adapted from Straus, SE, et al. Epstein-Barr virus infections: Biology, pathogenesis, and management. Ann Intern Med 118:45, 1993, with permission.
VCA = viral capsid antigen; EA = early antigen; EBNA = EBV nuclear antigen; IM = infectious mononucleosis

The clinical consequences of CMV infection are much more serious in the immunocompromised host, most notably organ-transplant recipients and patients with AIDS. CMV is the most important infectious agent associated with organ transplantation, with infections resulting from reactivation of CMV in the recipient or transmission of CMV from the donor.[66,67,69] CMV infection of a previously unexposed recipient from the donor organ poses a high risk for symptomatic disease, which can induce a variety of syndromes (e.g., fever and leukopenia, hepatitis, pneumonitis, gastrointestinal complications, and retinitis) and is associated with an increased risk for allograft failure. While combination antiretroviral therapy has reduced the incidence of CMV-related illness in patients with HIV infection, CMV remains a major opportunistic pathogen in patients with low CD4+ T cell counts, causing retinitis or disseminated disease involving the liver, lungs, gastrointestinal tract, or central nervous system.[66,68]

CMV is also the most common cause of congenital infections, occurring in approximately 1 percent of all neonates.[67,70,71] Transmission of the virus may occur through the placenta, by passage of the infant through an infected birth canal, or by postnatal contact with breast milk or other maternal secretions.[66] About 10 percent of infants with congenital CMV infection are symptomatic at birth.[71] Mothers who acquire primary CMV infection during their pregnancy have a significantly higher risk of giving birth to a symptomatic or severely affected infant than do women in whom CMV was reactivated during pregnancy. Symptomatic infants present with a multitude of symptoms that reflect platelet dysfunction and central nervous system involvement, including petechiae, jaundice, hepatosplenomegaly, and neurological abnormalities such as microcephaly and lethargy, with an associated mortality rate of about 5 percent.[65,67,71] Over one-half of the surviving infants will develop clinical sequelae, such as hearing loss, visual impairment, and mental retardation, in their early childhood years. While 90 percent of infants with congenital CMV infection are asymptomatic at birth, about 10 percent of these will develop sensorineural hearing loss that is slowly progressive during the first 5 to 10 years of life, and a smaller percentage may develop other abnormalities such as neuromuscular defects and chorioretinitis.[67,71]

Several laboratory methods have been developed to detect CMV infection, including viral culture, viral antigen assays, molecular assays, and serology. Isolation of the virus in culture, or demonstration of CMV antigens or DNA from appropriate clinical specimens, are the preferred diagnostic methods.[66,68] For example, the standard reference method for detecting congenital CMV infection is to isolate the virus from the urine or saliva of the neonate within 3 weeks of birth.[67,68] The traditional method of viral culture involves observing characteristic cytopathic effects (CPE) in human fibroblast cell lines inoculated with CMV-infected specimens. While this method provides definitive results when positive, it is limited, because CPE do not appear until a few days to several weeks after inoculation, depending on the viral titer. Implementation of the rapid centrifugation-enhanced (shell

vial) method has reduced the time of detection to 16 to 72 hours after inoculation.[72] This assay is an immunofluorescence method that uses monoclonal antibodies to detect immediate early CMV antigens in infected cells grown on coverslips in shell vials. Detection of the CMV lower matrix protein pp65 in CMV-infected leukocytes in the peripheral blood or cerebral spinal fluid by immunocytochemical or immunofluorescent staining has allowed for more rapid diagnosis and treatment of CMV infection in immunocompromised patients.[66,68,73]

Highly sensitive molecular methods are increasingly being used to detect CMV infection in conjunction with, or as an alternative to, culture methods.[68] PCR amplification of CMV DNA has been extremely useful for detecting CNS infections in immunodeficient hosts, for detecting CMV in amniotic fluid, and for establishing the diagnosis of CMV infection in transplant recipients.[67,72,74] Quantitative PCR, which detects CMV copy number in the peripheral blood, is used to monitor the effectiveness of antiviral treatment in immunocompromised hosts and to identify patients at risk for developing disseminated CMV disease.[67,68,74] The usefulness of this assay in predicting prognosis in congenital CMV infections is being investigated.[67,72]

While serology tests for CMV have been commercially available for many years, their clinical utility is limited. The serology methods performed most commonly are semi- or fully automated enzyme immunoassays (EIAs) that employ microtiter plates or microparticle systems.[68] Assays for CMV IgG are most useful in documenting a past CMV infection in healthy individuals, such as blood and organ donors, in order to reduce post-transfusion/post-transplant primary CMV infection in sero-negative recipients.[68] A fourfold rise in antibody titers of serial serum specimens in persons older than 6 months of age suggests a recent infection,[50,51] but rapid detection of infection is not possible by this process. Assays for IgM CMV antibodies have been developed but are limited in value because of the potential for false-negative results in newborns and immunocompromised patients and for false-positive results due to other infections or the presence of rheumatoid factor.[50-52] In addition, IgM antibodies may not necessarily indicate primary CMV infection, because they can also be produced as a result of CMV reactivation and may persist for up to 18 months.[47,50] Serological methods that use recombinant antigens to detect CMV antibodies of different avidities are being developed in an attempt to increase the sensitivity and specificity of tests for CMV disease.[47,51] Because of the limitations of serology testing, direct methods of detecting CMV infection are essential.

## Varicella–Zoster Virus

The **varicella-zoster virus (VZV)** is the cause of two distinct diseases: varicella, more commonly known as *chickenpox*, and herpes zoster, or shingles. The virus is transmitted primarily by inhalation of infected respiratory secretions or aerosols from skin lesions associated with the infection; transplacental transmission to the fetus may also occur.[75-77]

Primary infection with VZV results in chickenpox (i.e., varicella), a highly contagious illness characterized by a blisterlike rash with intense itching and fever.[75–78] Historically, the majority of varicella cases have occurred during childhood. In a typical infection, vesicular lesions first appear on the face and trunk, then spread to other areas of the body. Over a period of hours to a few days, the skin lesions evolve from maculopapules to fluid-containing vesicles and finally break down to form a scab. The illness is usually mild and self-limiting in healthy children but may in some cases produce complications, the most common of which are secondary bacterial skin infections due to scratching of the lesions. Primary infections in adults, neonates, or pregnant women tend to be more severe, with a larger number of lesions and a greater chance of developing other complications such as pneumonia. Varicella infection in pregnant women may also cause premature labor or congenital malformations if the infection is acquired during the first trimester of pregnancy or may cause severe neonatal infection if transmission of the virus occurs around the time of delivery.[75–78] Infections in immunocompromised patients are more likely to result in disseminated disease, with extensive skin rash, neurological conditions (e.g., encephalitis), pneumonia, or hepatitis.[75–78]

During the course of primary infection, VZV is thought to travel from the skin to the sensory nerve endings to the dorsal ganglion cells, where it establishes a latent state.[78] Reactivation of the virus occurs in 15 to 30 percent of persons with a history of varicella infection, probably as a result of a decrease in cell-mediated immunity; the number of cases increases with age or development of an immunocompromised condition.[79] Reactivation results in the virus moving down the sensory nerve to the dermatome supplied by that nerve, resulting in eruption of a painful vesicular rash known as herpes zoster, or shingles, in the affected area.[77–79] The rash may persist for weeks to months and is more severe in immunocompromised and elderly individuals. A significant number of patients with herpes zoster develop complications, the most common being postherpetic neuralgia, characterized by debilitating pain that persists weeks, months, or even years after resolution of the infection.[77,79] Life-threatening complications such as herpes ophthalmicus leading to blindness, pneumonia, and visceral involvement are more common in immunosuppressed persons.

In 1995, a vaccine consisting of a strain of live, attenuated varicella virus was licensed in the United States for use in children aged 12 months or older, adolescents, and adults. Implementation of the vaccine has resulted in a significant decline in the incidence of chickenpox and its associated complications.[77,80] However, breakthrough cases of varicella in vaccinated persons have been reported.[77,81] Although most patients experience mild illness, they are still contagious, and some individuals may experience more severe disease. This has prompted the CDC to recommend adding a booster dose of the vaccine to routine childhood immunization schedules.[77] In 2005, a vaccine was licensed for use in healthy children that combines the varicella vaccine with that for measles, mumps, and rubella.[77] In addition, a single-agent VZV vaccine was licensed in 2006 for prevention of herpes zoster in persons aged 60 or older, presumably by boosting the immune response.[79,82] Because these vaccines all contain a live agent, they are not recommended for use in immunocompromised persons. These patients should receive an antiviral drug or injections of varicella immune globulin within 96 hours after exposure to the virus.[77]

When varicella was commonplace in the United States, diagnosis of the disease was based primarily on clinical findings, and laboratory testing was usually unnecessary. Because the incidence of varicella has decreased as a result of immunization, laboratory diagnosis has become an increasingly important tool in recognizing the infection when it does occur.[83] Definitive diagnosis is based on identifying VSV or one of its products in skin lesions, tissue, or vesicular fluids. Rapid identification of the virus can be performed by microscopic examination of smears made from the base of the vesicles and stained with hematoxylin-eosin, Wright-Giemsa, toluidine blue, or Papanicolaou's stain to reveal multinucleated giant cells called *Tzanck cells;* however, this procedure cannot distinguish between VZV and **herpes simplex virus (HSV)**.[83,84] Culture of the virus and observation of characteristic CPE may be performed in a number of cell lines but is time-consuming and may not yield productive results if clinical specimens do not contain sufficient infectious virus.[83] Direct immunofluorescence staining of scrapings from vesicular lesions with monoclonal antibodies directed against VZV antigens provides a more rapid and sensitive means of detecting the virus.[83] The most accurate and sensitive method of detecting the infection is through the use of PCR to detect VZV DNA from clinical specimens.[83] PCR using cerebral spinal fluid is also helpful in detecting VZV in atypical manifestations of the infection involving the central nervous system.[85]

Serology testing is of limited use in detecting current infections, because accurate detection requires demonstration of a fourfold rise in antibody titer between acute and convalescent samples, a process that takes 2 to 4 weeks to perform.[75,83] In addition, testing for VZV IgM is not performed routinely for several reasons: IgM antibodies to VZV may not be detectable until the convalescent stage of illness, they cannot distinguish between primary and reactivated infection, and they may not be free of IgG antibodies when serum is processed for testing.[83,84]

Serology is most useful in determining immunity to VZV in individuals such as health-care workers and in identifying VSV-susceptible persons in outbreak settings who may benefit from prophylactic treatment.[83] Therefore, most serology tests detect total VZV antibody, which consists primarily of IgG. Several methods have been developed for this purpose. Rapid tests for point-of-care testing include latex agglutination and membrane-based EIAs. While these have good sensitivity, the latex bead method may be prone to false-positive results.[83] The most sensitive and reliable method of detecting VZV antibody is a fluorescent test called FAMA (fluorescent antibody to membrane antigen) that detects antibody to the envelope glycoproteins of the virus.[83] While FAMA is considered to be the reference method for VZV antibody, it requires live, virus-infected cells and is not suitable for large-scale routine testing. An ELISA method that detects an antibody to a highly purified solution of a VZV envelope glycoprotein has been developed and has a sensitivity and specificity comparable to FAMA.[83,86] This method is more sensitive than older ELISA methods that employ a whole antigen extract and is likely to be useful in clinical settings.

## VIRAL INFECTIONS OF CHILDHOOD

### Rubella

The **rubella virus** is a single-stranded, enveloped RNA virus of the genus *Rubivirus*, belonging to the family *Togaviridae*.[87–90] It is transmitted through respiratory droplets or through transplacental infection of the fetus during pregnancy.

This virus is the cause of the typically benign, self-limited disease that is also known as *German measles*. Prior to widespread use of the rubella vaccine, this was mainly a disease of young children. However, today it occurs most often in young, unvaccinated adults.[87,91] Following an incubation period of 12 to 23 days, the virus replicates in the upper respiratory tract and cervical lymph nodes, then travels to the bloodstream. It produces a characteristic erythematous, maculopapular rash, which appears first on the face, then spreads to the trunk and extremities and usually resolves in 3 to 5 days.[87–89] In adolescents and adults, this is usually preceded by a prodrome of low-grade fever, malaise, swollen glands, and upper respiratory infection lasting 1 to 5 days. However, up to 50 percent of rubella infections are asymptomatic.[72,88] The infection usually resolves without complications. A significant number of infected adult women experience arthralgias and arthritis, but chronic arthritis is rare.[87] Other clinical manifestations, including encephalitis, thrombocytopenia with hemorrhage, and neuritis, are infrequent.[87]

Rubella infection during pregnancy may have severe consequences, including miscarriage, stillbirth, or congenital rubella syndrome (CRS).[87–89,92] The likelihood of severe consequences increases when infection occurs earlier in the pregnancy, especially during the first trimester. Infants born with CRS may present with a number of abnormalities, the most common of which are deafness; eye defects, including cataracts and glaucoma; cardiac abnormalities; mental retardation; and motor disabilities. In mild cases, symptoms may not be recognized until months to years after birth.

A vaccine consisting of live, attenuated rubella virus was developed with the primary goal of preventing infection of pregnant women by preventing dissemination of the virus in the population as a whole.[88,93] The vaccine is part of the routine immunization schedule in infants and children and is usually given in combination with vaccines for measles and mumps (measles/mumps/rubella [MMR] vaccine) and possibly with varicella (MMRV). Following licensure of the

vaccine in 1969, the number of rubella infections and cases of CRS in the United States has dropped dramatically, with only limited outbreaks occurring, mostly among unvaccinated young immigrants to this country.

Laboratory testing is helpful in confirming suspected cases of German measles, whose symptoms may mimic those of other viral infections. It is essential in the diagnosis of CRS and in the determination of immune status in other individuals. Rubella virus can be grown in cultures inoculated with respiratory secretions or other clinical specimens; however, growth is slow and may not produce characteristic cytopathic effects upon primary isolation, requiring at least two successive subpassages.[72,89,90] Demonstration of the virus may also be accomplished by its ability to interfere with the growth of another virus added to the culture and by neutralization of this effect with specific rubella antibody; however, this method is also time-consuming and labor-intensive. For these reasons, viral culture is not routinely used to diagnose rubella infections, and serological testing is the method of choice.[72,89,90]

Several methods have been developed to detect rubella antibodies, including hemagglutination inhibition (HI), passive hemagglutination, complement fixation, latex agglutination, and immunoassays.[72,90] Although HI was once the standard technique for measuring rubella antibodies, the most commonly used method today is the ELISA because of its sensitivity, specificity, ease of performance, and adaptability to automation.[72,88,90] More specific solid-phase capture ELISAs can be used to detect IgM rubella antibodies. Newer immunoassays to detect rubella antibodies employ methods such as chemiluminescence and immunofluorescence and can be run on autoanalyzers.[90,94] EIAs that use dried venous blood spots or oral fluid samples have also been developed and may be useful in the diagnosis of CRS, especially in resource-poor countries.[95,96]

Serology tests can be used in both the diagnosis of rubella infections and in screening for rubella immunity. IgM and IgG antibodies to rubella appear as the rash of German measles begins to fade.[90] IgM antibodies generally decline by 4 or 5 weeks but may persist in low levels for a year or more in some cases.[72] IgG antibodies provide immunity and persist for life. Primary rubella infection is indicated by the presence of rubella-specific IgM antibodies or by a fourfold rise in rubella-specific IgG antibody titers between acute- and convalescent-phase samples.[87,88,90] Presence of IgG antibodies indicates immunity to rubella as a result of natural infection or immunization. An antibody level of 10 to 15 IU/mL is considered to be protective.[72]

While IgM assays have a high level of sensitivity and specificity,[90,94] false-positive results can occur in individuals with other viral infections, heterophile antibody, or rheumatoid factor, and in some cases, IgM titers may persist long after primary infection or immunization.[72,88] It has therefore been recommended that positive IgM results, particularly in pregnant women, be confirmed by a more specific test, such as an enzyme immunoassay that measures the avidity of rubella IgG antibodies, in order to distinguish between recent and past rubella infections.[72,97,98] In these assays, low antibody avidity indicates a recent infection, while high avidity is seen in past infections, reflecting the normal change in antibody avidity during the course of an immune response.

Laboratory diagnosis of congenital rubella infection begins with serological evaluation of the mother's antibodies and measurement of rubella-specific IgM antibodies in fetal blood, cord blood, or neonatal serum, depending on the age of the fetus/infant. To enhance the reliability of a CRS diagnosis, any positive IgM results should be confirmed by viral culture; by demonstration of persistently high titers of rubella IgG antibodies after 3 to 6 months of age; or, more commonly now, by reverse transcription and PCR-amplification of rubella nucleic acid (RT-PCR).[72] RT-PCR is a highly sensitive and specific aid in prenatal or postnatal diagnosis and can be used to detect rubella RNA in a variety of clinical samples, including chorionic villi, placenta, amniotic fluid, fetal blood, lens tissue, products of conception, pharyngeal swabs, spinal fluid, or brain tissue.[72,90,99]

## Rubeola

The **rubeola virus** is a single-stranded RNA virus belonging to the genus *Morbillivirus* in the *Paramyxoviridae* family.[89,100,101] It is spread by direct contact with aerosolized droplets from the respiratory secretions of infected individuals.

Rubeola virus is the cause of the disease commonly known as *measles*. Following an incubation period of about 10 to 12 days, the virus produces prodromal symptoms of fever, cough, coryza (runny nose), and conjunctivitis, which last 2 to 4 days.[89,100,101] During the prodromal period, characteristic areas known as *Koplik spots* appear on the mucous membranes of the inner cheeks or lips; these appear as gray-to-white lesions against a bright red background and persist for several days. The typical rash of measles appears about 14 days after exposure to the virus and is characterized by an erythematous, maculopapular eruption that begins on the face and head and spreads to the trunk and extremities, and lasts 5 to 6 days.

Measles is a systemic infection that can result in complications. These are most common in adults, children less than 5 years of age, and immunocompromised persons, and include diarrhea, otitis media, croup, bronchitis, pneumonia, and encephalitis.[89,100,101] Rarely, a fatal degenerative disease of the central nervous system, called *subacute sclerosing panencephalitis* (SSPE), can result from persistent replication of measles virus in the brain, with onset of symptoms typically appearing 7 to 10 years after primary measles infection.[101,102] Measles infection during pregnancy results in a higher risk of premature labor, spontaneous abortion, or low birth weight, but unlike rubella, it is not associated with a defined pattern of congenital malformations in the newborn.[101]

The incidence of measles has been greatly reduced in developed nations of the world since the introduction of a live, attenuated measles virus vaccine. A vaccine consisting of killed rubeola virus was originally licensed in 1963 but

was ultimately ineffective. A more effective vaccine consisting of live, attenuated rubeola virus was licensed in 1968 and is used in the routine immunization schedule of infants and children, either in combination with rubella and mumps (MMR) or in combination with rubella, mumps, and varicella (MMRV).[101] Recommended administration of the vaccine is in two doses, the first between the ages of 12 and 15 months and the second between ages 4 to 6. Administration of the first dose prior to the age of 12 months may result in vaccine failure, because the presence of maternal antibodies can interfere with the infant's immune response. Although measles continues to be a global concern, immunization against rubeola has resulted in a significant decrease in the number of cases in the United States, with most cases resulting from failure to immunize infants and young children due to religious or other reasons, or from cases brought into the United States by unvaccinated individuals from other countries.[101]

The diagnosis of measles has typically been based on clinical presentation of the patient. However, this basis for diagnosis has been complicated by physicians' decreased ability to recognize the clinical features of measles due to the reduction in the number of measles cases as a result of our immunization program.[89,101,103] In addition, atypical presentations of measles can occur in individuals who received the earlier form of measles vaccine, who have low antibody titers, or who are immunocompromised.[89,100,101] Laboratory tests are therefore of value in ensuring rapid, accurate diagnosis of sporadic cases; in addition, they are important for epidemiological surveillance and control of community outbreaks.[89,101,103]

Isolation of rubeola virus in conventional cell cultures is technically difficult and slow and is not generally performed in the routine diagnosis of measles, but it may be useful in epidemiological surveillance of measles virus strains.[101,103] The optimal time to recover measles virus from nasopharyngeal aspirates, throat swabs, or blood is from the prodrome period up to 3 days after rash onset. From urine, it is 1 week after appearance of the rash.[89,101]

Serological testing provides the most practical and reliable means of confirming a measles diagnosis.[89,101,103] In conjunction with clinical symptoms, a diagnosis of measles is indicated by the presence of rubeola-specific IgM antibodies or by a fourfold rise in the rubeola-specific IgG antibody titer between serum samples collected soon after the onset of rash and 10 to 30 days later.[101] SSPE is associated with extremely high titers of rubeola antibodies.[100,103] IgM antibodies are preferentially detected by an IgM capture ELISA method, which is highly sensitive and has a low incidence of false-positive results.[89,101] IgM antibodies become detectable 3 to 4 days after appearance of symptoms and persist for 8 to 12 weeks.[103] Samples collected before 72 hours may yield false-negative results, and repeat testing on a later sample is recommended in that situation.[101]

A variety of methods have been developed to detect IgG rubeola antibodies, including hemagglutination inhibition, microneutralization, plaque reduction neutralization, complement fixation, indirect fluorescent antibody tests, and

ELISA. The most commonly used is ELISA.[89,101,103] IgG antibodies become detectable 7 to 10 days after the onset of symptoms and persist for life.[103] Presence of rubeola-specific IgG antibodies indicates immunity to measles due to past infection or immunization.[89,103] Testing for IgG antibodies is therefore routinely performed by clinical laboratories in order to detect immune status of individuals such as health-care workers to the virus.

Molecular methods to detect rubeola RNA can be used in cases in which serological tests are inconclusive or inconsistent and can be used to genotype the virus in epidemiological studies.[103,104] The preferred molecular technique is reverse transcriptase PCR (RT-PCR), performed by traditional or real-time PCR methodologies. These assays are sensitive, can be performed on a variety of clinical samples or on infected cell cultures, and can detect viral RNA within 3 days of rash appearance.[103]

## Mumps

The **mumps virus,** like rubeola, is a single-stranded RNA virus that belongs to the *Paramyxoviridae family* (genus *Rubulavirus*). It is transmitted from person to person by infected respiratory droplets and possibly fomites, and replicates initially in the nasopharynx and regional lymph nodes.[103-108] Following an average incubation period of 14 to 18 days, the virus spreads from the blood to various tissues, including the meninges of the brain, salivary glands, pancreas, testes, and ovaries, producing inflammation at those sites.[106] Inflammation of the parotid glands, or parotitis, is the most common clinical manifestation of mumps, occurring in 30 to 40 percent of cases.[106] The swelling of parotitis results in earache and tenderness of the jaw, which can be bilateral or unilateral and resolves in 7 to 10 days.[105,106] Although parotitis is the classic symptom of mumps, about 20 percent of infections are asymptomatic, and another 40 to 50 percent have nonspecific or respiratory symptoms with no parotitis.[106]

Complications of mumps infections include asymptomatic meningitis (50 to 60 percent of cases); symptomatic meningitis (10 to 30 percent of cases); testicular inflammation, or orchitis (20 to 50 percent of postpubertal males); ovarian inflammation (in about 5 percent of postpubertal females); and deafness (in about 1 case per 20,000).[105-107] Prior to routine immunization, mumps was one of the most common causes of aseptic meningitis and sensorineural deafness in children.[106] Infrequent but important complications of mumps include pancreatitis, encephalitis, myocarditis, polyarthritis, and thrombocytopenia.[65,105-107] Mumps infection in pregnant women results in increased risk for fetal death when it occurs in the first trimester of pregnancy, but it is not associated with congenital abnormalities.[109] The number of mumps cases in the United States has declined significantly since the introduction of a live attenuated mumps virus vaccine in 1967 and its routine use in childhood immunization schedules in 1977.[107,109,110] The vaccine is most commonly combined with the vaccines for rubella and mumps (MMR) or is used in combination with the rubella, mumps, and varicella vaccines (MMRV).

The diagnosis of mumps is usually made on the basis of clinical symptoms, especially parotitis, and does not require laboratory confirmation.[89,105-107] However, laboratory testing is very useful in cases in which parotitis is absent or when differentiation from other causes of parotitis is required. Within the first few days of illness, mumps virus can be isolated from saliva, urine, cerebrospinal fluid, or swabs from the area around the excretory duct of the parotid gland. It can then be grown in shell vial cultures of rhesus monkey kidney cells or human embryonic lung fibroblasts and identified by staining with fluorescein-labeled monoclonal antibodies.[103,105] However, culture methods require experienced personnel and specialized reagents and may not be performed in the routine clinical laboratory.

Reverse transcriptase polymerase chain reaction (RT-PCR) methods have been developed to detect viral RNA in specimens collected from the buccal cavity, throat, cerebral spinal fluid, or urine of patients with a suspected mumps infection.[103,108,111] These methods have not been standardized but may be useful in confirming infection in cases where viral isolation is not successful.[103]

Serological testing provides the most simple and practical means of confirming a mumps diagnosis, when indicated.[89,103,106] Although a variety of methods have been developed to detect mumps antibodies, including complement fixation, hemagglutination inhibition, hemolysis in gel, neutralization assays, immunofluorescence assay, and ELISA, the latter two methods are used most commonly, because they are sensitive, specific, cost-effective, and readily performed by the routine clinical laboratory.[103,106] Use of solid-phase IgM capture assays reduces the incidence of false-positive results due to rheumatoid factor. Current or recent infection is indicated by the presence of mumps-specific IgM antibody in a single serum sample or by at least a fourfold rise in specific IgG antibody between two specimens collected during the acute and convalescent phases of illness.[103,105,106,108] Cross-reactivity between antibodies to mumps and related paramyxoviruses has been reported in tests for IgG but is usually not a problem because of differentiation in clinical symptoms.[89,103] IgM antibodies can be detected within 3 to 4 days of illness and can persist for at least 8 to 12 weeks.[103] IgG antibodies become detectable within 7 to 10 days and persist for years. The presence of specific IgG antibodies indicates immunity to mumps, either as a result of natural infection or immunization. In the United States, most serology tests for mumps are performed to evaluate immune status in health-care workers or in recipients of the mumps vaccine.[103]

## HUMAN T-CELL LYMPHOTROPIC VIRUSES

**Human T-cell lymphotropic virus** type I (HTLV-I) and human T-cell lymphotropic virus type II (HTLV-II) are closely related retroviruses. These viruses have RNA as their nucleic acid and an enzyme called *reverse transcriptase,* whose function is to transcribe the viral RNA into DNA. The DNA then becomes integrated into the host cell's genome as a provirus. The provirus can remain in a latent state within infected cells for a prolonged period of time. Upon activation of the host cell, the provirus can proceed to complete its replication cycle to produce more virions. Both HTLV-I and HTLV-II infect T lymphocytes, especially those that are CD4+, that cause T-cell proliferation, and that have the potential to establish persistent infection. HTLV-II can infect macrophages as well.[112]

Both viruses have three structural genes, called *gag, pol,* and *env,* and two major regulatory genes, called *tax* and *rev.*[113–115] The gag gene codes for the viral core proteins, the pol gene codes for the reverse transcriptase enzyme, and the env gene codes for the envelope glycoproteins.

HTLV-I and HTLV-II can be transmitted by three major routes: bloodborne (mainly through transfusions containing cellular components or through intravenous drug abuse), sexual contact, and mother-to-child (mainly through breastfeeding).[112–117] HTLV-I infection is endemic in southern Japan, the Caribbean islands, South and Central Africa, the Middle East, parts of South America, and Melanesia.[112–117] In the United States and Europe, infections result mainly from immigrants from endemic areas. HTLV-II infections are highest in various Native American populations and in intravenous drug abusers in North America and Europe.[112]

HTLV-I is associated with both malignant and nonmalignant disorders that have inflammatory or proliferative characteristics.[112–117] Most notably, infection with HTLV-I may lead to the development of adult T-cell leukemia/lymphoma (ATL), a spectrum of T-cell malignancies that can be classified into four different subtypes: acute, chronic, smoldering, and lymphoma type. The risk of developing ATL is highest in those who acquired the infection prior to adulthood, with the disease typically appearing at least 20 years after initial infection.[112,116] HTLV-I infection has also been associated with a 2 percent lifetime risk of developing a progressive neurological disorder called *HTLV-associated myelopathy/tropical spastic paraparesis (HAM/TSP),* a 2.5 percent risk of developing an intraocular inflammation of the eyes called *HTLV uveitis,* a greater risk of developing HTLV-I-associated sicca syndrome characterized by dry eyes and dry mouth, and an infective dermatitis in children associated with severe eczema.[112–117]

HTLV-II infection is thought to be associated with less severe disease, including a chronic encephalomyelopathy similar to HAM/TSP, various forms of generalized neurological dysfunction, recurrent bladder and kidney infections, fungal infections, and pneumonia.[112,118]

Serological testing plays an important role in detecting HTLV-I and HTLV-II infections, because culture of the viruses requires sophisticated techniques that cannot be performed in routine clinical laboratories. ELISA tests for HTLV-I and HTLV-II antibodies are used initially to detect HTLV infections in individuals and to screen blood donors.[112,117] These tests use a combination of HTLV-I and HTLV-II gag and env proteins as the source of antigen bound to a solid phase. Because false-positive results may also occur, any sample producing a reactive result in the initial ELISA screen is retested by ELISA and subsequently tested by a more specific, confirmatory method.

The confirmatory method of choice is the Western blot, which identifies antibodies to separate HTLV antigens. Specimens are considered positive for HTLV-I or HTLV-II by this test if bands representing antibodies to the gag protein p24 and the env glycoproteins of either virus are present.[112,114,117] Samples that are reactive by ELISA but negative by Western blot should be tested by the more sensitive radioimmunoprecipitation assay (RIPA).[112] PCR can be used to detect HTLV-I or HTLV-II RNA in various samples in order to clarify repeatedly indeterminate results, demonstrate the presence of virus in different tissues, and determine viral load in monitoring disease progression.[112,114]

## OTHER VIRAL INFECTIONS

See **Table 22–4** for laboratory methods used to detect infections with other viruses and their clinical significance.

## SUMMARY

Viruses are obligate intracellular parasites that can produce a wide range of diseases in humans. Viruses can exist as either free infectious virions or intracellular particles after they have infected host cells. These different states require the combined effort of innate, humoral, and cell-mediated immune responses to successfully defend the host against viral infections. Important innate defenses are carried out by interferons, which inhibit the replication of viruses, and NK cells, which release cytotoxic proteins that destroy virus-infected host cells. Antibodies directed against specific viral antigens can prevent the spread of viral infection in several ways: Antibodies can neutralize a virus and prevent it from binding to host cells, can opsonize a virus to make it more likely to be phagocytized, can activate complement-mediated mechanisms of destruction, and can agglutinate viruses. Cell-mediated immunity is required to eliminate intracellular viruses. This is accomplished by virus-specific CTL, which binds to virus-infected host cells and releases cytotoxic proteins that cause the cells to undergo apoptosis.

Despite these immunologic mechanisms, the immune system is not always successful in eliminating a viral pathogen from the host, because viruses have evolved several ways of evading the host's defenses. Many viruses accomplish this by undergoing frequent genetic mutations, which result in the production of new viral antigens that are not recognized by previous host responses. Some viruses can evade the action of interferons, complement, or other components of the immune system, or can cause suppression of the immune system by different means. Finally, some viruses are capable of integrating their nucleic acid into the host's genome and remaining inside the host cells

## Table 22–4. Laboratory Tests for Diagnosis of Other Viral Infections

| VIRUS | MODES OF TRANSMISSION | DISEASE ASSOCIATIONS | LABORATORY TESTS |
|---|---|---|---|
| Adenoviruses | Respiratory or fecal-oral | Febrile acute respiratory disease, gastroenteritis, myocarditis, pericarditis, keratoconjunctivitis, hemorrhagic cystitis | • Culture and confirmation with group-specific fluorescent-labeled antibodies<br>• Rapid methods to detect viral antigen or nucleic acid<br>• Serological tests to detect antibodies to human adenoviruses (EIA, IIF); a fourfold rise in antibody titer is diagnostic |
| Arbovirus | Arthropod-borne | Encephalitis | • IgM capture ELISA is preferred method for diagnosis; IIF also available<br>• Serum neutralization test used to confirm other serological test results<br>• Antigen capture ELISA used to detect current infection<br>• Immunohistochemical staining, in situ hybridization, and nucleic acid amplification tests also available |
| Herpes simplex (HSV) | HSV-1: close personal contact, perinatal<br>HSV-2: sexual, perinatal | HSV-1: gingivostomatitis, conjunctivitis, keratitis, herpetic whitlow, encephalitis<br>HSV-2: genital tract infection | • Diagnosis made by viral culture of swabs taken from mucocutaneous lesions and direct immunofluorescence for herpes antigens<br>• Serological tests require a significant rise in antibody titer to indicate current infection (EIA, indirect hemagglutination, immunoblotting, IFA, NT available)<br>• PCR for HSV nucleic acid is the method of choice for detecting active infection |
| Influenza | Inhalation of airborne droplets; contact with respiratory secretions | Respiratory illness, pneumonia | • Identification of influenza virus can be made by fluorescent antibody staining of viral antigens in epithelial cells from respiratory tract specimens by direct IFA, rapid immunoassays to detect influenza antigens in clinical samples, or culture of nose and throat swabs<br>• Serological tests (e.g., HI, EIA, microneutralization) can indicate infection by a fourfold rise in antibody titer when direct virus detection is not successful<br>• RT-PCR can be used to monitor genetic and antigenic characteristics of circulating strains |

*Continued*

| Table 22-4. | Laboratory Tests for Diagnosis of Other Viral Infections—Cont'd | | |
| --- | --- | --- | --- |
| **VIRUS** | **MODES OF TRANSMISSION** | **DISEASE ASSOCIATIONS** | **LABORATORY TESTS** |
| Parainfluenza | Inhalation of airborne droplets; contact with respiratory secretions | Respiratory illness, croup | • Virus isolation can be accomplished by culture of respiratory secretions in cell lines; nasal washes are the specimen of choice<br>• Rapid detection of virus antigens can be made by direct IFA or EIA using respiratory secretions or middle-ear effusions<br>• RT-PCR can be used to detect viral RNA in respiratory secretions<br>• Serological assays (e.g., ELISA, NT, direct IFA, IIF, CF, HI) can be used to assess immune status; recent infection is indicated by a four-fold rise in antibody titer |
| Parvovirus B19 | Respiratory route, blood transfusions, perinatal | Fifth disease, red cell aplasia in immunocompromised hosts, congenital anemia, hydrops fetalis, spontaneous abortion | • IFA, RIA, and ELISA used to detect B19 antigen and anti-B19 antibody<br>• B19 nucleic acid can be detected by PCR or in situ hybridization using tissues or cells |
| Respiratory syncytial virus (RSV) | Contact with respiratory secretions | Acute respiratory infection, bronchiolitis, pneumonia, croup | • Virus isolation can be accomplished by culture of respiratory secretions in cell cultures; nasal washes are the specimen of choice<br>• Rapid detection of virus antigens can be made by direct IFA or EIA using respiratory secretions or middle-ear effusions<br>• RT-PCR can be used to detect viral RNA in respiratory secretions<br>• Serological assays (e.g., ELISA, NT, direct IFA, IIF, CF, HI) can be used to assess immune status; recent infection is indicated by a four-fold rise in antibody titer |
| Rotavirus | Fecal-oral | Gastroenteritis, diarrhea | • EIA is used to detect rotavirus antibody and for serotyping<br>• EIA and latex agglutination can be used for detection of group A rotavirus antigen in fecal samples<br>• RT-PCR can detect rotavirus RNA |

CF = complement fixation; CNS = central nervous system; DNA = deoxyribonucleic acid; EIA = enzyme immunoassay; IFA = immunofluorescence assay; HI = hemagglutination inhibition; IIF = indirect immunofluorescence; NT = neutralization test; PCR = polymerase chain reaction; RNA = ribonucleic acid; RT-PCR = reverse transcriptase polymerase chain reaction; RIA = radioimmunoassay.

in a silent state for long periods of time before being reactivated at a later date.

Serological tests for viral antibodies are among the most important tests performed by the clinical immunology laboratory. These tests can be used to indicate current infections, congenital infections, and previous exposure to viruses or the vaccines used to prevent viral infections with subsequent immunity. Molecular methods have played an increasingly important role in the diagnosis and management of viral infections in recent years. These tests provide a sensitive means of rapidly detecting viral infections and of quantitating viral load to guide patient therapy. This chapter discussed the serological and molecular methods used by the clinical laboratory in the diagnosis and management of some of the most important viral infections.

The hepatitis viruses are those whose primary effect is inflammation of the liver. Hepatitis A and E are transmitted by the fecal-oral route, while hepatitis B, C, D, and G are transmitted primarily by the parenteral route. Hepatitis B, C, and D may lead to chronic infections. Serologic markers of hepatitis infections consist of virus-specific antibodies and antigens which are commonly detected by automated immunoassays. IgM anti-HAV antibodies indicate current or recent hepatitis A infection, while IgG antibodies indicate immunity to hepatitis A. Hepatitis B infection is indicated by the presence of the antigen HBsAg; HBeAg indicates high infectivity. IgM antibodies to hepatitis B core antigen are present in acute hepatitis B, while IgG anti-HBc is present during past or chronic hepatitis B infection. Antibodies to HBsAg can be present as a result of past hepatitis B infection or immunization with the hepatitis B vaccine and indicate immunity. Exposure to hepatitis C can be detected by ELISA measuring anti-HCV, with molecular tests being used to confirm infection in antibody-positive patients, to detect infection in antibody-negative patients, to detect perinatal infections, and to screen blood and organ donors for HCV. Hepatitis D occurs as a super- or co-infection with hepatitis B and is indicated by antibodies to hepatitis D or molecular tests to detect HDV RNA. Serological and molecular tests for hepatitis E have been developed but are not widely available.

There are eight human herpes viruses, including the Epstein-Barr virus, cytomegalovirus, and varicella-zoster virus. The Epstein-Barr virus is the cause of infectious mononucleosis, several hematologic and nonhematologic malignancies, and lymphoproliferative disorders in immuno-suppressed individuals. Most patients with infectious mononucleosis produce heterophile antibodies, which can react with antigens from beef, horse, or sheep red blood cells. Although these antibodies were once routinely screened for by the Monospot test, they are now commonly detected by rapid immunochromatographic or agglutination methods used to detect antibodies to bovine antigens. ELISA or immunofluorescence assay (IFA) tests for EBV-specific antigens are used to detect heterophile-negative cases of infectious mononucleosis and to diagnose other EBV-associated diseases. Molecular tests are useful in detecting EBV DNA in immunocompromised patients who may not develop a good antibody response and in monitoring viral load in patients with EBV-related malignancies during therapy.

CMV infection is asymptomatic in most healthy individuals but may produce a mononucleosis-like syndrome in some. The virus can remain latent for years and become reactivated later in life. CMV infection can have more serious consequences in immunocompromised individuals or congenitally infected infants. Active CMV infection is best detected by shell vial assays to identify CMV antigens by immunofluorescence, by CMV antigenemia assays for pp65

antigen, or by molecular assays to detect CMV viral load. Quantitative PCR is useful in determining the CMV DNA copy number in immunocompromised hosts undergoing antiviral treatment. Serological assays for CMV antibody are most helpful in documenting a past infection in potential blood and organ donors.

Primary infection with varicella virus causes chickenpox (varicella), while reactivation of the virus in nerve cells supplying the skin causes shingles (zoster). Diagnosis of current varicella virus infection is usually based on clinical findings, but detection of varicella virus antigens by shell vial assay and immunofluorescence or of varicella DNA by PCR may be helpful in some clinical settings. Serological methods, most commonly ELISA, are used mainly to document immunity to varicella virus.

Immunization programs have greatly reduced the incidence of three childhood infections: rubella, rubeola, and mumps. Rubella infection is the cause of German measles but can result in severe congenital abnormalities if it occurs during pregnancy. Rubeola viruses cause measles, a systemic infection that can cause complications in some individuals. Mumps virus is the cause of mumps, whose classic feature is swelling of the parotid glands; complications may occur. Although the diagnosis of these three infections is usually based on clinical findings, laboratory testing may be helpful in confirmation. Because culture of these viruses is slow and difficult, serology is most often used for this purpose. Current infections are indicated by the presence of IgM antibodies specific for the appropriate virus or by a fourfold rise in virus-specific IgG antibodies in two separate specimens collected during the acute and convalescent phases of disease. However, testing for IgG antibodies is most commonly performed to screen for immunity to these viruses. RT-PCR is a useful adjunct to serology in detecting viral RNA in patients with inconclusive serology or viral culture results, in epidemiological studies, and in the detection of congenital rubella infections.

The human T-cell lymphotropic viruses, HTLV-I and HTLV-II, are retroviruses that infect T lymphocytes. HTLV-I is the cause of adult T-cell leukemia/lymphoma, HTLV-I-associated myelopathy/tropical spastic paraparesis (HAM/TSP), and other inflammatory disorders. HTLV-II is thought to be associated with a HAM/TSP-like disease and several other disorders of neurological dysfunction. ELISA tests are used routinely to screen blood donors for antibodies to HTLV-I and HTLV-II and to detect exposure to HTLV in other individuals. Positive results are confirmed by Western blot. RIPA or PCR can be used to clarify indeterminate results.

Serological and molecular tests have also been developed to detect exposure to other viruses, including adenoviruses, arbovirus, herpes simplex-1 and -2, parainfluenza, parvovirus B19, respiratory syncytial virus, and rotavirus.

# CASE STUDIES

**1.** A 25-year-old male had been experiencing flulike symptoms, loss of appetite, nausea, and constipation for 2 weeks. His abdomen was tender, and his urine was dark in color. Initial testing revealed elevations in his serum alanine aminotransferase (ALT) and aspartate aminotransferase (AST) levels.

## Questions

a. What laboratory tests should be used to screen this patient for viral hepatitis?

b. If the patient tested positive for hepatitis B, which tests should be used to monitor his condition?

c. If the patient developed chronic hepatitis B, which markers would be present in his serum?

**2.** A 5-pound infant was born with microcephaly, purpuric rash, low platelet count, cardiovascular defects, and a cataract in the left eye. The infant's mother recalled experiencing flulike symptoms and a mild skin rash early in her pregnancy. She had not sought medical attention at the time. The infant's physician ordered tests to investigate the cause of the newborn's symptoms.

## Questions

a. What virus is the most likely cause of the infant's symptoms?

b. What laboratory tests would you suggest the doctor order on the mother to support your suggested diagnosis?

c. What tests should be performed on the infant's serum to support this diagnosis?

# EXERCISE

## TESTING FOR THE HETEROPHILE ANTIBODY OF INFECTIOUS MONONUCLEOSIS BY THE CLEARVIEW MONO® TEST*

A rapid test for the qualitative detection of infectious mononucleosis (IM) heterophile antibodies in whole blood, serum, and plasma for professional in vitro diagnostic use only.

### Intended Use

The Clearview Mono test is a rapid chromatographic immunoassay for the qualitative detection of infectious mononucleosis heterophile antibodies in whole blood, serum, or plasma to aid in the diagnosis of infectious mononucleosis.

### Summary

Infectious mononucleosis is caused by the Epstein-Barr virus, which is a member of the herpesvirus family. Symptoms of IM are fever, sore throat, and swollen lymph glands. In very rare cases, heart or central nervous system problems may occur. Diagnosis of IM is made based on the presence of heterophile antibodies. Infectious mononucleosis heterophile antibodies belong to the IgM class. They are present in 80 to 90 percent of acute IM cases and can be detected in 60 to 70 percent of patients during the first week of clinical illness.

The Clearview Mono test is simple and utilizes an extract of bovine erythrocytes to qualitatively and selectively detect IM heterophile antibodies in whole blood, serum, or plasma in just minutes.

### Principle

The Clearview Mono test is a qualitative, membrane-strip-based immunoassay that detects IM heterophile antibodies in whole blood, serum, or plasma. In this test procedure, bovine erythrocyte extracted antigen is coated on the test-line region of the device. The sample reacts with bovine erythrocyte extracted antigen-coated particles that have been applied to the label pad. This mixture migrates chromatographically along the length of the test strip and interacts with the coated bovine erythrocyte extracted antigen. If the sample contains IM antibodies, a colored line will appear in the test-line region, indicating a positive result. If the sample does not contain IM heterophile antibodies, a colored line will not appear in this region, indicating a negative result. To serve as a procedural control, a colored line will always appear at the control-line region, indicating that proper volume of specimen has been added and membrane wicking has occurred.

### Reagents

The test device contains bovine erythrocyte extracted antigen-coated particles and bovine erythrocyte extracted antigen-coated membrane.

### Sample Collection and Preparation

The Clearview Mono test can be performed using whole blood (from venipuncture or fingerstick), serum, or plasma.

### Materials Provided

Test devices

Disposable sample droppers

Disposable heparinized capillary tubes and dispensing bulbs

Positive control (diluted human plasma containing IM heterophil antibodies, 0.09 percent sodium azide)

Negative control (diluted human plasma, 0.09 percent sodium azide)

Sample buffer

Package insert

### Materials Required But not Provided

Sample-collection container (for venipuncture whole blood)

Lancet (for fingerstick whole blood only)

Centrifuge (for serum or plasma only)

Timer

### Procedure

Allow the test device, sample, buffer, and controls to reach room temperature (15°C to 30°C) before testing.

1. Remove the test device from the foil pouch and use it as soon as possible. For best results, perform the test immediately after opening the foil pouch.

2. Place the test device on a clean and level surface. (See **Fig. 22–5** for a diagram illustrating the procedure.)

**For whole blood (venipuncture) samples:** Hold the dropper upright and add two drops of whole blood (about 50 μL) to the sample well (S) of the test device. Then add one drop of sample buffer to the sample well. Start the timer.

**For whole blood (fingerstick) samples:** Add one capillary tube of blood (about 50 μL) to the sample well (S) of the test device. Then add one drop of sample buffer to the sample well. Start the timer.

**For serum or plasma samples:** Hold the dropper upright and add one drop of serum or plasma (about 25 μL) to the sample well (S) of the test device. Then add one drop of sample buffer to the sample well. Start the timer. Avoid trapping air bubbles in the sample well. (See Fig. 22–5.)

3. Wait for the red line(s) to appear. The result should be read at 5 minutes. The background should be clear before the result is read.

> **NOTE:** Low titers of IM heterophile antibodies might result in a weak line appearing in the test-line region (T) after a long period of time. Do not read the result after 10 minutes.

## Interpretation of Results

Refer to **Figure 22–6.**

### Positive*

**Two distinct red lines appear:** One line should be in the control-line region (C), and another line should be in the test-line region (T). A positive result means that IM heterophile antibodies were detected in the sample.

> ***NOTE:** The shade of the red color in the test line region (T) will vary based on the amount of IM heterophile antibodies in the sample. Any shade of red in the test line region (T) should be considered positive.

### Negative

**One red line appears in the control-line region (C):** No apparent red or pink line appears in the test-line region (T). A negative result means that IM heterophile antibodies were not found in the sample or are below the detection limit of the test.

### Invalid

**No line appears in the control-line region (C):** If this occurs, read the directions again and repeat the test with a new test device. If the result is still invalid, stop using the test kit and contact Inverness Medical Technical Support at (800) 637-3717.

## Internal Quality Control

Internal procedural controls are included in the test. A red line appearing in the control region (C) is an internal positive procedural control. It confirms sufficient sample volume and correct procedural technique. A clear background is an internal negative background control. If the test is working properly, the background in the result area should be white to light pink and should not interfere with the ability to read the test result.

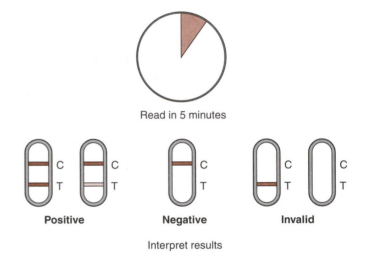

Read in 5 minutes

**Positive**          **Negative**          **Invalid**

Interpret results

**FIGURE 22–6.** Clearview Mono test results. © *2008 Inverness Medical. Used with permission.*

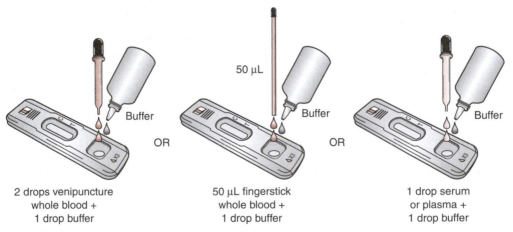

2 drops venipuncture whole blood + 1 drop buffer

OR

50 µL fingerstick whole blood + 1 drop buffer

OR

1 drop serum or plasma + 1 drop buffer

**FIGURE 22–5.** Clearview Mono test procedure. © *2008 Inverness Medical. Used with permission.*

*Reprinted with permission from Clearview Mono® whole blood serum, plasma kit package insert, Inverness Medical Professional Diagnostics, San Diego, CA, ©2006.

# EXERCISE

## TESTING FOR THE HETEROPHILE ANTIBODY OF INFECTIOUS MONONUCLEOSIS BY THE PAUL–BUNNELL TEST

### Principle

This test is used to determine the titer of the heterophile antibody in patients with infectious mononucleosis. Serial dilutions of patient serum are prepared and incubated with sheep red blood cells. The titer of the antibody is the reciprocal of the last dilution to show agglutination of the red blood cells.

### Reagents, Materials, and Equipment

0.9 percent saline solution

Sheep erythrocytes stored in Alsever's solution. Refrigerate until use.

Positive control serum containing heterophile antibody of infectious mononucleosis

Patient serum to be tested

13 × 100 mm glass test tubes

0.1 mL and 1.0 mL pipettes

### Procedure*

1. Inactivate complement in sera to be tested by heating in a 56°C water bath for 30 minutes.

2. Place sheep red blood cells into a tube and wash the cells three times in saline.

3. Prepare 5 mL of a 2 percent sheep red blood cell suspension by pipetting 0.1 mL of washed, packed red blood cells into 4.9 mL of saline.

4. Set up and label two rows of 10 test tubes in a rack. One row is for a positive-control serum and the other for the patient serum to be tested. Label the control tubes C1 through C10, and label the patient tubes P1 through P10.

5. Pipette 0.4 mL of saline in the first tube of each row and 0.25 mL of saline in each remaining tube.

6. Pipette 0.1 mL of positive control serum into tube 1 of the control row.

7. Mix and serially transfer 0.25 mL through tube 9, discarding 0.25 mL from tube 9. Tube 10 of this row contains no serum and serves as a negative control.

8. Obtain a sample of patient serum to be tested. Pipette 0.1 mL of patient serum into tube 1 of the patient row.

9. Mix and serially transfer 0.25 mL through tube 10, discarding 0.25 mL from tube 10.

10. Add 0.1 mL of the 2 percent sheep red blood cell suspension (prepared in step 3 above) to each tube in the control and patient rows.

11. Shake the tubes to obtain an even mixture. Cover the tubes with parafilm and incubate at room temperature for at least 15 minutes. A more accurate reading may be obtained by allowing the tubes to incubate for 2 hours.

12. Following the incubation period, read each tube individually for macroscopic agglutination, as follows: gently shake the tube to resuspend the red blood cells, tilt the tube, and hold up to light. Compare each tube to the negative control tube and record results.

### Interpretation of Results

The antibody titer is reported as the reciprocal of the dilution in the last tube, which shows visible agglutination (Fig. 22–7). Titers less than or equal to 56 are considered normal.

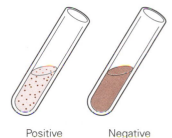

Positive          Negative

FIGURE 22–7. Interpretation of Paul-Bunnell test results.

---

*From Paul, JR, and Bunnell, WW. The presence of heterophile antibodies in infectious mononucleosis. Am J Med Sci 183:90, 1932.

# REVIEW QUESTIONS

1. An individual with hepatomegaly, jaundice, and elevated liver enzymes has the following laboratory results: IgM anti-HAV (negative), HBsAg (positive), IgM anti-HBc (positive), and anti-HCV (negative). These findings support a diagnosis of
   a. hepatitis A.
   b. acute hepatitis B.
   c. chronic hepatitis B.
   d. hepatitis C.

2. Which of the following hepatitis viruses is transmitted by the fecal-oral route?
   a. Hepatitis B
   b. Hepatitis C
   c. Hepatitis D
   d. Hepatitis E

3. Quantitative tests for HCV RNA are used to
   a. screen for hepatitis C.
   b. determine the HCV genotype.
   c. differentiate acute HCV infection from chronic HCV infection.
   d. monitor hepatitis C patients on antiviral therapy.

4. The serum of an individual who received all doses of the hepatitis B vaccine should contain
   a. anti-HBs.
   b. anti-HBe.
   c. anti-HBc.
   d. all of the above.

5. A 12-year-old girl presented to her physician with a sore throat, lymphadenopathy, and fatigue. Her laboratory results were 5000 lymphocytes/μL with 10 percent atypical lymphocytes, CMV antibody negative, and heterophile antibody screen negative. These laboratory results
   a. confirm a diagnosis of infectious mononucleosis.
   b. indicate that the diagnosis is not infectious mononucleosis, because the heterophile antibody screen is negative.
   c. suggest a diagnosis of infectious mononucleosis but should be followed by a heterophile antibody titer to strengthen the diagnosis.
   d. suggest a diagnosis of infectious mononucleosis but should be followed by a test for IgM anti-VCA to strengthen the diagnosis.

6. In the laboratory, heterophile antibodies are routinely detected by their reaction with
   a. B lymphocytes.
   b. bovine erythrocyte antigens.
   c. sheep erythrocyte antigens.
   d. Epstein-Barr virus antigens.

7. Presence of IgM anti-rubella antibodies in the serum from an infant born with a rash suggests
   a. a diagnosis of measles.
   b. a diagnosis of German measles.
   c. congenital infection with the rubella virus.
   d. passive transfer of maternal antibodies to the infant's serum.

8. A pregnant woman is exposed to a child with a rubella infection. She had no clinical symptoms but had a rubella titer performed. Her antibody titer was 1:8. Three weeks later, the test was repeated, and her titer was 1:128. She still had no clinical symptoms. Was the laboratory finding indicative of rubella infection?
   a. No, the titer must be greater than 256 to be significant.
   b. No, the change in titer is not significant if no clinical signs are present.
   c. Yes, a greater than fourfold rise in titer indicates early infection.
   d. Yes, but clinical symptoms must also correlate with laboratory findings.

9. The most common cause of congenital infections is
   a. CMV.
   b. rubella.
   c. VZV.
   d. HTLV-I.

10. A positive result on a screening test for HTLV-I antibody
    a. is highly specific for HTLV-I infection.
    b. should be followed by PCR.
    c. must be confirmed by Western blot.
    d. must be confirmed by viral culture.

# References

1. Kindt, TJ, Goldsby, RA, and Osborne, BA. Kuby Immunology, ed. 6. WH Freeman, New York, 2007, pp. 447–474.

2. Mak, TW, and Saunders, ME. The Immune Response: Basic and Clinical Principles. Elsevier Academic Press, Burlington, MA, 2006, pp. 664–680.

3. Williams, MA, and Bevan, MJ. Effector and memory CTL differentiation. Annu Rev Immunol 25:171–192, 2007.

4. Bendinelli, M, Pistello, M, Freer, G, Vatteroni, M, and Maggi, F. Viral hepatitis. In Detrick, B, Hamilton, RG, and Folds, JD (eds): Manual of Molecular and Clinical Laboratory Immunology, ed. 7. ASM Press, Washington, DC, 2006, pp. 724–745.

5. Dienstag, JL, and Isselbacher, KJ. Acute viral hepatitis. In Kasper, DL, Braunwald, E, Fauci, AS, et al. (eds): Harrison's online. Available at http://www.accessmedicine.com/content.aspx?aID=91413. Accessed June 13, 2007.

6. Kemmer, NM, and Miskovsky, EP. Hepatitis A. Infect Dis Clin North Am 14(3):605–615, 2000.

7. Wasley, A, Fiore, A, and Bell, BP. Hepatitis A in the era of vaccination. Epidemiol Rev 28:101–111, 2006.

8. Fiore, AE, Wasley, A, and Bell, BP. Prevention of hepatitis A through active or passive immunization. MMWR 55(RR07):1–23, 2006.

9. Nainan, OV, Xia, G, Vaughan, G, and Margolis, HS. Diagnosis of hepatitis A virus infection: A molecular approach. Clin Microbiol Rev 19(1):63–79, 2006.

10. Takahashi, M, Kusakai, S, Mizuo, H, et al. Simultaneous detection of immunoglobulin A (IgA) and IgM antibodies against hepatitis E virus (HEV) is highly specific for diagnosis of acute HEV infection. J Clin Microbiol 43(1):49–56, 2005.

11. Krawczynski, K. Hepatitis E vaccine—ready for prime time? N Eng J Med 356(9):949–951, 2007.

12. Dalton, HR, Hazeldine, S, Banks, M, Ijaz, S, and Bendall, R. Locally acquired hepatitis E in chronic liver disease. Lancet 369:1260, 2007.

13. Shrestha, MP, Scott, RN, Joshi, DM, et al. Safety and efficacy of a recombinant hepatitis E vaccine. N Eng J Med 356(9):895–903, 2007.

14. Krawczynski, K, Aggarwal, R, and Kamili, S. Hepatitis E. Infect Dis Clin N Amer 14(3):669–685, 2000.

15. Shepard, CW, Simard, EP, Finelli, L, Fiore, AE, and Bell, BP. Hepatitis B virus infection: Epidemiology and vaccination. Epidemiol Rev 28:112–125, 2006.

16. Alexander, J, and Kowdley, KV. Epidemiology of hepatitis B—Clinical implications. Med Gen Med8(2):13, 2006.

17. Hochman, JA, and Balistreri, JA. Chronic viral hepatitis. Pediatr Rev 24(12):309–410, 2003.

18. Mast, EE, Margolis, HS, Fiore, AE, et al. A comprehensive immunization strategy to eliminate transmission of hepatitis B virus infection in the United States. MMWR 54(RR16):1–23, 2005.

19. Befeler, AS, and Bisceglie, AM. Hepatitis B. Infect Dis Clinics of N Amer 14(3):617–663, 2000.

20. Ganem, D, and Prince, AM. Hepatitis B virus infection—natural history and clinical consequences. N Eng J Med 350(11):1118–1129, 2004.

21. Servoss, JC, and Friedman, LS. Serologic and molecular diagnosis of hepatitis B infection. Infect Dis Clin N Am 20:47–61, 2006.

22. Abbott Diagnostics. Hepatitis Products. Available at http://www.abbottdiagnostics.com/Products/Reagents_by_Condition/default.cfm?testcat=Hepatitis. Accessed June 21, 2007.

23. Ronsin, C, Pillet, A, Bali, C, and Denoyel, G-A. Evaluation of the COBAS AmpliPrep-total nucleic acid isolation-COBAS TaqMan hepatitis B virus (HBV) quantitative test and comparison to the Versant HBV DNA 3.0 assay. J Clin Microbiol 44(4):1390–1399, 2006.

24. de Franchis, R, Hadengue, G, Lau, G, et. al. EASL international consensus conference on hepatitis B. J Hepatol 39 (Suppl 1):S3–S25, 2003.

25. Pawlotsky, J-M. Hepatitis B virus (HBV) DNA assays (methods and practical use) and viral kinetics. J Hepatol 39 (Suppl 1):S31–S35, 2003.

26. Fang, CT. Blood screening for HBV DNA. J Clin Virol 36 (Suppl 1):S30–S32, 2006.

27. Allain, J-P. Occult hepatitis B virus infection. Transfus Clin Biol 11:18–25, 2004.

28. Sureau, C. The role of the HBV envelope proteins in the HDV replication cycle. Curr Top Microbiol Immunol 307:113–131, 2006.

29. Taylor JM. Hepatitis delta virus. Virology 344:71–76, 2006.

30. Farci, P. Delta hepatitis: An update. J Hepatol 39(Suppl 1):S212–S219, 2003.

31. Le Gal, F, Gordien, E, Affolabi, D, et al. Quantification of hepatitis delta virus RNA in serum by consensus real-time PCR indicates different patterns of virological response to interferon therapy in chronically infected patients. J Clin Microbiol 43(5):2363–2369, 2005.

32. Alter, MJ, Kruszon-Moran, D, Nainan, OV, et al. The prevalence of hepatitis C infection in the United States, 1988 through 1994. N Eng J Med 341:556–562, 1999.

33. Cheney, CP, Chopra, S, and Graham, C. Hepatitis C. Infect Dis Clin North Am 14(3):633–665, 2000.

34. Chou, PR. Hepatitis C virus: Epidemiology, diagnosis, and patient management. Lab Medicine 38(2):85–91, 2007.

35. Catalina, G, and Navarro, V. Hepatitis C: A challenge for the generalist. Hosp Prac 35(1):97–98, 101–104, 107–108, 2000.

36. Scott, JD, and Gretch, DR. Molecular diagnostics of Hepatitis C infection. JAMA 297:724–732, 2007.

37. Strader, DB, Wright, T, Thomas, DL, and Seeff, LB. Diagnosis, management, and treatment of hepatitis C. Hepatology 39:1147–1171, 2004.

38. Kim, AI, and Saab, S. Treatment of hepatitis C. Amer J Medicine 118(8):808–815, 2005.

39. Alter, MJ, Kuhnert, WL, and Finelli, L. Guidelines for laboratory testing and reporting of antibody to hepatitis C virus. MMWR 52(RR03):1–16, 2003.

40. Centers for Disease Control and Prevention. Reference for interpretation of HCV test results. Available at http://www.cdc.gov/ncidad/diseases/hepatitis/resource/PDFs/hcv_graph.pdf. Accessed June 13, 2007.

41. Jonas, G, Pelzer, C, Beckert, C, Hausmann, M, and Kapprell, H-P. Performance characteristics of the ARCHITECT Anti-HCV assay. J Clin Virology 34(2):97–103, 2005.

42. Sizmann, D, Boeck, C, Boelter, J, et al. Fully automated quantification of hepatitis C virus (HCV) RNA in human plasma and human serum by the COBAS AmpliPrep/COBAS Taqman system. J Clin Virol 38:326–333, 2007.

43. Davis, GL. Monitoring of viral levels during therapy of hepatitis C. Hepatology 36:S145–151, 2002.

44. Linnen, J, Wages, J, Zhang-Keck, Z-Y, et al. Molecular cloning and disease association of hepatitis G virus: A transfusion-transmissible agent. Science 271:505–508, 1996.

45. Simons, JN, Leary, TP, Dawson, TJ, et al. Isolation of novel virus-like sequences associated with human hepatitis. Nat Med 1:564–569, 1995.

46. Nishizawa, T, Okamoto, H, Konishi, K, et al. A novel DNA virus (TTV) associated with elevated transaminase levels in posttransfusion hepatitis of unknown etiology. Biochem Biophys Res Commun 241:92–97, 1997.

47. Lyra, AC, Pinho, JRR, Silva, LK, et al. HEV, TTV and GBV-C/HGV markers in patients with acute viral hepatitis. Brazilian J Med Biol Res 38:767–775, 2005.

48. Yang, J-F, Dai, C-Y, and Chuang, W-L. Prevalence and clinical significance of HGV/GBV-C infection in patients with chronic hepatitis B or C. Jpn J Infect Dis 59:25–30, 2006.

49. Abraham, A. TT viruses: How much do we know? Indian J Med Res 122:7–10, 2005.

50. Souza, IE, Allen, JB, Xiang, J, et al. Effect of primer selection on estimates of GB virus C (GBV-C) prevalence and response to antiretroviral therapy for optimal testing for GBV-C viremia. J Clin Microbiol 44(9):3105–3113, 2006.

51. Desai, MM, Pal, RB, and Banker, DD. Molecular epidemiology and clinical implications of TT virus (TTV) infection in Indian subjects. J Clin Gastroenterol 39(5):422–429, 2005.

52. Nauschuetz, WF. Clinical virology. In Mahon, CR, and Manuselis, G (eds): Textbook of Diagnostic Virology, ed. 2. WB Sanders, Philadelphia, 2000, pp. 866–870.

53. Hunt, R. Herpes viruses. In Microbiology and Immunology Online. Available at http://pathmicro.med.sc.edu/virol/herpes.htm. Accessed July 13, 2007.

54. Jenson, HB. Epstein-Barr virus. In Detrick, B, Hamilton, RG, and Folds, JD (eds): Manual of Molecular and Clinical Laboratory Immunology, ed. 7. ASM Press, Washington, DC, 2006, pp. 637–647.

55. Cohen, JI. Epstein-Barr virus infections, including infectious mononucleosis. In Kasper, DL, Braunwald, E, Fauci, AS, et al. (eds): Harrison's Online. Available at http://www.accessmedicine.com/content.aspx?aID=91413. Accessed July 13, 2007.

56. Junker, AK. Epstein-Barr virus. Pediatr Rev26(3):79–85, 2005.

57. Centers for Disease Control and Prevention. Epstein-Barr virus and infectious mononucleosis. Available at http://www.cdc.gov/ncidod/diseases/ebv.htm. Accessed June 26, 2007.

58. Hess, RD. Routine Epstein-Barr virus diagnostics from the laboratory perspective: Still challenging after 35 years. J Clin Microbiol 42(8):3381–3387, 2004.

59. Ebell, MH. Epstein-Barr virus infectious mononucleosis. Am Fam Physician 70(7):1279–1290, 2004.

60. Williams, H, and Crawford, DH. Epstein-Barr virus: The impact of scientific advances on clinical practice. Blood 107(3):862–869, 2006.

61. Feng, Z, Li, Z, Sui, B, Xu, G, and Xia, T. Serologic diagnosis of infectious mononucleosis by chemiluminescent immunoassay using capsid antigen p18 of Epstein-Barr virus. Clin Chim Acta 354:77–82, 2005.

62. Okano, M, Kawa, K, Kimura, H, et al. Proposed guidelines for diagnosing chronic active Epstein-Barr virus infection. Am J Hematol 80:64–69, 2005.

63. Gottschalk, S, Rooney, CM, and Heslop, HE. Post-transplant lymphproliferative disorders. Annu Rev Med 56:29–44, 2005.

64. Gulley, ML, Fan, H, and Elmore, SH. Validation of Roche LightCycler Epstein-Barr virus quantification reagents in a clinical laboratory setting. J Mol Diagn 8:589–597, 2006.

65. Adler, SP, and Marshall, B. Cytomegalovirus infections. Pediatr Rev 28(3):92–100, 2007.

66. Hirsch, MS. Cytomegalovirus and human herpesvirus types 6, 7, and 8. In Kasper, DL, Braunwald, E, Fauci, AS, et al. (eds): Harrison's online. Available at http://www.accessmedicine.com/content.aspx?aID=91413. Accessed July 13, 2007.

67. Ross, SA, and Boppana, SB. Congenital cytomegalovirus infection: Outcome and diagnosis. Semin Pediatr Infect Dis 16:44–49, 2004.

68. St. George, K, Hoji, A, and Rinaldo, CR. Cytomegalovirus. In Detrick, B, Hamilton, RG, and Folds, JD (eds): Manual of Molecular and Clinical Laboratory Immunology, ed. 7. ASM Press, Washington, DC, 2006, pp. 648–657.

69. Pereyra, F, and Rubin, RH. Prevention and treatment of cytomegalovirus infection in solid organ transplant recipients. Curr Opin Infect Dis 17:357–361, 2004.

70. Nigro, G, Adler, SP, La Torre, R, and Best, AM. Passive immunization during pregnancy for congenital cytomegalovirus infection. New Engl J Med. 353(13):1350-1362, 2005

71. Adler, SP, Nigro, G, and Pereira, L. Recent advances in the prevention and treatment of congenital cytomegalovirus infections. Semin Perinatol 31:10–18, 2007.

72. Mendelson, E, Aboudy, Y, Smetana, Z, Tepperberg, M, and Grossman, Z. Laboratory assessment and diagnosis of congenital viral infections: Rubella, cytomegalovirus (CMV), varicella-zoster virus (VZV), herpes simplex virus (HSV), parvovirus B19 and human immunodeficiency virus (HIV). Reprod Toxicol 21:350–382, 2006.

73. Landry, ML, and Ferguson, D. 2-Hour cytomegalovirus pp65 antigenemia assay for rapid quantitation of cytomegalovirus in blood samples. J Clin Microbiol 38(1):427–428, 2000.

74. DeBiasi, RL, and Tyler, KL. Molecular methods for diagnosis of viral encephalitis. Clin Microbiol Rev 17(4):903–925, 2004.

75. Whitley, RJ. Varicella-Zoster virus infections. In Kasper, DL, Braunwald, E, Fauci, AS, et al. (eds): Harrison's online. Available at http://www.accessmedicine.com/content.aspx?aID=91413. Accessed July 13, 2007.

76. Stover, BH, and Bratcher, DF. Varicella-zoster virus: Infection, control, and prevention. Am J Infect Control 26(3):369–381, 1998.

77. Marin, M, Gurtis, D, Chaves, SS, Schmid, S, and Seward, JF. Prevention of varicella: Recommendations of the Advisory Committee on Immunization Practices (ACIP). MMWR 56(RR-4):1–40,2007.

78. McCrary, ML, Severson, J, and Trying, SK. Varicella zoster virus. J Am Acad Dermatol 41:1–14, 1999.

79. Kimberlin, DW, and Whitley, RJ. Varicella-zoster vaccine for the prevention of herpes zoster. N Engl J Med 356:1338–1343, 2007.

80. Zhou, F, Harpaz, R, Jumaan, AO, Winston, CA, and Shefer, A. Impact of varicella vaccination on health care utilization. JAMA 294(7):797–802, 2005.

81. Chaves, SS, Garguillo, P, Zhang, JX, et al. Loss of vaccine-induced immunity to varicella over time. N Engl J Med 356:1121–1129, 2007.

82. Oxman, MN, Levin, MJ, Johnson, GR, et al. A vaccine to prevent herpes zoster and postherpetic neuralgia in older adults. N Engl J Med 343:222, 2000.

83. Schmid, DS, and Loparev, V. Varicella virus. In Detrick, B, Hamilton, RG, and Folds, JD (eds): Manual of Molecular and Clinical Laboratory Immunology, ed. 7. ASM Press, Washington, DC, 2006, pp. 631–636.

84. Breuer, J, Harper, DR, and Kangro, HO. Varicella zoster. In Zuckerman, AJ, Banatvala, JE, and Pattison, JR. Principles and Practice of Clinical Virology, ed. 4. John Wiley & Sons, Chichester, England, 2000, pp. 47–77.

85. Schvoerer, E, Frechin, V, Fritsch, S, et al. Atypical symptoms in patients with herpesvirus DNA detected by PCR in cerebrospinal fluid. J Clin Virol 35:458–462, 2006.

86. Sauerbrei, A, and Wutzler, P. Serological detection of varicella-zoster virus-specific immunoglobulin G by an enzyme-linked immunosorbent assay using glycoprotein antigen. J Clin Microbiol 44(9):3094–3097, 2006.

87. Gershon, A. Rubella (German measles). In Kasper, DL, Braunwald, E, Fauci, AS, Hauser, SL, Longo, DL, Jameson, JL, and Isselbacher, KJ, (eds): Harrison's online. Available at http://www.accessmedicine.com/content.aspx?aID=91413. Accessed July 13, 2007.

88. Centers for Disease Control and Prevention. Rubella. In: The Pink Book. Available at http://www.cdc.gov/vaccines/pubs/pinkbook/downloads/rubella.pdf. Accessed August 7, 2007.

89. Hodinka, RL, and Moshal, KL. Childhood infections. In Storch, GA: Essentials of Diagnostic Virology. Churchill Livingstone, New York, 2000, pp. 167–186.

90. Mahony, JB. Rubella virus. In Detrick, B, Hamilton, RG, and Folds, JD (eds): Manual of Molecular and Clinical Laboratory Immunology, ed. 7. ASM Press, Washington, DC, 2006, pp. 712–718.

91. Meissner, HC, Reef, SE, and Cochi, S. Elimination of rubella from the United States: A milestone on the road to global elimination. Pediatrics 117(3):933–935, 2006.

92. DeSantis, M, Cavaliere, AF, Straface, G, and Caruso, A. Rubella infection in pregnancy. Reprod Toxicol 21:390–398, 2006.

93. Centers for Disease Control and Prevention. Elimination of rubella and congenital rubella syndrome—United States, 1969–2004. MMWR 54(11):279–282, 2005.

94. Dimech, W, Panagiotopoulos, L, Marler, J, Laven, N, Leeson, S, and Dax, EM. Evaluation of three immunoassays used for detection of anti-rubella virus immunoglobulin M antibodies. Clin Diagn Lab Immunol 12(9):1104–1108, 2005.

95. Karapanagiotidis, T, Riddell, M, and Kelly, H. Detection of rubella immunoglobulin M from dried venous blood spots using a commercial enzyme immunoassay. Diagn Microbiol and Infect Dis 53:107–111, 2005.

96. Vijaylakshmi, P, Muthukkaruppan, VR, Rajasundari, A, et al. Evaluation of a commercial rubella IgM assay for use on oral fluid samples for diagnosis and surveillance of congenital rubella syndrome and postnatal rubella. J Clin Virol 37: 265–268, 2006.

97. Hamkar, R, Javilvand, S, Mokhtari-Azad, T, et al. Assessment of IgM enzyme immunoassay and IgG avidity assay for distinguishing between primary and secondary immune response to rubella vaccine. J Virol Meth 130:59–65, 2005.

98. Mubareka, S, Richards, H, Gray, M, and Tipples, GA. Evaluation of commercial rubella immunoglobulin G avidity assays. J Clin Microbiol 45(1):231–233, 2007.

99. Mace, M, Cointe, D, Six, C, et al. Diagnostic value of reverse transcription-PCR of amniotic fluid for prenatal diagnosis of congenital rubella infection in pregnant women with confirmed primary rubella infection. J Clin Microbiol 42(10): 4818–4820, 2004.

100. Gershon, A. Measles (Rubeloa). In Kasper, DL, Braunwald, E, Fauci, AS, et al. (eds): Harrison's online. Available at http://www.accessmedicine.com/content.aspx?aID=91413. Accessed August 2, 2007.

101. Centers for Disease Control and Prevention. Measles. In: The Pink Book. Available at http://www.cdc.gov/vaccines/pubs/pinkbook/downloads/meas.pdf. Accessed August 7, 2007.

102. Bellini, WJ, Rota, JS, Lowe, LE, et al. Subacute sclerosing panencephalitis: More cases of this fatal disease are prevented by measles immunization than was previously recognized. J Infec Dis 192:1686–1693, 2005.

103. Leland, DS. Measles and mumps. In Detrick, B, Hamilton, RG, and Folds, JD (eds): Manual of Molecular and Clinical Laboratory Immunology, ed. 7. ASM Press, Washington, DC, 2006, pp. 707–711.

104. Hummel, KB, Lowe, L, Bellini, WJ, Rota, PA. Development of quantitative gene-specific real-time RT-PCR assays for detection of measles virus in clinical specimens. J Virol Meth 132:166–173, 2006.

105. Gershon, A. Mumps. In Kasper, DL, Braunwald, E, Fauci AS, et al. (eds): Harrison's online. Available at http://www.accessmedicine.com/content.aspx?aID=91413. Accessed August 2, 2007.

106. Centers for Disease Control and Prevention. Mumps. In: The Pink Book. Available at http://www.cdc.gov/vaccines/pubs/pinkbook/downloads/meas.pdf. Accessed August 7, 2007.

107. Shanley, JD. The resurgence of mumps in young adults and adolescents. Cleveland Clinic J Med 74(1):42–48, 2007.

108. Kyaw, MH, Bellini, WJ, and Gustavo, HD. Mumps surveillance and prevention: Putting mumps back on our radar screen. Cleveland Clinic J Med 74(1):13–15, 2007.

109. Centers for Disease Control and Prevention. Measles, mumps, and rubella—vaccine use and strategies for elimination of measles, rubella, and congenital rubella syndrome and control of mumps: Recommendations of the advisory committee on immunization practices (ACIP). MMWR 47(RR-8):1, 1998.

110. Centers for Disease Control and Prevention. Updated recommendations of the advisory committee on immunization practices (ACIP) for the control and elimination of mumps. MMWR 55(22):629–630, 2006.

111. Krause, CH, Eastick, K, and Ogilvie, MM. Real-time PCR for mumps diagnosis on clinical specimens—comparison with

results of conventional methods of virus detection and nested PCR. J Clin Virol 37:184–189, 2006.

112. Nyland, SB, Loughran, TP, and Ugen, K. Human T-cell lymphotropic virus types 1 and 2. In Detrick, B, Hamilton, RG, and Folds JD (eds): Manual of Molecular and Clinical Laboratory Immunology, ed. 7. ASM Press, Washington, DC, 2006, pp. 798–802.

113. Manns, A, Hisada, M, and Grenade, LL. Human T-lymphotropic virus type I infection. Lancet 353(9168): 1951–1958, 1999.

114. Verdonck, K, Gonzalez, E, Van Dooren, SV, Vandamme, A-M, Vanham, G, and Gatuzzo, E. Human T-lymphotropic virus I: Recent knowledge about an ancient infection. Lance Infect Dis 7:266–281, 2007.

115. Lal, RB. Delineation of immunodominant epitopes of human T-lymphotropic viruses types I and II and their usefulness in developing serologic assays for detection of antibodies to HTLV-I and HTLV-II. J AIDS Hum Retro 13(suppl 1):S170–S178, 1996.

116. Proietti, FA, Carneiro-Proietti, ABF, Catalan-Soares, BC, and Murphy, EL. Oncogene 24:6058–6068, 2005.

117. Thorstensson, R, Albert, J, and Andersson, S. Strategies for diagnosis of HTLV-I and -II. Transfusion 42:780–791, 2002.

118. Araujo, A, and Hall, WW. Human T-lymphotropic virus type II and neurological disease. Ann Neurol 56:10–19, 2004.

# Laboratory Diagnosis of HIV Infection

23

*Linda E. Miller, PhD, I, MP(ASCP)SI*

## LEARNING OBJECTIVES

*After finishing this chapter, the reader will be able to:*

1. Explain conditions under which transmission of human immunodeficiency virus (HIV) can occur.
2. Describe the makeup of the HIV particle.
3. Differentiate the three main structural genes of HIV and their products.
4. Describe replication of the HIV virus.
5. Describe the effects of HIV on the immune system.
6. Discuss antiretroviral treatments and the impact they have had on HIV infection.
7. Discuss flow cytometric methods for CD4 T-cell enumeration.
8. Discuss the roles of various laboratory tests in diagnosing and monitoring HIV infection.
9. Compare first-generation, second-generation, third-generation, and fourth-generation enzyme-linked immunosorbent assay (ELISA) tests for HIV antibody.
10. Give reasons for false positives and false negatives in HIV antibody testing.
11. Define *positive predictive value* and relate this to HIV antibody testing.
12. Describe the Western blot test.
13. Interpret a Western blot test, given the types of reactive bands.
14. Discuss advantages and disadvantages of p24 antigen testing.
15. Differentiate between reverse transcriptase polymerase chain reaction (RT-PCR), real-time RT-PCR, branched DNA (bDNA) amplification, and nucleic acid sequence-based amplification (NASBA) testing for HIV nucleic acid.
16. Discuss the clinical utility of HIV viral load testing and drug-resistance testing.
17. Discuss the protocol for HIV testing of infants and children younger than 18 months of age.

## KEY TERMS

___ AIDS
___ Amplicon
___ Branched chain DNA
___ CD4 T cell
___ ELISA
___ Env
___ Flow cytometry
___ Gag
___ HAART
___ HIV
___ Hybridization
___ NASBA
___ p24 antigen
___ Pol
___ Positive predictive value
___ Reverse transcriptase
___ Seroconversion
___ Viral load tests
___ Western blot test

# CHAPTER OUTLINE

Human immunodeficiency virus (**HIV**) is the etiologic agent of the acquired immunodeficiency syndrome, or **AIDS,** a disease that has posed one of the greatest medical challenges worldwide. According to the World Health Organization, in 2007, an estimated 33.2 million people were living with HIV infection, 2.5 million people became newly infected, and 2.1 million people died of AIDS.[1] Although the majority of infected persons reside in developing countries, HIV infection has also created a significant problem in developed nations. For example, in the United States, over 1 million cases of AIDS and more than 565,000 AIDS-related deaths were reported from 1981 (when the first cases of AIDS were identified) through the year 2006.[2] Accurate diagnosis is essential for early intervention and halting the spread of the disease. This chapter emphasizes techniques for laboratory diagnosis of HIV infection, presents some characteristics of the virus, and outlines immunologic manifestations of the disease.

The virus that is responsible for causing AIDS, HIV-1, was identified independently by the laboratories of Luc Montagnier of France and Robert Gallo and Jay Levy of the United States in 1983 and 1984 respectively.[3–5] It was formerly called *human T-cell lymphotrophic virus-type III (HTLV-III), lymphadenopathy-associated virus (LAV),* and *AIDS-associated retrovirus (ARV).* Isolates of HIV-1 have been classified into three groups: group M (the main or major group), group N (the non-M/non-O, or new group), and group O (the outlier group).[6,7] Group M viruses are responsible for the majority of HIV-1 infections worldwide. This group contains nine subtypes or clades, designated A through D, F through H, J, and K.[8] Subtype C is the most predominant subtype worldwide, and subtype B is the most prevalent subtype in the United States and Europe.[8–10] Groups N and O are largely confined to Central Africa.

A related but genetically distinct virus, HIV-2, was discovered in 1986.[9] The majority of HIV-2 infections have occurred in West Africa, although the virus has also been identified in patients in other parts of the world.[8] HIV-2 is transmitted in the same manner as HIV-1 and may also cause AIDS, but it is less pathogenic and has a lower rate of transmission.[6,8] Although this chapter discusses the differences between the two viruses, our focus is on HIV-1, because it is much more prevalent throughout the world. In this chapter, the term *HIV* is used to refer to HIV-1, and HIV-2 is so named.

## HIV TRANSMISSION

Transmission of HIV occurs by one of three major routes: (1) intimate sexual contact; (2) contact with blood or other body fluids; or (3) perinatally, from infected mother to infant.[10–12] The majority of cases of HIV infection have occurred by sexual transmission, through either vaginal or anal intercourse. Worldwide, about 85 percent of cases of HIV infection can be attributed to heterosexual contact, while in the United States, the largest number of cases has resulted from anal intercourse in homosexual males.[2,10–13] The presence of other sexually transmitted diseases such as syphilis, gonorrhea, or genital herpes increases the likelihood of transmission by disrupting protective mucous membranes and increasing immune activation in the genital areas.[10,12,13]

The second route of transmission is by parenteral exposure to infected blood or body fluids. This has occurred through the sharing of contaminated needles by intravenous drug users, blood transfusions or the use of clotting factors by hemophiliacs, occupational injuries with needle sticks or other sharp objects, or by mucous membrane contacts in health-care workers exposed to infectious fluids.[12,14,15] The virus has also been acquired by transplantation of infected tissue. Screening of blood and organ donors for HIV has dramatically decreased the incidence of infection in recipients of blood transfusions, clotting factors, and organ transplants to an estimated one transmission per 2 million blood donations.[13,16] Studies by the Centers for Disease Control and Prevention (CDC) have estimated the average risk of transmission to health-care workers to be approximately 0.3 percent after a percutaneous exposure to

HIV-infected blood and about 0.09 percent after a mucous membrane exposure. Body fluids considered to be potentially infectious include blood, semen, vaginal secretions, cerebral spinal fluid, synovial fluid, pleural fluid, peritoneal fluid, pericardial fluid, amniotic fluid, and other fluids containing visible blood. Saliva, sputum, nasal secretions, tears, sweat, urine, vomitus, and feces are not considered to be infectious unless they contain visible blood.[14,15,17]

The third route of transmission is perinatal, from infected mother to her fetus or infant. Transmission by this route can occur during pregnancy, by transfer of blood during delivery, or through breastfeeding.[10,18] Perinatal transmission has been markedly reduced through HIV screening during pregnancy, administration of antiretroviral drugs to HIV-positive pregnant women and their newborn babies, and use of infant formula by mothers who are infected with the virus. These measures have reduced the rate of perinatal transmission to less than 2 percent, as compared to rates of 25 to 30 percent in untreated mothers.[18]

## CHARACTERISTICS OF HIV

### Composition of the Virus

HIV belongs to the genus *Lentivirinae* of the virus family *Retroviridae*.[11,12,19] It is classified as a retrovirus, because it contains ribonucleic acid (RNA) as its nucleic acid and a unique enzyme, called **reverse transcriptase,** that transcribes the viral RNA into DNA, a necessary step in the virus's life cycle. HIV is a spherical particle, 100 to 120 nm in diameter, which contains an inner core with two copies of single-stranded RNA, surrounded by a protein coat or capsid and an outer envelope of glycoproteins embedded in a lipid bilayer.[11,12,19,20] The glycoproteins are knoblike structures that are involved in binding the virus to host cells during infection. **Figure 23–1** shows the structure of the HIV virion.

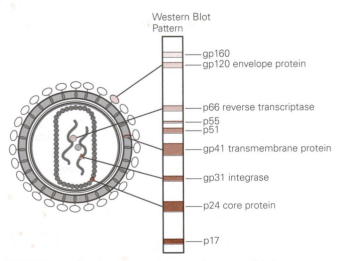

**FIGURE 23–1.** Structure of HIV virion, showing some of the major components. (*Modified from Sloand, E, et al. HIV testing: State of the art. JAMA 266:2862, 1991, with permission.*)

## Structural Genes

The genome of HIV includes three main structural genes—gag, env, and pol—and a number of regulatory genes. **Figure 23–2** shows the relative locations of the major HIV genes and indicates their gene products. The **gag** gene codes for p55, a precursor protein with a molecular weight of 55 kd, from which four core structural proteins are formed: p6, p9, p17, and p24.[12,19] All four are located in the nucleocapsid of the virus. The capsid that surrounds the internal nucleic acids contains p24, p6, and p9, while p17 lies in a layer between the protein core and the envelope, called the *matrix*, and is actually embedded in the internal portion of the envelope.[19]

The **env** gene codes for the glycoproteins gp160, gp120, and gp41, which are found in the viral envelope. Gp160 is a precursor protein that is cleaved to form gp120 and gp41. Gp120 forms the numerous knobs or spikes that protrude from the outer envelope, while gp41 is a transmembrane glycoprotein that spans the inner and outer membrane and attaches to gp120. Both gp120 and gp41 are involved with fusing and attaching HIV to receptors on host cells.[11,12,19]

The third structural gene, **pol,** codes for enzymes necessary for HIV replication,[11,12,19] namely p66 and p51. These are subunits of reverse transcriptase p31, or integrase, which mediates integration of the viral DNA into the genome of infected host cells, and of p10, a protease that cleaves protein precursors into smaller active units. The p66 protein is also involved in degradation of the original HIV RNA. These proteins are located in the core, in association with the HIV RNA.

Several other genes in the HIV genome code for products that have regulatory or accessory functions.[11,12,19] Although these products are not an integral part of the viral structure, they serve important functions in controlling viral replication and infectivity. The tat (transactivator) gene codes for p14, a regulatory protein that activates transcription of HIV proviral genes. Rev (which regulates expression of virion proteins) codes for p19, a protein that transports viral RNA out of the nucleus and into the cytoplasm for translation. Nef codes for p27, which has multiple functions, including modification of the host cell to enhance viral replication and make it less likely to be destroyed by the immune system. Vpu (viral protein "U") codes for p16, a protein with multiple roles, including efficiently assembling and budding the virions off infected host cells and promoting host cell death. Vpr (viral protein "R") codes for p15, which helps integrate HIV DNA into the host cell nucleus. Vif codes for p23, which acts as a viral infectivity factor by stabilizing newly synthesized HIV DNA and facilitating its transport to the nucleus. **Table 23–1** summarizes the major HIV-1 genes, their products, and their functions.

HIV-2 has gag, env, pol, and regulatory/accessory genes that have similar functions to those seen in HIV-1. The homology between the genomes of the two viruses is approximately 50 percent.[19,21] The gag and pol regions are most similar, while the env region differs greatly. Thus, the viruses can most easily be distinguished on the basis of antigenic differences in their env proteins.

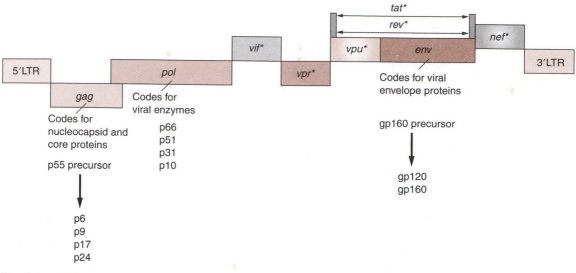

**FIGURE 23–2.** The HIV-1 genome. The relative locations of the major genes in the HIV-1 genome are indicated, as well as their gene products.

| Table 23–1. | Major HIV Genes and Their Products | |
|---|---|---|
| **GENE** | **PROTEIN PRODUCT** | **FUNCTION** |
| gag | p17 | Inner surface of envelope |
|  | p24 | Core coat for nucleic acids |
|  | p9 | Core-binding protein |
|  | p7 | Binds to genomic RNA |
| env | gp120 | Binds to CD4 on T cells |
|  | gp41 | Transmembrane protein associated with gp120 |
| pol | p66 | Subunit of reverse transcriptase; degrades original HIV RNA |
|  | p51 | Subunit of reverse transcriptase |
|  | p31 | Integrase; mediates integration of HIV DNA into host genome |
|  | p10 | Protease that cleaves gag precursor |
| tat | p14 | Activates transcription of HIV provirus |
| rev | p19 | Transports viral mRNA to the cytoplasm of the host cell |
| nef | p27 | Enhance HIV replication |
| vpu | p16 | Viral assembly and budding |
| vpr | p15 | Integration of HIV DNA into host genome |
| vif | p23 | Infectivity factor |

RNA = ribonucleic acid

## Viral Replication

The first step in the reproductive cycle of HIV is the virus attaching to a susceptible host cell. This interaction is mediated through the host-cell CD4 antigen, which serves as a receptor for the virus by binding the gp120 glycoprotein on the outer envelope of HIV. T helper cells are the main target for HIV infection, because they express high numbers of CD4 molecules on their cell surface and bind the virus with high affinity.[12] Other cells such as macrophages, monocytes, dendritic cells, Langerhans cells, and microglial brain cells can also be infected with HIV, because they have some surface CD4. HIV viruses that preferentially infect T cells are known as *T-tropic* or *X4* strains, while those strains that can infect both macrophages and T cells are called *M-tropic* or *R5* strains.

Entry of HIV into the host cells to which it has attached requires an additional binding step involving coreceptors that promote fusion of the HIV envelope with the plasma cell membrane. These coreceptors belong to a family of proteins known as *chemokine receptors*, whose main function is to direct white blood cells to sites of inflammation. The chemokine receptor CXCR4 is required for HIV to enter T lymphocytes, while the chemokine receptor CCR5 is required for entry into macrophages.[11,12,19] Binding of the coreceptors allows for HIV entry by inducing a conformational change in the gp41 glycoprotein, which mediates fusion of the virus to the cell membrane.

After fusion occurs, the viral particle is taken into the cell, and uncoating of the particle exposes the viral genome.[11,12,19] Action of the enzyme reverse transcriptase produces complementary DNA from the viral RNA. This DNA becomes integrated into the host cell's genome and is called a *provirus* (**Fig. 23–3**). The provirus can remain in a latent

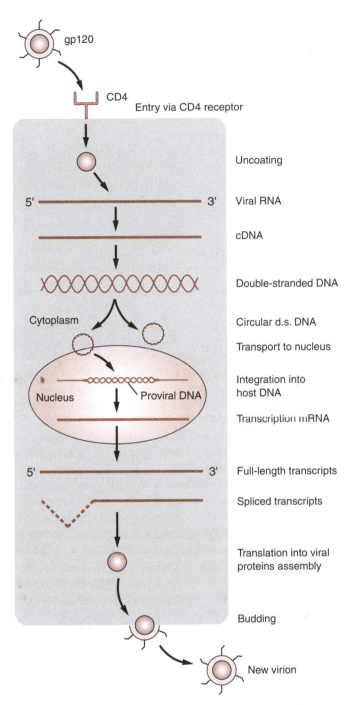

gp120

CD4
Entry via CD4 receptor

Uncoating

5'  3'  Viral RNA

cDNA

Double-stranded DNA

Cytoplasm

Circular d.s. DNA

Transport to nucleus

Integration into
host DNA

Nucleus      Proviral DNA

Transcription mRNA

5'  3'  Full-length transcripts

Spliced transcripts

Translation into viral
proteins assembly

Budding

New virion

**FIGURE 23–3.** Replication cycle of HIV. *(From Crowe, S, and Mills, J. Virus infections of the immune system. In Parslow, TG, et al: Medical Immunology. Lange Medical Books, McGraw-Hill, New York, NY, 2001, p. 646, with permission.)*

state for a long period of time, during which viral replication does not occur. Eventually, expression of the viral genes is induced when the infected host cell is activated by binding to antigen or by exposure to cytokines. Viral DNA within the cell nucleus is then transcribed into genomic RNA and messenger RNA (mRNA), which are transported to the cytoplasm. Translation of mRNA occurs, with production of viral proteins and assembly of viral particles. The intact virions

bud out from the host cell membrane and acquire their envelope during the process. These viruses can then proceed to infect additional host cells. Viral replication occurs to the greatest extent in antigen-activated T helper cells. Because viral replication occurs very rapidly, and the reverse transcriptase enzyme lacks proofreading activity, genetic mutations commonly occur, producing distinct isolates that exhibit antigenic variation. These isolates can vary in their susceptibility to the host's immune responses.[19]

## IMMUNOLOGIC MANIFESTATIONS

### Immune Responses to HIV

When HIV infects a healthy individual, there is typically an initial burst of viral replication followed by a slowing down of virus production as the host's immune response develops and keeps the virus in check.[12,19–21] This initial viral replication can be detected in the laboratory by the presence of increased levels of **p24 antigen** and viral RNA in the host's bloodstream (see discussion later). As the virus replicates, some of the viral proteins produced within host cells form complexes with major histocompatibility complex (MHC) class I antigens and are transported to the cell surface, where they stimulate lymphocyte responses. While HIV can stimulate both humoral and cell-mediated immune responses, the interactions between HIV and the immune system are complex, and the relevance of the responses generated to clearing the virus are not completely understood,[20,21] as will be discussed below.

B lymphocytes are stimulated to produce antibodies to HIV, which can usually be detected in the host's serum by 6 weeks after primary infection.[19–21] The first antibodies to be detected are directed against the gag proteins such as p24, followed by production of antibodies to the envelope, pol, and regulatory proteins. The most immunogenic proteins are in the viral envelope and elicit the production of neutralizing antibodies. These antibodies appear within the first 6 months of infection and prevent the virus from infecting neighboring cells. Antibodies to the envelope proteins have also been shown to bind to Fc receptors on NK cells and participate in ADCC-mediated killing of HIV-infected cells. However, the in vivo role of these antibodies is unclear, as they are unable to completely eliminate the virus from the host, for reasons that are discussed below.

T cell–mediated immunity is thought to play an important role in the immune response to HIV, as it does in other viral infections.[19–23] CD8+ cytotoxic T lymphocytes, also known as *cytolytic T cells (CTLs)*, appear within weeks of HIV infection and are associated with a decline in the amount of HIV in the blood during acute infection. While antibodies can attach only to virions circulating freely outside of host cells, CTLs can attack host cells harboring viruses internally. This process involves the binding of CTL containing HIV-specific antigen receptors to HIV proteins associated with MHC class I molecules on the surface of infected host cells. HIV-specific CTL are stimulated to develop into mature, activated clones through the effects of cytokines released by activated CD4 T helper cells, a process that is common to immune responses against other viruses (see Chapter 5 for details). After the CTLs bind to HIV-infected host cells, cytolytic enzymes are released from their granules and destroy the target cells. Free virions are released from the damaged cells and can be bound by antibodies. CTL can also suppress replication and spreading of HIV by producing cytokines like interferon-γ, which have antiviral activity.

## Effects of HIV Infection on the Immune System

Although the humoral and cell-mediated immune responses of the host usually reduce the level of HIV replication, they are generally not sufficient to completely eliminate the virus. This is because HIV has developed several mechanisms by which it can escape immune responses.[19-22,24] CTL and antibody responses to HIV are hindered by the virus's ability to undergo rapid genetic mutations, generating escape mutants with altered antigens toward which the host's initial immune responses are ineffective. In addition, HIV can downregulate the production of MHC class I molecules on the surface of the host cells it infects, protecting them from CTL recognition. HIV can also be harbored as a silent provirus for long periods by numerous cells in the body, including resting CD4 T cells, dendritic cells, cells of the monocyte/macrophage lineage, and microglial cells in the brain. In this proviral state, HIV is protected from attack by the immune system until cell activation stimulates the virus to multiply and display its viral antigens.

The ability of HIV to evade the immune response results in a persistent infection that can destroy the immune system. Because the virus's prime targets are the CD4 T helper cells, these cells are most severely affected, and a decrease in this cell population is the hallmark feature of HIV infection.[25] CD4 T helper cells are killed or rendered nonfunctional as a result of HIV infection. These effects occur from a variety of mechanisms, including loss of plasma membrane integrity due to viral budding, destruction by HIV-specific CTL, and viral induction of apoptosis.[19,22] Infected T cells turn over much more rapidly than they can be replaced, having a half-life of 12 to 36 hours.[22] In addition to reducing T-cell numbers, HIV also causes abnormalities in T helper cell function and impairment of memory T helper cell responses.[12,19,21,25]

Because T helper cells play a central role in the immune system by regulating the activities of B and T lymphocytes (see Chapter 5), destruction of these cells results in decreased effectiveness of both antibody- and cell-mediated immune responses. HIV proteins actually stimulate polyclonal activation of B cells, resulting in maturational and functional defects, with increased circulating immunoglobulin levels, immune complexes, and auto-antibodies.[12,19,21,26] However, B cells in HIV-infected individuals have a reduced ability to mount antibody responses after exposure to specific antigens, due to the decrease in T-cell help.[12,19,21]

Cell-mediated immunity is also affected by the reduction in T helper activity, resulting in a decline in CTL activity and delayed-type hypersensitivity responses to specific antigens.[12,19,21,22,24] Altered production of cytokines and chemokines have also been seen, including increases in the levels of some cytokines during the early stages of disease, followed by declining levels of IL-2 and interferon-γ and a shift in the cytokine profile from Th1 to Th2 as the infection progresses toward development of AIDS.[12,19,22] Other immunologic abnormalities, including defective antigen presentation and oxidative burst by monocytes/macrophages and decreased natural killer (NK) cell activity, have also been observed in AIDS patients.[19,21,22,25]

## CLINICAL SYMPTOMS

HIV infection causes a chronic infection that is characterized by a progressive decline in the immune system. Although the manifestations of the disease vary in individual patients, the infection progresses through a clinical course that begins with primary, or acute, infection, followed by a period of clinical latency and eventually culminating in AIDS.[19,21,23] The acute, or early, stage of infection is characterized by a rapid burst of viral replication prior to the development of HIV-specific immune responses. In this stage, high levels of circulating virus, or viremia, can be seen in the blood of infected individuals, and HIV begins to disseminate to the lymphoid organs. As the immune system becomes activated, an acute retroviral syndrome may develop. This syndrome, which has been noted in 50 to 70 percent of patients with primary HIV infection, is characterized by flulike or infectious mononucleosis-like symptoms, such as fever, lymphadenopathy, sore throat, arthralgia, myalgia, fatigue, rash, and weight loss.[19,21,23,27] Symptoms of the primary stage usually appear 3 to 6 weeks after initial infection and resolve within a few days to a few weeks. Some patients are asymptomatic during this stage.

As HIV-specific immune responses develop, they begin to curtail replication of the virus, and patients enter a period of clinical latency. This stage is characterized by a decrease in viremia as the virus is cleared from the circulation, and clinical symptoms are subtle or absent.[19,21,23,27] However, studies have demonstrated that the virus is still present in the plasma, albeit at lower levels, and more so in the lymphoid tissues, where it causes a gradual deterioration of the immune system. The period of clinical latency can vary widely but has a median length of 10 years in untreated patients.[21] A small proportion of HIV-infected individuals, termed long-term nonprogressors (LTNP), have normal or mildly depressed CD4+ T cell counts, low viral loads, and remain asymptomatic for more than 10 years in the absence of antiretroviral therapy.[19,28] The factors that influence this slower rate of progression are not completely understood but appear to be associated with certain HLA types, prevalence of the R5 strain of HIV, and infection at a younger age.[19]

Untreated individuals will ultimately progress to the final stage of HIV infection, AIDS, which is characterized by profound immunosuppression, a resurgence of viremia, and life-threatening infections and malignancies. The rate at which individuals progress to the development of AIDS varies, but progression typically occurs within a median time of 10 years after initial infection.[23,25] The rate of progression has been dramatically decreased with the use of antiretroviral therapies (see the section on treatment).

The CDC first defined AIDS as "a disease, at least moderately predictive of a defect in cell mediated immunity, occurring in a person with no known cause for diminished resistance to that disease."[29] The definition has been revised several times over the years as more information has been acquired about HIV and as additional laboratory tests for HIV have been developed. In the 1993 case definition, the CDC classified HIV-infected adults and adolescents into nine categories (A1 through C3), based on CD4 T-cell counts, in association with clinical conditions found in HIV infection (Table 23–2).[30] According to this definition, HIV-infected individuals are classified as having AIDS if they have an absolute CD4 T lymphocyte count of less than 200/μL or certain opportunistic infections or malignancies indicative of AIDS (Table 23–3). Individuals with AIDS are classified in categories A3, B3, C1, C2, or C3.

In addition to opportunistic infections and malignancies, HIV-infected individuals often demonstrate neurological symptoms resulting from the ability of HIV to infect cells in the brain. In early HIV infection, these symptoms may manifest as forgetfulness, poor concentration, apathy, psychomotor retardation, and withdrawal, while progression to late disease may result in confusion, disorientation, seizures, dementia, gait disturbances, ataxia, or paraparesis.[21,31]

The CDC has also published a separate case definition for AIDS in children.[32] Symptoms of AIDS in infants include failure to thrive, persistent oral candidiasis, hepatosplenomegaly, lymphadenopathy, recurrent diarrhea, or recurrent bacterial infections.[33,34] In addition, abnormal neurological findings may be present. The rate by which HIV infection progresses in children varies and may be influenced by factors such as maturity of the immune system at the time of infection, the dose of virus to which the child was exposed, and the route of infection.[34]

Since the advent of new antiretroviral therapies that have delayed progression to AIDS (see discussion in "Treatment" section), the CDC now tracks individuals who are HIV-positive but who have not developed AIDS in addition to following people with AIDS. As a result, they published a revised surveillance case definition for HIV infection in 1999.[35] According to this definition, adults, adolescents, and children aged 18 months or older are considered to be HIV-infected if they meet the previously published clinical criteria[30] or if they demonstrate positive test results on screening and confirmatory tests for HIV antibody or on an HIV virological test (i.e., HIV nucleic acid detection, HIV p24 antigen test, or HIV isolation in culture). The principles of these tests will be discussed in the "Laboratory Testing for HIV Infection" section.

## TREATMENT

Treatment of HIV infection involves supportive care of the infections and malignancies and administration of antiretroviral drugs to suppress the virus's replication. Several classes of antiretroviral drugs have been developed to treat HIV infection: nucleoside analogue reverse transcriptase inhibitors, nonnucleoside reverse transcriptase inhibitors, protease inhibitors, fusion inhibitors, coreceptor antagonists, and integrase inhibitors.[21,36–38] These drugs block various steps of the HIV replication cycle.

| Table 23–2. | 1993 Revised Classification System for HIV Infection and Expanded AIDS Surveillance Case Definition for Adolescents and Adults | | |
|---|---|---|---|
| | **CLINICAL CATEGORIES** | | |
| | **(A)** | **(B)** | **(C)** |
| **CD4+ T-CELL CATEGORIES** | **ASYMPTOMATIC, ACUTE (PRIMARY) HIV OR PGL*** | **SYMPTOMATIC, NOT (A) OR (C) CONDITIONS** | **AIDS-INDICATOR CATEGORIES CONDITIONS** |
| (1) ≥500/μL | A1 | B1 | C1§ |
| (2) 200–499/μL | A2 | B2 | C2§ |
| (3) <200/μL (AIDS-indicator T-cell count) | A3§ | B3§ | C3§ |

*PGL = persistent generalized lymphadenopathy. Clinical Category A includes acute (primary) HIV infection.
§These cells illustrate the expanded AIDS surveillance case definition. Persons with AIDS-indicator conditions (Category C) as well as those with CD4+ T lymphocyte counts <200/μL (Categories A3 or B3) are reportable as AIDS cases in the United States and Territories, effective January 1, 1993. (For more information, see Centers for Disease Control and Prevention: 1993 revised classification system for HIV infection and expanded surveillance case definition for AIDS among adolescents and adults. MMWR 41 (RR-17):1–19, 1992.)

## Table 23-3. Clinical Categories of HIV Infection

### Category A

One or more of the conditions listed following in an adolescent (≥13 years) or adult with documented HIV infection. Conditions listed in Categories B and C must not have occurred.

- Asymptomatic HIV infection
- Persistent generalized lymphadenopathy
- Acute (primary) HIV infection with accompanying illness or history of acute HIV infection

### Category B

Symptomatic conditions in an HIV-infected adolescent or adult that are not included among conditions listed in Category C and that meet at least one of the following criteria: (1) conditions are attributed to HIV infection or are indicative of a defect in cell-mediated immunity or (2) conditions considered by physicians to have a clinical course or require management that is complicated by HIV infection. Examples include:

- Bacillary angiomatosis
- Candidiasis, oropharyngeal (thrush)
- Candidiasis, vulvovaginal; persistent, frequent, or poorly responsive to therapy
- Cervix dysplasia (moderate or severe)/cervix carcinoma in situ
- Constitutional symptoms, such as fever (38.5°C) or diarrhea lasting >1 month
- Hairy leukoplakia, oral
- Herpes zoster (shingles), involving at least two distinct episodes or more than one dermatome
- Idiopathic thrombocytopenic purpura
- Listeriosis
- Pelvic inflammatory disease
- Peripheral neuropathy

### Category C

- Candidiasis of bronchi, trachea, or lungs
- Candidiasis, esophageal
- Cervical cancer, invasive
- Coccidiomycosis, disseminated or extrapulmonary
- Cryptococcosis, extrapulmonary
- Cryptosporidiosis, chronic intestinal (>1 month's duration)
- Cytomegalovirus (other than liver, spleen, or nodes)
- Cytomegalovirus retinitis (with loss of vision)
- Encephalopathy, HIV-related
- Herpes simplex: chronic ulcer(s) (>1 month's duration); or bronchitis, pneumonitis, or esophagitis
- Histoplasmosis, disseminated or extrapulmonary
- Isosporiasis, chronic intestinal (>1 month's duration)
- Kaposi's sarcoma
- Lymphoma, Burkitt's
- Lymphoma, immunoblastic
- Lymphoma, primary, of brain
- *Mycobacterium avium* complex or *M. kansasii*, disseminated or extrapulmonary
- *Mycobacterium tuberculosis*, any site
- *Mycobacterium*, other species or unidentified species, disseminated or extrapulmonary
- *Pneumocystis carinii* pneumonia
- Pneumonia, recurrent
- Progressive multifocal leukoencephalopathy
- Salmonella septicemia, recurrent
- Toxoplasmosis of brain
- Wasting syndrome due to HIV

For more information, see Reference 30.

The nucleoside analogue reverse transcriptase inhibitors are similar in structure to nucleosides and inhibit further action of the reverse transcriptase enzyme when they incorporate themselves into the viral DNA being generated. This class of drugs includes zidovudine (also known as ZDV or azidothymidine [AZT]), lamivudine (deoxythiacytidine or 3TC), didanosine (dideoxyinosine or ddI), abacavir (ABC), and tenofovir (TDF). Another class of drugs, the nonnucleoside reverse transcriptase inhibitors, stops reverse transcriptase from transcribing RNA into DNA by binding directly to the enzyme and rendering it inactive. This class of drugs includes nevirapine (NVP), delavirdine (DLV), and efavirenz (EFV) and etravirine. The protease inhibitors prevent the cleavage of precursor proteins necessary for the assembly and release of HIV virions during the last stage of the viral reproductive cycle. These drugs include saquinavir (SQV), indinavir (IDV), ritonavir (RTV), nelfinavir (NFV), fosamprenavir, and lopinavir. Fusion inhibitors, such as enfuvirtide (T20), block entry of HIV into host cells by preventing fusion of the HIV membrane with the target cell membrane. Coreceptor antagonists like maraviroc (MVC) block the binding of HIV to the chemokine coreceptor necessary for penetration of the host cell. Integrase inhibitors such as raltegravir inhibit integration of HIV DNA into the host genome. New drugs continue to be developed as advances in this area are made. (Updated guidelines on the use of these drugs are available in reference 38.)

Studies have shown that treatment with multiple drugs is more effective in killing the virus and avoiding viral resistance than treatment with a single drug. Potent regimens involving a combination of drugs from at least two of the drug classes mentioned earlier are the standard of treatment and are referred to as **HAART,** or highly active antiretroviral therapy.[36,38] Currently preferred treatment protocols use combinations of two nucleoside reverse transcriptase inhibitors and either a nonnucleoside reverse transcriptase inhibitor or a protease inhibitor.[38] The goal of this therapy is to reduce the patient's HIV viral load, consequently boosting the patient's level of immunocompetence. This is most likely to be achieved if treatment is started early in the course of infection and the patient can adhere to the treatment as prescribed.[23,36]

HAART has had a dramatic effect on the clinical course of HIV infection, as evidenced by a significant decline in the incidence of opportunistic infections, a delay in progression to AIDS, and decreased mortality in patients who have received this multidrug treatment.[38–40] Retroviral drugs have also had a significant impact in reducing perinatal transmission of HIV, as discussed previously in this chapter.[18] In 1994, investigators from the United States and France published the results of a large clinical trial demonstrating that ZDV administered to HIV-positive women during pregnancy and labor and to the newborn during his or her first few weeks of life reduced transmission of HIV to the infant by two-thirds.[41] As a result of this and subsequent studies, antiretroviral drugs and advice to avoid breastfeeding are recommended routinely for pregnant women who are HIV-positive.[18]

Although antiretroviral drugs and HAART have significantly improved morbidity and mortality in HIV-infected patients, they cannot be considered a cure for AIDS. Research has shown that while blood levels of the virus are greatly reduced in patients treated with antiretroviral drugs, HIV is still harbored in lymphoid organs throughout the body and still progressively destroys the immune system.[19,21] Viral resistance to the drugs may also develop, and some patients may be unable to take the drugs because they cannot tolerate the side effects.

Therefore, many approaches for dealing with this virus have been directed toward measures to prevent initial infection from occurring. Community-based education aimed at high-risk groups such as homosexual males and intravenous drug users has provided beneficial information on reducing transmission of the virus. In addition, the CDC and the Occupational Safety and Health Administration have published precautions to prevent transmission of HIV and other bloodborne pathogens in health-care workers.[42,43] Prophylactic therapy with antiretroviral drugs is also offered to health-care workers who may have been exposed to HIV through percutaneous or mucous membrane contact with potentially infected blood or body fluids, in hope that early treatment will prevent infection.[44]

The ultimate means of preventing HIV infection is the development of an effective vaccine. Some of the strategies used in developing an HIV vaccine include subunit vaccines, which consist of recombinant HIV envelope glycoproteins; live vector-based vaccines, which use other viruses that have been genetically altered to carry HIV genes; and DNA vaccines produced from DNA that codes for HIV proteins.[45–47] Much research has been directed in this area, but the task has been very difficult for many reasons, including the ability of HIV to rapidly mutate and escape immune recognition, the capability of HIV to persist despite vigorous immune responses of the host, genetic variability in HIV clades, the need to induce mucosal immunity because HIV is usually transmitted through mucosal surfaces, the need to induce potent CTL and antibody responses, and the lack of an ideal animal model.[20,21,45–47] If research is unable to produce a vaccine that can prevent HIV infection in the traditional sense, it is possible that a less-than-perfect vaccine may provide some benefits by prolonging the disease-free period and reducing transmission of this devastating virus.[20]

## LABORATORY TESTING FOR HIV INFECTION

Four types of laboratory tests have been used in diagnosing and monitoring HIV infection: CD4 T-cell enumeration, antibody detection, antigen detection, and testing for viral nucleic acid. Culturing for the virus, although a definitive method of demonstrating HIV infection, has been used primarily in research settings. Principles of each of these methods are discussed along with their particular applicability to diagnosis at various stages of the disease.

### CD4 T–Cell Enumeration

Destruction of the CD4 T lymphocytes is central to the immunopathogenesis of HIV infection, and CD4 lymphopenia has long been recognized as the hallmark feature of AIDS. Therefore, enumeration of **CD4 T cells** in the peripheral blood has played a central role in evaluating the degree of immune suppression in HIV-infected patients for several years. In untreated patients, there is a progressive decline in the number of CD4 T cells during the course of infection **(Fig. 23–4).** As discussed earlier, the CDC has used CD4 T-cell counts to classify patients into various stages of HIV infection, with those whose counts are below 200/μL being classified as having AIDS.[30] In addition, CD4 T-cell counts are used routinely to monitor the effectiveness of antiretroviral therapy. It is recommended that CD4 T-cell measurements be performed every 3 to 6 months in HIV-infected patients to guide physicians in determining when antiviral therapy should be initiated, whether a change in therapy is necessary, and if prophylactic drugs for certain opportunistic infections should be administered.[21,48–50] According to published guidelines, antiretroviral therapy should be initiated in patients whose CD4 T-cell count is less than 350/μL; therapy should be changed if CD4 T-cell counts decline more than 25 percent.[21,49]

The gold standard for enumerating CD4 T cells is immunophenotyping with data analysis by **flow cytometry.** The basic principle of this method involves incubating whole peripheral blood with a panel of fluorescent-labeled monoclonal antibodies, removing the erythrocytes by lysis, and stabilizing the leukocytes by fixation with paraformaldehyde.[50–52] The results are analyzed via histograms that display the patterns of light scatter and fluorescence emitted by individual cell populations. The CDC has published guidelines to standardize the performance of CD4 T-cell determinations by flow cytometry.[50,51] Early guidelines referred to a dual platform technology in which both a flow cytometer and a hematology analyzer are required to make CD4 T-cell measurements. According to this protocol, the percentage of CD4 T cells in a sample is determined by dividing the number of lymphocytes positive for the CD4 marker by the total number of lymphocytes counted by the flow cytometer, according to the following equation:

$$\% \text{ CD4 T cells} = \frac{\# \text{ CD4 lymphocytes}}{\text{total } \# \text{ lymphocytes}} \times 100$$

In this determination, three- or four-color immunofluorescence assays are used in which the lymphocytes are differentiated from other cell types in the sample by their side scatter and CD45 staining properties. Lymphocytes are identified on the basis of their low side scatter (which represents the amount of cell complexity as determined by properties such as granularity and membrane irregularity) and their ability to stain brightly with fluorescent-labeled antibody to the CD45 marker, which is present on all white blood cells. The percentage of CD4 T cells obtained for the patient sample is compared to a reference range established by the laboratory performing the test.

Absolute numbers of CD4 T cells are calculated by multiplying the absolute number of lymphocytes (determined by the whole blood cell [WBC] count and differential from a hematology analyzer) by the percentage of CD4 T cells in the sample, according to the following equation:

$$\text{Absolute } \# \text{ CD4 T cells} = \text{WBC} \\ \text{count} \times \% \text{ Lymphocytes} \times \% \text{ CD4 T cells}$$

The absolute CD4 T-cell count is then compared to the reference range, which is typically from 500 to 1300 cells/μL peripheral blood.[53]

Newer technologies employ three- or four-color monoclonal antibody panels in a single-platform approach, which allows CD4 T-cell percentages and absolute numbers to be obtained from one tube using a single instrument, the flow cytometer.[49,50] This is made possible by counting CD4+ T cells in a precisely measured blood volume or by incubating the sample with a known number of commercially available fluorescent microbeads, which function as an internal calibrator. The counts can then be determined by specific flow cytometry software, according to the following equation:[50]

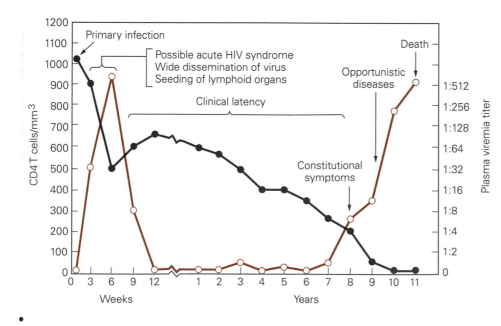

**FIGURE 23–4.** Typical CD4 T cells numbers and plasma viremia during the natural course of HIV infection. *(From Pantaleo, G, Graziosi, C, and Fauci, AS. The immunopathogenesis of human immunodeficiency virus infection. N Engl J Med 328:327–335, 1993.)*

$$\dfrac{\dfrac{\text{\# of events in the bright CD45 region}}{\text{\# of events in the microfluorosphere region}}}{\dfrac{\text{Total \# microspheres added}}{\text{Volume of blood added}}} \times$$

As with the dual-platform technology, lymphocytes are selected for analysis (or "gated") on the basis of their low side scatter and ability to stain brightly with CD45 antibody.

In addition to CD4+ T-cell percentages and absolute numbers, the ratio of CD4 T cells to CD8 T cells may be reported to assess the dynamics between the two T-cell populations. In HIV-infected patients, particularly those with AIDS, the large decrease in the number of CD4 T cells, along with a possible increase in CD8 + cytotoxic T cells, results in an inverted ratio, or a ratio that is less than 1:1.

While flow cytometry is the accepted gold standard for enumeration of CD4+ T cells, it is a costly method that requires the need for highly skilled personnel. Less expensive methods of lower complexity have also been developed to determine CD4 T-cell measurements. These include microcapillary flow cytometry, flow cytometry dedicated for CD4/CD8 measurements, a latex bead-based method read by light microscopy, magnetic bead cell isolation with fluorescent or light microscopy, CD4/CD8 enumeration with an automated hematology analyzer, and an ELISA that measures CD4 protein in lysed whole blood.[49,54-56] Some of these methods may be suitable for resource-limited laboratories, particularly those in developing countries.

## Detection of HIV Antibody

Serological tests for HIV antibody have many important purposes.[57] Since 1985, these tests have played a critical role in screening the donor blood supply to prevent transmission of the virus through blood transfusions or administration of blood products. In addition, serological tests are typically used in the initial diagnosis of HIV infection, because most individuals will develop antibody to the virus within 1 to 2 months after exposure.[57,58] Serological tests are also used in epidemiology studies to provide health officials with information about the extent of the infection in high-risk populations; these groups can then be targeted for counseling, treatment, vaccine trials, and their medical or social concerns can be addressed.

HIV antibody tests can be divided into two groups: (1) screening tests, whose goal is to detect all infected persons, and (2) confirmatory tests, performed on samples giving a positive result on a screening test, to differentiate true-positive from false-positive results. The standard screening method for HIV antibody has been the ELISA, and the standard confirmatory test is the Western blot. In addition to the standard tests, rapid tests have been developed that can detect HIV antibody within minutes, making them an attractive alternative to the ELISA in certain situations. Modifications of these tests, which use saliva or urine or are available as home test kits, have also been developed. The principles of these methods are discussed below.

## Screening Tests Using ELISA Methodology

### Principles of ELISA

Using **ELISAs** (enzyme-linked immunosorbent assays) to detect HIV antibody was first implemented in the United States in 1985 in response to the need to screen donated blood to curtail spread of the infection. ELISAs have been the cornerstone of screening procedures for HIV, because they are easy to perform, can be adapted to test a large number of samples, and are highly sensitive and specific.[21,57,58] Several manufacturers have developed commercial kits that are useful in screening blood products and in diagnosing and monitoring patients.[59] Over the years, technical advances have been made in these ELISAs, resulting in improved sensitivity and specificity.

The first-generation of ELISAs was developed based on a solid-phase, indirect-assay system that detected antibodies to only HIV-1.[57,58] (See Chapter 10 for general principles of ELISA.) In these tests, HIV antibodies in patient serum were detected after binding to a solid support coated with viral lysate antigens from HIV-1 cultured in human T-cell lines, followed by adding an enzyme-labeled conjugate and substrate. These first-generation assays were prone to false-positive results caused by reactions with HLA antigens or other components from the cells used to culture the virus, and they were unable to detect antibodies to HIV-2.[57,58]

The second-generation ELISAs, introduced in the late 1980s, were indirect binding assays that used highly purified recombinant (i.e., genetically engineered) or synthetic antigens from both HIV-1 and HIV-2, rather than crude cell lysates.[57,58] These assays demonstrated improved specificity and sensitivity overall and were able to detect antibodies to both HIV-1 and HIV-2. However, decreased sensitivity resulted when samples containing antibodies to certain subtypes of HIV that lacked the limited antigens used in the assays were tested.

Third-generation assays use the sandwich technique, based on the ability of antibody to bind with more than one antigen.[57,58] In this method, antibodies in patient serum or plasma bind to recombinant HIV-1 and HIV-2 proteins coated onto the solid phase. After washing, enzyme-labeled HIV-1 and HIV-2 antigens are added and bind to the already bound HIV-specific patient antibodies. After substrate is added, color development is proportional to the amount of antibody in the test sample. This format improved sensitivity by simultaneously detecting HIV antibodies of different immunoglobulin classes, including IgM. Enhancements of this method have increased sensitivity further by detecting low affinity antibodies and antibodies to group O HIV-1 and the more common group M. These enhancements resulted in a diagnostic sensitivity of 100 percent and diagnostic specificity of 99.9 percent.[60]

Most recently, fourth-generation assays have been developed that can simultaneously detect HIV-1 antibodies, HIV-2 antibodies, and p24 antigen.[57,58] These combination assays allow for slightly earlier detection of HIV infection than the third-generation assays, because they include the p24 antigen (see following). One study evaluating such a kit found that the fourth-generation assay could detect HIV infection 6.3 days earlier than an established third-generation assay.[61]

In addition, ELISAs with reduced sensitivity, known as "detuned" assays, have been used to differentiate a recent HIV infection from a more established infection. Individuals with a more recent infection (less than 4 months) will give a positive result only with a standard, highly sensitive ELISA test and a negative result with the less sensitive, detuned assay, while persons with a more established infection will give positive results in both assays.[21,57,58,62]

## Interpretation of ELISA Results

While ELISAs have a high level of sensitivity and specificity, they may sometimes give erroneous results. False-negative results occur infrequently but may be due to the collection of the test serum prior to the patient developing HIV antibodies (i.e., prior to **seroconversion**), to administration of immunosuppressive therapy or replacement transfusion, to conditions of defective antibody synthesis such as hypogammaglobulinemia, or to technical errors attributed to improper handling of kit reagents.[58,63] False-negative results may also occur if the patient harbors a genetically diverse, recombinant strain of HIV, or an HIV-1 group O strain that is tested for by an assay that does not detect antibody to group O virus. The likelihood of false negatives occurring because the assay was performed prior to seroconversion has been reduced by the technical advances of the newer generation ELISAs, which can detect HIV antibodies 3 to 6 weeks after infection.[63]

False-positive results may also occur in HIV-antibody ELISA tests. These can result from several factors, including heat inactivation of serum prior to testing, repeated freezing/thawing of specimens, presence of autoreactive antibodies, history of multiple pregnancies, severe hepatic disease, passive immunoglobulin administration, recent exposure to certain vaccines, and certain malignancies.[58] The rate of false positives is substantially higher in low-risk populations than in high-risk populations; in other words, in low-risk populations, the ELISAs have a low **positive predictive value,** or probability that the patient truly has the disease if the test result is positive. For example, the positive predictive value of a repeatedly reactive HIV ELISA was estimated to be only 13 percent in a large study done by the American Red Cross on low-risk blood donors, meaning that only 13 percent of all positives were true positives, and 87 percent were false positives in this population.[58,64] Any positive results obtained by ELISA must therefore be confirmed by additional testing.

According to a commonly accepted testing algorithm established by the CDC, when a sample screened for HIV antibody by ELISA yields a positive result, it should be retested in duplicate by the same ELISA test. If two out of the three specimens are reactive, then the results must be confirmed by a more specific method, usually Western blot (see following).[58,65] Repeatedly reactive units of blood are not used for transfusion, regardless of results of confirmatory testing.

## Rapid Screening Tests

While ELISAs are ideal screening tests for HIV antibodies in clinical laboratories that perform large-volume batch testing, they require complex instrumentation and skilled personnel with technical expertise, and typically have a turn-around time of a few days. To overcome these limitations and to encourage more patients to be tested, advances in technology have led to the development of rapid and simpler methods to screen for HIV antibody. Because these tests are highly sensitive, simple to perform, and provide results in less than 30 minutes, they are used throughout the world. Rapid tests are ideal for use in resource-limited settings in developing nations and in situations in which fast notification of test results is desired.[57,63,66] For example, rapid results are important in guiding decisions to begin prophylactic therapy with antiretroviral drugs following occupational exposures, as this therapy appears to be most effective when administered in the first few hours following exposure. Other situations in which rapid tests are very beneficial include testing women whose HIV status is unknown during labor and delivery, and testing patients in sexually transmitted disease clinics or emergency departments who are unlikely to make a return visit for their test results.

Studies conducted by the CDC and the World Health Organization have shown that the rapid tests for HIV antibody have a high level of sensitivity and specificity, comparable to that of the standard ELISA tests.[67,68] At the time of this writing, there are six rapid tests commercially available in the United States that are approved by the FDA.[69] These kits can be used to test serum, plasma, whole blood, and oral fluid (in one method). While each test has unique features, all are lateral flow or flow-through immunoassays that produce a colorimetric reaction in the case of a positive result. The flow-through assays require multiple steps in which the sample and reagents are added to a solid support encased in a plastic device, while the lateral-flow assays involve a one-step procedure in which the patient sample migrates along the test strip by capillary action. With either procedure, the patient's sample is applied to a test strip or membrane containing HIV antigens. The antigen–antibody complexes bind to an enzyme-labeled conjugate or an antibody-binding (protein A) colloidal gold conjugate and are detected by a colorimetric reaction that produces a colored line or dot in the case of a positive result.[57,58,66,69] Interpretation of the results is made through visual observation of the test device and does not require instrumentation. A reactive result is reported as a preliminary positive and, like the standard ELISA, requires confirmation by a more specific test like the Western blot because of the possibility of false-positive results.[63,66]

## Other Screening Tests

Methods that can test urine for HIV antibody have been developed but are not as accurate as the blood or saliva tests and must be confirmed with a standard serological test.[58,63] In addition, the FDA has approved the use of home test kits for individuals who prefer this format to being tested by a clinic or private physician. In this test system, individuals are provided with written information about HIV and AIDS, obtain a small blood sample by performing a fingerstick with a sterile lancet, and apply the sample to a designated area on a test card.[58,63] The card is then mailed to a certified laboratory, in which traditional ELISA testing for HIV antibody is performed, followed with confirmation by Western blot. The results can be obtained by telephone using a personal identification number.

## Confirmatory Tests

Because of the possibility of obtaining false-positive results, as discussed earlier, all positive samples from HIV screening tests must be referred for testing with a more specific confirmatory method. A variety of different confirmatory methods have been developed for this purpose. The most widely used confirmatory test for HIV antibody, and the standard test in use today, is the Western blot test.

### Western Blot Testing

**Principles** The **Western blot test,** or immunoblot, for HIV antibodies was introduced in 1984 and has been used for systematic confirmation of positive ELISA results since 1985. This technique is more technically demanding than ELISA but can provide an antibody profile of the patient sample that reveals the specificities to individual HIV antigens present. Several commercial kits are available for this type of testing and can provide results within a few hours.[57,58,70]

Western blot kits are prepared commercially as nitrocellulose or nylon strips containing individual HIV proteins that have been separated by polyacrylamide gel electrophoresis and blotted onto the test membrane. The protein antigens are derived from HIV virus grown in cell culture. Antigens with low molecular weight migrate most rapidly and are therefore positioned toward the bottom of the test strip, while antigens of high molecular weight remain toward the top of the membrane.

The testing laboratory then reacts the test strip with patient serum. During the incubation period, any HIV antibodies present will bind to their corresponding antigen on the test membrane, and unbound antibody is removed by washing. Next, an antihuman immunoglobulin with an enzyme label (i.e., the conjugate) is added directly to the test strip and binds to specific HIV antibodies from the patient sample. Unbound conjugate is removed by washing, and bound conjugate is detected after adding the appropriate substrate, which produces a chromogenic reaction. Colored bands appear in the positions where antigen-specific HIV antibodies are present. Separate HIV-1- and HIV-2-specific Western blot tests must be used to test for antibodies to each virus.[57,58,70]

In HIV-1 infection, antibodies to the gag proteins p24 and p55 antigens appear relatively early after exposure to the virus but tend to decrease or become undetectable as clinical symptoms of AIDS appear.[71] Antibodies to the envelope proteins gp41, gp120, and gp160 appear slightly later but remain throughout all disease stages in an HIV-infected individual, making them a more reliable indicator of the presence of HIV.[72] Other antibodies commonly detected by this method are those directed against pol proteins p51 and p66, while antibodies against the regulatory gene products are usually not detectable by conventional methods.[58,71] The bands produced by the test sample are examined visually for the number and types of antibodies present. Densitometry can also be performed to quantitate the intensity of the bands, which would reflect the amount of each antibody produced. Patients can be followed over time to determine whether there is a change in the antibody pattern.

Because Western blot testing is highly dependent on the laboratorian's technical skill and subjective interpretation, it should be performed only in laboratories that have an adequate proficiency testing program. The inclusion of positive and negative control sera in the test run provides quality control for the Western blot. For the test to be valid, the negative control should produce no bands, and the positive control should be reactive with p17, p24, p31, gp41, p51, p55, p66, and gp120/160. In addition, a vigorous external proficiency program should be in place.

**Interpretation of Western Blot Results** A negative test result is reported if either no bands are present or if none of the bands present correspond to the molecular weights of any of the known viral proteins.[58]

Criteria for determining a positive test result have been published by the Association of State and Territorial Public Health Laboratory Directors and CDC, the Consortium for Retrovirus Serology Standardization, the American Red Cross, and the FDA.[58,70-72] Although some controversy exists as to what banding pattern constitutes a positive result, most laboratories follow the criteria of the Association of State and Territorial Public Health Laboratory Directors and CDC.[58] According to these criteria, a result should be reported as positive if at least two of the following three bands are present: p24, gp41, and gp120/gp160[71] **(see Figure 23–5).**

Specimens that have some of the characteristic bands present but do not meet the criteria for a positive test result are considered to be *indeterminate.* This result may be produced if the test serum is collected in the early phase of seroconversion or if the serum contains antibodies that cross-react with some of the immunoblot antigens, producing false-positive results. False positives may be caused by antibodies produced to contaminants from the cells used to culture HIV to prepare the antigens for the test; to autoantibodies, including those directed against HLA, nuclear, mitochondrial, or T-cell antigens; or to antibodies produced after vaccinations.[57,58,63]

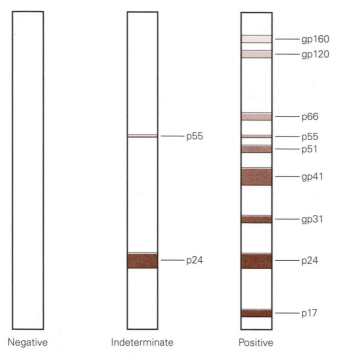

**FIGURE 23–5.** Western blot, showing results from a negative sample, an indeterminate sample, and a positive sample.

The use of recombinant antigens instead of viral lysates has reduced the incidence of false-positive results. If an indeterminate test result is obtained, it is recommended that the test be repeated with the same or a fresh specimen; if the test is still indeterminate, testing may be performed with a new specimen obtained a few weeks later, and if the pattern converts to positive, it can be concluded that the first specimen was obtained during the early phase of seroconversion. Failure of an indeterminate test pattern to convert to positive after a few weeks strongly suggests that the pattern is due to a false-positive test rather than HIV infection.[21,58] During this period, additional tests that detect components of the virus, such as HIV nucleic acid or p24 protein, can be performed to provide more conclusive results (see below).

Because of the possibility of false-positive results, the level of technical difficulty, and the time-consuming nature of the Western blot, this test is inappropriate for use as an initial screen for HIV infection. In the standard testing algorithm described earlier, in which samples determined to be repeatedly reactive by ELISA are then tested by Western blot, the Western blot has a positive predictive value greater than 99 percent for both low-risk and high-risk populations.[58]

### Other Confirmatory Tests

Other confirmatory tests, including IFA, RIPA, line immunoassays, and rapid confirmatory tests, have also been developed.[57,58] These assays may be used as an alternative to the Western blot in the initial confirmation of HIV infection or in cases where the Western blot yields indeterminate results.[73] In the IFA (indirect immunofluorescence assay), antibodies are detected to HIV antigens expressed on

the surface of infected T-cell lines fixed onto a glass slide. This assay has the advantage of being able to detect antibodies to many HIV antigens but requires a well-maintained fluorescent microscope and subjective interpretation of the results. RIPA (radioimmunoprecipitation assay) uses minimally denatured antigens but requires radioactive materials; its use is limited to research laboratories that can maintain HIV in cell cultures. Line immunoassays are similar to Western blots except that recombinant or synthetic HIV proteins are applied to the test strips, rather than being electrophoresed from cultured virus preparations. These assays have allowed for easier interpretation because of fewer bands and false-positive results. In addition, several rapid or simple confirmatory assays have been developed, which may be suitable for use in resource-limited countries that do not have sophisticated instrumentation or stable electricity.[57] Such countries may also use confirmatory strategies other than the traditional screening by ELISA/confirmation by Western blot, including an ELISA followed by a rapid test, testing with two different ELISAs, and testing with two different rapid assays.[57]

## Detection of HIV Antigen

### p24 Antigen Testing

This test detects p24 antigen from the core of the HIV-1 virion. Levels of this antigen in the circulation are thought to correlate with the amount of HIV replication, because they are high in the initial weeks of infection during the early burst of viral replication, then become undetectable as antibody to p24 develops, and then rise again during the later stages of infection when impairment of the immune system allows the virus to replicate.

Testing for the p24 antigen played an important role in HIV testing in the United States prior to the development of more sensitive tests that detect nucleic acid of the virus (see below). The rationale behind using the p24 test is that the antigen appears about 1 week before the appearance of HIV antibody during the acute stage of infection, allowing for slightly earlier detection of the virus.[74] For this reason, the p24 antigen test was used in the United States from 1996 to 1999, along with the tests for HIV antibody to screen blood and plasma donors, until nucleic acid testing was implemented.[70]

This marker has also been used to achieve earlier diagnosis, detect HIV infection in newborns, and monitor patients on antiretroviral therapy. Today, p24 antigen testing is used most commonly in laboratories with limited resources, because it is less expensive and easier to perform than the HIV nucleic acid tests, which have largely replaced tests for p24 antigen in developed nations.[70]

### Test Principles

The p24 antigen is detected by a solid-phase antigen capture enzyme immunoassay[58] (see Chapter 10 for details of capture assays). In this method, a solid support coated with monoclonal anti-HIV-1 antibody is incubated with patient serum or plasma. After washing to remove any unbound antigens, a second anti-HIV-1 antibody conjugated with an enzyme label is added to the reaction. When substrate is added, color development indicates the presence of captured antigen. Optical density can be measured against a standard curve to make a quantitative determination of antigen present.

All positive results should be confirmed by a neutralization assay. This is accomplished by preincubating the patient specimen with human anti-HIV-1 antibody prior to performing the antigen assay. If p24 antigen is present, the neutralizing antibody will form immune complexes and will prevent the antigen from binding to the HIV antibody on the solid support. In a positive test, absorbance should decreased by at least 50 percent.[58]

Because p24 antigen becomes undetectable as the host produces antibody and binds the antigen in immune complexes, the p24 antigen test cannot replace the ELISA test for HIV antibody as the primary screening test for HIV-1 infection. The overall sensitivity of the p24 test is less than that of the ELISA for HIV antibody, with only 20 to 30 percent of asymptomatic HIV-infected individuals showing detectable serum levels of p24 antigen.[58] This lack of sensitivity is partially due to complexing of free antigen with p24 antibody. Sensitivity may be improved by dissociating these immune complexes by treatment with heat or acid prior to the assay.[58,70]

More recently, combination tests have been developed that simultaneously detect p24 antigen and HIV antibody through a series of steps in an enzyme immunoassay or a random access system.[58,61] A procedure combining p24 antigen detection by EIA and HIV RNA by PCR has also been developed.[70] It is hoped that combination assays such as these will allow for detection of HIV infection in situations in which antibody is not detectable or yields indeterminate results.

## Nucleic Acid Testing

Tests for HIV nucleic acid have been incorporated into routine clinical practice and have had an important impact on the management of HIV-infected patients. These tests are used to determine the amount of virus present in patients and to determine whether and what type of drug resistance has developed. Quantitative tests for HIV nucleic acid, also known as **viral load tests,** are used routinely to help predict disease progression, predict response to antiretroviral therapy, and monitor effects of the therapy.[70,75–78] Viral load testing is performed by nucleic acid amplification methods. Tests for drug resistance can be performed by genotypic or phenotypic assays.

### Viral Load Assays

Viral load assays are based on amplification methods that increase the number of HIV RNA copies (or their derivatives) in test samples to detectable levels. Several amplification methods have been developed for this purpose, including the reverse transcriptase polymerase chain reaction (RT-PCR) and real-time PCR, which amplify complementary DNA generated from HIV RNA; the **branched chain DNA** assay (bDNA), which amplifies a labeled signal bound to the test plate; and nucleic acid sequence-based amplification (**NASBA**), which amplifies HIV RNA. The basic principles of each of these methods are discussed briefly here and are covered in more detail in Chapter 11.

### Polymerase Chain Reaction (PCR)

Two kinds of polymerase chain reaction methods have been developed to detect HIV nucleic acid: the reverse-transcriptase polymerase chain reaction (RT-PCR) and more recently, real-time PCR.

A commercial RT-PCR was the first assay to be licensed by the FDA for quantitative measurement of circulating HIV nucleic acid. The basic principle of this test is to amplify a DNA sequence that is complementary to a portion of the HIV RNA genome.[70,75,77,79] In this assay, HIV RNA is isolated from patient plasma by lysis of the virions and precipitation with alcohol. The RNA is treated with a thermostable DNA polymerase enzyme that has both reverse transcriptase activity and the ability to initiate DNA synthesis in the presence of the appropriate reagents; the enzyme is also stable at high temperatures. The reverse transcriptase activity of the enzyme transcribes the HIV RNA into complementary DNA (cDNA). The cDNA is then amplified by standard polymerase chain reaction (PCR) methodology. In this process, double-stranded cDNA molecules are separated into single strands by heating, and each can then serve as a template for synthesis of a new DNA strand. The separated strands are incubated with primers, or short pieces of DNA that are complementary to the ends of a highly conserved region of the HIV-1 gag gene. Cooling of the reaction allows the primers to bind to the cDNA at the appropriate sites. The reaction is heated again, and the region in between the primers is synthesized in the presence of the DNA polymerase enzyme and the four deoxynucleoside triphosphates. This series of steps, referred to as one cycle, generates a copy of the selected portion of the cDNA, called an **amplicon.** This process is repeated for several cycles in an automated thermocycler, resulting in exponential growth in the number of amplicons produced. After the amplification process is complete, the amplicons are chemically denatured into single strands, bound to microtiter plates, and quantitated by the addition of an enzyme-labeled probe, followed by a substrate. The amount of color change produced in each well (i.e., the optical density of the sample) is proportional to the amount of HIV RNA contained in the specimen.

The standard RT-PCR method can detect 400 to 750,000 copies of HIV-1 RNA per mL of plasma, while an ultrasensitive version of the test quantitates HIV-1 RNA over a range of 50 to 100,000 copies/mL.[70,76,77] Both versions of the test must be performed for samples whose values fall outside of the dynamic range. Technical care must be taken when performing the RT-PCR, because this assay is susceptible to cross-contamination of test samples with amplicon, target DNA, or target RNA.[77] To minimize cross-contamination, physically separate work areas should be designated for reagent preparation, sample preparation, amplification, and detection, and the work should flow in one direction only.

More recently, real-time RT-PCR assays have been developed to quantitate HIV RNA.[70,76,79,80] In these assays, the amplicons are analyzed at the same time they are produced (i.e., in real time). This is accomplished by adding a fluorescent marker that is incorporated into the amplicon during the reaction. The fluorescent signal produced is proportional to the amount of amplicon generated and is compared to a standard curve to produce a quantitative result. The reaction is carried out in a closed tube, minimizing the risk of carryover contamination with other amplicons. Real-time PCR is highly sensitive and is capable of detecting a broad range of RNA copies, from 40 to 10 million copies/mL.[70,76,80] The test is also capable of detecting all subtypes of groups M, N, O, and recombinant strains of HIV.[76,80] Because of these advantages, real-time RT-PCR is likely to replace standard RT-PCR methods to detect HIV RNA in many laboratories in the future.[70]

### Branched-Chain DNA (bDNA) Assay

In contrast to RT-PCR, the bDNA method is based on amplifying the detection signal generated rather than amplifying the HIV target sequence. This is accomplished by using a solid-phase sandwich **hybridization** assay that incorporates multiple sets of oligonucleotide probes and hybridization steps to create a series of "branched" molecules.[70,75,77,79] First, RNA isolated from lysed virions in patient plasma is captured on wells of a microtiter plate coated with a number of probes. The captured RNA is then hybridized with branched amplifier probes and incubated with an enzyme-labeled probe that will bind to the DNA branches. Finally, a chemiluminescent substrate is added, and color change is measured with a luminometer. Quantitative results are generated from a standard curve.

The bDNA test can detect 50 to 500,000 copies of HIV RNA/mL of plasma.[76,77] As compared to the RT-PCR, the bDNA has higher upper limits in its detection ranges, does not require separate rooms for its various steps because amplification of the target is not involved, and is better at detecting all known subtypes of HIV; however, it is more conducive for laboratories with higher testing volumes and requires a larger sample volume.[70,77]

### Nucleic Acid Sequence-Based Amplification (NASBA)

NASBA is a target amplification assay based on amplification of HIV RNA.[70,75,79] In this procedure, HIV viral RNA is isolated from the clinical specimen to be tested and is initially treated with reverse transcriptase to form cDNA. An RNase H enzyme is used to remove RNA from the RNA:cDNA hybrid formed, and the cDNA generated serves as a template to generate new RNA molecules in the presence of RNA polymerase, primers specific for a region of the gag gene, and the ribonucleotide triphosphates. All steps of the reaction are performed at a constant temperature; thus, a thermocycler is not required. The amplicons produced are captured onto probes bound to magnetic beads, which are in turn hybridized with chemiluminescent probes and attached to the surface of an electrode, where an electrochemiluminescent reaction occurs. The amount of light generated is proportional to the amount of amplicon in the sample, and quantitative results are obtained via internal calibrators that are used to produce a standard curve.

The NASBA method has a wide detection range: 176 to 3.4 million copies of HIV-1 RNA/mL of specimen.[70,76] It requires a small volume of specimen, making it conducive to testing neonates and children, and it can be used for a variety of specimens in addition to plasma, including cerebrospinal fluid, whole blood, semen, cervical washings, and sputum.[75,76] However, NASBA is a more technically complex method to perform than RT-PCR or bDNA and may be best suited for research laboratories.

### Clinical Utility of Viral Load Tests

Viral load tests play an essential role in helping physicians determine when to initiate antiretroviral therapy, monitoring patient responses to therapy, and predicting time of progression to AIDS.[70,78] They may also be helpful in establishing a diagnosis of HIV infection in cases where the HIV antibody tests are negative or indeterminate.[70,78]

The amount of HIV RNA, or the viral load, in a patient's plasma reflects the natural history of HIV infection in that individual.[12,81] HIV RNA levels become detectable about 11 days after infection and rise to very high levels shortly thereafter, during the initial burst of viral replication. Typically, over a period of a few months, the viral load drops as the individual's immune system clears viral particles from the circulation, and a stable level of plasma HIV RNA, known as the "set point" is achieved (see Fig. 23–4). In untreated individuals, this level can persist for a long time and then rise again later as the immune system deteriorates and the patient progresses to AIDS. Successful therapy with antiretroviral drugs will result in a drop in the viral load level.

Therefore, viral load tests are used routinely to monitor patients during the course of HIV infection and play a critical role in the clinical management of these individuals. Studies performed by the Multicenter AIDS Cohort and other groups have demonstrated that information obtained from viral load tests has prognostic value.[48,81–83] These studies have shown that baseline plasma viral load values obtained in patients prior to the start of antiretroviral therapy are an important predictor of disease progression, in that a higher number of HIV RNA copies/mL of plasma is associated with more rapid development of an AIDS-defining illness or AIDS-related death.

In addition, viral load values have been instrumental in monitoring patients during the course of antiretroviral therapy. Patients who attain a lower number of HIV-RNA copies/mL of plasma are more likely to achieve a longer treatment response.[38,48,81,82] The optimal goal of therapy is to reach undetectable levels of HIV RNA (i.e., <50 to 80 copies/mL, depending on the assay).[38,70] Patients who fail to achieve a significant decrease in viral load after receiving antiretroviral drugs may not be adhering to the appropriate drug administration schedule or may have problems absorbing the drugs, while patients whose viral loads increase over a period may have developed viral resistance to the drugs.[48]

The U.S. Department of Health and Human Services recommends that plasma HIV RNA testing be performed before antiretroviral therapy begins, to obtain a baseline value; testing should then be done 2 to 8 weeks after the initiation of therapy and every 3 to 4 months thereafter to determine the effectiveness of the therapy.[38,70,78] In order to obtain an accurate assessment of viral load dynamics in a single patient, it is recommended that the same assay be used for these viral load measurements, because values may differ between different molecular tests.[70] A change in viral load is considered to be significant if there is at least a threefold or 0.5 log increase or decrease in the number of copies/mL.[38,70] Initiation of antiretroviral therapy or a change in the therapy protocol is recommended for patients whose HIV RNA levels and CD4 T-cell counts reach critical values (200 to 350 cells/mm³).[38,81] Viral load testing is also recommended for individuals who develop symptoms consistent with primary HIV infection, who develop a clinically significant opportunistic infection, or whose CD4 T-cell counts drop unexpectedly.

Although molecular methods are not approved by the FDA for the diagnosis of HIV infection, these tests can be helpful in identifying the infection in certain individuals, such as those who are HIV-antibody-negative or who have equivocal antibody test results (e.g., those tested prior to seroconversion, infants).[70,78]

## Drug-Resistance Testing

Because HIV has high replication and mutation rates and because no treatment completely eradicates the virus, it is possible for drug-resistant subpopulations to emerge during the course of antiretroviral therapy. Two types of laboratory methods can be used to test for drug resistance: genotype resistance assays and phenotype resistance assays.[38,48,70,77,84,85] Genotype resistance assays are performed more frequently than phenotype resistance assays, because they are less expensive, are more widely available, and have a shorter turnaround time.[70]

Genotype resistance assays detect mutations in the reverse transcriptase and protease genes of HIV. In these tests, RNA is isolated from patient plasma, the desired genes are amplified by RT-PCR, and the products are analyzed for mutations associated with drug resistance by automated DNA sequencing or hybridization.[38,48,70,77,84] Commercial kits for genotyping assays are available, and there are online services to assist in interpreting the results.[38,70,77,84] The tests may also be performed and interpreted by reference laboratories. While genotyping tests are less expensive and have a shorter turnaround time than phenotypic methods, they can identify only known mutations and cannot assess the effects of combinations of individual mutations on drug resistance.[84]

Phenotype resistance assays determine the ability of clinical isolates of HIV to grow in the presence of antiretroviral drugs.[38,48,70,77,84,85] These assays are technically complex and are performed only by highly specialized reference laboratories. In these assays, recombinant viruses are created by inserting the reverse transcriptase and protease gene sequences from HIV RNA in the patient's plasma into a laboratory reference strain of HIV and transfecting the recombinant virus into mammalian cells. Varying concentrations of antiviral drugs are incubated with the transfected cells, and the $IC_{50}$ values, or drug concentrations needed to suppress the replication of the patient's viral isolate by 50 percent, are calculated. These values are then compared to the $IC_{50}$ values of cells transfected with a reference strain of HIV in order to determine drug resistance.[38,48,84] The major advantage of phenotypic assays is that they measure drug susceptibility directly, on the basis of all mutations present in the patient's isolate. However, they involve sophisticated technologies that are not widely available, are expensive, and have a long turnaround time.[84]

Both genotypic and phenotypic assays require that a viral load of at least 500 to 1000 copies of HIV RNA/mL be present in the test sample and for the resistant virus to constitute more than 20 percent of the total viral population in the patient to be detected.[48,70,84] Despite these limitations, studies have shown that patients undergoing drug-resistance testing, particularly by genotyping methods, have a better chance of receiving antiretroviral therapy regimens that are more likely to result in greater reductions in viral load.[48,85-88] Therefore, the U.S. Department of Health and Human Services recommends that drug-resistance testing be performed in individuals prior to initiating antiretroviral therapy, in patients in whom HAART has failed or viral load values have not been optimally reduced by antiretroviral therapy, and in all HIV-positive pregnant women.[38,70]

## Virus Isolation

Definitive evidence of HIV infection can be provided through the use of cell culture techniques to isolate viral particles from patient cells and tissues. A cocultivation system has been used in which cells from patients are mixed with T-cell lines or peripheral blood mononuclear cells from HIV-seronegative donors that have been stimulated with phytohemagglutinin and interleukin-2.[70,89] The best patient sample is peripheral blood, but virus can be isolated from other body fluids, such as cerebrospinal fluid, saliva, cervical secretions, semen, and tears, and from organ biopsies.[88]

Samples other than peripheral blood, however, have varying levels of virus, which makes culture less efficient.

Infection can be confirmed by detecting reverse transcriptase activity or p24 antigen in the culture supernatant, detecting the HIV genome by molecular methods, or observing characteristic cytopathic effects.[90] Presence of the virus can also be demonstrated by using fluorescent-labeled monoclonal anti-HIV antibody. Typically, culture results become positive within 2 weeks of incubation, but periods of up to 60 days may be required for some samples.[89] Viral culture can also be used in drug-resistance assays and to determine the viral replicative capacity in isolates from patients undergoing antiretroviral therapy.[70]

Viral culture is laborious, time-consuming, and costly, and it may be hazardous to laboratory personnel involved in the testing process. Because of these reasons, it is not suitable for implementation in the clinical laboratory and is employed primarily in research. In most cases, information regarding HIV infection can be obtained in a more practical manner by performing tests that detect HIV components, such as RT-PCR and p24 antigen.

## Testing of Infants and Young Children

The traditional algorithm for laboratory diagnosis of HIV infection in adults, as discussed above, involves screening individuals using an ELISA or rapid test for HIV antibody and confirming positive results by Western blot. However, serological tests are not reliable in detecting HIV infection in children younger than 18 months of age because of placental passage of IgG antibodies from an infected mother to her child. These maternal antibodies persist in the bloodstream of the infant during the first year of life (or longer in a small proportion of infants) and can confuse the interpretation of serological results from infant samples.[91,92] Thus, a child born to an HIV-positive mother may test positive for HIV antibody during the first 18 months of life even though the child is not infected.

Because of the difficulties with serological testing, HIV infection in infants is best diagnosed using molecular methods. A qualitative HIV-1 DNA PCR test is the preferred method for this purpose. This test, which detects proviral DNA within the infants' peripheral blood mononuclear cells, has a sensitivity of 90 to 100 percent and a specificity of 95 to 100 percent in infants older than 1 month of age.[91,92] Alternatively, quantitative HIV RNA assays may be used to diagnose HIV infection in infants and young children and are more likely to detect infections with strains other than subtype B.[91,92] Testing for p24 antigen is not recommended, as it has a low sensitivity in infants.[91,93]

It is recommended that nucleic acid tests for HIV be performed in infants with known perinatal exposure at the ages of 14 to 21 days, 1 to 2 months, 4 to 6 months, and possibly at birth.[94] A positive test result should be confirmed by repeat testing. Negative test results provide presumptive evidence for the absence of HIV infection and should be confirmed by serological tests at 12 to 18 months of age.[91,92] The HIV status of breastfed infants, who are continually exposed to the virus, cannot be determined accurately until breastfeeding is stopped.[92]

Increased emphasis on screening pregnant women for HIV infection should also help in the identification of HIV-positive infants.[95] Rapid tests for HIV antibody should be performed on women whose HIV status is unknown and on their newborn infants soon after birth.[92] Prompt detection of HIV infection in newborns is important, because infected infants have a better prognosis when HAART is started early and can benefit from treatment with prophylactic drugs for opportunistic infections.[91,94]

## SUMMARY

Human immunodeficiency virus type 1 (HIV-1) is responsible for the majority of AIDS cases throughout the world. A related virus, HIV-2, may also cause AIDS but is generally less pathogenic. These viruses belong to the retrovirus family, which contains RNA as the genetic material from which DNA is transcribed. Transmission of HIV occurs by three major routes: through intimate sexual contact, through contact with contaminated blood or body fluids, or through vertical transmission from infected mother to her fetus or infant.

The three main structural genes of HIV are gag, env, and pol. The gag gene codes for the core proteins of the virus, including p24 antigen, the first to appear during infection. Products of the pol gene are the enzymes reverse transcriptase, integrase, and protease. The env gene codes for the envelope proteins gp120 and gp41, which facilitate attachment of the virus to the CD4 receptor and chemokine coreceptors on susceptible host cells. Several other genes are present that function to regulate replication of the virus.

After HIV binds to a host cell, fusion occurs, and the viral particle is taken inside the cell. Reverse transcriptase produces DNA from the viral RNA, and HIV is incorporated into the host-cell DNA as a provirus. A burst of viral replication occurs after initial infection. This is followed by a period of latency that begins as an immune response to the virus develops and can last for 10 years or more as viral replication is held in check. The prime targets of HIV infection are the T helper cells, which have large numbers of CD4 molecules on their cell surface. Untreated HIV infection results in a progressive destruction of these cells, with resumption of high rates of viral replication and development of profound immunosuppression in the host.

Clinical symptoms of HIV infection are associated with the levels of viral replication and helper T cell destruction in the host. The infection progresses through an acute stage, followed by a latent stage, and eventual progression to AIDS. During the latent period, the virus is harbored in the lymphoid tissues, where it causes gradual destruction of the immune system. In untreated patients, this will eventually result in AIDS, which is characterized by an increase in viral reproduction, with profound immunosuppression and host susceptibility to several opportunistic infections and malignancies. The use of HAART, a combination of antiretroviral drugs that inhibit HIV replication, has resulted in improved immune function in infected individuals, with a decline in the incidence of opportunistic infections and a delay in progression to AIDS. Antiretroviral drugs have also played an important role in decreasing perinatal transmission.

The main laboratory tests for HIV infection are CD4 T-cell enumeration, HIV antibody detection, p24 antigen detection, and testing for HIV nucleic acid. The standard method for CD4 T-cell enumeration is multicolor immunofluorescence staining, followed by analysis with flow cytometry. CD4 T-cell counts are routinely monitored in HIV-infected individuals and provide important information regarding likelihood of disease progression and development of opportunistic infections, and effectiveness of antiretroviral therapy. These counts are also used in the CDC classification system for HIV infection and AIDS.

Detection of HIV antibodies is performed with an initial ELISA screening test. Third-generation ELISAs employ a sandwich technique in which HIV antibodies in patient serum or plasma are sandwiched between two sets of HIV antigens, one bound to a solid phase and a second containing an enzyme label. ELISA testing is sensitive but is subject to false-positive reactions created by cross-reactivity of antibodies produced in a number of other conditions. Therefore, confirmatory testing of positive specimens is necessary. The Western blot is the most commonly used confirmatory test. In this test, patient serum is reacted with a nitrocellulose strip containing separate areas of distinct HIV antigens. HIV antibodies to specific antigens on the strip are detected after addition of an enzyme-labeled antihuman immunoglobulin and substrate. Colored bands develop in the areas on the strip where HIV antibodies have bound. A positive test result is indicated by the presence of two of the following three major bands: p24, gp41, or gp120/160.

Detection of p24 antigen was designed to identify HIV infection during the window period before antibody is detectable. This test may be used to detect infection in patients whose antibody status is negative or indeterminate. An antigen capture or sandwich assay is employed, which uses a solid-phase antibody to capture p24 in the patient specimen. A second labeled antibody is added and adheres only to antigen caught on the solid phase.

Nucleic acid testing for HIV is used to determine the amount of virus harbored by patients and the development of drug-resistant strains of virus. Quantitative tests for HIV nucleic acid are known as *viral load tests*. These tests have had an important impact on the clinical management of HIV-infected patients by allowing physicians to predict disease progression, to predict response to antiretroviral therapy, and to monitor effects of the therapy. Viral load tests are performed by one of three molecular methods: reverse transcriptase polymerase chain reaction (RT-PCR), a method that converts HIV RNA into cDNA and then amplifies the cDNA generated; branched chain DNA assay (bDNA), which amplifies a labeled signal bound to a test plate; and nucleic acid sequence-based amplification (NASBA), which amplifies HIV RNA. Drug-resistance testing can be performed by genotypic assays that use molecular methods or by phenotypic assays in which HIV replication in clinical isolates is assessed in the presence of varying concentrations of antiretroviral drugs.

Isolation of HIV in culture represents another technique for identifying HIV infection. Because it is time-consuming, costly, and hazardous to workers, it is not used to a great extent.

Diagnosis of HIV in neonates is more complex than testing in adults. The presence of maternally acquired antibody in newborns makes ELISA tests for HIV antibody unreliable until a child is over 18 months old. The preferred method for testing infants and children younger than 18 months is a PCR that detects HIV proviral DNA in the patient's peripheral blood mononuclear cells. Careful monitoring of HIV-infected mothers and early testing of infants at risk is being implemented to facilitate prompt medical intervention.

# CASE STUDY

A young woman recently discovered that her boyfriend tested HIV-positive. She was concerned that she may have also contracted the infection, because she had experienced flulike symptoms 1 month ago. She decided to visit her physician for a medical evaluation.

## Questions

a. What initial laboratory tests should be performed on the young woman to determine if she has been exposed to HIV?

b. If the woman tests positive in the initial evaluation, how can it be determined whether her test results are truly positive because of HIV infection or if they represent a false-positive result?

c. If the woman's test results are truly positive, what tests can be done to monitor her over time?

# EXERCISE

## SIMULATION OF HIV-1 DETECTION

### Principle: An HIV Screening Simulation

Enzyme linked immunosorbent assay (ELISA) tests were originally developed for antibody measurement. These immunoassays have also been adapted to successfully detect samples that contain antigens. This HIV ELISA simulation experiment has been designed to detect a hypothetical patient's circulating IgG directed toward the viral (HIV) antigen. ELISAs are done in microtiter plates that are generally made of polystyrene or polyvinyl chloride. The plates are somewhat transparent and contain many small wells, in which liquid samples are deposited.

The following are the basic steps of the ELISA reaction.

1. Antigens are added to the wells, where some remain adsorbed to the wells by hydrophobic bonds. Antigens can be from whole HIV lysates, specific HIV proteins, or a mixture of the two. There is no specificity involved with the adsorption process to the wells, although some substances may exhibit differential binding. In certain cases, the antigens can be covalently cross-linked to the plastic using UV light.

2. Wells are washed to remove unadsorbed antigens.

3. Block the unoccupied sites on the walls of the plastic wells with proteins, typically gelatin or bovine serum albumin.

4. Infection by HIV-1 causes the individual to mount an antibody response that eventually results in plasma IgG molecules that bind to different HIV proteins (or different areas or the same protein). If these antibodies are present, as in the plasma sample of an HIV-positive patient, they will bind to the adsorbed antigens in the well and will remain there after washing. If the antibody (from an HIV-positive patient) remains bound to the antigen in the well, then the secondary antibody will bind to it and remain attached after washing. If the patient is negative for HIV, there will be no primary antibody to bind to the antigen and, in turn, no secondary antibody binding. Secondary antibodies are usually raised in rabbits and goats immunized with human IgG fractions. Secondary antibodies (anti-HIV-IgG) are purified and covalently cross-linked to horseradish peroxidase. This modification does not usually affect the binding specificity and affinity of the antibody or the enzymatic activity of the peroxidase.

5. Wells are washed to remove unbound secondary antibody.

6. After washing, a solution containing hydrogen peroxide and aminosalicylate is added to each well. Peroxidase possesses a high catalytic activity and can exceed turnover rates of 106 per second. Consequently, amplification of an HIV-positive sample can occur over several orders of magnitude. Many hydrogen donor cosubstrates can be used by peroxidase. These cosubstrates include o-dianisidine, aminoantipyrine, aminosalicylic acid, and numerous phenolic compounds that develop color upon oxidation. The substrate solution used for the ELISA reaction is nearly colorless. Peroxidase converts the peroxide to $H_2O + O_2$ using the salicylate as the hydrogen donor. The oxidized salicylate is brown and can be easily observed in wells containing anti-HIV-1 IgG (positive plasma). It should be noted that polyclonal antibody preparations to a given antigen can have variable binding affinities due to differences in the immunologic responses between animals. Different immunizations with the same antigen in the same animal can also produce variable binding affinities. The use of monoclonal antibodies directed against a single epitope eliminates this variability. Western blot analysis of positive ELISA samples is used to confirm the presence of HIV in a patient.

### Reagents, Materials, and Equipment

EDVOTEK Kit #271: AIDS Kit 1—Simulation of HIV-1 Detection, containing the following:

HIV antigens (simulated)

Positive control (primary antibody)

Donor 1 serum (simulated)

Donor 2 serum (simulated)

Anti-IgG-peroxidase conjugate (secondary antibody)

Hydrogen peroxide, stabilized

Aminosalicylic acid (peroxide cosubstrate)

Phosphate buffered saline concentrate

Microtiter plates

Transfer pipettes

Microtest tubes with attached caps

1 mL pipettes

Plastic tubes, 50 mL

This experiment does not contain HIV virus or its components. None of the components have been prepared from human sources.

### Additional Materials Required

Distilled or deionized water

Beakers

37°C incubation oven

Disposable lab gloves

Safety goggles

Automatic micropipettes and tips recommended

Make sure glassware is clean, dry, and free of soap residue.

## Experiment Objective

The objective of this experiment is to understand the molecular biology of HIV and the pathogenesis of AIDS. The experimental concepts and methodology involved with enzyme linked immunosorbent (ELISA) assays will be introduced in the context of the clinical screening of serum samples for antibodies to the virus.

## Laboratory Safety

1. Exercise extreme caution when working with equipment that is used in conjunction with the heating or melting of reagents.

2. Do not mouth pipette reagents—use pipette pumps or bulbs.

3. Gloves and goggles should be worn routinely as good laboratory practice.

## Procedure*

### General Instructions and Procedures

#### Labeling The Microtiter Plate

• Mark the microtiter plate with your initials or lab group number and number the rows 1 to 4 down the side.

  Label 5 transfer pipets as follows:

• − (negative)

• + (positive)

• DS 1 (donor serum 1)

• DS 2 (donor serum 2)

• PBS (phosphate buffered saline)

  Use the appropriately labeled plastic transfer pipette for liquid removals and washes.

## Instructions for Adding Liquids and Washing Wells

Adding reagents to wells:

• For adding reagents to the wells, use the same 1 ml pipette.

• Rinse the pipette thoroughly with distilled water before using it for adding the next reagent.

#### Liquid Removal and Washes

When instructed in the experimental procedures, remove liquids with the appropriately labeled transfer pipette, and then wash the wells as follows:

1. Use the transfer pipette labeled "PBS" to add PBS buffer to the wells in all rows. Add PBS buffer until each well is almost full. The capacity of each well is approximately 0.2 ml. Do not allow the liquids to spill over into adjacent wells.

2. With the appropriately labeled transfer pipette, remove all the liquid (PBS buffer) from the wells in each row. Dispose the liquid in the beaker labeled "waste."

## Experimental Steps for the Elisa

1. To all 12 wells, add 100 µl of "HIV" (viral antigens).

2. Incubate for 5 minutes at room temperature.

3. Remove all the liquid (viral antigens) with a transfer pipette.

4. Wash each well once with PBS buffer as described in "Liquid Removal and Washes." Wear safety goggles and gloves. In research labs, following this step, all sites on the microtiter plate are saturated with a blocking solution consisting of a protein mixture, such as BSA. We have designed this experiment to eliminate this step to save time.

5. Add reagents as outlined below:

  Remember to rinse the 1 ml pipette thoroughly with distilled water before adding a new reagent. If you are using automatic micropipettes, use a clean micropipette tip for each reagent.

• Add 100 µl of PBS buffer to the three wells in row 1. (This is the negative control.)

• Add 100 µl of + (positive) to the three wells in row 2. (This is the positive control.)

• Add 100 µl of donor serum "DS1" to the three wells in row 3.

• Add 100 µl of donor serum "DS2" to the three wells in row 4.

6. Incubate at 37°C for 15 minutes.

7. Remove all the liquid from each well with the appropriately labeled transfer pipette.

8. Wash each well once with PBS buffer (as described under "Liquid Removal and Washes").

9. Add 100 µl of the anti-IgG peroxidase conjugate (2°Ab) to all 12 wells.

10. Incubate at 37°C for 15 minutes. At this time you can obtain the substrate to be used in step 13. Since the substrate must be prepared just prior to use, your instructor will prepare it toward the end of the incubation in step 10.

11. Remove all the liquid from each well with the appropriately labeled transfer pipette.

> **Quick Reference:** The positive control, which contains IgG directed against HIV antigens, is the primary antibody. Positive serum samples will also contain anti-HIV IgG, while negative serum samples will not contain anti-HIV IgG.

---

* Permission granted to reproduce the following information by EDVOTEK—The Biotechnology Education Company (edvotek@aol.com).

12. Wash each well once with PBS buffer (as described under "Liquid Removal and Washes").

13. Add 100 µl of the substrate to all 12 wells.

14. Incubate at 37°C for 5 minutes.

15. Remove the plate for analysis.

16. If color is not fully developed after 5 minutes, incubate at 37°C for a longer period of time.

## Interpretation of Results

The positive control, which contains IgG directed against HIV antigens, is the primary antibody. Positive serum samples will also contain anti-HIV IgG. Wells containing positive control or positive serum samples will develop a brown color. Negative serum samples will not contain anti-HIV IgG and will remain colorless.

# REVIEW QUESTIONS

1. All of the following apply to HIV *except*

   a. it possesses an outer envelope.
   b. it contains an inner core with p24 antigen.
   c. it contains DNA as its nucleic acid.
   d. it is a member of the retrovirus family.

2. Which of the following genes is responsible for the coding of reverse transcriptase?

   a. Env
   b. Pol
   c. Gag
   d. Tat

3. HIV virions bind to host T cells through which receptors?

   a. CD4 and CD8
   b. CD4 and the IL-2 receptor
   c. CD4 and CXCR4
   d. CD8 and CCR2

4. Antibodies to which of the following viral antigens are usually the first to be detected in HIV infection?

   a. gp120
   b. gp160
   c. gp41
   d. p24

5. Which of the following is typical of the latent stage of HIV infection?

   a. Proviral DNA is attached to cellular DNA.
   b. Large numbers of viral particles are synthesized.
   c. A large amount of viral RNA is synthesized.
   d. Viral particles with no envelope are produced.

6. The decrease in T-cell numbers in HIV-infected individuals is due to

   a. lysis of host T cells by replicating virus.
   b. fusion of the T cells to form syncytia.
   c. killing of the T cells by HIV-specific cytotoxic T cells.
   d. all of the above.

7. The most common means of HIV transmission worldwide is through

   a. blood transfusions.
   b. intimate sexual contact.
   c. sharing of needles in intravenous drug use.
   d. transplacental passage of the virus.

8. All of the following are likely immunologic manifestations of HIV infection *except*

   a. decreased CD4 T-cell count.
   b. increased CD8 T-cell count.
   c. increased response to vaccine antigens.
   d. increased serum immunoglobulins.

9. The drug zidovudine is an example of a

   a. nucleoside analogue reverse transcriptase inhibitor.
   b. nonnucleoside reverse transcriptase inhibitor.
   c. protease inhibitor.
   d. fusion inhibitor.

10. Which of the following methods is used in third-generation ELISA tests for HIV antibody?

    a. Binding of patient antibody to solid-phase recombinant HIV antigens followed by addition of enzyme-labeled antihuman immunoglobulin
    b. Binding of patient antibody to solid-phase recombinant HIV antigens, followed by addition of enzyme-labeled HIV-specific antibodies
    c. Binding of patient antibody to solid-phase recombinant HIV antigens, followed by addition of enzyme-labeled HIV antigens
    d. Binding of patient antibody to a solid-phase coated with antigens purified from HIV viral lysates, followed by addition of enzyme-labeled antihuman immunoglobulin

11. If a test has a high positive predictive value, which of the following is true?

    a. There will be no false negatives.
    b. Most positives are true positives.
    c. It is not a good screening test.
    d. The number of true positives will vary with the population.

12. False-negative test results in the ELISA test for HIV antibody may occur because of

    a. heat inactivation of the serum prior to testing.
    b. collection of the test sample prior to seroconversion.
    c. interference by autoantibodies.
    d. recent exposure to certain vaccines.

13. Which of the following combinations of bands would represent a positive Western blot for HIV antibody?

    a. p24 and p55
    b. p24 and p31
    c. gp41 and gp120
    d. p31 and p55

14. Which of the following tests would give the least reliable results in a 2-month-old infant?

    a. CD4 T-cell count
    b. ELISA for HIV antibody
    c. RT-PCR for HIV nucleic acid
    d. NASBA for HIV nucleic acid

15. The RT-PCR is a highly sensitive method that involves

    a. direct amplification of HIV RNA.
    b. amplification of a label attached to HIV RNA.
    c. amplification of a complementary DNA sequence to a portion of the HIV RNA.
    d. DNA sequencing of a portion of HIV RNA.

# References

1. World Health Organization. Global HIV prevalence has leveled off. Available at http://who.int/mediacentre/news/releases/ 2007/pr61/en/print.html. Accessed January 30, 2008.

2. Centers for Disease Control and Prevention. HIV/AIDS surveillance report, 2006, vol. 18, rev. ed. U.S. Department of Health and Human Services, Centers for Disease Control and Prevention, Atlanta, 2007, pp. 1–55.

3. Barre-Sinoussi, F, et al. Isolation of a T-lymphotropic retrovirus from a patient at risk for acquired immunodeficiency syndrome (AIDS). Science 220:868–870, 1983.

4. Gallo, RC, et al. Human T-lymphotropic retrovirus, HTLV-III isolated from AIDS patients and donors at risk for AIDS. Science 224:500–503, 1984.

5. Levy, JA, et al. Isolation of lymphocytopathic retroviruses from San Francisco patients with AIDS. Science 225:840–842, 1984.

6. Schupbach, J, and Gallo, RC. Human retroviruses. In Spector, S, Hodinka, RL, and Young, SA (eds): Clinical Virology Manual, ed. 3. ASM Press, Washington, DC, 2000, pp. 513–560.

7. Weiss, RA, Dalgleish, AG, and Loveday, C. Human immunodeficiency viruses. In Zuckerman, AJ, Banatvala, JE, and Pattison, JR (eds): Principles and Practice of Clinical Virology, ed. 4. John Wiley & Sons, Chichester, England, 2000, pp. 659–693.

8. Kandathil, AJ, Ramalingam, S, Kannangai, R, David, S, and Sridharan, G. Molecular epidemiology of HIV. Indian J Med Res 121:333–344, 2005.

9. Clavel, F, et al. Isolation of a new human retrovirus from West African patients. Science 223:343–346, 1986.

10. Karim, SS, Karim, QA, Gouws, E, and Baxter C. Global epidemiology of HIV-AIDS. Infect Dis Clin N Am 21:1–17, 2007.

11. Collier, L, and Oxford, J. Human Virology, ed. 3. New York, Oxford University Press, 2006, pp. 179–188.

12. Kindt, TJ, Goldsby, RA, and Osborne, BA. Kuby Immunology, ed. 6. WH Freeman, New York, 2007, pp. 504–521.

13. Centers for Disease Control and Prevention. Twenty-five years of HIV/AIDS—United States, 1981–2006. MMWR 55:585–589, 2006.

14. Centers for Disease Control and Prevention. Public health service guidelines for the management of health-care worker exposures to HIV and recommendations for postexposure prophylaxis. MMWR 47:211–215, 1998.

15. Centers for Disease Control and Prevention. Updated U.S. public health service guidelines for the management of occupational exposures to HIV and recommendations for postexposure prophylaxis. MMWR 54(RR09):1–17, 2005.

16. Dodd, RY, Notari, EP, and Stramer, SL. Current prevalence and incidence of infectious disease markers and estimated window period risk in the American Red Cross blood donor population. Transfusion 42:975–979, 2002.

17. Centers for Disease Control and Prevention. Updated U.S. public health service guidelines for the management of occupational exposures to HBV, HCV, and HIV and recommendations for postexposure prophylaxis. MMWR 54(RR09):1–17, 2005.

18. Centers for Disease Control and Prevention. Achievements in Public Health: Reduction in perinatal transmission of HIV infection—United States, 1985–2005. MMWR 55(21):592–597, 2006.

19. Mak, TW, and Saunders, ME. The Immune Response: Basic and Clinical Principles. Elsevier Academic Press, Boston, MA, 2006, pp. 785–823.

20. Johnston, MI, and Fauci, AS. An HIV vaccine—evolving concepts. New Eng J Med 356:2073–2081, 2007.

21. Fauci, AS, and Lane, C. Human immunodeficiency virus disease: AIDS and related disorders. Harrison's Principles of Internal Medicine, ed. 17. McGraw-Hill, 2008. Available at http://www.accessmedicine.com.libproxy1.upstate.edu/content.aspx?aID=2904810&searchStr=hiv#2904810. Accessed May 12, 2008.

22. Paranjape, RS. Immunopathogenesis of HIV infection. Indian J Med Res 121:240–255, 2005.

23. Zetola, NM, and Pilcher, CD. Diagnosis and management of acute HIV infection. Infect Dis Clin N Am 21:19–48, 2007.

24. Collins, KL. Resistance of HIV-infected cells to cytotoxic T lymphocytes. Microbes Infect 6:494–500, 2004.

25. Lane, HC, and Fauci, AS. Immunologic abnormalities in the acquired immunodeficiency syndrome. Annu Rev Immunol 3:477–500, 1985.

26. Frost, SDW, Trkola, A, Gunthard, HF, and Richman, DD. Curr Opin HIV AIDS 3:45–51, 2008.

27. Pantaleo, G, Graziosi, C, and Fauci, AS. The immunopathogenesis of human immunodeficiency virus infection. N Engl J Med 328(5):327–335, 1993.

28. Rodes, B, Toro, C, Paxinos, E, et al. Differences in disease progression in a cohort of long-term non-progressors after more than 16 years of HIV-1 infection. AIDS. 18(8):1109–1116, 2004.

29. Centers for Disease Control and Prevention. Update on acquired immunodeficiency syndrome (AIDS)—United States. MMWR 31:507–514, 1982.

30. Centers for Disease Control and Prevention. 1993 revised classification system for HIV infection and expanded surveillance case definition for AIDS among adolescents and adults. MMWR 41(RR-17):1–19, 1992.

31. Price, RW, et al. The brain in AIDS: Central nervous system HIV-1 infection and AIDS dementia complex. Science 239:586–592, 1988.

32. Centers for Disease Control and Prevention. 1994 revised classification system for human immunodeficiency virus infection in children less than 13 years of age. MMWR 43 (RR-12):1–19, 1994.

33. European Collaborative Study. Children born to women with HIV-1 infection: Natural history and risk of transmission. Lancet 337:253–260, 1991.

34. Peckham, C, and Gibb, D. Mother-to-child transmission of the human immunodeficiency virus. N Eng J Med 333(5):298–302, 1995.

35. Centers for Disease Control and Prevention. Appendix: Revised surveillance case definition for HIV infection. MMWR 48(RR13):29–31, 1999.

36. Chen, LF, Hoy, J, and Lewin, SR. Ten years of highly active antiretroviral therapy for HIV infection. MJA 186(3):146–151, 2007.

37. Hammer, SM, et al. Treatment for adult HIV infection: 2006 recommendations of the International AIDS Society—USA panel. JAMA 296(7):827–843,2006.

38. U.S. Department of Health and Human Services. Clinical guidelines portal. Available at http://aidsinfo.nih.gov/Guidelines/Default.aspx. Accessed May 15, 2008.

39. Tashima, KT, and Flanigan, TP. Antiretroviral therapy in the year 2000. Infect Dis Clin North Am 14(4):827–849, 2000.

40. Hammer, SM. Clinical practice. Management of newly diagnosed HIV infection. N Eng J Med 353:1702–1710, 2005.

41. Connor, EM, et al. Reduction of maternal-infant transmission of human immunodeficiency virus type 1 with zidovudine treatment. N Engl J Med 331:1173–1180, 1994.

42. Centers for Disease Control and Prevention. Recommendations for prevention of HIV transmission in health-care settings. MMWR 36 (suppl no. 2S):1S–17S, 1987.

43. OSHA. The OSHA bloodborne pathogens standard 29 CFR 1910.1030. Available at http://www.osha.gov/pls/oshaweb/owadisp.show_document?p_table=STANDARDS&p_id=10051. Accessed May 16, 2008.

44. Panlilio, AL, Cardo, DM, Grohskopf, LA, Heneine, W, and Ross, CS. Updated U.S. Public Health Service guidelines for the management of occupational exposures to HIV and recommendations for postexposure prophylaxis. MMWR 54(RR09):1–17, 2005.

45. Kim, D, Elizaga, M, and Duerr, A. HIV vaccine efficacy trials: Toward the future of HIV prevention. Infect Dis Clin N Am 21:201–217, 2007.

46. Sahloff, EG. Current issues in the development of a vaccine to prevent human immunodeficiency virus. Pharmacotherapy 25(5):741–747, 2005.

47. Yuki, Y, Nichi, T, and Kiyono, H. Progress towards an AIDS mucosal vaccine: An overview. Tuberculosis 87:S35–S44, 2007.

48. Urban, AW, and Graziano, FM. Laboratory monitoring in the management of HIV infection. Lab Med 33(3):193–202, 2002.

49. Pattanapanyasat, K, and Thakar, MR. CD4+ T cell count as a tool to monitor HIV progression & anti-retroviral therapy. Indian J Med Res 121:539–549, 2005.

50. Centers for Disease Control and Prevention. Guidelines for performing single-platform absolute CD4+ T cell determinations with CD45 gating for persons infected with human immunodeficiency virus. MMWR 52(RR-2):1–13, 2003.

51. Centers for Disease Control and Prevention. 1997 revised guidelines for performing CD4+ T-cell determinations in persons infected with human immunodeficiency virus. MMWR 46(RR-2):1–29, 1997.

52. Stevens, RA, et al. General immunologic evaluation of patients with human immunodeficiency virus infection. In Detrick, B, Hamilton, RG, and Folds, JD (eds): Manual of Molecular and Clinical Laboratory Immunology, ed. 7. ASM Press, Washington, DC, 2006, pp. 847–861.

53. Cohen, PT. Understanding HIV disease. In Cohen, PT, Sande, MA, and Volberding, PA (eds): The AIDS Knowledge Base, ed. 3. Lippincott Williams & Wilkins, Philadelphia, 1999, pp. 175–194.

54. Balakrishnan, P, Solomon, S, Kumarasamy, N, and Mayer, KH. Low-cost monitoring of HIV infected individuals on highly active antiretroviral therapy (HAART) in developing countries. Indian J Med Res 121:345–355, 2005.

55. Didier, J-M, et al. Comparative assessment of five alternative methods for CD4+ T lymphocyte enumeration for implementation in developing countries. J Acquir Immune Defic Syndr 26:193–195, 2001.

56. Hagihara, K, et al. Evaluation of an automated hematology analyzer (Cell-Dyn 4000) for counting CD4+ T helper cels at low concentrations. Ann Clin Lab Sci 35(1):31–36, 2005.

57. Constantine, NT, and Zink, H. HIV testing technologies after two decades of evolution. Indian J Med Res 121:519–538, 2005.

58. Dewar, R, Highbarger, H, Davey, R, and Metcalf, J. Principles and procedures of human immunodeficiency virus serodiagnosis. In Detrick, B, Hamilton, RG, and Folds, JD (eds): Manual of Molecular and Clinical Laboratory Immunology, ed. 7. ASM Press, Washington, DC, 2006, pp. 834–846.

59. U.S. Food and Drug Administration. Donor screening assays for infectious agents and HIV diagnostic assays. Available at http://fda.gov/cber/products/testkits.htm. Accessed May 29, 2008.

60. Schappert, J, et al. Multicenter evaluation of the Bayer ADVIA Centaur HIV 1/O/2 enhanced (EHIV) assay. Clin Chim Acta 372:158–166, 2006.

61. Yeom, J-S, et al. Evaluation of a new fourth generation enzyme-lined immunosorbent assay, the LG HIV Ag-Ab Plus, with a combined HIV p24 antigen and anti-HIV-1/2/O screening test. J Virol Meth 137:292–297, 2006.

62. Kothe, D, et al. Performance characteristics of a new less sensitive HIV-1 enzyme immunoassay for use in estimating HIV seroincidence. J AIDS 33:625, 2003.

63. Barlett, JG. Serologic tests for the diagnosis of HIV infection. Available at http://www.uptodate.com. Accessed May 27, 2008.

64. Houn, HY, Pappas, AA, and Walker, Jr., EM. Status of current clinical tests for human immunodeficiency virus (HIV): Applications and limitations. Ann Clin Lab Sci 17:279–285, 1987.

65. Centers for Disease Control and Prevention. Update: Serologic testing for antibody to human immunodeficiency virus. MMWR 36:833, 843, 1998.

66. Greenwald, JL, Burstein, GR, Pincus, J, and Branson, B. A rapid review of rapid HIV antibody tests. Curr Infect Dis Reports 8:125–131, 2006.

67. Delaney, KP, et al. Performance of an oral fluid rapid HIV-1/2 test: Experience from four CDC studies. AIDS 20:1655–1660, 2006.

68. Dewsnap, C, McCowan, A, Rossi, M, and Mandalia, S. Introducing HIV point-of-care testing. AIDS Hepatitis Dig 106:5–7, 2005.

69. Centers for Disease Control and Prevention. General and laboratory considerations: Rapid HIV tests currently available in the United States. Available at http://www.cdc.gov/hiv/topics/ testing/resources/factsheets/print/rt-lab.htm. Accessed May 21, 2008.

70. Griffith, BP, Campbell, S, and Mayo, DR. Human immunodeficiency viruses. In Murray, PR, Baron, EJ, Jorgensen, JH, Landry, ML, and Pfaller, MA (eds): Manual of Clinical Microbiology, ed. 9. ASM Press, Washington, DC, 2007, pp. 1308–1329.

71. Centers for Disease Control and Prevention. Interpretation and use of the Western blot assay for serodiagnosis of human immunodeficiency virus type I infections. MMWR 38(S-7):1–7, 1989.

72. Consortium for Retrovirus Serology Standardizations. Serologic diagnosis of human immunodeficiency virus infection by Western blot testing. JAMA 260:674–679, 1988.

73. Uneke, CJ, Alo, MN, Ogbonnaya, O, and Ngwu, BAF. Western blot—indeterminate results in Nigerian patients HIV serodiagnosis: The clinical and public health implication. AIDS Patient Care STDs 21(3):169–176, 2007.

74. Centers for Disease Control and Prevention. U.S. public health service guidelines for testing and counseling blood and plasma donors for human immunodeficiency virus type-1 antigen. MMWR 45 (RR2):1–9, 1996.

75. Weikersheimer, PB. Viral load testing for HIV: Beyond the CD4 count. Lab Med 30(2):102–108, 1999.

76. Caliendo, AM. Techniques and interpretation of HIV-1 RNA quantitation. Available at http://www.uptodate.com. Accessed June 3, 2008.

77. Elbeik, T, Highbarger, H, Dewar, R, Natarajan, V, Imamichi, H, and Imamichi, T. Quantitation of viremia and determination

of drug resistance in patients with human immunodeficiency virus infection. In Detrick, B, Hamilton, RG, and Folds, JD (eds): Manual of Molecular and Clinical Laboratory Immunology, ed. 7. ASM Press, Washington, DC, 2006, pp. 862–877.

78. Hill, CE, and Caliendo, AM. Viral load testing. In Persing, DH, et al. (eds): Molecular Microbiology: Diagnostic Principles and Practice. ASM Press, Washington, DC, 2004, pp. 475–487.

79. Nolte, FS, and Caliendo, AM. Molecular detection and identification of microorganisms. In Murray, PR, Baron, EJ, Jorgensen, JH, Landry, ML, and Pfaller, MA (eds): Manual of Clinical Microbiology, ed. 9. ASM Press, Washington, DC, 2007, pp. 218–244.

80. Schumacher, W, Frick, E, Kauselmann, M, Maier-Hoyle, V, van der Vliet, R, and Babiel, R. Fully automated quantification of human immunodeficiency virus (HIV) type 1 RNA in human plasma by the COBAS AmpliPrep/COBAS TaqMan system. J Clin Virol 38:304–312, 2007.

81. Mylonakis, E, Paliou, M, and Rich, JD. Plasma viral load testing in the management of HIV infection. Am Fam Physician 63:483–490, 495–496, 2001.

82. Mellors, JW, et al. Plasma viral load and CD4+ lymphocytes as prognostic markers of HIV-1 infection. Ann Intern Med 126:946–954, 1997.

83. Mellors, JW, et al. Prognosis in HIV-1 infection predicted by the quantity of virus in plasma. Science 272:1167–1170, 1996.

84. Demeter, LM. Overview of HIV drug resistance testing assays. Available at http://www.uptodate.com. Accessed June 12, 2008.

85. Petropolous, CJ. Phenotypic testing of human immunodeficiency virus type 1 drug susceptibility. In Persing, DH, et al. Molecular Microbiology: Diagnostic Principles and Practice. ASM Press, Washington, DC, 2004, pp. 501–528.

86. Hirsch, M, et al. Antiretroviral drug resistance testing in adult HIV-1 infection. Recommendations of an International AIDS Society—USA panel. JAMA 28:2417–2426, 2000.

87. Baxter, J, et al. A randomized study of antiretroviral management based on plasma genotypic antiretroviral resistance testing in patients failing therapy. AIDS 14:F83–93, 2000.

88. Durant, J, et al. Drug-resistance genotyping in HIV-1 therapy. Lancet 353:2195–2199, 1999.

89. Constantine, NT, Callahan, JD, and Watts, DM. Retroviral Testing: Essentials for Quality Control and Laboratory Diagnosis. CRC Press, Boca Raton, FL, 1992.

90. Weiss, RA, Dalgleish, AG, and Loveday, C. Human immunodeficiency viruses. In Zuckerman, AJ, Banatvala, JE, and Pattison, JR (eds): Principles and Practice of Clinical Virology, ed. 4. John Wiley & Sons, Chichester, England, 2000, pp. 659–693.

91. Schwarzwald, H. Diagnostic testing for HIV infection in infants and young children. Available at http://www.uptodate.com. Accessed June 12, 2008.

92. Read, JS, and the Committee on Pediatric AIDS. Diagnosis of HIV-1 infection in children younger than 18 months in the United States. Pediatrics 120:e1547–e1562, 2007.

93. King, SM, and the Committee on Pediatric AIDS. Evaluation and treatment of the human immunodeficiency virus-1-exposed infant. Pediatrics 114:497–505, 2004.

94. Working Group on Antiretroviral Therapy and Medical Management of HIV Infected Children. Guidelines for the use of antiretroviral agents in pediatric HIV infection. Available at http://aidsinfo.nih.gov/contentfiles/PediatricGuidelines.pdf. Accessed June 12, 2008.

95. Centers for Disease Control and Prevention. Revised recommendations for HIV testing of adults, adolescents, and pregnant women in health care settings. MMWR 55(RR-14):1–17, 2006.

**Accelerated rejection:** A form of rejection that occurs within 1 to 5 days after second exposure to tissue antigens based on reactivation of B- and T-cell responses.

**Accuracy:** The ability of a test to actually measure what it claims to measure.

**Acquired immunity:** See *adaptive immune response.*

**Activation unit:** The combination of complement components C1, C4b, and C2b that form the enzyme C3 convertase, whose substrate is C3.

**Acute cellular rejection:** A type of rejection that occurs days to weeks after transplantation due to cellular mechanisms and antibody formation.

**Acute GVHD:** Graft-versus-host disease, which occurs shortly after immunocompetent cells are transplanted into a recipient. It is characterized by skin rashes, diarrhea, and increased susceptibility to infection.

**Acute phase reactants:** Normal serum proteins that increase rapidly as a result of infection, injury, or trauma to the tissues.

**Acute phase response:** Proteins and cells in the blood that increase rapidly in response to an infectious agent. It is considered part of natural immunity.

**Acute rheumatic fever:** A disease that develops as a sequel to group A streptococcal pharyngitis, characterized by the presence of antibodies that cross-react with heart tissue.

**Adaptive immune response:** Host response to foreign agents that depends on T and B lymphocytes and is characterized by specificity, memory, and recognition of self versus nonself.

**Adaptive T regulatory 1 cells (TR1):** CD4+ T cells induced from antigen-activated naïve T cells under the influence of interleukin-10. They exert suppressive activities.

**Adjuvant:** A substance administered with an immunogen that enhances and potentiates the immune response.

**Affinity:** The initial force of attraction that exists between a Fab site on an antibody and one epitope or a determinant site on the corresponding antigen.

**Agglutination:** The process by which particulate antigens such as cells aggregate to form large complexes when specific antibody is present.

**Agglutination inhibition reaction:** An agglutination reaction based on competition between antigen-coated particles and soluble patient antigens for a limited number of antibody-combining sites. Lack of agglutination is a positive test result.

**Agglutinin:** An antibody that causes clumping or agglutination of the cells that triggered its formation.

**AIDS:** Acquired immunodeficiency syndrome, a disease affecting the immune system caused by the human immunodeficiency virus (HIV).

**Allele:** A different form of a gene that codes for a slightly different form of the same product.

**Alloantigen:** An antigen that is found in another member of the host's species and that is capable of eliciting an immune response in the host.

**Allograft:** Tissue transferred from an individual of one species into another individual of the same species.

**Allotype:** A minor variation in amino acid sequence in a particular class of immunoglobulin molecule that is inherited in Mendelian fashion.

**Alternative pathway:** A means of activating complement proteins without antigen–antibody combination. This pathway is triggered by constituents of microorganisms.

**Amplicon:** A copy of a select portion of DNA that is obtained by the polymerase chain reaction.

**Analyte:** The substance being measured in an immunoassay.

**Anaphylatoxin:** A small peptide formed during complement activation that causes increased vascular permeability, contraction of smooth muscle, and release of histamine from basophils and mast cells.

**Anaphylaxis:** A life-threatening response to an allergen characterized by the systemic release of histamine.

**Anaplastic:** Tumors that are poorly differentiated and are similar to fetal or embryonic tissue.

**Aneuploidy:** Any deviation from the normal number of chromosomes.

**Antibodies:** Serum factors in the blood formed in response to foreign substance exposure. Antibodies are also known as *immunoglobulins.*

**Antibody conjugates:** Antibody that is attached to toxins or radioisotopes to help specifically destroy cancer cells.

**Antibody-dependent cell cytotoxicity:** The process of destroying antibody-coated target cells by natural killer cells, monocytes, macrophages, and neutrophils, all of which have specific receptors for antibody.

**Antibody screen:** The process of testing recipient serum for the presence of antibodies to HLA antigens on potential donor transplant cells.

**Anti-DNase B:** An antibody directed against DNase B, which is secreted by group A streptococci.

**Antigenic variation:** Result of the process of antigen switching.

**Antigens:** Macromolecules that are capable of eliciting formation of immunoglobulins (antibodies) or sensitized cells in an immunocompetent host.

**Antigen switching:** A protecting mechanism used by parasites that involves varying synthesis of surface antigens to evade an immune response by the host.

**Anti-HBc:** Antibody to hepatitis B core antigen.

**Anti-Hbe:** Antibody to hepatitis B capsid antigen.

**Anti-HBs:** Antibody to hepatitis B surface antigen.

**Antinuclear antibody (ANA):** Antibody produced to different components of the nucleus during the course of several autoimmune diseases. Examples include anti-DNA, antideoxyribonucleoprotein, and antiribonuclear protein antibodies, all of which occur in systemic lupus erythematosus.

**Apoptosis:** Programmed cell death.

**Arthus reaction:** A type III hypersensitivity reaction that occurs when an animal has a large amount of circulating antibody and is exposed to the antigen intradermally, resulting in localized deposition of immune complexes.

**ASO titer:** A test for the diagnosis of poststreptococcal sequelae, based on the neutralization of streptolysin 0 by antistreptolysin 0 found in patient serum.

**Aspergillosis:** An opportunistic fungal infection predominantly caused by *Aspergillus fumigatus.*

**Ataxia-telangiectasia (AT):** An autosomal recessive syndrome that results in a combined defect of both cellular and humoral immunity. The defect is in a gene responsible for recombination of immunoglobulin superfamily genes.

**Atopy:** An inherited tendency to respond to naturally occurring allergens; it results in the continual production of IgE.

**Autoantigen:** One that belongs to the host and is not capable of eliciting an immune response under normal circumstances.

**Autocrine:** Produced by the cell that stimulates the same cell to grow.

**Autograft:** Tissues removed from one area of an individual's body and reintroduced in another area in the same individual.

**Autoimmune disease:** A condition in which damage to body organs results from the presence of autoantibodies or autoreactive cells.

**Autoimmune thyroid disease:** A disease that affects the function of the thyroid and is due to formation of antibody or sensitized cells.

**Automatic sampling:** Automatic pipetting of a sample that is programmed into an instrument for testing of that sample.

**Avidity:** The strength with which a multivalent antibody binds a multivalent antigen.

**Batch analyzer:** An instrument that permits analysis of several different samples at the same time.

**Bence Jones proteins:** Proteins found in the urine of patients with multiple myeloma. They are now recognized as monoclonal immunoglobulin light chains.

**Benign:** Tissue that is not malignant.

**Biohazardous:** Hazards caused by infectious organisms.

**Body substance isolation (BSI):** A modification of Universal Precautions not limited to bloodborne pathogens that considers all body fluids and moist body substances to be potentially infectious.

**Bone marrow:** The largest tissue in the body, located in the long bones. Its role is the generation of hematopoietic cells.

***Borrelia burgdorferi:*** A spirochete that is the causative agent of Lyme disease.

**Branched chain signal amplification (bDNA):** A technique used to detect a small amount of DNA via several hybridization steps that create a branching effect with several nucleic acid probes.

**Bruton's agammaglobulinemia:** An X-linked recessive immunodeficiency disease that results in a lack of mature B lymphocytes and immunoglobulins of all classes.

**Bystander lysis:** A phenomenon that occurs in complement activation when C3b becomes deposited on host cells, making them a target for destruction by phagocytic cells.

**C1 inhibitor (C1NH):** A glycoprotein that acts to dissociate C1r and C1s from C1q, thus inhibiting the first active enzyme formed in the classical complement cascade.

**C4-binding protein (C4BP):** A protein in the complement system that serves as a cofactor for factor 1 in the inactivation of C4b.

**Candidiasis:** An opportunistic fungal infection caused by *Candida albicans* and other *Candida* species.

**Capture assay:** An enzyme immunoassay using two antibodies: The first binds the antigen to solid phase, and the second contains the enzyme label and acts as an indicator.

**CD4 T cell:** Type of lymphocyte that provides help to B cells to initiate antibody production.

**Cell flow cytometry:** An automated system for identifying cells based on the scattering of light as cells flow single file through a laser beam.

**Central tolerance:** Destruction of potentially self-reactive T and B cells as they mature in either the thymus or the bone marrow.

**Chain of infection:** A continuous link between three elements—a source, a method of transmission, and a susceptible host.

**Chancre:** The initial lesion that develops on the external genitalia in syphilis.

**Chemiluminescence:** The production of light energy by a chemical reaction.

**Chemokines:** A large family of homologous cytokines.

**Chemotaxin:** A protein or other substance that acts as a chemical messenger to produce chemotaxis.

**Chemotaxis:** The migration of cells in the direction of a chemical messenger.

**Chronic granulomatous disease (CGD):** A trait inherited in either an X-linked or autosomal recessive fashion that results in a defect in the microbicidal function of neutrophils.

**Chronic GVHD:** Graft-versus-host disease that occurs over time when transplanted immunocompetent cells react with recipient cells. It is characterized by involvement of skin, eyes, mouth, and other mucosal surfaces.

**Chronic rejection:** Rejection of a graft that usually occurs after the first year and results from progressive fibrosis of blood vessels in the grafted tissue.

**Class I MHC (HLA) molecules:** Proteins coded for by genes at three loci (A, B, C) in the major histocompatibility complex. They are expressed on all nucleated cells and are important to consider in the transplantation of tissues.

**Class II MHC (HLA) molecules:** Proteins coded for by the DR, DP, and DQ loci of the major histocompatibility complex. They are found on B cells, macrophages, activated T cells, monocytes, dendritic cells, and endothelium.

**Classical pathway:** A means of activating complement that begins with antigen–antibody combination.

**Class switching:** The production of immunoglobulins other than IgM by daughter cells of antigen-exposed B lymphocytes.

**Clonal selection theory:** A theory postulated to explain the specificity of antibody formation, based on the premise that each lymphocyte is genetically programmed to produce a specific type of antibody and is selected by contact with antigen.

**Clusters of differentiation (CD):** Antigenic features of leukocytes that are identified by groups of monoclonal antibody expressing common or overlapping activity.

**Coagglutination:** An agglutination reaction using bacteria as the inert particle to which antibody is attached.

**Coccidioidomycosis:** A fungal disease caused by *Coccidioides immitis* that is endemic to the southwestern United States and may be characterized by primary pulmonary infection.

**Cold autoagglutinin:** Antibodies that react below 30°C, typically formed in response to diseases such as *Mycoplasma* pneumonia and certain viral infections.

**Colony stimulating factor (CSF):** A protein in human serum that promotes monocyte differentiation.

**Common variable immunodeficiency:** A heterogeneous group of immunodeficiency disorders that usually appears in patients between the ages of 20 and 30 years. It is characterized by a deficiency of one or more classes of immunoglobulins.

**Competitive immunoassay:** An immunoassay in which unlabeled and labeled antigen compete for a limited number of binding sites on reagent antibody.

**Complement:** A series of proteins that are normally present in serum and whose overall function is mediation of inflammation.

**Complement-dependent cytotoxicity (CDC):** Killing of cells that results from attachment of antibody with activation of complement.

**Conformational epitope:** Key antigenic site that results from the folding of one chain or multiple chains, bringing certain amino acids from different segments of a linear sequence or sequences into close proximity with each other so they can be recognized together.

**Congenital syphilis:** The transfer of syphilis from an infected mother to the fetus during pregnancy. It results in disease or death.

**Conidia:** Asexual reproductive structures produced by fungi at the tip of hyphae; also known as *spores*.

**Constant region:** The carboxy-terminal segment (half of immunoglobulin light chains or three-quarters of heavy chains) of antibody molecules that consist of a polypeptide sequence found in all chains of that type.

**Contact dermatitis:** A delayed hypersensitivity reaction caused by T-cell sensitization to low molecular weight compounds, such as nickel and rubber, that come in contact with the skin.

**C-reactive protein:** A trace constituent of serum that increases rapidly following infection or trauma to the body and acts as an opsonin to enhance phagocytosis.

**Cross-immunity:** The phenomenon in which exposure to one infectious agent produces protection against another agent.

**Crossmatch:** Incubation of donor lymphocytes with recipient serum to determine the presence of antibodies, which would indicate rejection of a potential transplant.

**Cross-reactivity:** A phenomenon that occurs when an antibody reacts with an antigen that is structurally similar to the original antigen that induced antibody production.

**Cryoglobulins:** Immunoglobulins of the IgM class that precipitate at cold temperatures, causing occlusion of blood vessels in the extremities if a patient is exposed to the cold.

**Cryptococcosis:** A fungal disease caused by *Cryptococcus neoformans* and characterized as a pulmonary infection that may spread to the central nervous system and the brain.

**Cyst:** Inactive form of a parasite that can transmit infection.

**Cytogenics:** The branch of genetics devoted to the study of chromosomes.

**Cytokine:** Chemical messenger produced by stimulated cells that affects the function or activity of other cells.

**Cytomegalovirus:** A virus in the herpes family that is responsible for infection, ranging from a mononucleosis-like syndrome to a life-threatening illness in immunocompromised patients.

**Decay-accelerating factor (DAF):** A glycoprotein found on peripheral red blood cells, endothelial cells, fibroblasts, and epithelial cell surfaces that is capable of dissociating C3 convertases formed by both the classical and alternative pathways.

**Delayed hypersensitivity:** An immune response in which antibody production plays a minor role. It is primarily caused by activated T cells.

**Deoxyribonucleic acid (DNA):** The nucleic acid whose sugar is deoxyribose. It is the primary genetic material of all cellular organisms and DNA viruses.

**Diapedesis:** The process by which cells are capable of moving from the circulating blood to the tissues by squeezing through the wall of a blood vessel.

**DiGeorge anomaly:** A congenital defect of the third and fourth pharyngeal pouches that affects thymic development, leading to a T-cell deficiency. Patients are subject to recurring viral and fungal infections.

**Diluent:** One of two entities needed for making up a solution. It is the medium into which the solute is added.

**Direct agglutination:** An antigen–antibody reaction that occurs when antigens are naturally found on a particle.

**Direct allorecognition:** Pathway in which recipient T cells recognize intact HLA molecules on donor cells.

**Direct antiglobulin test:** A technique to determine in vivo attachment of antibody or complement to red blood cells, using antihuman globulin to cause a visible agglutination reaction.

**Direct immunofluorescent assay:** A technique to identify a specific antigen using an antibody that has a fluorescent tag attached.

**Dissemination:** Tumor cells that have traveled throughout the body by means of the bloodstream or lymphatics.

**DNA sequencing:** Determining the order of nucleotides in a segment of DNA.

**Dot-blot:** A serological test that uses microparticles of antigen using an antibody that has a fluorescent tag attached.

**Dual-parameter dot plot:** Grouping of cells based on two different characteristics, one of which is plotted on the x-axis and the other on the y-axis.

**Dysplasia:** Abnormal cell growth.

**Electrophoresis:** The separation of molecules in an electrical field based on differences in charge and size.

**ELISA:** See *enzyme-linked immunosorbent assay*.

**Endocrine:** Internal secretion of substances such as hormones or cytokines directly into the bloodstream that cause systemic effects.

**Endogenous pyrogen:** A substance produced by the body that causes fever. Interleukin-1 is an example.

**Endosmosis:** The movement of the buffer particles during electrophoresis.

**Env:** A structural gene of HIV that codes for envelope proteins gp160, gp120, and gp41.

**Enzyme-linked immunosorbent assay (ELISA):** An immunoassay that employs an enzyme label on one of the reactants.

**Eosinophil chemotactic factor:** A preformed mediator released from basophils and mast cells during an allergic reaction. It is responsible for attracting eosinophils to the area.

**Epitope:** The key portion of the immunogen against which the immune response is directed; also known as the *determinant site*.

**Epstein-Barr virus:** A DNA virus of the herpesvirus family.

**Erythema chronicum migrans:** A rash associated with Lyme disease. It begins as a small red papule and expands to form a large ring with a central clear area.

**Erythropoietin:** A colony stimulating factor that increases red blood cell production in the bone marrow.

**Exoantigen:** An antigen excreted by a bacterial or fungal cell as it metabolizes.

**External defense system:** Structural barriers that prevent most infectious agents from entering the body.

**Extrinsic parameter:** A parameter that is not an inherent part of the cell. Specific cell surface proteins that are analyzed through attachment of fluorescent antibodies.

**F(ab)2:** Fragment of an immunoglobulin molecule obtained by pepsin cleavage that consists of two light chains and two heavy chain halves held together by disulfide bonding. This piece has two antigen-binding sites.

**Fab fragment:** Fragment of an immunoglobulin molecule obtained by papain cleavage that consists of a light chain and one-half of a heavy chain held together by disulfide bonding.

**Factor H:** A control protein in the complement system. It acts as a cofactor with factor I to break down C3b formed during complement activation.

**Factor I:** A serine protease that cleaves C3b and C4b formed during complement activation. A different cofactor is required for each of these reactions.

**FC fragment:** Fragment of an immunoglobulin molecule obtained by papain cleavage that consists of the carboxyterminal halves of two heavy chains. These two halves are held together by disulfide bonds. This fragment spontaneously crystallizes at 4°C.

**Flocculation:** The formation of downy masses of precipitate that occurs over a narrow range of antigen concentration.

**Flow cytometer:** An automated system in which single cells in a fluid are analyzed in terms of intrinsic light scattering characteristics as well as extrinsic properties.

**Flow cytometry:** See *cell flow cytometry.*

**Fluorescence:** Results from compounds that have the ability to absorb energy from an incident light source and convert that energy into light of a longer wavelength.

**Fluorescence polarization immunoassay (FPIA):** An immunoassay based on the change in polarization of fluorescent light emitted from a labeled molecule when it is bound by antibody.

**Fluorescent antinuclear antibody (FANA) testing:** Testing to identify the presence of antibody to nuclear antigens, using animal cells and a fluorescent labeled antihuman immunoglobulin.

**Forward angle light scatter:** Light scattered at an angle of less than 90 degrees, which indicates the size of a cell.

**FTA-ABS test:** Fluorescent treponemal antibody absorption test, a confirmatory test for syphilis, which detects antibodies to *Treponema pallidum* by using antihuman immunoglobulin with a fluorescent label.

**Fungi:** Organisms made up of eukaryotic cells with rigid walls composed of chitin, mannan, and sometimes cellulose.

**Gag:** A structural gene of HIV that codes for three core proteins: p1S, p17, and p24.

**Gel electrophoresis:** Method of separating either proteins or DNA based on their size and electrical charge. Samples are placed in wells on the gel and exposed to an electrical current.

**Genotype:** Actual alleles, for a particular trait, that are inherited.

**Germinal center:** The interior of a secondary follicle where blast transformation of B cells takes place.

**Graft-versus-host disease (GVHD):** A condition that results from transplantation of immunocompetent cells into an immunodeficient host. The transfused cells attack the tissues of the recipient within the first 100 days post-transplant.

**Graft-versus-leukemia:** Transfer of allogenic T cells to destroy recipient leukemia cells.

**Granulocyte-CSF:** A cytokine produced by fibroblasts and epithelial cells that enhances the production of neutrophils.

**Granulocyte-macrophage-CSF:** A cytokine produced by T cells and other cell lines that stimulates an increased supply of granulocytic cells and macrophages.

**Graves' disease:** An autoimmune disease characterized by hyperthyroidism caused by the presence of antibody to thyroid-stimulating hormone receptors. Antigen–antibody combination results in continual release of thyroid hormones.

**Group A streptococci:** Gram-negative, catalase-negative cocci often found in pairs or chains that are responsible for diseases ranging from pharyngitis to necrotizing fasciitis.

**Gummas:** Localized areas of granulomatous inflammation on bones, skin, and subcutaneous tissue caused by tertiary syphilis.

**HAART:** Highly active antiretroviral therapy, a multidrug regimen that is the standard of treatment for HIV infection.

**Hairy cell leukemia:** Chronic leukemia characterized by the formation of large mononuclear cells with irregular cytoplasmic projections found in bone marrow.

**Haplotype:** A set of genes that are located close together on a chromosome and are usually inherited as a single unit.

**Hapten:** A simple chemical group that can bind to antibody once it is formed but that cannot stimulate antibody formation unless tied to a larger carrier molecule.

**Hashimoto's thyroiditis:** An autoimmune disease that results in hypothyroidism caused by the presence of antithyroglobulin and antimicrosomal antibodies, which progressively destroy the thyroid gland.

**HbeAg:** Antigen associated with the capsid of hepatitis B virus.

**HbsAg:** The surface antigen of hepatitis B virus, the first marker to appear in hepatitis B infection.

**Heavy (H) chain:** One of the polypeptide units that makes up an immunoglobulin molecule. Each immunoglobulin monomer consists of two heavy chains paired with two light chains.

*Helicobacter pylori:* A gram-negative spiral bacterium that is a major cause of gastric and duodenal ulcers.

**Hemagglutination:** An antigen–antibody reaction that results in the clumping of red blood cells.

**Hemagglutination inhibition reaction:** A test for detecting antibodies to certain viruses, based on lack of agglutination as a result of antibody neutralizing the virus.

**Hemolytic disease of the newborn (HDN):** A cytotoxic reaction that destroys an infant's red blood cells because of placental transfer of maternal antibodies to Rh antigens.

**Hemolytic titration (Ch50) assay:** An assay that measures complement activating ability by determining the amount of patient serum required to lyse 50 percent of a standardized concentration of antibody-sensitized sheep erythrocytes.

**Hepatitis:** Inflammation of the liver caused by radiation, exposure to chemicals, autoimmune disease, or viruses.

**Hepatitis B virus (HBV):** DNA virus responsible for acute hepatitis, transmitted by parenteral route or sexual contact.

**Hepatitis C virus (HCV):** Virus responsible for both acute and chronic hepatitis, transmitted sexually or through contaminated blood or needles.

**Hereditary angioedema:** A disease characterized by swelling of the extremities, the skin, the gastrointestinal tract, and other mucosal surfaces as a result of a deficiency in the complement inhibitor C1NH.

**Herpes simplex virus:** A DNA virus, found as type I and type II, that causes acute infection characterized by the development of small fluid-filled vesicles on the skin or mucous membranes.

**Heteroantigen:** An antigen of a species different from that of the host, such as other animals, plants, or microorganisms.

**Heterogeneous enzyme immunoassay:** Immunoassay in which enzyme is used as a label and which requires a separation step to separate free from bound analyte.

**Heterophile antigen:** An antigen that exists in unrelated plants or animals but that is either identical or closely related, so that antibody to one will cross-react with antibody to the other.

**High-dose hook effect:** Limitation of antibody-based assays due to massive amounts of tumor marker antigens present.

**Hinge region:** The flexible portion of the heavy chain of an immunoglobulin molecule that is located between the first and second constant regions. This allows the molecule to bend to let the two antigen-binding sites operate independently.

**Histamine:** A vasoactive amine released from mast cells and basophils during an allergic reaction.

**Histocompatibility antigens:** Antigens found on cells that are highly polymorphic and elicit a transplant response.

**Histocompatibility tests:** Laboratory testing to determine individual histocompatibility antigens on donor and recipient cells involved in a transplant.

**HIV:** Human immunodeficiency virus, a retrovirus that is the etiological agent of AIDS.

**HLA genotype:** Actual alleles, for HLA antigens, that are inherited.

**HLA match:** The pairing up of donor and recipient in a transplant on the basis of similar HLA antigens.

**HLA phenotype:** The expression of HLA genes that actually appear as proteins on cells.

**Hodgkin's lymphoma (HL):** A malignant disease that typically begins in one lymph node and is characterized by the presence of Reed-Sternberg cells, giant multinucleate cells that are usually transformed B lymphocytes.

**Homogeneous enzyme immunoassay:** An immunoassay in which no separation step is necessary. It is based on the principle of a decrease in enzyme activity when specific antigen–antibody combination occurs.

**Host-versus-graft response (HvGR):** Recognition by the host of nonself histocompatibility antigens on grafts that may result in rejection.

**Human immunodeficiency virus (HIV):** See *HIV.*

**Humoral immunity:** Protection from disease resulting from substances in the serum.

**Hybridization:** Specific binding of two single-stranded DNA segments, as in binding of a probe with a known nucleic acid sequence to an unknown piece of DNA.

**Hybridoma:** A cell line resulting from the fusion of myeloma cell and a plasma cell. These can be maintained in tissue culture indefinitely and can produce a very specific type of antibody known as *monoclonal antibody.*

**Hyperacute rejection:** Rejection of tissue that occurs within minutes or hours following transplantation, because of antibodies, already present, to ABO and HLA antigens.

**Hypersensitivity:** A heightened state of immune responsiveness.

**Hyphae:** Filamentous tubular branching structures characteristic of some fungi.

**Hyposensitization:** A treatment for allergies that involves the buildup of IgG antibodies to block the effects of IgE.

**Idiotype:** The variable portion of light and heavy immunoglobulin chains that is unique to a particular immunoglobulin molecule. This region constitutes the antigen-binding site.

**IgM anti-HBc:** Antibody that is the first to appear in hepatitis B infection. It is of the IgM class and is directed against core antigen on the virus particle.

**Immediate hypersensitivity:** Reaction to an allergen that occurs in minutes and can be life-threatening.

**Immune adherence:** The ability of phagocytic cells to bind complement-coated particles.

**Immunity:** The condition of being resistant to infection.

**Immunoblotting:** A technique used to identity antibodies to complex antigens and consisting of electrophoresis of the antigen mix followed by transfer of the pattern to nitrocellulose paper for reaction with patient serum.

**Immunoediting:** The ability of tumor cells to escape immune surveillance through suppression of immunogenicity.

**Immunoelectrophoresis:** A semiquantitative gel precipitation technique in which proteins are first separated by electrophoresis and then subjected to double diffusion with antibodies directed against the individual proteins.

**Immunofixation electrophoresis:** A semiquantitative gel precipitation technique similar to that of immunoelectrophoresis, except that antibody is added directly to the surface of the gel after electrophoresis has taken place.

**Immunofluorescent assay (IFA):** Identification of antigens on cells using an antibody with fluorescent tag.

**Immunogen:** Any substance that is capable of inducing an immune response.

**Immunoglobulin (Ig):** Glycoproteins in the serum portion of the blood that are considered part of humoral immunity.

**Immunohistochemistry:** The use of labeled antibodies to directly detect tumor markers in tissue.

**Immunology:** The study of the reactions of a host when foreign substances are introduced into the body.

**Immunophenotyping:** Identifying cells according to their surface antigen expression.

**Immunosuppressive agent:** An agent used to suppress an anti-graft immune response to transplanted tissue.

**Immunosurveillance:** The mechanism by which the body rids itself of transformed or abnormal cells.

**Immunotherapy:** The stimulation of a patient's own immune system to fight a tumor.

**Immunotoxins:** Antibodies conjugated to toxins to help destroy cancer cells.

**Indirect allorecognition pathway:** Presentation of processed donor HLA peptides bound to HLA class II molecules to CD4+lymphocytes. This results in antibody formation against the donor graft.

**Indirect antiglobulin test:** A technique to determine in vitro antigen–antibody combination. Antihuman globulin is used to cause a visible agglutination reaction with antibody-coated red blood cells.

**Indirect immunofluorescent assay:** A technique to identify antigen by using two antibodies: one that is specific to the antigen and a second that is an antihuman immunoglobulin with a fluorescent tag.

**Induction:** Phase where cells are exposed to a variety of environmental insults.

**Inflammation:** Cellular and humor mechanisms involved in the overall reaction of the body to injury or invasion by an infectious agent.

**Innate immune response:** See *natural immunity.*

**In situ:** Within the tissue itself.

**In situ hybridization:** Binding of a nucleic acid probe to target DNA located in intact cells.

**Interferons:** Cytokines produced by T cells and other cell lines that inhibit viral synthesis or act as immune regulators.

**Interleukins (IL):** Cytokines or chemical messengers produced by leukocytes that affect the inflammatory process through an increase in soluble factors or cells.

**Internal defense system:** Defense mechanism inside the body in which both cells and soluble factors play essential parts.

**Intrinsic parameter:** Light scattering properties that are a part of the cell, such as size and granularity.

**Invariant chain:** A protein that associates with HLA class II antigens shortly after they are synthesized to prevent interaction of their binding sites with any endogenous peptides in the endoplasmic reticulum.

**Invasion:** Infiltration and destruction of surrounding tissue by a malignant tumor.

**Isohemagglutinin:** Antibody that agglutinates red blood cells of other individuals of the same species.

**Isotype:** A unique amino acid sequence that is common to all immunoglobulin molecules of a given class in a given species.

**Joining (J) chain:** A glycoprotein with a molecular weight of 15,000 that serves to link immunoglobulin monomers together. These are found only in IgM and secretory IgA molecules.

**Kappa (K) chain:** One of two types of immunoglobulin light chains that are present in approximately two-thirds of all immunoglobulin molecules.

**Lambda (λ) chain:** One of two types of immunoglobulin light chains that are present in approximately one-third of all immunoglobulin molecules.

**Lancefield group:** A means of classifying streptococci on the basis of differences in the cell wall carbohydrate.

**Laser light source:** Used in cell flow cytometry to identify properties of a cell such as size and granularity. It is also used with antibody conjugated with a fluorochrome to determine particular cell surface antigens.

**Lattice formation:** The combination of antibody and multivalent antigen to produce a stable network that results in a visible reaction.

**Law of mass action:** A law used to mathematically describe the equilibrium relationship between soluble reactants and insoluble products. It can be applied to antigen–antibody relationships.

**Lectin pathway:** A pathway for the activation of complement based on binding of mannose binding protein to constituents on bacterial cell walls.

**Leukemia:** A progressive malignant disease of blood-forming organs, characterized by proliferation of leukocytes and their precursors in the bone marrow.

**Ligand:** A molecule that binds to a specific receptor.

**Ligase chain reaction (LCR):** A means of increasing signal probes through the use of an enzyme called a *ligase*, which joins two pairs of probes only after they have bound to a complementary target sequence.

**Light (L) chain:** Small chain in an immunoglobulin molecule that is bound to the larger chain by disulfide bonds. The two types of light chains are called *kappa* and *lambda*.

**Linear epitope:** Amino acids following one another on a single chain that act as a key antigenic site.

**Low ionic strength saline:** Used to enhance agglutination reactions by decreasing the surface charge on red blood cells.

**Lymph node:** A secondary lymphoid organ that is located along a lymphatic duct and whose purpose is to filter lymphatic fluid from the tissues and act as a site for processing of foreign antigen.

**Lymphoma:** Cancer of the lymphoid cells that tends to proliferate as a solid tumor.

**Macrophage-monocyte-CSF:** A cytokine that induces growth of hematopoietic cells destined to become monocytes and macrophages.

**Major histocompatibility complex (MHC):** The genes that control expression of a large group of proteins originally identified on leukocytes but now known to be found on all nucleated cells in the body. These proteins regulate the immune response and play a role in graft rejection.

**Mannose-binding lectin (MBL):** Normally present protein in the blood that binds to mannose on bacterial cells and initiates the lectin pathway for complement activation.

**Mass spectrometry (MS):** An analytical technique that identifies the chemical composition of a sample on the basis of the mass-to-charge ratio of charged particles.

**Material Safety Data Sheet (MSDS):** An MSDS contains information on physical and chemical characteristics, fire, explosion reactivity, health hazards, primary routes of entry, exposure limits and carcinogenic potential, precautions for safe handling, spill clean-up, and emergency first aid information.

**Membrane attack complex:** The combination of complement components C5b, C6, C7, CS, and C9 that becomes inserted into the target cell membrane, causing lysis.

**Memory cell:** Progeny of an antigen-activated B or T cell that is able to respond to antigen more quickly than the parent cell.

**Metastasis:** When malignant cells travel through the body causing new foci of malignancy.

**Mixed lymphocyte response (MLR):** A means of measuring the proliferation of responder CD8+ T cells to nonself antigens in a potential transplant.

**Mold:** A filamentous growth form found in fungi.

**Molecular mimicry:** The similarity between an infectious agent and a self-antigen that causes antibody formed in response to the former to cross-react with the latter.

**Monoclonal antibody:** Very specific antibody derived from a single antibody-producing cell that has been cloned or duplicated.

**Monoclonal gammopathy:** A clone of lymphoid cells that cause overproduction of a single immunoglobulin component called a *paraprotein*.

**Multiple myeloma:** A malignancy of mature plasma cells that results in a monoclonal increase in an immunoglobulin component. The most common component increased is IgG.

**Multiple sclerosis:** An autoimmune disease in which the myelin sheath of axons becomes progressively destroyed by antibodies to myelin proteins.

**Mumps virus:** A single-stranded RNA virus that is the causative agent of mumps, a disease characterized by swelling of the parotid glands.

**Myasthenia gravis:** An autoimmune disease characterized by progressive muscle weakness caused by formation of antibody to acetylcholine receptors.

**Mycelium:** A dense mat formed by some fungi that is made up of intertwined hyphae.

**Mycoplasma pneumoniae:** A small gram-negative bacterium that lacks a cell wall and is the cause of upper respiratory infections.

**Mycoses:** Diseases produced by fungus.

**NASBA:** Nucleic acid sequence-based amplification, a method for increasing the number of copies of RNA in viral load testing for HIV infection.

**Natural immunity:** The ability of the individual to resist infection by means of normally present body functions.

**Natural T regulatory cells (Treg):** A subclass of CD4+ T cells that play a key role in establishing tolerance to self-antigens, allergens, tumor cells, and transplant antigens.

**Negative selection:** The process by which T cells that can respond to self-antigen are destroyed in the thymus.

**Neoplasia:** Abnormal cell growth that results in a tumor.

**Nephelometry:** A technique for determining the concentration of particles in a solution by measuring the light scattered at a particular angle from the incident beam as it passes through the solution.

**Neutrophil chemotactic factor:** A preformed mediator released from mast cells and basophils during an allergic reaction whose function is to attract neutrophils to the area.

**Noncompetitive assay:** An assay in which an excess of binding sites is present so that all the patient analyte can be bound and measured.

**Non-Hodgkin's lymphoma (NHL):** A wide range of cancers of the lymphoid tissue, of which B-cell lymphomas represent the majority.

**Nontreponemal tests:** Serological tests for syphilis that detect antibody to cardiolipin and not specific antitreponemal antibody.

**Northern blot:** Technique for the identification of specific RNA sequences by separating short RNA molecules electrophoretically, denaturing them, transferring the pattern to a nitrocellulose membrane, and incubating with a labeled probe that is specific for the sequence of interest.

**Nucleic acid probe:** Short strand of DNA or RNA of a known sequence used to identify a complementary nucleic acid strand in a patient specimen.

**Nucleic acid sequence based amplification (NASBA):** A technique for amplifying RNA by first making a DNA copy and then making RNA transcripts from it.

**Occupational Safety and Health Administration (OSHA):** Monitors and enforces safety regulations for workers.

**Oncofetal antigens:** Antigens that are expressed in the developing fetus and in rapidly dividing tissue, such as that associated with tumors, but that are absent in normal adult tissue.

**Oncogene:** Gene that encodes a protein capable of inducing cellular transformation.

**Oncopeptidomics:** Protein profiling in cancer patients to determine the presence of new tumor markers or proteins that are consistent with cancer.

**Opsonins:** Serum proteins that attach to a foreign substance and enhance phagocytosis (from the Greek word meaning "to prepare for eating").

**Ouchterlony double diffusion:** A qualitative gel precipitation technique in which both antigen and antibody diffuse out from wells cut in the gel. The pattern obtained indicates whether or not antigens are identical.

**Oxidative burst:** An increase in oxygen consumption in phagocytic cells, which generate oxygen radicals used to kill engulfed microorganisms.

**p24 antigen:** A structural core antigen that is part of the human immunodeficiency virus (HIV).

**Paracrine:** Secretions such as cytokines that affect only target cells in close proximity.

**Paraprotein:** A single immunoglobulin component produced by a malignant clone of lymphoid cells in lymphoproliferative diseases.

**Paroxysmal nocturnal hemoglobinuria (PNH):** A disease characterized by complement-mediated hemolysis of erythrocytes resulting from a deficiency of decay-accelerating factor on the red blood cells.

**Particle-counting immunoassay (PACIA):** A technique for measuring residual nonagglutinating particles in a specimen using nephelometry to determine the amount of forward light scatter. Antigen–antibody combination decreases light scatter so that the amount of patient antigen present is indirectly proportional to the amount of light scattered.

**Passive agglutination:** A reaction in which particles coated with antigens not normally found on their surfaces clump together because of combination with antibody.

**Passive cutaneous anaphylaxis:** An allergic skin reaction produced when serum containing IgE against a particular allergen is injected under the skin and that individual is later exposed to the allergen.

**Passive immunodiffusion:** A precipitation reaction in a gel in which antigen–antibody combination occurs by means of diffusion.

**Periarteriolar lymphoid sheath:** White pulp of splenic tissue, which is made up of lymphocytes, macrophages, plasma cells, and granulocytes. It is found surrounding central arterioles.

**Peripheral tolerance:** Destruction or repression of lymphocytes in the peripheral lymphoid organs that could respond to self-antigens.

**Personal protective equipment (PPE):** Items such as gowns, masks, gloves, and face shields, used to protect the body from infectious agents.

**Phagocytosis:** From the Greek word *phagein*, meaning "cell eating." The engulfment of cells or particulate matter by leukocytes, macrophages, or other cells.

**Phagolysosome:** The structure formed by the fusion of cytoplasmic granules and a phagosome during the process of phagocytosis.

**Phagosome:** A vacuole formed within a phagocytic cell as pseudopodia surround a particle during the process of phagocytosis.

**Plasma cell:** A transformed B cell that actively secretes antibody.

**Plasma cell dycrasias:** Immunoproliferative diseases characterized by overproduction of a single immunoglobulin component by a clone of lymphoid cells.

**Pleiotropy:** Many different actions of a single cytokine. It may affect the activities of more than one kind of cell and have more than one kind of effect on the same cell.

**Pol:** A structural gene of HIV that codes for reverse transcriptase and an endonuclease.

**Polymerase chain reaction (PCR):** A means of amplifying tiny quantities of nucleic acid using a heat-stable polymerase enzyme and a primer that is specific for the DNA sequence desired.

**Population gating:** Selection of a particular cell population on the basis of certain characteristics such as forward or side light scatter.

**Positive predictive value:** The percent of all positives in a serological test that are true positives.

**Positive selection:** The process of selecting immature T lymphocytes for survival on the basis of expression of high levels of CD3 and the ability to respond to self-MHC antigens.

**Postexposure prophylaxis:** Course of preventative treatment used following exposure to potentially infectious organisms.

**Poststreptococcal glomerulonephritis:** A condition that damages the glomeruli of the kidney due to an initial immune response to a streptococcal infection.

**Postzone phenomenon:** Lack of a visible reaction in an antigen–antibody reaction caused by an excess of antigen.

**Precipitation:** The combination of soluble antigen with soluble antibody to produce visible insoluble complexes.

**Precision:** The ability to consistently reproduce the same result upon repeated testing of the same sample.

**Primary follicle:** A cluster of B cells that have not yet been stimulated by antigen.

**Primary response:** The initial response to a foreign antigen.

**Primer:** Short sequences of DNA, usually 20 to 30 nucleotides long, used to hybridize specifically to a particular target DNA to help initiate replication of the DNA.

**Properdin:** A protein that stabilized the C3 convertase generated in the alternative complement pathway.

**Proteomics:** The field of study that involves identification and quantification of the array of proteins present in a sample.

**Proto-oncogenes:** Regulatory genes that promote cell division.

**Prozone:** See *prozone phenomenon*.

**Prozone phenomenon:** Lack of a visible reaction in antigen–antibody combination caused by the presence of excess antibody. This may result in a false-negative reaction.

**Purine:** Nitrogenous bases adenine and guanine incorporated into DNA and RNA, which represent part of the genetic code.

**Purine-nucleoside phosphorylase (PNP) deficiency:** Lack of the enzyme purine nucleoside phosphorylase. The deficiency is inherited as an autosomal recessive trait. Accumulation of a purine metabolite is toxic to T cells, leading to a defect in cell-mediated immunity.

**Pyrimidine:** Nitrogenous bases cytosine and thymidine in DNA and cytosine and uracil in RNA, which form part of the genetic code.

**Radial immunodiffusion:** A single-diffusion technique in which antibody is incorporated into a gel and antigen is measured by the size of a precipitin ring formed when it diffuses out in all directions from a well cut into the gel.

**Radioimmunoassay (RIA):** A technique used to measure small concentrations of an analyte, using a radioactive label on one of the immunologic reactants.

**Random access analyzer:** An analyzer that can run multiple tests on multiple samples using multiple analytes.

**RAST:** A technique used to measure antigen-specific IgE by means of a noncompetitive solid-phase immunoassay.

**Reagin:** An antibody formed during the course of syphilis that is directed against cardiolipin and not against *Treponema pallidum* itself.

**Real-time PCR:** A sensitive technique for measuring amplification of DNA by using fluorescent dyes or probes to take readings after each cycle instead of waiting until all cycles have been completed.

**Recognition unit:** The complement component that consists of the C1qrs complex. This must bind to at least two Fc regions to initiate the classical complement cascade.

**Redundancy:** Different cytokines that have the same effect.

**Respiratory burst:** An increase in oxygen consumption that occurs within a phagocytic cell as it begins to engulf particulate matter.

**Restriction endonuclease:** Enzymes that cleave DNA at specific recognition sites that are typically 4 to 6 base pairs long.

**Restriction fragment length polymorphisms (RFLPs):** Variations in nucleotides within DNA that change where restriction enzymes cleave the DNA. Where mutations occur, different-size pieces of DNA are obtained, resulting in an altered electrophoretic pattern.

**Reverse passive agglutination:** A reaction in which carrier particles coated with antibody clump together because of a combination with antigen.

**Reverse transcriptase:** An enzyme produced by certain RNA viruses to convert viral RNA into DNA.

**Rheumatoid arthritis (RA):** An autoimmune disease that affects the synovial membrane of multiple joints. It is characterized by the presence of an autoantibody called *rheumatoid factor*.

**Rheumatoid factor (RF):** An antibody of the IgM class produced by patients with rheumatoid arthritis that is directed against IgG.

**Ribonucleic acid (RNA):** The nucleic acid containing the sugar ribose. It is the primary genetic material of RNA viruses and plays a role in the transcribing of genetic information in cells.

**Rickettsiae:** Small gram-negative fastidious bacteria that are obligate intracellular parasites and are responsible for diseases such as Rocky Mountain spotted fever and typhus.

**Right angle, side angle, light scatter:** Light scattered at 90 degrees in a flow cytometer that indicates the granularity of a cell.

**RIST:** Radioimmunosorbent test. A technique to measure total IgE using a solid-phase immunoassay with anti-IgE.

**Rocket immunoelectrophoresis:** A technique used to quantify antigens on the basis of the height of a rocket-shaped precipitin band obtained when radial immunodiffusion is combined with electrophoresis.

**Rosetting:** A daisy pattern created by sheep red blood cells, which adhere to CD2 antigens found on T cells.

**RPR test:** Rapid plasma reagin test; a slide flocculation test for syphilis that detects the antibody called *reagin*.

**Rubella virus:** An RNA virus that causes German, or 3-day, measles.

**Rubeola virus:** A single-stranded RNA virus that causes measles.

**Sandwich hybridization:** A nucleic acid detection method using two probes, one of which is placed on a solid support, such as a membrane or microtiter plate, to capture the target DNA. A second labeled probe, which binds to a second site on the target DNA, is added to detect specific gene sequences.

**Sandwich immunoassays:** Immunoassays based on the ability of antibody to bind with more than one antigen.

**Secondary follicle:** A cluster of B cells that are proliferating in response to a specific antigen.

**Secretory component (SC):** A protein with a molecular weight of 70,000 that is synthesized in epithelial cells and added to IgA to facilitate transport of IgA to mucosal surfaces.

**Sensitivity:** The lowest amount of an analyte that can be measured.

**Sensitization:** (1) The combination of antibody with a single antigenic determinant on the surface of a cell without agglutination. (2) Induction of an immune response.

**Serial dilution:** A method of decreasing the strength of an antibody solution by using the same dilution factor for each step.

**Seroconversion:** The change of a serological test from negative to positive as a result of developing the measurable antibodies in response to infection or immunization.

**Serology:** The study of a noncellular portion of the blood known as *serum*.

**Serum sickness:** A type III hypersensitivity reaction that results from the buildup of antibodies to animal serum used in passive immunization.

**Severe combined immunodeficiency (SCID):** An inherited deficiency of both cell-mediated and antibody-mediated immunity. It results in death in infancy caused by overwhelming infections.

**Single diffusion:** A precipitation reaction in which one of the reactants is incorporated in the gel, while the other diffuses out from the point of application.

**Single-parameter histogram:** Plot of a chosen parameter or measurement on the x-axis against the number of events on the y-axis.

**Solute:** One of the two entities needed for making a dilution.

**Southern blot:** Technique for the identification of specific DNA sequences in which DNA is cleaved into fragments by enzymes, separated electrophoretically, denatured, transferred to a nitro-cellulose membrane, and incubated with a labeled probe that is specific for the sequence of interest.

**Spherule:** A saclike funnel structure that is filled with endospores when mature.

**Spleen:** The largest secondary lymphoid organ in the body, located in the upper left quadrant of the abdomen. Its function is to filter out old cells and foreign antigens.

**Spotted fever:** A group of rickettsiae that produce diseases characterized by nausea, vomiting, headache, fever, and a rash.

**S protein:** A control protein in the complement cascade that interferes with binding of the C5b67 complex to a cell membrane, thus preventing lysis.

**Standard Precautions:** Guidelines describing personnel protection that should be used for the care of all patients, including handwashing, gloves, mask, eye protection, face shield, gown, patient-care equipment, environmental control, linens, taking care to prevent injuries, and patient placement.

**Strand displacement amplification:** A method for amplifying DNA by using a DNA primer that is nicked by an endonuclease, allowing for displacement of the amplified strands.

**Streptolysin O:** A protein capable of lysing red and white blood cells, which is given off by some groups of streptococci as they grow.

**Streptozyme:** A serological test for infection with group A streptococci that detects five different antibodies to streptococcal products.

**Stringency:** Conditions that affect the ability of a probe to correctly bind to a specific target DNA sequence. These include temperature, salt concentration, and concentration of formamide or urea.

**Susceptibility genes:** Genes associated with an increased risk of developing a certain disease or cancer.

**Syngenic graft:** The transfer of tissue or organs between genetically identical individuals such as identical twins.

**Systemic lupus erythematosus (SLE):** A chronic inflammatory autoimmune disease characterized by the presence of antinuclear antibodies. Symptoms may include swelling of the joints, an erythematous rash, and deposition of immune complexes in the kidneys.

**Tertiary syphilis:** The last stage of syphilis that appears months to years after secondary infection. It is characterized by granulomatous inflammation, cardiovascular disease, and central nervous system involvement.

**T helper cells (Th):** Lymphocytes that express the CD4 antigen. Their function is to provide help to B cells in recognizing foreign antigen and producing antibody to it.

**Thermal dimorphism:** A phenomenon found in some fungi in which the organism reproduces as a mold at 25°C to 30°C and as a yeast at 35°C to 37°C.

**Thymocyte:** Immature lymphocyte, found in the thymus, that undergoes differentiation to become a mature T cell.

**Thymus:** A small, flat, bilobed organ found in the thorax of humans, which serves as the site for differentiation of T cells.

**Thyroid-stimulating hormone (TSH):** A hormone produced by the thyroid gland that binds to specific receptors, causing thyroglobulin to be broken down into secretable T3 and T4.

**Thyroid-stimulating hormone receptor antibody (Trab):** An antibody that is directed against the receptor for thyroid-stimulating hormone. It is associated with Graves' disease and results in overstimulation of the thyroid gland.

**Thyrotoxicosis:** A condition caused by overproduction of thyroid hormones, as seen in Graves' disease.

**Titer:** A figure that represents the relative strength of an antibody. It is the reciprocal of the highest dilution in which a positive reaction occurs.

**TMN system:** A classification system for tumors based on the size of the primary tumor (T), involvement of adjacent lymph nodes (N), and detection of metastasis (M).

**Toxoplasmosis:** A parasitic disease that is usually transmitted to humans by cysts found in contaminated soil, cat litter, or improperly cooked pork.

**Transcription:** The process of generating a messenger RNA strand from DNA. This is used to code for protein.

**Transcription-mediated amplification (TMA):** Method of increasing target DNA through the use of two enzymes, an RNA polymerase and a reverse transcriptase, to make new strands of DNA.

**Transforming growth factor beta (TGF-b):** A cytokine that induces antiproliferative activity in a variety of cell types and down-regulation of the inflammatory response.

**Transient hypogammaglobulinemia:** A condition characterized by low immunoglobulin levels that occur in infants around 2 to 3 months of age. It is believed to be caused by delayed maturation of one or more components of the immune system and usually corrects itself spontaneously.

**Translation:** The process by which messenger RNA is used to make functional proteins.

**Transporters associated with antigen processing (TAP):** Proteins that are responsible for the ATP-dependent transport of newly synthesized short peptides from the cytoplasm to the lumen of the endoplasmic reticulum for binding to class I HLA antigens.

**Treponema pallidum:** A spirochete that is the causative agent of syphilis.

**Treponemal tests:** Serological tests for syphilis that detect antibodies directed against *Treponema pallidum* itself.

**Tumor-associated antigens:** Antigens found on tumor cells that are not unique to such cells but that can still be used to distinguish them from normal cells.

**Tumor infiltrating lymphocyte (TIL):** Lymphocytes within a tumor mass that are able to react with antigens on tumor cells to help destroy them.

**Tumor necrosis factor (TNF):** A major mediator of the innate defense against gram-negative bacteria.

**Tumor suppressor genes:** Genes that inhibit the growth of tumors.

**Turbidimetry:** A technique for determining the concentration of particles in a solution based on the change in absorbance caused by the scattering of light that occurs when an incident beam is passed through the solution.

**Type I diabetes mellitus:** A chronic autoimmune disease characterized by insufficient insulin production due to progressive destruction of the beta cells of the pancreas.

**Typhus:** A group of rickettsiae that cause endemic and epidemic typhus, diseases characterized by fever, rash, and a cough.

**Universal Precautions (UP):** Guidelines stating that all body fluids are capable of transmitting diseases and recommending wearing gloves, face shields, and disposing of all needles and sharp objects in puncture-resistant containers without recapping.

**Urease:** An enzyme that breaks down urea to form ammonia and bicarbonate. Presence of urease is used as an indicator of *Helicobacter pylori.*

**Variable region:** The amino-terminal region of an immunoglobulin molecule (half of a light chain or quarter of a heavy chain) that has a unique amino acid sequence for each different immunoglobulin molecule. This part is responsible for the specificity of a particular immunoglobulin molecule.

**Varicella-zoster virus:** A herpes virus that is responsible for chicken pox and zoster, or shingles.

**VDRL test:** A flocculation test for reagin antibody found in syphilis; designed by the Venereal Disease Research Laboratories.

**Viral load tests:** Quantitative tests for HIV nucleic acid that are used to predict disease progression and to monitor the effects of antiretroviral therapy.

**Waldenström's macroglobulinemia:** An immunoproliferative disease caused by a malignancy of lymphocytes that results in production of IgM paraproteins.

**Warm autoimmune hemolytic anemia:** An autoimmune disease that results in the destruction of red blood cells caused by formation of IgG antibody that reacts at 37°C.

**Western blot:** A confirmatory test for HIV based on separation of HIV antigens by electrophoresis followed by transfer or blotting of the antigen pattern to a supporting medium for reaction with test serum.

**Wiskott-Aldrich syndrome (WAS):** A rare X-linked recessive syndrome characterized by immunodeficiency, eczema, and thrombocytopenia.

**Xenograft:** The transfer of tissue from an individual of one species to an individual of another species, such as animal tissue transplanted to a human.

**Yeast:** A unicellular form of certain fungi that reproduce asexually by budding, in which the parent cell divides into two unequal parts.

**Zone of equivalence:** The point in an antigen–antibody reaction at which the number of multivalent sites of antigen and antibody are approximately equal, resulting in optimal precipitation.

# Answer Key

## CHAPTER 1

### Answers to Review Questions

1. a    2. d    3. c    4. d    5. c    6. c    7. a
8. d    9. d    10. b    11. c    12. d    13. a    14. c
15. a

### Answers to Case Studies

**1.** Although the cholesterol levels were within normal limits for both HDL and total cholesterol, recent studies indicate that an increase in CRP has been associated with a greater risk of a future heart attack. Increased fibrinogen levels are also associated with an increased risk for a future cardiovascular event, although it is not as great a risk factor as increased CRP. A rise in both of these acute phase reactants indicates an underlying chronic inflammatory process. Such a process is associated with atherosclerosis, a condition that damages coronary blood vessels. Rick's wife should help him by encouraging him to follow a healthy diet and to lose weight through exercise.

**2.** CRP is one of the first indicators of a possible infection. If the infection was bacterial, an increase in the white blood cell count should have been seen. This increase would mainly be due to recruitment of neutrophils to help fight the invading organism. However, if an infection is due to a virus, there is typically no apparent increase in the white blood cell count. As an acute phase reactant, CRP levels increase dramatically within 24 hours, long before specific antibody can be detected. Thus, an increase in CRP supports the likelihood that an infection is present. The mono test being indeterminate probably indicates a small amount of antibody present but not enough for a definite positive test. Repeating the mono test in a few days will allow a detectable level of antibody to form.

## CHAPTER 2

### Answers to Review Questions

1. c    2. a    3. d    4. a    5. c    6. b    7. a
8. c    9. a    10. b    11. b    12. d    13. b    14. d

### Answers to Case Study

The normal CD19+ cells indicate that there is not a lack of B cells, which are presumably capable of responding to antigen and producing antibody. The population most affected is T cells, which carry CD3 on their surface. T helper cells are necessary for a B-cell response, especially

IgG. Thus, this indicates an immunodeficiency due to a low number of T cells, most likely T helper (CD4+) cells. The lack of ability to produce IgG results in recurrent bacterial infections, such as pneumonia.

## CHAPTER 3

### Answers to Review Questions

1. d    2. b    3. a    4. c    5. d    6. b    7. b
8. d    9. c    10. c

### Answers to Case Study

**a.** Since every child inherits one haplotype of packet of genes from the mother and one from the father, 50 percent of the HLA antigens would match the mother and 50 percent would match the father. It will never be more than that unless the mother and father have at least one antigen in common. **b.** According to the law of independent assortment, there would be a 1:4 chance that a sister would be an exact match, a 1:2 chance that a sister would share half of the same alleles, and a 1:4 chance that a sister would share no alleles, having received the opposite haplotype from each parent. **c.** It is possible that a cadaver kidney may actually be a better match, if neither sister is an exact match. The most important alleles to match are HLA A, B, and DR. If a cadaver match has more than one allele in common with the recipient at each of these loci, then it would be a closer match.

## CHAPTER 4

### Answers to Review Questions

1. a    2. a    3. d    4. b    5. c    6. d    7. a
8. c    9. b    10. a    11. c    12. d    13. b    14. b
15. c    16. b

### Answers to Case Studies

**1. a.** Presence of IgM only is an indicator of an early acute infection. IgM is the first antibody to appear, followed by IgG. In a reactivated case of mono, a small amount of IgM might be present, but IgG would also be present. The memory cells created by the first exposure to the virus would trigger production of IgG in a much shorter time. Thus, this patient is encountering the virus for the first time.

**2. a.** Chronic respiratory infections may be due to a decrease or lack of IgA, but this is not the case here. Normal IgG, IgM, and IgA levels indicate that this child is not immunocompromised. The increase in IgE is an indicator that the cold symptoms may actually be due to allergy. This is especially evident in the springtime, when pollen is at high levels. The child should be tested for specific allergies to determine what is causing the symptoms. Treatment with antihistamine and avoidance of the allergen will help to relieve the symptoms.

## CHAPTER 5

### Answers to Review Questions

1. b    2. a    3. d    4. c    5. c    6. d    7. d
8. b    9. c    10. d

### Answers to Case Study

**a.** G-CSF stimulates the growth and differentiation of neutrophils. It is best to treat with the factor that is most specific to the problem, rather than with a growth factor that would increase all cell lines. **b.** IFN-$\gamma$, IL-2, IL-12, IL-18 **c.** IL-10, IL-4, IL-5, IL-13

## CHAPTER 6

### Answers to Review Questions

1. b    2. c    3. d    4. d    5. c    6. a    7. d
8. a    9. d    10. a    11. b    12. c    13. b    14. d
15. c    16. d

### Answers to Case Studies

**1. a.** A decreased $Ch_{50}$ indicates a problem with the classical pathway. The decreased radial hemolysis with a buffer that chelates calcium indicates a problem with the alternative pathway as well. **b.** Levels of C3 and C4 are normal, indicating that a deficiency of one or more of the membrane attack components is involved. While a lack of C1q or C2 cannot absolutely be ruled out, the fact that the alternative pathway is also affected is a second indicator that the common components C5 through C9 are the ones involved. Since defense against encapsulated bacteria such as meningococci is reduced if there is a decrease in C5 through C9, the patient's symptoms are in accord with this conclusion. **c.** In order to confirm the actual deficiency, testing for the individual components C5 through C9 should be performed. Since this type of deficiency reduces the overall functioning of the complement system, patients should receive prompt therapy when signs of infection are noted.
**2. a.** While the abdominal pain and vomiting could be due to several infectious agents, the normal white blood cell count decreases the likelihood of a bacterial infection. The accompanying swelling of the hands and legs may be an indicator of a possible inflammatory problem associated with continuous activation of the complement system. Since this has been a recurring problem, the likelihood of an immune problem is increased. Because total serum protein is within

the normal range, it is unlikely that the deficiency is from lack of antibody production. A decrease of one complement component would not be apparent on a total protein determination. **b.** Reduced levels of both C4 and C2 could be from inheritance of defective genes for both components. However, the probability of that is extremely rare. A more plausible explanation is that the deficiency of both C2 and C4 is due to overconsumption rather than a lack of production. **c.** A lack of C1-INH would result in overconsumption of C4 and C2. As this is the most common deficiency of the complement system, this represents a likely explanation for the symptoms, and should be determined by testing for this component.

## CHAPTER 7

### Answers to Review Questions

1. c    2. a    3. a    4. c    5. c    6. c    7. b
8. d    9. a    10. c    11. b

### Answers to Case Study

Gloves should never be removed when working with patient specimens. When they are, hands should be washed right away using the correct procedure. Any contamination of the lab bench should be treated with sodium hypochlorite, and the paper towels should be disposed of in the regulated medical waste. Since the supervisor's lab coat was disposable and became contaminated, it should be discarded in the regulated medical waste and replaced with a new coat. Pipetting should have been done behind a Plexiglas shield, and this would have prevented the spill onto the lab coat.

## CHAPTER 8

### Answers to Review Questions

1. c    2. d    3. b    4. d    5. b    6. a    7. a
8. b    9. c    10. a    11. d    12. d    13. a    14. c

### Answers to Case Study

**a.** The results indicate normal levels of IgG and IgM but a decreased level of IgA. This most likely indicates a selective IgA deficiency, the most common genetic immunodeficiency. Selective IgA deficiency occurs in approximately 1:1000 individuals. **b.** A decrease in serum IgA most likely indicates a decrease in secretory IgA, the immunoglobulin that is found on mucosal surfaces. Individuals with a selective IgA deficiency are more prone to respiratory tract and gastrointestinal tract infections, since this represents the first line of defense against organisms that invade mucosal surfaces. **c.** Nephelometry is a more sensitive method for measuring immunoglobulin levels. It is able to detect small quantities of immunoglobulins present. Results are obtained faster than for RID, and since the process is automated, it is not subject to human error in reading the results. Other errors that may occur in radial immunodiffusion include overfilling or underfilling of wells, nicking of wells, and inaccurate incubation time or temperature. Therefore, nephelometry has largely replaced RID for measurement of immunoglobulin levels.

# CHAPTER 9

## Answers to Review Questions

1. b    2. c    3. a    4. c    5. a    6. b    7. c
8. c    9. b    10. d    11. c    12. d

## Answers to Case Study

**a.** The positive test on an undiluted patient specimen indicates that at least 10 IU/ml of rubella antibody is present. This indicates immunity to the virus if the patient was tested immediately after exposure to the disease. **b.** The presence of antibody indicates that the patient will not likely be reinfected with the virus. Therefore, she does not have to be concerned about possible consequences for the fetus. **c.** The antibodies detected are most likely due to vaccination and not the disease itself. If there is any question about how soon after exposure the patient was tested, a serum sample should be frozen. An additional specimen should be collected if any clinical symptoms appear or after 30 days. Both specimens should be tested simultaneously using the semiquantitative procedure. A fourfold increase in titer would indicate recent infection.

# CHAPTER 10

## Answers to Review Questions

1. c    2. a    3. c    4. b    5. b    6. c    7. b
8. c    9. b    10. d    11. d    12. d

## Answers to Case Study

**a.** A negative finding only means that no parasites were observed for that particular specimen at that particular time. It does not automatically rule out the possibility of parasites being present. **b.** Capture enzyme immunoassays that are specific for parasites such as *Giardia* and *Cryptosporidium* are available. Typically, a solid phase such as microtiter wells is coated with specific antibody, and very small amounts of antigen can be detected. If a parasite is suspected, and traditional test results are negative, this would be the next step. **c.** Capture enzyme immunoassays are very sensitive and are capable of detecting minute amounts of parasitic antigens that may be present. This is important in testing a stool culture, because large amounts of parasitic antigens may not be present at any one time. Many of these organisms such as *Giardia* and *Cryptosporidium* are extremely small and may not be easily found on a stained slide preparation. **d.** In addition to the increased sensitivity, enzyme immunoassays are simple to perform and are less time-consuming than traditional testing for parasites. Since instrumentation is

usually used, the results are more easily interpreted with less subjectivity than stained smears.

# CHAPTER 11

## Answers to Review Questions

1. d    2. a    3. d    4. b    5. d    6. a    7. a
8. d    9. a    10. b    11. a    12. d

## Answers to Case Study

**a.** This is likely a case of acute HIV infection or acute retroviral syndrome where patients often report flulike symptoms following HIV infection, prior to the development of detectable antibodies. Symptoms often include fever, fatigue, pharyngitis, weight loss, myalgias (body aches), rash, and headache. **b.** Repeat the HIV serology to detect antibodies for HIV. At the time of the patient's first visit, an antibody response would not have developed; however, at the time of his second visit, which is now 28 days from exposure, the patient may well have developed antibodies to HIV that can be detected by ELISA. **c.** HIV PCR to detect viral RNA can be detected as early as 9 days after infection, before antibody response has developed. Viral loads early in infection are usually very high (millions of copies/mL).

# CHAPTER 12

## Answers to Review Questions

1. a    2. c    3. b    4. c    5. a    6. b    7. c
8. b    9. b    10. c

## Answers to Case Studies

**1. a.** This may represent an error of specificity, in that the newer instrument is getting positive results on specimens that were negative by the older method. However, the newer instrument could actually be more sensitive than the older one, and these could actually be positive samples. **b.** To resolve this discrepancy, known positive and negative controls should be run. The positive controls need to include those at the lower limit of detection, as well as more highly positive samples. This would help to determine if the new instrument is actually more sensitive rather than lacking in specificity.
**2. a.** The flow pattern in A indicates that the majority of lymphocytes are B cells, since they are CD19+. The population most affected appears to be CD3, which are T cells. Pattern B indicates that of the CD3+ lymphocytes, the majority are CD8+, or cytotoxic T cells. The CD4+ count is very low. **b.** T helper cells are necessary to provide help to B cells so they can respond by making antibody. Thus, she is unable to make IgG in response to potential pathogens she might encounter in the environment. **c.** This child should be tested for HIV. That would explain the decrease in CD4+ T cells.

## CHAPTER 13

### Answers to Review Questions

| 1. c | 2. b | 3. d | 4. b | 5. d | 6. a | 7. b |
|------|------|------|------|------|------|------|
| 8. d | 9. d | 10. c | 11. a | 12. c | 13. a | 14. b |

### Answers to Case Studies

**1. a.** An increase in eosinophils is typically found in allergic individuals. Interleukins released by stimulated Th1 cells are involved in the recruitment of eosinophils from the bone marrow. While there are other causes of eosinophilia, such as a parasitic infection, an increased number most often indicates an allergic reaction. **b.** IgE levels of greater than 333 IU are considered to be abnormally elevated if the patient is over the age of 14. In this case, the young age of the patient plus the accompanying symptoms all point to the likelihood that an allergic tendency is present. **c.** Allergen-specific testing, either in the form of RAST testing or skin testing, would be indicated to determine specific allergens. Skin testing is considered to be more sensitive, but in vitro testing is easier on the patient. In either case, specific allergens need to be identified in order for treatment to be successful.

**2. a.** A positive DAT indicates that the red cells are coated with either antibody or complement components. The destruction of some red cells is the reason for the man's symptoms. **b.** The most likely cause of the positive DAT is the presence of an antibody of the IgM class. It might be an anti-I, triggered by *Mycoplasma pneumoniae*. This is a cold-reacting antibody. **c.** A DAT that is only positive with anti-C3d indicates that only complement products are present on the red cells. This is a further indication that the antibody is an IgM antibody, as it does not remain on the cells at 37°C but does trigger complement activation, which can cause the cell destruction.

## CHAPTER 14

### Answers to Review Questions

| 1. a | 2. c | 3. d | 4. a | 5. c | 6. d | 7. c |
|------|------|------|------|------|------|------|
| 8. a | 9. b | 10. b | 11. a | 12. c | | |

### Answers to Case Studies

**1. a.** In systemic lupus erythematosus, a low titer rheumatoid factor is often present. Conversely, a low titer of antinuclear antibodies can be associated with rheumatoid arthritis. Thus, these two cannot be differentiated on the basis of the slide agglutination test results. **b.** The decreased red cell count may be due to the presence of a low-level autoantibody directed against red cells, often associated with lupus. **c.** A fluorescent antinuclear antibody (FANA) test is a good screening tool to help distinguish between these two conditions. A homogeneous pattern or a peripheral pattern would be indicative of lupus, while a speckled pattern can sometimes be found in rheumatoid arthritis or lupus. Therefore, if a speckled pattern is obtained, more specific testing such as an immunodiffusion assay should be done. Presence of anti-Sm antibody would be diagnostic for lupus. This is what was found in this case.

**2. a.** The low T4 level, enlarged thyroid gland, and presence of antithyroglobulin antibody are all indicators of Hashimoto's thyroiditis. **b.** Antithyroglobulin antibodies progressively destroy thyroglobulin produced by the thyroid. Thyroglobulin is normally cleaved in the thyroid to produce secretable hormones triiodothyronine (T3) and thyroxine (T4). Presence of antithyroglobulin antibodies causes enlargement of the thyroid due to the immune response, and hypothyroidism results, characterized by tiredness and weight gain. **c.** Graves' disease is also an autoimmune illness that affects the thyroid, but it is characterized by hyperthyroidism. In this disease, antibodies to thyroid-stimulating hormone receptors are produced, sending a signal to the thyroid to constantly produce T3 and T4. Symptoms include nervousness, insomnia, restlessness, and weight loss, exactly opposite to characteristics of Hashimoto's thyroiditis.

## CHAPTER 15

### Answers to Review Questions

| 1. b | 2. c | 3. a | 4. c | 5. d | 6. a | 7. b |
|------|------|------|------|------|------|------|
| 8. b | 9. c | | | | | |

### Answers to Case Study

**a.** The patient has evidence of anemia and pneumonia. The elevated erythrocytic sedimentation rate (ESR) is a nonspecific indicator of inflammation or elevated serum proteins. Based upon these findings, the physician requested the measurement of serum immunoglobulins. Elevated serum immunoglobulins can produce an elevated ESR. The extremely high IgG levels indicate a monoclonal gammopathy. The patient is most likely suffering from multiple myeloma. The infiltration of cancerous myeloma cells into the bone marrow is responsible for the patient's anemia, and despite having pneumonia, the white blood cell count is only slightly elevated. The back pain could also be due to infiltration of myeloma cells into the vertebra. The age of the patient is appropriate for the diagnosis of multiple myeloma. Patients with Waldenström's macroglobulinemia can present with similar symptoms. However, Waldenström's macroglobulinemia is typically characterized by elevated IgM levels, while elevated IgG levels are more often associated with multiple myeloma. The diagnosis could be confirmed by detecting Bence Jones proteins in the urine.

# CHAPTER 16

## Answers to Review Questions

1. c    2. c    3. d    4. b    5. a    6. a    7. a
8. d

## Answers to Case Studies

**1. a.** The constant bacterial infections coupled with laboratory results indicate an immunodeficiency disease, likely Bruton's agammaglobulinemia or severe combined immunodeficiency syndrome (SCIDS). **b.** Both conditions are inherited as an X-linked recessive gene, which affects males almost exclusively. **c.** To differentiate between the two immunodeficiency states, several types of testing are recommended. Measurement of serum IgA, IgM, and IgG levels should be performed to determine if, in fact, all classes of antibody are absent. Enumeration of classes of lymphocytes should also be determined by flow cytometry. In SCIDS, both T- and B-cell development is affected, and both lymphocyte populations would be deficient, while in Bruton's agammaglobulinemia, only B-cell development is affected. Since the differential indicates that some lymphocytes are present, this would point to Bruton's agammaglobulinemia. Flow cytometry findings confirming the presence of T cells only validate this diagnosis.

**2. a.** The decrease in the T-cell population coupled with facial abnormalities indicate DiGeorge syndrome. The weak gamma band indicates that some antibody production is occurring but is decreased due to low numbers of T helper cells. **b.** DiGeorge syndrome, unlike most other immunodeficiency diseases, is due to abnormal embryonic development rather than an inherited genetic deficiency. The third and fourth pharyngeal pouches fail to develop normally, affecting development of the thymus and causing possible mental retardation and facial anomalies. **c.** Treatment depends upon the severity of the T-cell deficit. This condition can be treated with fetal thymus transplantation or with thymic hormones if there is some thymic function.

**3. a.** The patient's specimen is seen in region 4. Note the faint, diffuse IgG and light chain bands. No IgA or IgM bands are visible. Specimen 1 is a normal control. Specimen 2 contains a monoclonal IgG kappa protein. Specimen 3 is a concentrated 24-hour urine specimen that contains albumin. **b.** Her history and the SPE results indicate that she is immunocompromised and producing very little antibody at all. The faint IgG band would confirm this.

# CHAPTER 17

## Answers to Review Questions

1. b    2. c    3. d    4. d    5. b    6. b    7. a
8. d

## Answers to Case Study

Friend 2. Sibling 1 has the B35 antigen for which the patient possesses HLA antibody. Sibling 2 also has the B35 antigen and is also ABO incompatible. Friend 1 is ABO incompatible. Friend 2 is ABO identical and does not express the HLA-B235 antigen and is thus the most appropriate donor.

## Answers to Exercise

**1.** Child 1 could only inherit DQ2, DR17, B8, Cw7, and A24 from the father, since these antigens do not occur in the mother. Therefore, the tentative haplotype assignments for the father are:

DQ2, DR17, B8, Cw7, A24
DQ2 or X, DR13, B8 or X, Cw7 or X, A1

The second haplotype of child 1 must be DQ1, DR1, B35, Cw4, and A3. Therefore, the tentative maternal haplotypes are:

DQ1, DR1, B35, Cw4, A3
DQ1, DR13, B60, Cw3, A2

**2.** The following haplotypes can now be assigned to the children:

Child 1: (a) DQ2, DR17, B8, Cw7, A24
DQ1, DR1, B35, Cw4, A3
Child 2: (a) DQ2, DR17, B8, Cw7, A24
DQ1, DR13, B60, Cw3, A2
Child 3: (a\b) DQ2, DR17, B8, Cw7, A1 Cross-over
 between (a) locus C and (b) locus A
(d) DQ1, DR13, B60, Cw3, A2
Child 4: (b) DQ2, DR13, B8, Cw7, A1
(d) DQ1, DR13, B60, Cw3, A2 Homozygous DR13
Child 5: (b) DQ2, DR13, B8, Cw7, A1
(c) DQ1, DR1, B35,Cw4, A3

Note: Children 4 and 5 resolve the question on the (b) haplotype of whether the DQ and B loci are null alleles (blanks, X) or were expressed DQ2 and B8. In both Child 4 and Child 5, they were expressed as DQ2 and B8.

**3.** There are no genotypically identical sibling donors for Child 1, the patient who is genotype (a,c).

Child 2 (a,d) is mismatched for 1 DR, 1 B, and 1 A antigen; 3 antigen mismatch if HLA-C is not included.
Child 3 (a\b,d) is mismatched for 1DR, 1 B, and 2 A antigens because of the recombinant haplotype; 3 antigen mismatch.
Child 4 (b,d) is mismatched for 1 DR, 1 B, and 2A antigens because of a 2 haplotype mismatch; 3 antigen mismatch.
Child 5 (b,c) is mismatched for 1 DR and 1 A antigen because of a 1 haplotype mismatch; 2 antigen mismatch. If a sibling became the organ donor, Child 5 would be the best available match among these siblings.

# CHAPTER 18

## Answers to Review Questions

1. d    2. b    3. a    4. c    5. a    6. d    7. b
8. a    9. d    10. b    11. d    12. e    13. a    14. b
15. a

## Answers to Case Study

**1. a.** If no further CA-15.3 is being produced by tumor tissue, levels will decrease at the rate of biological half-life for the molecule. Since CA-15.3 levels are not decreasing at this rate, residual tumor is suspected. **b.** HER-2/neu overexpression indicates that therapy with the monoclonal antibody Herceptin may be successful. **c.** Since the tumor lacks estrogen and progesterone receptors, hormone-suppressing therapy is unlikely to improve prognosis.

**2. a.** TG assays are almost always inaccurate in the presence of anti-TG antibodies in the patient. Since no antibodies were detected, there is increased confidence in the TG measurement. **b.** TSH stimulates thyroid tissue to produce hormones, and TG is required to produce these hormones. Resting tissue will produce less TG, so to detect residual cancer, TSH must be elevated. In this case, when the patient discontinued her thyroid replacement hormones, the TSH rose. TSH can also be given artificially. **c.** The increase in TG indicates that there may be residual cancer.

**3. a.** No other tissues in men are known to produce PSA, so another source is extremely unlikely. **b.** PSA velocity is the rate of PSA increase between determinations. Since PSA increases with age and prostatic enlargement, examining PSA velocity is an attempt to separate benign and malignant conditions, as velocity is higher in malignancy. Current recommendations for biopsy are for PSA velocities that exceed 0.5 ng/mL per year. **c.** Although the total PSA has increased to above the reference interval, the proportion of free PSA remains within the interval associated with benign disease. Further, his PSA velocity did not exceed 0.5 ng/mL per year, and the digital rectal exam did not detect any obvious sign of malignancy. Given the man's age, benign prostatic hypertrophy is likely, and further PSA testing after a waiting period may be warranted in lieu of a biopsy. **d.** Once a man's life expectancy is less than 10 years, PSA testing is no longer recommended.

# CHAPTER 19

## Answers to Review Questions

1. d    2. c    3. b    4. b    5. d    6. a    7. b
8. d    9. c    10. c    11. a    12. c

## Answers to Case Studies

**1. a.** Poststreptococcal glomerulonephritis. **b.** Group A *Streptococcus pyogenes.* **c.** Immune complexes resulting from the combination of streptococcal antigen–antibody combinations are deposited in the glomeruli of the kidney. These immune complexes stimulate an inflammatory response in the area, causing tissue damage and impaired kidney function. **d.** The organism is no longer present in the throat, and it is not present in the urine. The disease is caused by accumulation of antibodies and not by the organism itself.

**2. a.** *Mycoplasma pneumoniae.* **b.** *Mycoplasma pneumoniae* grows only on specialized media, and it grows very slowly. **c.** The cold agglutinin titer is not specific for *Mycoplasma.* Something else may have triggered production of anti-I antibody. Additionally, any tube titer is accurate only to +/− one tube.

# CHAPTER 20

## Answers to Review Questions

1. d    2. c    3. d    4. a    5. a    6. b    7. d
8. d    9. c    10. d    11. a    12. b    13. b    14. c
15. a    16. b    17. c    18. c    19. a

## Answers to Case Study

**a.** It cannot be determined by the test results available whether the baby has congenital toxoplasmosis. The IgG antibodies in the baby may be totally the result of the mother's antibodies that crossed the placenta. **b.** Since newborns have underdeveloped immune systems and limited ability to produce IgG antibodies, it would be better to test the child for IgM antibodies to *T. gondii*. A single test with an elevated IgM level would indicate a current infection in the baby. Testing for *T. gondii* IgM allows the fastest diagnosis. If only a *T. gondii* IgG test is available, the baby must be tested again for IgG antibodies in 10 days to 2 weeks. If the titer is at least four times greater than the initial titer, the baby is infected.

# CHAPTER 21

## Answers to Review Questions

1. c    2. d    3. d    4. b    5. d    6. b    7. c
8. c    9. d    10. b    11. b    12. d    13. c    14. b
15. c    16. b    17. b

## Answers to Case Studies

**1. a.** Almost 25 percent of individuals with Lyme disease do not exhibit the characteristic rash. Its presence is a good indicator of Lyme disease, but absence of the rash does not rule out possibility of the disease. **b.** There are several false-positive results in EIA testing, including syphilis, other treponemal diseases, infectious mononucleosis, and autoimmune diseases such as rheumatoid arthritis. Thus, low levels of antibody might indicate one of these other diseases. However, false-negative results in Lyme disease are also possible due to a low level of antibody production. Therefore, an indeterminate test neither rules out nor confirms the presence of Lyme disease. **c.** If there is a history of tick bite and patient symptoms are consistent with Lyme disease, then a confirmatory Western blot should be performed. The Western blot is fairly specific for Lyme disease. If 5 of 10 protein bands specific for *Borrelia burgdorferi* are positive, this confirms presence of Lyme disease.

**2. a.** While it is possible that the mother's positive RPR test could be a false positive, it is also likely that the mother is in the latent stage of syphilis, with no obvious signs of the disease. Although syphilis is not sexually transmitted during this stage, it can be transmitted from a mother to her unborn child. Many infants do not exhibit clinical signs of the disease at birth, but if infected and untreated, a large percentage of babies develop later symptoms, including neurological deficits such as blindness and mental retardation. **b.** A positive RPR on cord blood could be from transplacental passage of mother's IgG antibodies. A titer should be performed on the cord blood and a serum sample obtained from the infant in several weeks. If infection is present in the infant, the titer will remain the same or increase. An IgM capture assay could also be performed. Presence of specific antitreponemal IgM would indicate that the infant had been exposed to *Treponema pallidum*, since IgM antibodies do not cross the placenta. **c.** Since there is a good chance that the infant is at risk for congenital syphilis, immediate treatment with penicillin can prevent any further neurological consequences.

## CHAPTER 22

### Answers to Review Questions

1. b    2. d    3. d    4. a    5. d    6. b    7. c
8. c    9. a    10. c

### Answers to Case Study

**1. a.** The patient's clinical symptoms and increase in liver function enzymes indicate inflammation of the liver. In order to determine whether this inflammation is due to viral hepatitis and to identify the cause, the following tests should be ordered: (1) IgM anti-HAV to screen for hepatitis A, (2) HBsAg to screen for hepatitis B, (3) IgM anti-HBc to screen for hepatitis B in the core window period when HBsAg is absent, and (4) anti-HCV to screen for hepatitis C. **b.** In order to monitor hepatitis B infection, testing for HBsAg and HBeAg should be performed periodically to determine how long the infection is persisting and the relative infectivity of the patient. Tests for anti-HBe and anti-HBs are performed to indicate whether the infection has resolved, and whether immunity has been established, respectively. **c.** In chronic hepatitis B, HBsAg persists in the serum for more than 6 months. Total anti-HBc is also present, and HBeAg may or may not be present, depending on the degree of disease progression. Anti-HBe and anti-HBs are usually not present, but may have a delayed appearance in those individuals who eventually recover.

**2. a.** Many viruses can produce congenital abnormalities in an infant born to a mother infected during pregnancy. These include cytomegalovirus, rubella virus, and varicella zoster virus. The infant's symptoms and mother's history suggest infection with rubella virus. **b.** Ideally, the mother would have been tested at the time of her illness during her pregnancy for rubella antibodies. Demonstration of rubella-specific IgM antibody, seroconversion from negative to positive for rubella antibody, or a four-fold rise in antibody titer would have indicated an active rubella infection. However, since this was not done, the mother could be tested for rubella-specific IgG antibody; this would indicate rubella exposure in the past, but would not provide information as to when the exposure occurred. **c.** The infant's serum should be tested for rubella-specific IgM antibody, preferably with an IgM antibody capture enzyme immunoassay. IgM antibodies, which cannot pass through the placenta, would have been produced by the fetus as a result of active rubella infection. IgG antibodies, on the other hand, are derived mainly from the mother's serum as a result of passive transfer through the placenta.

## CHAPTER 23

### Answers to Review Questions

1. c    2. b    3. c    4. d    5. a    6. d    7. b
8. c    9. a    10. c    11. b    12. b    13. c    14. b
15. c

### Answers to Case Studies

**1. a.** The standard test used in screening for HIV infection is the ELISA test for HIV antibody. This test has a high level of sensitivity and detects over 99 percent of HIV infections. If the woman tests negative, her physician would likely recommend that she be retested in a few weeks, given her high risk for infection, in order to exclude the possibility that she may have been tested in the short window period prior to development of HIV-specific antibodies. **b.** While the ELISA is a sensitive test, it has resulted in a high number of false-positive results from cross-reacting antibodies that can be present in the test specimen. If the woman tests positive by the initial ELISA test, in order to help reduce the possibility that her result represents a false positive, the standard testing algorithm for HIV antibody should be performed. According to this algorithm, a fresh specimen should be collected from the woman and tested by ELISA in duplicate. If a least two out of the three samples tested in both runs are determined to be positive, then her sample should be referred for confirmatory testing by the Western blot method. This method is more specific in that it tests for antibodies to individual HIV antigens. The woman's specimen would be reported as HIV-positive if her specimen produced at least 2 out of the 3 characteristic bands for this test (p24, gp41, and gp120/gp160). While a chance that the result is false positive still exists after a positive Western blot is obtained, it would be very small. If equivocal results are produced in the Western blot test, her specimen may be referred for molecular testing to detect HIV nucleic acid. **c.** If it has been determined that the woman is truly infected with HIV, then it would be important for her physician to monitor her immune status by periodically measuring her peripheral blood CD4 T cell counts. Immunofluorescence staining and analysis by flow cytometry is the standard method in use for this measurement. CD4 T cells, which are the primary target of HIV infection, are known to progressively decrease in number as the infection progresses. This decrease can leave HIV-infected individuals susceptible to developing a variety of opportunistic infections and malignancies. If such testing reveals a significant decrease in CD4 T cell numbers, the woman's physician may recommend that she begin antiretroviral therapy in order to limit replication of the virus and the damage it can cause to the immune system. Once this therapy has begun, it would be important to monitor its effectiveness by continuing periodic evaluations of the CD4 T cell counts, and by performing viral load tests to quantitate the amount of HIV being harbored in the body. Viral load tests are performed using one of the following molecular methods: RT-PCR, bDNA, or NASBA. A depression in the number of HIV RNA copies/mL of plasma would indicate that the therapy was effective, while an increase in the number of HIV RNA copies would indicate ineffectiveness of the drugs being used, and the need to change the patient's therapeutic regimen. This change can be facilitated by performance of drug resistance assays to identify the presence of isolates of HIV that may be resistant to certain antiretroviral drugs.

# Index